Fundamentals of Anatomy and Physiology for Student Nurses

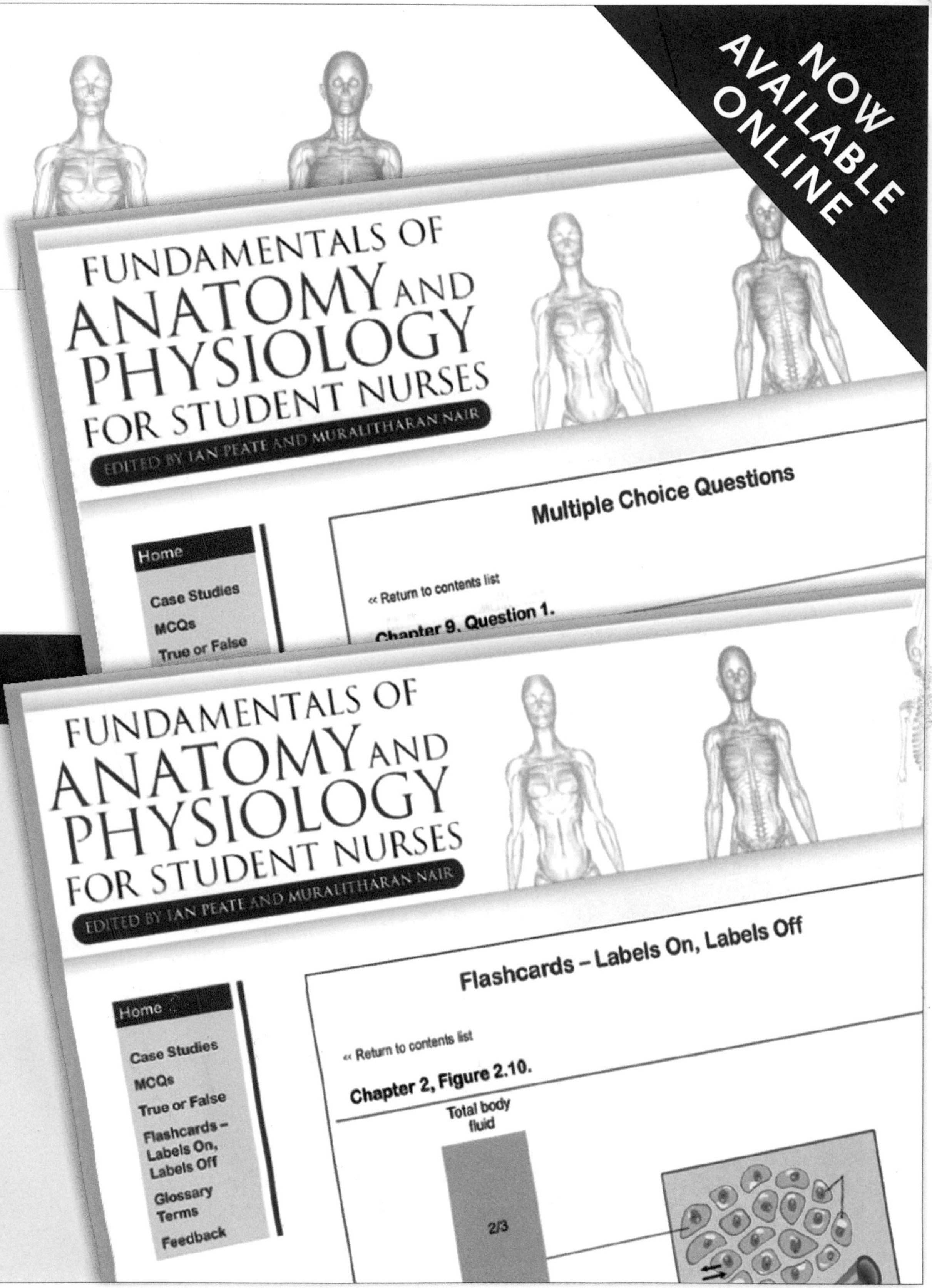

NOW AVAILABLE ONLINE
FUNDAMENTALS OF ANATOMY AND PHYSIOLOGY FOR STUDENT NURSES
EDITED BY IAN PEATE AND MURALITHARAN NAIR
Multiple Choice Questions
Home
Case Studies
MCQs
True or False
« Return to contents list
Chapter 9, Question 1.
FUNDAMENTALS OF ANATOMY AND PHYSIOLOGY FOR STUDENT NURSES
EDITED BY IAN PEATE AND MURALITHARAN NAIR
Flashcards – Labels On, Labels Off
Home
Case Studies
MCQs
True or False
Flashcards – Labels On, Labels Off
Glossary Terms
Feedback
« Return to contents list
Chapter 2, Figure 2.10.
Total body fluid
2/3

Fundamentals of Anatomy and Physiology for Student Nurses

Edited by

Ian Peate

EN(G) RGN DipN (Lond) RNT BEd(Hons) MA(Lond) LLM
Professor of Nursing
Head of School
School of Nursing, Midwifery and Healthcare
University of West London

and

Muralitharan Nair

SRN, RMN, DipN (Lond) RNT, Cert Ed., BSc (Hons) MSc (Surrey), Cert in Counselling, FHEA
Senior Lecturer
School of Nursing, Midwifery and Social Work
Faculty of Health and Human Sciences
University of Hertfordshire

WILEY-BLACKWELL
A John Wiley & Sons, Inc., Publication

This edition first published 2011

Blackwell Publishing was acquired by John Wiley & Sons in February 2007. Blackwell's publishing program has been merged with Wiley's global Scientific, Technical and Medical business to form Wiley-Blackwell.

Registered office: John Wiley & Sons Ltd, The Atrium, Southern Gate, Chichester, West Sussex, PO19 8SQ, UK

Editorial offices: 9600 Garsington Road, Oxford, OX4 2DQ, UK
The Atrium, Southern Gate, Chichester, West Sussex, PO19 8SQ, UK
2121 State Avenue, Ames, Iowa 50014-8300, USA

For details of our global editorial offices, for customer services and for information about how to apply for permission to reuse the copyright material in this book please see our website at www.wiley.com/wiley-blackwell.

Library of Congress Cataloging-in-Publication Data

Fundamentals of anatomy and physiology for student nurses / edited by Ian Peate and Muralitharan Nair.
p. ; cm.
Includes bibliographical references and index.
ISBN 978-1-4443-3443-2 (pbk. : alk. paper)
1. Human physiology. 2. Human anatomy. 3. Nursing. I. Peate, Ian. II. Nair, Muralitharan.
[DNLM: 1. Anatomy–Nurses' Instruction. 2. Physiology–Nurses' Instruction. QS 4]
QP34.5.F862 2011
612–dc22
2010040972

A catalogue record for this book is available from the British Library.

Set in 10/12pt Calibri by Toppan Best-set Premedia Limited

Printed and bound in Malaysia by Vivar Printing Sdn Bhd

1 2011

Short contents

Contributors xx
Acknowledgements xxiii
Copyright acknowledgements xxiv
Introduction xxv

Chapter 1
Basic scientific principles of physiology **1**
Peter S Vickers

Chapter 2
Cells: cellular compartment, transport system, fluid movements **32**
Muralitharan Nair

Chapter 3
The immune system **62**
Peter S Vickers

Chapter 4
Tissue **102**
Anthony Wheeldon

Chapter 5
The skin **130**
Ian Peate

Chapter 6
The nervous system **154**
Louise McErlean and Janet G Migliozzi

Chapter 7
The endocrine system **190**
Carl Clare

Chapter 8
The skeletal system **224**
Ian Peate

Chapter 9
The muscular system **258**
Janet G Migliozzi

Chapter 10
The cardiac system **294**
Carl Clare

Chapter 11
The respiratory system **328**
Anthony Wheeldon

Chapter 12
The circulatory system **366**
Muralitharan Nair

Chapter 13
The digestive system and nutrition **406**
Louise McErlean

Chapter 14
The renal system **446**
Muralitharan Nair

Chapter 15
The reproductive systems **476**
Ian Peate

Chapter 16
The special senses **510**
Carl Clare

Chapter 17
Genetics **550**
Peter S Vickers

Index 585

www.wiley.com/go/peate

Contents

Contributors xx
Acknowledgements xxiii
Copyright acknowledgements xxiv
Introduction xxv

Chapter 1 Basic scientific principles of physiology **1**
Peter S Vickers

Introduction 2
Levels of organisation 2
Characteristics of life 2
Bodily requirements 4
Atoms 4
Atomic number 6
Carbon atom 6
Molecules 7
Chemical bonds 7
Ionic bonding of atoms 7
Ions 7
Covalent bonds 8
Polar bonds 9
Electrolytes 9
Elements 10
Properties of elements 13
Compounds 13
Chemical equations/chemical reactions 13
Acids and bases (pH) 16
Blood and pH values 18
Homeostasis 18
Organic and inorganic substances 19
Examples of organic substances 19
Examples of inorganic substances 20
Units of measurement 20
Conclusion 23
Glossary 23
References 25
Activities 26

Chapter 2 Cells: cellular compartment, transport system, fluid movements **32**
Muralitharan Nair

Introduction 34
Cell membrane 35
Functions of the cell membrane 37
Transport systems 38
Active transport system 41
Endocytosis 42
Exocytosis 43
Fluid compartments 43

Composition of body fluid 46
Effects of water deficiency 47

Electrolytes 47
Functions of electrolytes 47
Hormones that regulate fluid and electrolytes 50

Conclusion 51
Glossary 52
References 53
Activities 53

Chapter 3 The immune system **62**

Peter S Vickers

Introduction 64

Blood cell development 64

Organs of the immune system 67
The thymus 67

The lymphatic system 68
Lymph nodes 70
Lymphoid tissue 70
The spleen 71

Types of immunity 72
The innate immune system 72
Physical barriers 72
Mechanical barriers 73
Chemical barriers 73
Blood cells 73
Blood cells of the immune system 73
Phagocytosis 74
Cytotoxicity 76
Inflammation 76

The acquired immune system 79
Cell-mediated immunity (T-cell lymphocytes) 79
Humoral immunity (B-cell lymphocytes) 80

Immunoglobulins (antibodies) 83

Types of immunoglobulins 83
Immunoglobulin G 83
Immunoglobulin A 83
Immunoglobulin M 84
Immunoglobulin E 84
Immunoglobulin D 84
Role of immunoglobulins 84
Natural killer cells 86

Primary and secondary response to infection 86
Primary immune response 86
Secondary immune response 88

Immunisations 89
Passive immunisation 89
Active immunity 90

Conclusion 91
Glossary 92
References 95
Activities 96

Chapter 4 Tissue **102**

Anthony Wheeldon

Introduction *104*

Epithelial tissue **104**
Simple epithelia 105
Stratified epithelia 108
Glandular epithelia 110

Connective tissue **110**
Connective tissue proper 113
Loose connective tissue 113
Dense connective tissue 113
Cartilage 114

Bone **115**

Liquid connective tissue **115**

Membranes **115**
Cutaneous membrane 115
Mucous membranes 115
Serous membranes 117
Synovial membranes 118

Muscle tissue **118**

Nervous tissue **118**

Tissue repair **119**

Conclusion *121*
Glossary *122*
References *123*
Activities *124*

Chapter 5 The skin **130**

Ian Peate

Introduction *132*

The structure of skin **132**

The epidermis **132**
Keratinocytes 133
Melanocytes 133
Langerhans cells 133
Merkel cells 133
Stratum basale 134
Stratum spinosum 135
Stratum granulosum 135
Stratum lucidum 136
Stratum corneum 136

The dermis **137**
The papillary and reticular aspects 138

The accessory skin structures **139**
The hair 139

Skin glands **140**
Eccrine glands 140
Apocrine glands 141

Nails **141**

The functions of the skin **142**
Sensation 143
Thermoregulation 143
Protection 143
Excretion and absorption 144
Synthesis of vitamin D 145

Conclusion *145*
Glossary *146*
References *147*
Activities *148*

Chapter 6 The nervous system **154**

Louise McErlean and Janet G Migliozzi

Introduction *156*

Organisation of the nervous system **156**

Sensory division of the peripheral nervous system **157**

Central nervous system **157**

Motor division of the peripheral nervous system **157**
Somatic nervous system 157
Autonomic nervous system 157
Neurones 157
Dendrites 158
Cell body 158
Axons 158
Myelin sheath 158
Sensory (afferent) nerves 160
Motor (efferent) nerves 160
The action potential 160
Simple propagation of nerve impulses 161
Saltatory conduction 161
The refractory period 161

Neurotransmitters **161**

Neuroglia **163**

The meninges **163**

Cerebrospinal fluid (CSF) **164**

The brain **166**

The peripheral nervous system **170**
Cranial nerves 170

The spinal cord **170**
Functions of the spinal cord 172
Spinal nerves 173

The autonomic nervous system **176**
Sympathetic division (fight or flight) 176
Parasympathetic division (rest and digest) 178

Conclusion *178*
Glossary *180*
References *182*
Activities *183*

Chapter 7 The endocrine system **190**

Carl Clare

Introduction *192*

The endocrine organs **193**

Hormones **194**
Effects of hormones 196
Destruction and removal of hormones 197

Control of hormone release 197

The physiology of the endocrine organs **198**
The hypothalamus and the pituitary gland 198
Hormones released by the anterior pituitary gland 199

Growth hormone 200
Prolactin 200
Follicle stimulating hormone and luteinising hormone (gonadotrophins) 201
Thyroid stimulating hormone (TSH) 201
Adrenocorticotrophic hormone (ACTH) 201

The thyroid gland **202**

The parathyroid glands **205**

The adrenal glands **205**
Adrenal medulla 206
Adrenal cortex 207

Mineralocorticoids **208**

Glucocorticoids **208**

Pancreas **211**

Insulin **211**

Glucagon **212**

Somatostatin **213**

Conclusion *213*
Glossary *214*
References *216*
Activities *216*

Chapter 8 The skeletal system **224**

Ian Peate

Introduction *226*

The axial and appendicular skeleton **226**
The axial skeleton 226
The appendicular skeleton 226

Bone and its functions **226**
Support 229
Movement 229
Storage 229
Protection 229
Production 229

Bone formation and growth (ossification) **230**

Embryonic formation **231**
Intramembranous ossification 231
Endochondral ossification 231
Bone length and thickness 234
Bone remodelling 234

Bone fractures **235**

Bone structure and blood supply (histology) **236**
Blood supply 237

Organisation of bone based on shape **237**
Long bones 237
Short bones 238
Flat bones 238
Irregular bones 241
Sesamoid bones 241

Joints **241**
Fibrous joints 242
Cartilaginous joints 242
Synovial joints 243

Conclusion *243*
Glossary of terms *247*
References *249*
Activities *250*

Chapter 9 The muscular system **258**

Janet G Migliozzi

Introduction *260*

Types of muscle tissue **260**
Smooth 260
Cardiac 260
Skeletal 260

Functions of the muscular system **260**
Maintenance of body posture 261
Production of movement 261
Stabilisation of joints 261
Protection and control of internal tissue structures/organs 261
Generation of heat 261

Composition of skeletal muscle tissue **261**

Gross anatomy of skeletal muscles **262**

Microanatomy of skeletal muscle fibre **263**
The sarcolemma and transverse tubules 264
The sarcoplasm 264
The myofibrils 264
The sarcomeres 264

Types of muscle fibres **264**

Blood supply **265**

Skeletal muscle contraction and relaxation **266**

Energy sources for muscle contraction **267**

Aerobic respiration **269**

Oxygen debt **269**

Muscle fatigue **269**

Organisation of the skeletal muscular system **270**

Skeletal muscle movement **271**

The effects of ageing **285**

Conclusion *285*
Glossary *286*
References *286*
Activities *287*

Chapter 10 The cardiac system **294**

Carl Clare

Introduction *296*

Size and location of the heart **296**

The structures of the heart **297**
Heart wall 297
The heart chambers 299

The blood supply to the heart **302**

Blood flow through the heart **304**

The electrical pathways of the heart **306**

The cardiac cycle **309**

Factors affecting cardiac output **312**

Regulation of stroke volume **313**
Preload 313
Force of contraction 313
Afterload 314

Regulation of heart rate **314**
Autonomic nervous system activity 314
Baroreceptors and the cardiovascular centre 315
Hormone activity 315
Conclusion *315*
Glossary *317*
References *321*
Activities *321*

Chapter 11 The respiratory system **328**
Anthony Wheeldon

Introduction *330*
Organisation of the respiratory system **330**
The upper respiratory tract **330**
The lower respiratory tract **331**
Larynx 332
Trachea 333
Bronchial tree 334
Blood supply **336**
Respiration **336**
Pulmonary ventilation **337**
Mechanics of breathing 337
Work of breathing **339**
Volumes and capacities **340**
Control of breathing **342**
External respiration **343**
Gaseous exchange 343
Factors affecting diffusion 344
Ventilation and perfusion **345**
Transport of gases **345**
Transport of oxygen (O_2) 345
Transport of carbon dioxide (CO_2) 347
Acid base balance **348**
Internal respiration **350**
Conclusion *350*
Glossary *352*
References *357*
Activities *357*

Chapter 12 The circulatory system **366**
Muralitharan Nair

Introduction *368*
Composition of blood **368**
Properties of blood and plasma **369**
Blood plasma **370**
Water in plasma 371
Functions of blood **371**
Transportation 372
Formation of blood cells **374**
Red blood cells **374**
Haemoglobin 375
Formation of red blood cells 375
Life cycle of the red blood cell 376
Transport of respiratory gases 377

White blood cells **378**
Neutrophils 379
Eosinophils 379
Basophils 380
Monocytes 380
Lymphocytes 380

Platelets **382**

Haemostasis **382**
Vasoconstriction 382
Platelet aggregation 382
Coagulation 383

Blood groups **384**

Blood vessels **385**
Structure and function of arteries and veins 385
Capillaries 388

Blood pressure **389**
Physiological factors regulating blood pressure 389
Control of arterial blood pressure 390

Lymphatic system **391**
Lymph 391
Lymph capillaries and large lymph vessels 391
Lymph nodes 394

Lymphatic organs **394**
Spleen 394
The thymus gland 394

Functions of the lymphatic system **394**

Conclusion *396*
Glossary *397*
References *398*
Activities *398*

Chapter 13 The digestive system and nutrition **406**

Louise McErlean

Introduction *408*

The activity of the digestive system **408**
The mouth (oral cavity) 409
Tongue 409
Palate 409
Teeth 409
Salivary glands 410
Pharynx 413
Swallowing (deglutition) 413
Oesophagus 414

The structure of the digestive system **414**
Stomach 416
Small intestine 418

The pancreas **421**

The liver and production of bile **423**
The functions of the liver 424

The gall bladder **425**

The large intestine **425**

Digestive tract hormones **427**

Nutrition, chemical digestion and metabolism **427**
Nutrients 428
Balanced diet 428
Nutrient groups 429

Conclusion *431*
Glossary *435*
References *439*
Activities *439*

Chapter 14 The renal system **446**

Muralitharan Nair

Introduction *448*

Renal system **448**

Kidneys – external structures **449**

Kidneys – internal structures **450**
Nephrons 451

Functions of the kidney **455**

Blood supply of the kidney **456**

Urine formation **457**
Filtration 457
Selective reabsorption 457
Secretion 459
Hormonal control of tubular reabsorption and secretion 460

Composition of urine 461
Characteristics of normal urine 462

Ureters **463**

Urinary bladder **464**

Urethra **466**
Male urethra 466
Female urethra 467

Micturition **467**

Conclusion *468*
Glossary *469*
References *470*
Activities *470*

Chapter 15 The reproductive systems **476**

Ian Peate

Introduction *478*

The male reproductive system **478**
The testes 479
Spermatogenesis 482
Sperm 483
The testes and hormonal influences 484
The scrotum 484
The penis 486
Epididymis 487
The vas deferens, ejaculatory duct and spermatic cord 488
The prostate gland 488

The female reproductive system **488**
The ovaries 489
The ovarian cortex 490
Graafian follicles 490

Corpus luteum 490
The ovarian medulla 490
Oogenesis 490
The role of the female sex hormones 490
The menstrual cycle 492

The internal organs **494**
The uterus 494
The fallopian tubes 495
The vagina 496
The cervix 496
The external genitalia 497
The breasts 497

Conclusion *497*
Glossary *498*
References *501*
Activities *502*

Chapter 16 The special senses **510**

Carl Clare

Introduction *512*

The chemical senses **512**

The sense of smell (olfaction) **512**
Olfactory receptors 513
The olfactory pathway 514
Olfactory discrimination 514

The sense of taste **516**
Taste buds 516
The taste receptor 517
The gustatory pathway 519

The special senses of equilibrium and hearing **520**
The structure of the ear 520
Equilibrium 523
Pathways for the equilibrium sensations 526

Hearing **527**
The hearing process 529

The special sense of sight **530**
Lacrimal apparatus 531

The eye **531**
The wall of the eye 531
Neural tunic (retina) 533
The chambers of the eye 535

Focusing images onto the retina **536**
Refraction 536
Myopia, hyperopia and presbyopia 538

The processing of visual information **539**
Central processing of visual information 540

Conclusion *540*
Glossary *540*
References *543*
Activities *543*

Chapter 17 Genetics **550**

Peter S Vickers

Introduction *552*

The double helix **552**
Nucleotides 553
Bases 553

Chromosomes **554**

From DNA to proteins **557**
Protein synthesis 557
Transcription 557
Translation 559
Protein synthesis 559
Summary of protein synthesis 562

The transference of genes **563**
Mitosis 563
Interphase 564
Prophase 565
Metaphase 565
Anaphase 565
Telophase 565
Cell division 565
Meiosis 565

First meiotic division 567
Second meiotic division 568

Mendelian genetics 569
Dominant genes and recessive genes 570
Autosomal dominant inheritance and ill health 571
Autosomal recessive inheritance and ill health 571
Morbidity and mortality of dominant versus recessive disorders 573
X-linked recessive disorders 574

Spontaneous mutation 575

Conclusion 575
Glossary 575
References 578
Activities 579

Index 585

www.wiley.com/go/peate

Contributors

About the editors

Ian Peate
Professor of Nursing
Head of School
School of Nursing, Midwifery and Healthcare
University of West London

EN(G), RGN, DipN (Lond), RNT, Bed (Hons), MA(Lond), LLM
Ian began his nursing a career in 1981 at Central Middlesex Hospital, becoming an enrolled nurse working in an intensive care unit. He later undertook three years student nurse training at Central Middlesex and Northwick Park Hospitals, becoming a staff nurse then a charge nurse. He has worked in nurse education since 1989. His key areas of interest are nursing practice and theory, men's health, sexual health and HIV/AIDS. He is currently Head of School.

Muralitharan Nair
Senior Lecturer
School of Nursing, Midwifery and Social Work
University of Hertfordshire

SRN, RMN, DipN (Lond) RNT, Cert Ed., BSc (Hons) MSc (Surrey), Cert in Counselling, FHEA
Muralitharan commenced his nursing a career in 1971 at Edgware General Hospital becoming a Staff Nurse. In 1975 he commenced his mental health nurse training at Springfield Hospital and worked as a Staff Nurse for approximately 1 year. He has worked at St Mary's Hospital Paddington and Northwick Park Hospital returning to Edgware General Hospital to take up the post of Senior Staff Nurse and then Charge Nurse. He has worked in nurse education since 1989. His key interests include physiology, diabetes, surgical nursing and nurse education. Muralitharan has published in journals and written a chapter on elimination and published a textbook on pathophysiology. He is a fellow of the Higher Education Academy.

About the contributors

Louise McErlean
Senior Lecturer
School of Nursing, Midwifery and Social Work
University of Hertfordshire

RGN, BSc(Hons), MA (Herts)

Louise began her nursing career in 1986 at the Victoria Infirmary in Glasgow, becoming a registered general nurse. She later completed the intensive care course for RGNs while working in Belfast as a staff nurse. She then worked as a junior sister at the Royal Free Hospital and has worked in nurse education since 2005. Her key areas of interest are pre-registration nurse education and intensive care nursing.

Janet G Migliozzi
Senior Lecturer
School of Nursing , Midwifery and Social Work
Faculty of Health and Human Sciences
University of Hertfordshire

RGN, BSc (Hons), MSc (London), PGDEd, FHEA

Janet commenced her nursing career in London becoming a staff nurse in 1988. She has worked at a variety of hospitals across London, predominately in vascular, orthopaedic and high dependency surgery before specialising in infection prevention and control. Janet has worked in nurse education since 1999 and her key interests include microbiology particularly in relation to healthcare associated infections, vascular/surgical nursing, health informatics and nurse education. Janet is currently a senior lecturer and a member of the Infection Prevention Society.

Carl Clare
Senior Lecturer
School of Nursing, Midwifery and Social Work
University of Hertfordshire

RN, DipN, BSc (Hons), MSc (Lond), PGDE (Lond)

Carl began his nursing a career in 1990 as a nursing auxiliary. He later undertook three years student nurse training at Selly Oak Hospital (Birmingham), moving to The Royal Devon and Exeter Hospitals, then Northwick Park Hospital, and finally The Royal Brompton and Harefield NHS Trust as a resuscitation officer and honorary teaching fellow of Imperial College (London). He has worked in nurse education since 2001. His key areas of interest are physiology, sociology, cardiac care and resuscitation. Carl has previously published work in cardiac care, resuscitation and pathophysiology.

Peter S Vickers
Visiting Fellow
School of Nursing and Midwifery
University of Hertfordshire

Cert Ed, Dip CD, SRN, RSCN, BA, PhD, FHEA

Following a career in teaching, Peter commenced his nursing career in 1980 at the York District Hospital, followed shortly afterwards by studying and working at the Hospital for Sick Children, Great Ormond Street, London. He later obtained his first degree in Biosciences and Health Studies and then obtained a doctorate in his specialty, immunology nursing, concentrating on the long-term development of children with SCID in the UK and Germany. He has worked in nurse education for several years, and has recently completed a research study into adult palliative care. The author of books on children's responses to early hospitalisation, and research methodology/

proposals, he has also written chapters for several nursing bioscience and pathophysiology books, as well as presented papers at many national and international conferences. His key areas of interest are all aspects of immunology and immunology nursing, infectious diseases, genetics, and research. Although officially retired, he continues to work part-time at the University of Hertfordshire, as well as continuing with his writing and presenting at conferences.

Anthony Wheeldon
School of Nursing, Midwifery and Social Work
Faculty of Health and Human Sciences
University of Hertfordshire

MSc (Lond), PGDE, BSc(Hons), DipHE, RN
After qualification in 1995 Anthony worked as a staff nurse and senior staff nurse in the Respiratory Directorate at the Royal Brompton and Harefield NHS Trust. He began teaching on post-registration courses in 2000 before moving into full-time nurse education at Thames Valley University in 2002. Anthony has a wide range of nursing interests including cardiorespiratory nursing, anatomy and physiology, respiratory assessment and nurse education. Anthony has previously published work on respiratory assessment and pathophysiology. He is currently a senior lecturer at the University of Hertfordshire.

Acknowledgements

We would like to thank all of our colleagues and students for their help, support, comments and suggestions.

Muralitharan would like to thank his wife, Evangeline, and his daughters, Samantha and Jennifer, for their continued support and patience.

Ian would like to thank his partner, Jussi Lahtinen, for all of his continued support and encouragement.

Thank you to Anthony Peate who contributed to some of the illustrations.

Copyright acknowledgements

The following figures were produced with the kind permission of the copyright holders.

Tortora, G.J. and Derrickson, B.H. (2009) *Principles of Anatomy and Physiology*, 12th edn. Hoboken, NJ: John Wiley & Sons.
1.1, 1.4, 1.5, 1.6, 1.7, 1.8, 1.9, 2.1, 2.3, 2.5, 2.6, 2.7, 3.1, 3.2, 3.3, 3.8, 3.10, 3.11, 3.12, 3.13, 4.1, 4.2, 4.3, 4.4, 4.5, 4.6, 4.7, 4.8, 4.9, 4.10, 4.11, 4.12, 4.14, 4.15, 4.16, 5.1, 5.2, 6.2, 6.3, 6.5, 6.6, 6.7, 6.8, 6.9, 6.11, 6.12, 6.14, 6.15, 6.16, 7.1, 7.7, 7.9, 8.1, 8.2, 8.3, 8.5, 8.8, 8.9, 9.1, 9.3, 9.4, 9.5, 9.10, 9.11, 10.1, 10.2, 10.5, 10.6, 10.8, 10.9, 10.11, 11.1, 11.2, 11.3, 11.4, 11.6, 11.11, 11.12, 11.14, 11.15, 12.1, 12.2, 12.5, 12.6, 12.8, 12.9, 12.10, 12.11, 12.12, 12.13, 12.14, 12.16, 12.18, 12.19, 12.21, 12.22, 13.1, 13.2, 13.3, 13.4, 13.5, 13.6, 13.7, 13.8, 13.9, 13.11, 13.12, 13.13, 13.14, 13.15, 14.1, 14.3, 14.4, 14.5, 14.6, 14.7, 14.9, 15.1, 15.2, 15.3, 15.4, 15.5, 15.6, 15.8, 15.9, 15.10, 15.11, 15.13, 16.1, 16.2, 16.3, 16.4, 16.5, 16.6, 16.7, 16.8, 16.9, 16.10, 16.12, 16.13, 16.14, 16.15, 16.16, 16.18, 16.19, 16.20, 17.1, 17.2, 17.3, 17.5, 17.6, 17.7, 17.9, 17.10.

Nair, M. and Peate, I. (2009) *Fundamentals of Applied Pathophysiology: An Essential Guide for Nursing Students*. Oxford: Wiley-Blackwell.
2.2, 2.4, 2.10, 2.12, 3.4, 5.3, 5.4, 5.5, 5.6, 7.5, 7.10, 7.11, 7.12, 7.13, 11.5, 11.9, 11.10, 13.16, 14.8, 15.12.

Jenkins G.W., Kemnitz C.P. and Tortora G.J. (2007) *Anatomy and Physiology: From Science to Life*. Hoboken, NJ: John Wiley & Sons.
4.13, Unnumbered illustration from clinical application, Pessary insertion box

Tortora, G.J. (2008) *A Brief Atlas of the Skeleton*. Hoboken, NJ: John Wiley & Sons.
8.6, 8.7.

Tortora, G.J. and Derrickson, B. (2010) *Essentials of Anatomy and Physiology*, 8th edn. New York: John Wiley & Sons.
6.4, 13.10.

Lister Hill National Center for Biomedical Communications (2010) *Genetics Home Reference: Your Guide to Understanding Genetic Conditions,* p.19. http://ghr.nlm.nih.gov/handbook.pdf
17.4.

National Heart Lung and Blood Institute
Unnumbered illustration in Clinical application: Myocardial Infarction box

Peate, I. (2009) *Men's Health*. Oxford: Wiley-Blackwell.
15.7.

Introduction

The contributors to this text are all committed to the provision of high quality care. The authors are all experienced academics working in higher education, with many years of clinical experience, knowledge and skills, teaching a variety of students at various academic levels. We are confident that after you have gained a sound understanding of the anatomy and physiology of the various bodily systems you will be able to understand better the needs of the people you have the privilege to care for. High quality care for all is something we should be striving to provide but it is not possible to do this effectively if we do not fully appreciate the whole being, the whole person. This text has been formulated in such a way that we hope you enjoy reading it, and more importantly that you are hungry to learn more, that you will be tempted to delve deeper and that you grow and develop.

The companion to this book, *The Fundamentals of Applied Pathophysiology* (Nair & Peate 2009) will aid in your development and understanding. It is essential in any programme of study related to the provision of care that you are confident and competent in this field of study. It is not enough that you remember all of the facts (and there are many of these) that are associated with anatomy and physiology; you must be able to relate these to the people you care for. Some of these people may be vulnerable and at risk of harm; you have a duty to ensure that you are knowledgeable. *Fundamentals of Anatomy and Physiology for Student Nurses* will help you. The Standards for Pre Registration Nursing Education (Nursing and Midwifery Council, 2010) make it clear that you must be competent in a number of spheres in order to register successfully with the Nursing and Midwifery Council.

The human body is as beautiful on the inside as it is on the outside; the mind and the body when working in harmony is a fantastic machine capable of extraordinary things. Healthcare students work and study both in the hospital and the community setting where they will meet and care for patients with diverse altered anatomical and physiological problems. Using a fundamental approach with a sound anatomical and physiological understanding will provide healthcare students with an essential basis on which to offer care.

Anatomy and physiology

Anatomy can be defined simply as the science related to the study of the structure of biological organisms; many dictionaries use such a definition. *Fundamentals of Anatomy and Physiology for Student Nurses* focuses on human anatomy, and the definition for the purposes of this text is a study of the structure and function of the human body. This allows for reference to function as well as structure; in all biological organisms structure and function are closely interconnected. The human body operates through interrelated systems.

The term anatomy is Greek in origin and means 'to cut up' or 'to dissect'. While the first scientifically based anatomical studies (attributed to a 16th-century Flemish anatomist, doctor and artist, Vesalius) were based on observations of cadavers (dead bodies), modern approaches to human anatomy differ as they include other ways of observation, for example, with the aid of a microscope and other imaging tools. Subdivisions are now affiliated within the broader field of anatomy; the word anatomy is often preceded with an adjective that identifies the method of observation, for example, gross anatomy (the study of body parts visible to the naked eye, for example, the heart or the bones) or microanatomy (where body parts, for example, cells or tissues are only visible with the use of a microscope).

Living systems can be defined from a number of perspectives:

- At the very smallest level, the chemical level, atoms, molecules and the chemical bonds connecting atoms provide the structure upon which living activity is based.
- The smallest unit of life is the cell. Specialised bodies – organelles – within the cell carry out particular cellular functions. Cells may be specialised, for example, bone cells and muscle cells.
- Tissue is a group of cells that are similar and they perform a common function. Muscle tissue, for example, is made up of muscle cells.
- Organs are groups of different types of tissues performing together to carry out a specific activity. The stomach is an organ made up of muscle, nerve and tissues.
- A system is two or more organs working together to carry out a particular activity. The digestive system, for example, comprises the coordinated activities of a number of organs, including the mouth, stomach, intestines, pancreas and liver.
- Another system that possesses the characteristics of living things is an organism; this has the capacity to obtain and process energy, the ability to react to changes in the environment and the ability to reproduce.

As anatomy is associated with the function of a living organism it is almost always inseparable from physiology. Physiology can be described as the science which deals with the study of the function of cells, tissues, organs and organisms.

Physiology is concerned with how an organism carries out its many activities, considering how it moves, how it is nourished, how it adapts to changing environments – human and animal, hostile and friendly. It is the study of life.

Physiology is the foundation upon which we build our knowledge of what life is; it can help us to decide how to treat disease as well as helping us to adapt and manage changes imposed on our bodies by new and changing surroundings – internal and external. Studying physiology will help you understand disease (pathophysiology) arising from this; physiologists are able to develop new ways for treating diseases.

Just as there are a number of branches of anatomical study, so too are there a number of physiological branches that can be studied, for example, endocrinology, neurology and cardiology.

The chapters

There are 17 chapters. The text is not intended to be read from cover to cover, but you may find reading the first three chapters will help you come to terms with some of the complex concepts; we encourage you to delve in and out of the book. The chapters use simple and generously sized full colour art work to assist you in understanding and appreciating the complexities associated with the human body from an anatomical and physiological perspective. There are many features contained within each chapter that assist you to build upon and develop your knowledge base; we would encourage you to get the most out of this book.

Getting the most out of your copy of *Fundamentals of Anatomy and Physiology for Student Nurses*

The text takes the reader from the microscopic to macroscopic level in the study of anatomy and physiology. The contents demonstrate the movement from cells and tissues through to systems. This approach to teaching is a tried and tested approach when helping learners understand a topic area that can sometimes be seen as complex.

This book has been written with these key principles in mind, to help inform your practice as well as your academic work. A number of features are provided to help bring to life the fascinating subject of human anatomy and physiology.

Each chapter begins with several questions that are posed to test your current knowledge and which will allow you to pre-test. Learning outcomes are provided. These will cover the content within the chapter but only you can do the learning; these outcomes are what are expected of you after reading and absorbing the information. This is a minimum of what you can learn; do not be constrained by the learning outcomes, they are only there to guide you. Where appropriate an anatomical map is provided; the anatomical map is related to the chapter you are reading, this allows you to visualise the anatomy being discussed.

Another feature in the chapter that is provided to help you consider people you care for, to help you make clinical links, are the boxes in most of the chapters called Clinical considerations. These boxes demonstrate the application to your learning citing specific care issues that you may come across when working with people in clinical settings.

At the end of the chapter you are provided with a bank of multiple choice questions that are based on the content of the chapter. Some of the answers to the questions are not found in the text; in this case you are encouraged to seek out the answers helping to develop your learning further.

Other features provided will help you measure the learning that has taken place, for example, true or false, label the diagram, find out more, crosswords or word searches; they are meant to be fun but they also aim to pull together the content of the chapter.

The feature called Conditions provides you with a list of conditions that are associated with the topics discussed in the chapter. You are encouraged to take some time to write notes about each of the conditions that have been described; this will help you relate theory to practice. You can make notes taken from other textbooks or other resources, for example, people you work with in a clinical area, or you may make the notes as a result of people you have cared for. It is important however that if you are making notes about people you have cared for you must ensure that you adhere to the rules of confidentiality.

A glossary of terms is provided at the end of every chapter. We present this to facilitate the learning of difficult words or phrases; understanding these words and phrases is important to your success as a healthcare student. When you have mastered the words your medical vocabulary will have grown and you will be in an ideal position to develop it further.

Patient notes are provided as an accompaniment to the text as a part of the web resources feature. These notes can be read at the beginning of the chapter as this will enable you to relate the issues being discussed to the people you may care for. We would suggest you revisit the patient notes several times as you work your way through each chapter – making a link from theory to practice and practice to theory. The patient notes are there merely to help you visualise, contextualise and to think about the application of theory to practice.

The use of computers and other electronic resources now play a central role in education as well as the education of nurses and other healthcare students with many universities using virtual learning environments. The electronic resources associated with this book are designed to help enhance your learning; they are varied and informative and are visually stimulating.

The text is accompanied by a raft of electronic resources that will support your learning. These resources can be used in your own place at your own pace. The aim is to encourage further learning and to build upon what you know already. There are also links to other resources. Using the electronic resources alongside the book as well as the human resources you will meet in practice will enhance the quality of your learning. The electronic resources available cannot replace the more conventional face to face learning with other students, lecturers, registered nurses and patients; they complement it.

What's in a name?

The use of terminology is important. Sometimes the term 'the patient' has been used in this text; universally the term is used because it is easier to do so and it is commonly understood. There are some possible dangers with this as it implies the person is in receipt of medical care and this can then mean that the care provider has the upper hand. This suggestion must be avoided at all costs as those in receipt of care are participants and the person offering care should be acting as advocate.

Throughout this text we have chosen to use a multitude of words that may be used to describe the people you care for, for example, patient, person, service user. These words (and many more) are used in everyday practice and you will come across them when you are in clinical and healthcare settings. The most important thing to remember is that the people being cared for are people, not labels or names attached to them. The Patients Association (2009) suggest: 'Patients not numbers ... People not statistics'.

When you are caring for people on an individual basis you must ask them what they would prefer you to call them. Some people are content with you addressing them by their first name, others may not be and you must, from the beginning of the therapeutic relationship, determine what the individual prefers; this demonstrates respect.

Just because a person becomes ill, prone to illness or vulnerable, they do not lose all their own values and beliefs, their sense of self as mother, father, lover, partner, brother or sister. How a person is addressed can impact on their health and wellbeing.

You may also note that we have used a variety of words to describe you, the reader. We have done this because we know that many people from a variety of backgrounds will read and use this text. All of us are learners and this is the perspective that we have used when writing this text.

The provision of a world-class health and social care service

The National Health Service (NHS) is the main provider (but not the only one) of health care in the United Kingdom (UK); the NHS belongs to all of us. There are thousands of healthcare workers employed by the NHS; most of them provide hands-on care – the NHS aims to deliver world-class care. This includes engaging people cared for and empowering them and their communities; as well as this you are an important part of this aim, you are central to ensuring that this intention is realised.

The provision of care and access to services – how it is provided, where it is provided, when it is provided and who provides it is changing all of the time. Accessibility of services is important, so too is the prevention of illness and disability with the intention of helping people to stay active and healthy – mind and body.

The four countries of the UK have planned the way services are provided in their own countries. The people of these four countries deserve the very best and they should settle for nothing less. You must also strive to deliver world-class care along with other health and social care workers, for example, physiotherapists, speech and language therapists, doctors, midwives, dieticians, paid carers, informal carers, social services and the people you care for themselves.

We wish you much success with your studies be they in the classroom or in the multitude of care areas that you might find yourself working.

References

Nair, M. and Peate, I. (2009) *Fundamentals of Applied Pathophysiology: An Essential Guide for Nursing Students*. Oxford: Wiley-Blackwell.

Nursing and Midwifery Council (2010) *Standards for Pre Registration Nursing Education*. London: NMC.

Patients Association (2009) *Patients not Numbers ... People not Statistics*. London: Patients Association.

1

Basic scientific principles of physiology

Peter S Vickers

Contents

Introduction 2

Levels of organisation 2

Characteristics of life 2

Bodily requirements 4

Atoms 4
Atomic number 6
Carbon atom 6
Molecules 7
Chemical bonds 7
Ionic bonding of atoms 7
Ions 7
Covalent bonds 8
Polar bonds 9
Electrolytes 9

Elements 10
Properties of elements 13

Compounds 13

Chemical equations/chemical reactions 13

Acids and bases (pH) 16

Blood and pH values 18

Homeostasis 18

Organic and inorganic substances 19
Examples of organic substances 19
Examples of inorganic substances 20

Units of measurement 20

Conclusion 23
Glossary 23
References 25
Activities 26

Fundamentals of Anatomy and Physiology for Student Nurses, First Edition. Edited by Ian Peate, Muralitharan Nair.

Test your knowledge

- What are the three basic components of an atom?
- What are the essential requirements of all organisms (including humans)?
- Why is it important for atoms to be able to bind together?
- What is a pH scale?

Learning outcomes

On completion of this chapter, the reader will be able to:

- Describe the levels of organisation of a body
- Describe the characteristics of life
- Understand and explain an atom and how it relates to molecules
- Describe and understand the ways in which atoms can bind together
- Describe elements and their characteristics
- Understand how to read chemical equations
- Describe the pH scale and its importance to life
- List the differences between organic and inorganic substances
- List the various ways in which we measure things.

Introduction

Learning about the physiology of the body is very much like learning a foreign language – there is new vocabulary, new grammar and new concepts to learn and understand. This first chapter introduces you to this new language so that you can then use your knowledge to understand the physiology of the different parts of the body that are discussed in all the other chapters of this book.

First of all there are two terms to learn and understand – namely, anatomy and physiology:

- **Anatomy** is the study of structure
- **Physiology** is the study of function.

However, structure is always related to function because the structure determines the function, which in turn determines how the body/organ, etc. is structured – the two are interdependent.

Levels of organisation

The body is a very complex organism which consists of many components, starting with the smallest of them – the atom – and concluding with the many organs that are found within the body (Figure 1.1). Starting from the smallest component and working towards the largest, the body is organised in this way:

- The atom – e.g. hydrogen, carbon
- The molecule – e.g. water, glucose
- The macromolecule (large molecule) – e.g. protein, DNA
- The organelle (found in the cell) – e.g. nucleus, mitochondrion
- The tissues – bone, muscle
- The organs – e.g. heart, kidney
- The organ system – e.g. skeletal, cardiovascular
- The organism – e.g. human, cat.

Characteristics of life

All living organisms have certain characteristics in common. Although these characteristics may differ from organism to organism, they are important for the maintenance of life. These characteristics are:

- Reproduction – both at the micro- and the macro-level, reproduction is essential. At the macro-level it is the reproduction of the organism and at the micro-level it is the reproduction of new cells to maintain the efficiency and growth of the organism
- Growth – essential for the growth and development of an organism
- Movement – both change in position and motion are parts of movement. This characteristic is essential to allow the organism to seek out nutrition and partners for reproduction, as well as to escape predators

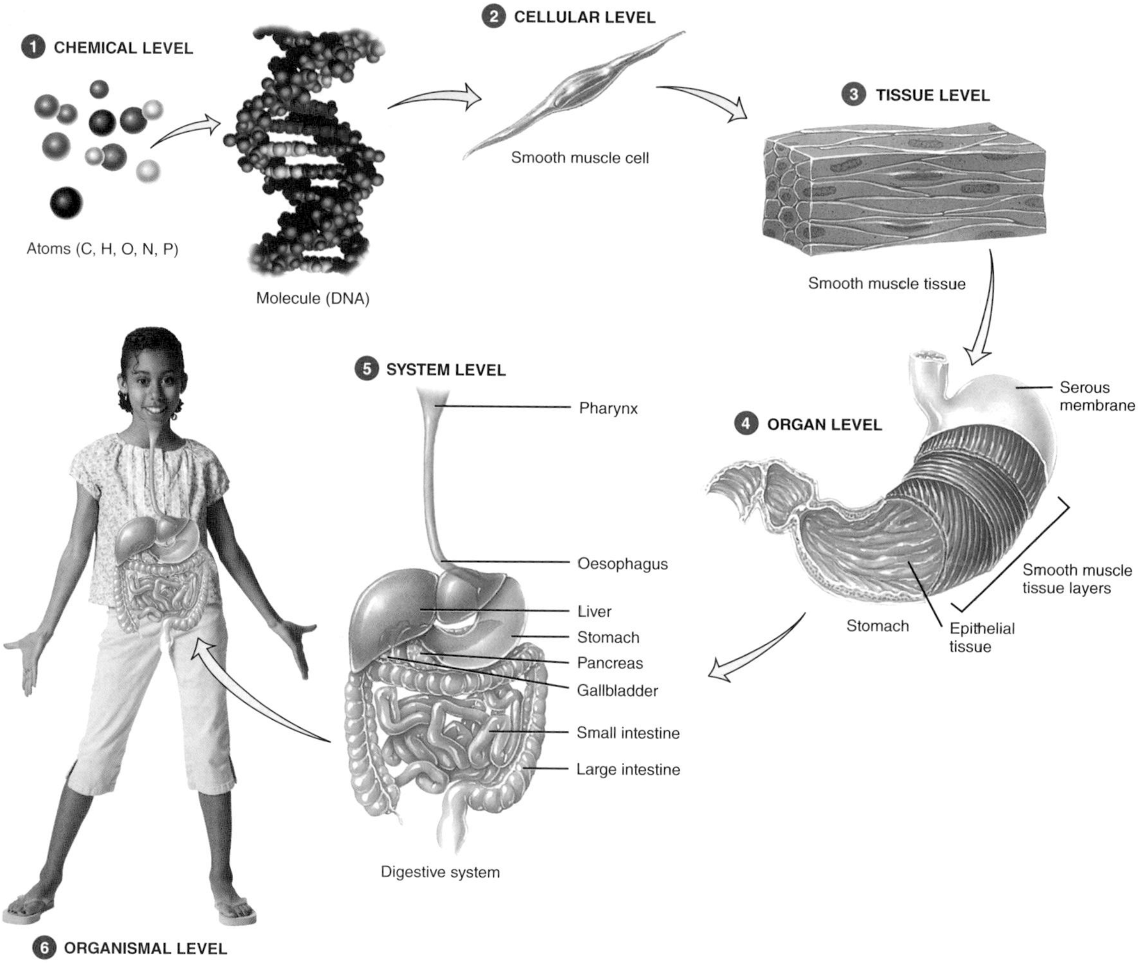
1 CHEMICAL LEVEL
Atoms (C, H, O, N, P)
Molecule (DNA)
2 CELLULAR LEVEL
Smooth muscle cell
3 TISSUE LEVEL
Smooth muscle tissue
4 ORGAN LEVEL
Serous membrane
Smooth muscle tissue layers
Stomach
Epithelial tissue
5 SYSTEM LEVEL
Pharynx
Oesophagus
Liver
Stomach
Pancreas
Gallbladder
Small intestine
Large intestine
Digestive system
6 ORGANISMAL LEVEL

Figure 1.1 Levels of organisation of the body (Tortora and Derrickson 2009)

- Respiration – respiration is important for obtaining oxygen and releasing carbon dioxide (or obtaining carbon dioxide and releasing oxygen if a green plant), known as external respiration, as well as releasing energy from foods (internal respiration)
- Responsiveness – this allows the organism to respond to changes, for example in the environment or to other stimuli
- Digestion – this is the breakdown of food substances, so that the organism can produce the energy necessary for life
- Absorption – the movement of substances (including digested food) through membranes and into body fluids, including blood and lymph, which then carry the substances to the parts of the organism requiring them
- Circulation – the movement of substances through the body in the body fluids

Atomic number

All atoms are designated a number, known as the atomic number, and the atomic number of an atom is the same as the number of protons in that atom. Consequently, the atomic number of a carbon atom is 6. Similarly, the sodium atom has 11 protons and therefore its atomic number is 11, whilst a chlorine atom has 17 protons and so has an atomic number of 17.

Carbon atom

A look at a very important atom, namely carbon, will demonstrate the makeup of an actual atom. Carbon is very important in bioscience because we are all carbon-based entities.

As you can see from Figure 1.4, carbon has six electrons orbiting around the nucleus which is made up of six protons and six neutrons, therefore having the same numbers of electrons, protons and neutrons. This is unusual, because whilst, as explained below, it is normal to have the same number of electrons and protons, usually the number of neutrons differs from the numbers of electrons and protons in an atom.

A basic principle of the atom is that the number of electrons is equal to the number of protons in each atom, and this is all to do with electricity. As mentioned above, protons carry a positive electrical charge, electrons carry a negative electrical charge and neutrons carry a neutral charge (i.e. they carry no charge), and the aim of all atoms is to remain electrically stable, i.e. electrically neutral. Therefore, as neutrons carry no electrical charge, it is important that electrons and protons are equal in number to maintain the stability/neutrality.

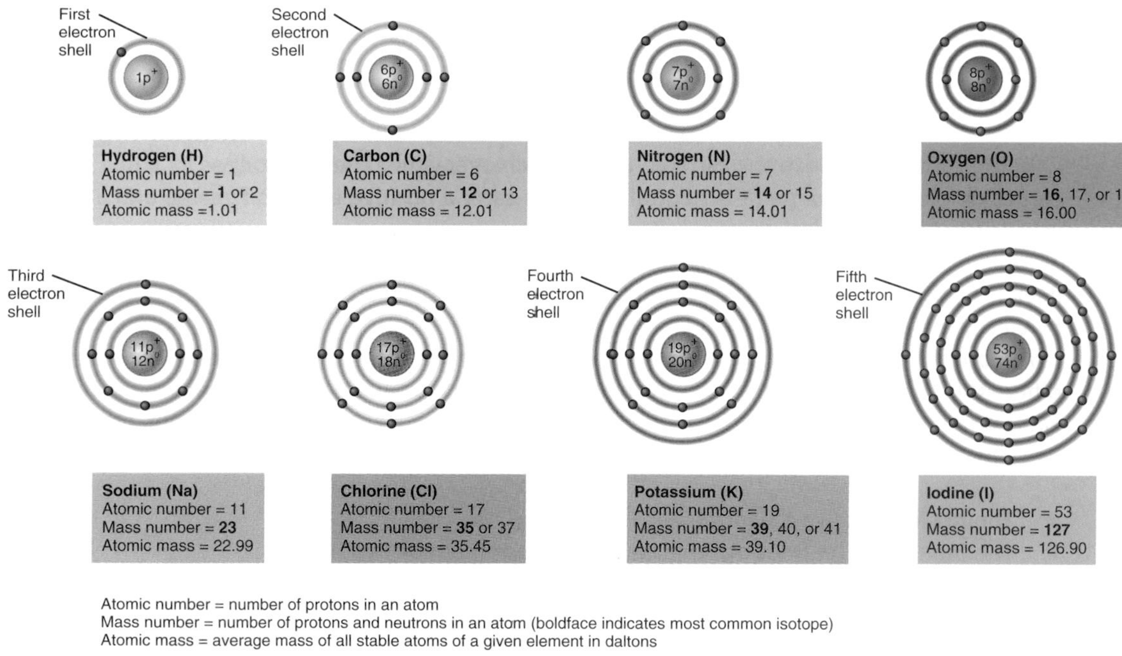

First electron shell
1p+
Hydrogen (H)
Atomic number = 1
Mass number = 1 or 2
Atomic mass =1.01
Second electron shell
6p+ 6n0
Carbon (C)
Atomic number = 6
Mass number = 12 or 13
Atomic mass = 12.01
7p+ 7n0
Nitrogen (N)
Atomic number = 7
Mass number = 14 or 15
Atomic mass = 14.01
8p+ 8n0
Oxygen (O)
Atomic number = 8
Mass number = 16, 17, or 18
Atomic mass = 16.00
Third electron shell
11p+ 12n0
Sodium (Na)
Atomic number = 11
Mass number = 23
Atomic mass = 22.99
17p+ 18n0
Chlorine (Cl)
Atomic number = 17
Mass number = 35 or 37
Atomic mass = 35.45
Fourth electron shell
19p+ 20n0
Potassium (K)
Atomic number = 19
Mass number = 39, 40, or 41
Atomic mass = 39.10
Fifth electron shell
53p+ 74n0
Iodine (I)
Atomic number = 53
Mass number = 127
Atomic mass = 126.90
Atomic number = number of protons in an atom
Mass number = number of protons and neutrons in an atom (boldface indicates most common isotope)
Atomic mass = average mass of all stable atoms of a given element in daltons

Figure 1.4 Carbon atom (Tortora and Derrickson 2009)

To understand how this works, the carbon atom carries six electrons, six protons and six neutrons, and therefore the electrical charges of the electrons and protons cancel one another out. Consequently, overall, the atom is neutrally charged and it is said to be in a state of equilibrium.

Molecules

This need for the atom to be in equilibrium is the driving force behind the combining of atoms to make molecules (the next stage in the building of life forms). A molecule can be defined as the smallest particle of an element or compound which exists independently. It contains atoms that have bonded together. For example, sodium chloride (NaCl) is a molecule containing one atom of sodium (also known as natrium – symbol Na) which has bonded to one atom of chlorine (symbol Cl). Similarly, the molecule H_2O is made up of two atoms of hydrogen (H) bonded to one atom of oxygen (O). H_2O is better known as water.

Chemical bonds

A chemical bond is the way in which atoms bind to one another by the atoms attaining a lower energy state by losing, gaining or sharing their outer shell electrons with other atoms. A chemical bond is the 'attractive' force that holds atoms together. This interaction results in the formation of atoms or ions that are in a lower energy state than the original atoms.

The formation of chemical bonds also results in the release of energy previously contained in the atoms, as shown in the following formula:

$$\text{atom} + \text{atom} \rightarrow \text{atom-atom} + \text{energy}$$

The combining power of atoms is known as **valence**. Because the only shell that is important in bonding is the outermost shell, this shell is known as the valence shell (Marieb and Hoehn 2009).

There are several types of chemical bonds that occur between atoms, namely:

- Ionic bonds
- Covalent bonds
- Polar bonds/hydrogen bonds.

Ionic bonding of atoms

It has been remarked above that atoms prefer always to be in a state of equilibrium, but sometimes an atom which has a stable structure may lose an electron, in which case it becomes unstable. For example, a sodium (Na) atom is an atom that may lose an electron and in this case, in order to become stable again, it must connect with an atom which can accept an electron – for example, chlorine (Cl). So consequently, when sodium atoms and chlorine atoms are mixed together, one electron of each sodium atom will move to an equivalent atom of chlorine – as depicted in Figure 1.5 – thus forming the molecule sodium chloride (NaCl), also known as common salt. This is known as **ionic bonding**, because **ions** are involved.

Ions

Ions are atoms which are no longer in an electrically neutral state, but are either negatively or positively electrically charged. In the example above, sodium and chlorine have positive and

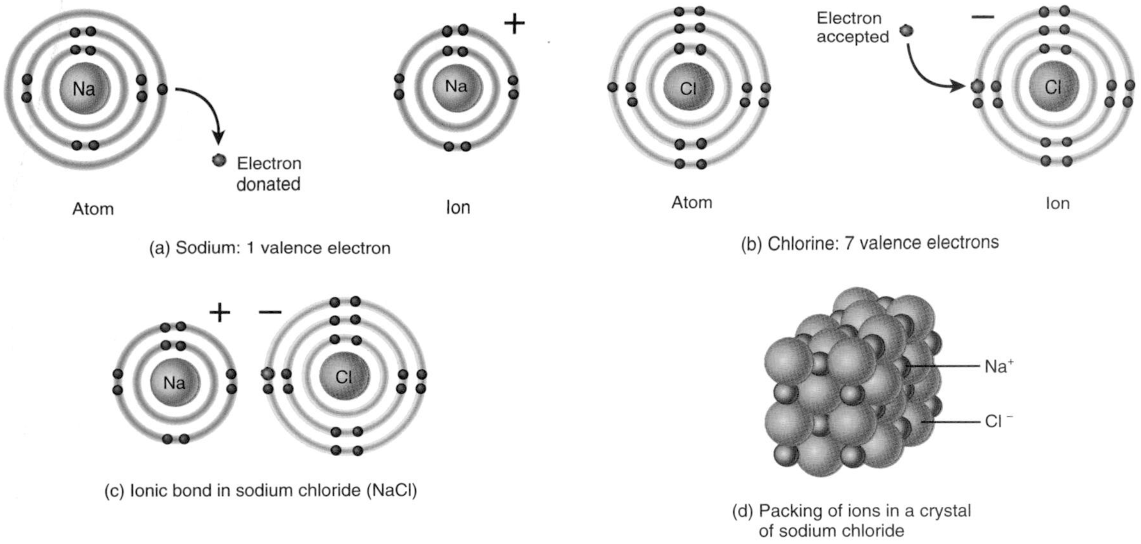
Atom
Electron donated
Ion
+
(a) Sodium: 1 valence electron
Atom
Electron accepted
Ion
(b) Chlorine: 7 valence electrons
Na
Cl
(c) Ionic bond in sodium chloride (NaCl)
Na⁺
Cl⁻
(d) Packing of ions in a crystal of sodium chloride

Figure 1.5 Ionic bonding of a sodium and a chlorine atom to form a sodium chloride molecule (Tortora and Derrickson 2009)

negative electrical charges respectively due to the interchange of electrons, so they are now ions, and we depict them as:

- Na^+ (sodium positive)
- Cl^- (chlorine negative).

However, we write the resultant sodium chloride molecule as NaCl because the positive (+) and the negative (–) have attracted each other, but as the charges are non-directional an ionic lattice is formed. An ionic lattice is a structure that is made up of millions of atomic formations, composed of an ionic substance. It is put together like building blocks, so that the end product is a single, three-dimensional structure.

- Ions which carry a positive electrical charge are known as **cations**
- Ions which carry a negative electrical charge are known as **anions**.

To summarise, an ionic bond is a bond that is formed between ions, some of which are positively charged and some of which are negatively charged. These atoms are known as ions and are attracted to, and stabilise, each other, but they neither transfer nor share electrons between themselves. Consequently this can be seen more as an interaction between atoms rather than as a bond between them (Fisher and Arnold 2004).

Covalent bonds

Unlike ionic bonding, covalent bonding does involve the sharing of valence electrons with compatible adjacent electrons. In this way, none of the atoms involved in this type of bonding actually loses or gains electrons. Instead, electrons are shared between them so that each of the atoms will have a complete valence shell (i.e. outermost shell) for at least part of the time (Marieb and Hoehn 2009).

Covalent bonding occurs when two atoms are close to one another and an overlapping of the outer shell electrons occurs. Following this overlapping, each outer shell becomes attracted to the other's nucleus (Figure 1.6). This type of bonding does not require positive and negative electrical charges as ionic bonding does.

There are three types of covalent bonding, depending upon the number of electrons that are shared between the bonded atoms:

(1) Single covalent bonds (one electron from each atom is shared in the outermost shell), e.g. hydrogen molecule
(2) Double covalent bonds (two electrons from each atom are shared), e.g. oxygen molecule
(3) Triple covalent bonds (three electrons from each atom are shared), e.g. nitrogen molecule.

Polar bonds

Sometimes, molecules do not share electrons equally and so there is a separation of the electrical charge into positive or negative. This is called **polarity**, and because of this separation of electrical charge, there is an additional weak bond. However, this bond is NOT between **atoms**, but is between the **molecules** themselves. Just as with ionic bonding, this polar bonding comes about because of the electrical rule that **opposites attract**. Thus the small opposite charges from different polar molecules can be attracted to each other. Polar bonding only occurs with molecules that contain the atom hydrogen – so a polar bond is also known as a **hydrogen bond**. (See Figure 1.7).

The fact that polar molecules can bond (albeit only weakly) is very important in determining the structure and function of physiologically active substances such as:

- Enzymes
- Antibodies
- Genetic molecules
- Pharmacological agents (drugs).

Electrolytes

A further development of bonding is the production of electrolytes. Electrolytes are substances that move to oppositely charged electrodes in fluids, and occur in this way. If molecules that are bonded together ionically (see ionic bonding above) are dissolved in water within the body cells, then they undergo a process where the ions separate, i.e. they become dissociated. These ions are now known as electrolytes.

However, this does not apply to molecules that are produced by other types of bonding (e.g. covalent bonding). Molecules that are produced as a result of other types of bonding are called non-electrolytes, and these include most organic compounds, such as glucose, urea and creatinine.

Electrolytes are particularly important for three things within the body:

(1) Many are essential minerals.
(2) They control the process of osmosis.
(3) They help to maintain the acid base balance, which is necessary for normal cellular activity.

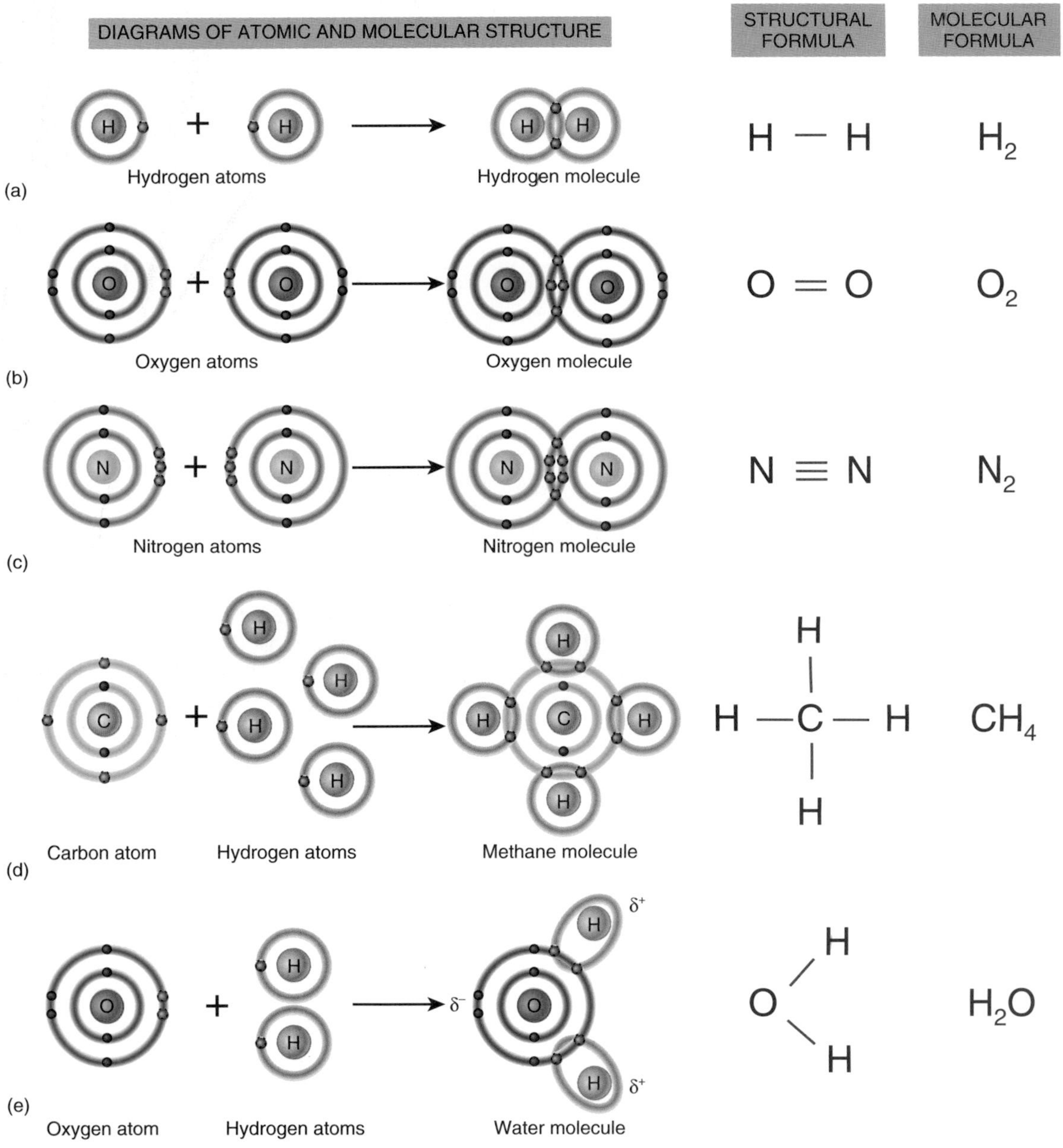
DIAGRAMS OF ATOMIC AND MOLECULAR STRUCTURE
STRUCTURAL FORMULA
MOLECULAR FORMULA
(a)
Hydrogen atoms
Hydrogen molecule
H — H
H2
(b)
Oxygen atoms
Oxygen molecule
O = O
O2
(c)
Nitrogen atoms
Nitrogen molecule
N ≡ N
N2
(d)
Carbon atom
Hydrogen atoms
Methane molecule
CH4
(e)
Oxygen atom
Hydrogen atoms
Water molecule
δ+
δ−
H2O

Figure 1.6 Covalent bond (Tortora and Derrickson 2009)

Elements

A chemical element is a pure chemical substance which cannot be broken down into anything simpler by chemical means. Each element consists of just one type of atom, which is distinguished by its atomic number (which in turn is determined by the number of protons in the nucleus of an

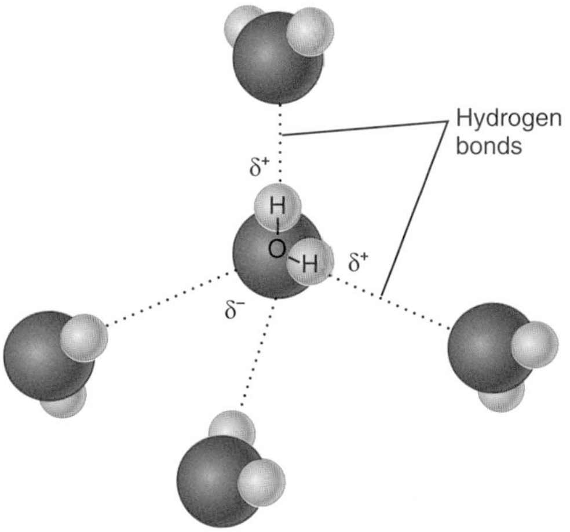
Hydrogen bonds
δ+
H
O
H
δ+
δ−

Figure 1.7 Hydrogen bonds and water (Tortora and Derrickson 2009)

atom – see above). If the number of protons in the nucleus of an atom changes, then we have a new element, not the original one. This, of course, is different from the electrons in which the number can change but the atom remains basically the same – although it is now an **ion**. Some common examples of elements found in the body include:

- Iron
- Hydrogen
- Carbon
- Nitrogen
- Oxygen
- Calcium
- Potassium
- Sodium
- Chlorine
- Sulphur
- Phosphorous.

By 2008, a total of 117 elements had been observed; these are usually presented as a **Periodic Table**. All chemical matter consists of these elements, although new elements of higher atomic number are discovered from time to time – but only as a result of artificial nuclear reactions and so are not found in the body.

There are three classes of elements:

(1) Metals (e.g. iron – symbol 'Fe' from ferrum).
(2) Non-metals (e.g. oxygen – symbol 'O').
(3) Metalloids (e.g. arsenic – symbol 'As').

These three classes of elements all have certain characteristics that define them:

Characteristics of metals, non-metals and metalloids:

Metals	Non-metals	Metalloids
They conduct heat and electricity. They donate electrons (to other atoms to make molecules) At normal temperatures they are all solids – with the exception of mercury (symbol 'Hg')	They are poor conductors of heat and electricity They accept electrons (from donor atoms) They may exist as a solid, a liquid or a gas	They are neither metals nor non-metals – they are sometimes referred to as semi-metals They tend to have the physical properties of metals whilst having the chemical properties of both metals and non-metals depending upon their oxidation state. However, they are not relevant to biochemistry, so will not be discussed in this book

Usually metals bond with non-metals (electron donors with electron acceptors).

Below are examples of elements important for the body that are metals and some examples of non-metals.

Metals	Non-Metals
Calcium – Ca	Chlorine – Cl
Potassium – K	Nitrogen – N
Sodium – Na	Oxygen – O
	Carbon – C
	Sulphur – S
	Phosphorus – P

As well as sodium chloride – NaCl (met previously in this chapter) – some other important compounds that a nurse will need to know about include:

- Sodium bicarbonate – NaHCO3
- Potassium chloride – KCl.

An interesting element is hydrogen (H), because hydrogen actually has properties of both metals and non-metals. As a consequence, water (H_2O) is an example of a substance that, although made up of two gases – oxygen (1 molecule) and hydrogen (2 molecules) – becomes a liquid once these gases have bonded together, due to the process of hydrogen bonding between molecules.

Properties of elements

All substances have certain individual properties, particularly in the way that they react (i.e. behave):

- Physical properties – include such characteristics as colour, density, boiling point, melting point, solubility, hardness, etc.
- Chemical properties – include whether or not a substance is a metal or non-metal (or even metalloid), whether it reacts with an acid or an alkaline substance, or whether it dissolves in water or alcohol.

Compounds

'Compound' is a new term with which to become acquainted; a compound is a pure substance which is made up of two or more elements chemically bonded together. The properties of a compound are totally different from the individual properties of the elements that are bonded together to make that compound. In addition, compounds can be broken down chemically, whilst elements cannot. Examples of compounds include:

- Water (H_2O)
- Salt (NaCl)
- Carbon dioxide (CO_2).

Note that when the symbol for an atom has a small lower number after it, then that denotes that there are that number of that particular atom in the molecule. So, water (H_2O) is made up of two atoms of hydrogen and one atom of oxygen, whilst carbon dioxide (CO_2) consists of one atom of carbon and two atoms of oxygen. This will be discussed again later in this chapter.

Chemical equations/chemical reactions

Any mention of chemical equations and most non-chemists/non-scientists immediately start to panic and quickly turn the page. Not to worry, however, because if anyone is capable of doing simple addition sums, then they are capable of working through chemical equations. Everyone has worked through simple mathematical equations, such as:

- $1 + 1 = 2$
- $2 + 2 = 4$
- $4 + 4 = 8$
- $1 + 1 + 2 + 2 + 2 = 8$
- $1 + 1 + 2 + 2 + 2 = 4 + 3 + 1$

and so on.

Chemical equations work on the same basic principles. When a chemical reaction occurs (which is depicted by an equation), then a new substance is formed, which is called the **product** (as with a mathematical equation). However, in a chemical equation, this new substance (product) will have different properties from the individual substances involved in the reaction (called the reactants).

As discussed above, when atoms are combined they form elements or molecules, and symbols are used to describe this process. This look at chemical equations will start with a very simple example, namely the production of water (Figure 1.8). As discussed above, two atoms of hydrogen (H_2) combined with one atom of oxygen (O) produce one molecule of water (H_2O). The chemical equation for this process is

$$2H + 2H + 2O \rightarrow 2H_2O$$

$$\text{hydrogen} + \text{hydrogen} + \text{oxygen} \rightarrow \text{water}$$

In this equation (of a chemical reaction) there are four atoms of hydrogen and two atoms of oxygen on the left hand side, and there are four atoms of hydrogen and two atoms of oxygen on the right hand side. However, on the right, because of a chemical reaction, the same six atoms of gas have created water – a liquid.

Thus, a chemical equation is just a shorthand way of describing a chemical reaction. Note that the equals sign in a mathematical equation is replaced by an arrow, meaning 'leads to', in a chemical equation. Basically, all chemical equations are as simple as this. There may be more reactants and products, but there are similar basic principles involved in chemical equations as in mathematical equations.

A very important basic principle is that when chemical reactions occur, the amount of each substance must be the same after the reaction has occurred as was present before the reaction. The two sides of a chemical reaction (and therefore a chemical equation) – the reactants and the products – must balance. In other words, no atoms/molecules are lost in a chemical reaction, they are just organised differently. Another thing to be aware of with chemical reactions is that although the numbers of atoms are the same before and after the reaction, during a chemical reaction, something extra is produced every time – namely, heat. This is known as an exothermic reaction, which is a process/reaction that gives out energy in the form of heat.

In a chemical equation, the reactants and the product may be separated by a single arrow ($\rightarrow$) as in the example of H_2O above. This indicates that the reaction occurs only in one direction, namely in the direction that the arrow is pointing.

Sometimes the reactants and product may be separated by two arrows – one above the other and pointing in different directions ($\rightleftharpoons$). This indicates that the chemical reaction can be reversed.

If the reactants and the products are separated by an equals sign '=' (which is a symbol used in mathematics to indicate a state of equality), instead of single or double arrows, this indicates that a state of chemical equilibrium exists.

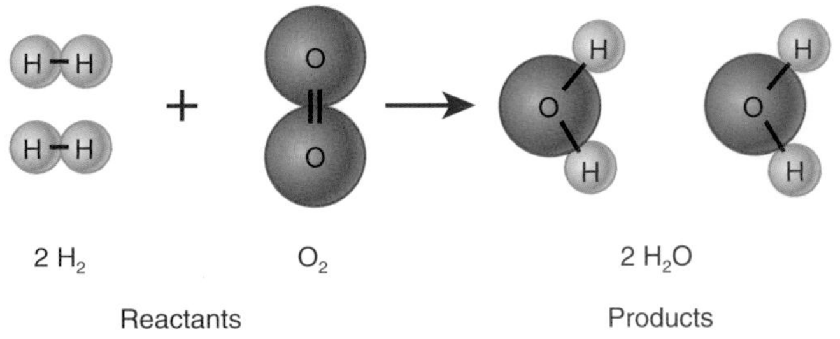
H–H
H–H
+
O
O
O
H
H
O
H
H
2 H2
O2
2 H2O
Reactants
Products

Figure 1.8 Pictorial depiction of the chemical equation (reaction) producing water (Tortora and Derrickson 2009)

Another important principle to be aware of as regards chemical reactions and equations is that a chemical equation has to be consistent. The elements cannot be changed into other elements by chemical means.

If electrical charges are involved (as occurs with the involvement of **ions**), the net charge on both sides of the equation must be equal – i.e. they must balance.

So, to summarise, all equations must balance (i.e. the number of reactants and their electrical charges must equal the number of products and their electrical charges). However, balancing a chemical equation (and thus a reaction) may require the altering of the quantity of molecules.

Now to turn to a more complicated chemical reaction/equation – but the principles still hold for this.

$$Zn + 2HCl \longrightarrow ZnCl_2 + H_2$$

$$\text{Zinc} + \text{hydrogen chloride} \longrightarrow \text{zinc chloride} + \text{hydrogen}$$

Note – mention has been made previously in this chapter of the principle that when using the chemical symbols of substances – elements, compounds, molecules, etc. – if a small number comes after an atom as in H_2O, then that number applies to the atom immediately before it. In other words H_2O is composed of two atoms of hydrogen and one atom of oxygen. However, if an an atom or molecule is preceded by a large number, then that applies to everything immediately afterwards until another mathematical symbol (e.g. +, →, etc.) occurs. For example 2HCl means that there are two atoms of hydrogen and two atoms of chlorine bonded together to make two molecules of hydrogen chloride.

In this chemical reaction/equation, two molecules of hydrogen chloride – in the form of two ions of chloride (Cl^-) and two ions of hydrogen (H^+) – along with one atom of zinc have been changed to one molecule of zinc chloride ($ZnCl_2$) and one molecule of hydrogen (H_2). So, even though the original atoms have now been combined differently following the chemical reaction, the balance between the two sides of the equation in terms of numbers and types of atoms and electrical charge has not been altered.

With this even more complicated chemical reaction/equation, it is a good idea to take some time and work out just what is going on here before reading on:

$$HCl + NaHCO_3 \longrightarrow NaCl + H_2CO_3$$

$$\text{Hydrochloric acid} + \text{sodium bicarbonate} \longrightarrow \text{sodium chloride} + \text{carbonic acid}$$

Also in this reaction, H_2CO_3 can be broken down further

$$H_2CO_3 \rightleftharpoons CO_2 + H_2O$$

The reactants on the left-hand side are duplicated on the right-hand side (the products) but in different combinations. Note the double arrow – what does this mean?

The presence of the double-headed arrow means that the equation is capable of being reversed, so that the products become the reactants, and the reactants the products. Note that sodium bicarbonate is made up of one atom each of sodium, hydrogen and carbon and three atoms of oxygen, whilst carbonic acid is composed of two atoms of hydrogen, one atom of carbon and three atoms of oxygen. Counting the numbers and types of each atom on both sides demonstrates again that nothing is added and nothing deleted when the reaction takes place – everything is just rearranged in such a way that elements that can be used by the body are produced (along with any waste elements which are then excreted).

This is the end of the section on chemical equations, and as can be seen, if someone can do simple arithmetic sums, then they can understand and work with chemical equations (remembering that the equations are a depiction of chemical reactions that are taking place within the body all the time).

Acids and bases (pH)

This next section may initially appear complicated because it is quite scientific, but it is important to understand **pH** values, alkalinity and acidity, as our bodies (indeed our very lives) depend upon the relationship between acidity and alkalinity.

- An **acid** is any substance which donates hydrogen ions (H^+) into a solution.
- An **alkali** (also known as a **soluble base**) is any substance which donates hydroxyl ions (OH^-) into a solution or accepts H^+ ions from a solution.

The more OH^- ions that have been donated or H^+ ions accepted, the greater the alkalinity of a substance, and conversely, the greater the number of H^+ ions that are released, the more acidic is the solution. Obviously, whenever the numbers of H^+ and OH^- ions are the same, then a **neutral** solution exists.

The chemical equation for the slight ionisation of water is shown as

$$H_2O \leftrightarrow H^+ + OH^-$$

In other words, water contains hydrogen and hydroxyl ions, and in 1 litre of pure water, 10^{-14} **moles** of water are dissociated into H^+ ions and OH^- ions. If there are 10^{-7} moles of H^+ ions and 10^{-7} moles of OH^- ions in 1 litre, then they are balanced and the water is neutral (neither acidic nor alkaline).

- Note that a **mole** in chemistry is a unit of amount of substance (it is a unit of measurement for chemicals) and is defined as the mass of substance that contains as many elements (atoms, molecules, etc.) as there are atoms in 12 grams of carbon-12 (International Bureau of Weights and Measures 2006).

  The concept of a mole in chemistry is quite complicated, but it is only necessary in this chapter to use it in relation to acid base balance.
- The concept of 10^{-14} is an arithmetic one and denotes a very small number – $10^{-14} = 0.00000000000001$ of a mole.
- In biochemistry, **dissociation** is the separation of a substance into two or more simpler substances – such as a molecule into atoms or ions – by the action of heat or a chemical process. This process is usually reversible.

The properties of water are such that the minimum concentration of H^+ ions and OH^- ions is 10^{-14} mol/l (moles per litre), whilst the maximum concentration of H^+ ions and OH^- ions is 1 mole/litre or 1.00 mol/l. Thus, the dissociation of properties of water restricts the concentration of H^+ ions and OH^- ions to the range of 10^{-14} to 10^0 mol/l.

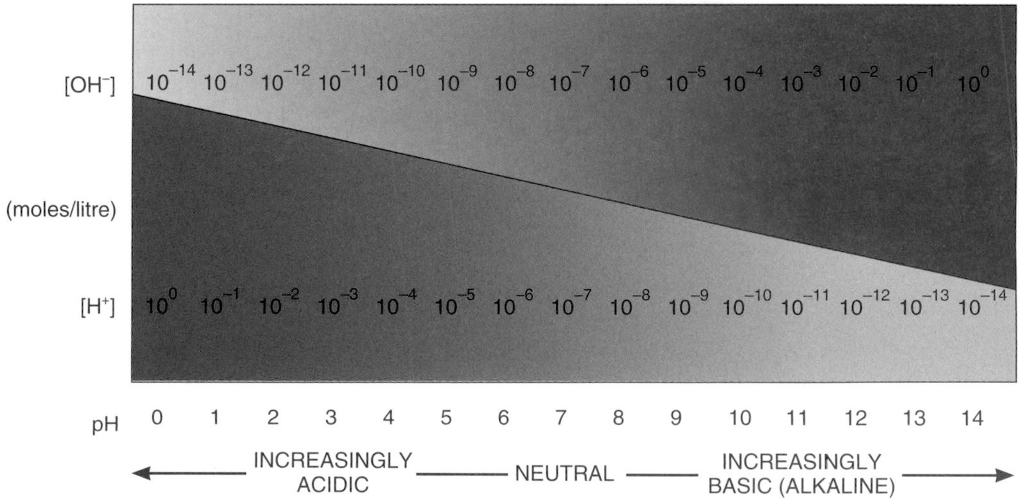

[OH⁻]
10^{-14} 10^{-13} 10^{-12} 10^{-11} 10^{-10} 10^{-9} 10^{-8} 10^{-7} 10^{-6} 10^{-5} 10^{-4} 10^{-3} 10^{-2} 10^{-1} 10^{0}
(moles/litre)
[H⁺]
10^{0} 10^{-1} 10^{-2} 10^{-3} 10^{-4} 10^{-5} 10^{-6} 10^{-7} 10^{-8} 10^{-9} 10^{-10} 10^{-11} 10^{-12} 10^{-13} 10^{-14}
pH 0 1 2 3 4 5 6 7 8 9 10 11 12 13 14
INCREASINGLY ACIDIC
NEUTRAL
INCREASINGLY BASIC (ALKALINE)

Figure 1.9 pH scale (Tortora and Derrickson 2009)

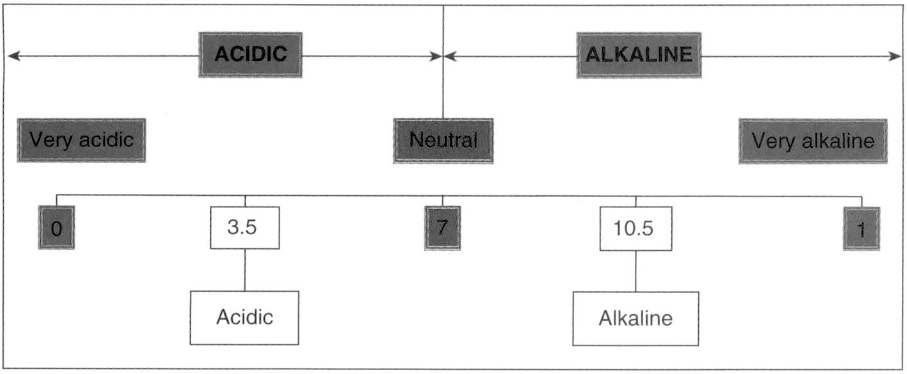

ACIDIC
ALKALINE
Very acidic
Neutral
Very alkaline
0
3.5
7
10.5
1
Acidic
Alkaline

Figure 1.10 Simplified diagram of a pH scale

A scale of acidity and alkalinity has been devised that uses this range of 10^{-14} to 10^{0} mol/l of H^{+} and OH^{-} ions – known as the **pH scale** (see Figure 1.9 and Figure 1.10). Consequently, the addition of H^{+} ions to pure water results in a proportionate decrease of OH^{-} ions from the initial concentration of 10^{-7} mol/l. Similarly, a H^{+} ion concentration of 10^{-8} mol/L results in a OH^{-} concentration of 10^{-8} mol/l. In this way, the combined totals of H^{+} and OH^{-} molecules will always equal 10^{-14}. The pH scale represents the powers of 10 of H^{+} ions from 10^{-14} to 10^{0}, but for convenience, the scale uses positive numbers, so the scale is from pH 14 to pH 0.

At pH 7 an equal number of H^+ ions and OH^- ions occur, whilst solutions with a pH that is lower than 7 are **acids** and those with a pH that is greater than 7 are **bases/alkaline.** The further away from a pH of 7 a solution becomes the more acidic or alkaline it is.

The pH scale is a logarithmic scale so consequently each whole pH value below 7 is ten times more acidic than the next higher value. For example, a solution with a pH 3 value is ten times more acidic than a solution with a pH 4 value. In addition, it is 100 times (i.e. times 10) more acidic than solution with a pH 5, and 1,000 times (i.e. 10 times 10 times 10) more acidic than a solution that has a pH value of 7 (i.e. a neutral solution). Exactly the same applies to pH values that are above 7 (i.e. alkaline solutions), in that each is 10 times more alkaline than the next lowest value. For example, a solution with a pH of 10 is 10 times more alkaline than one with a pH of 9, 100 times (10 times 10) more alkaline than a solution with a pH of 8, and so on.

This last concept of logarithmic values and pH is very important for us, as can be seen in the next section which looks at pH values and blood.

Blood and pH values

In blood, the physiologically normal pH range is 7.35–7.45, i.e. it is slightly alkaline. However, a blood pH lower than 7.35 is considered to be acidic, whereas a pH greater than 7.45 is alkaline, and when either of these events occurs, it can have a serious effect on the body, as is discussed in other chapters within this book. The reason for this is that because the scale is a logarithm, then just a small change in pH indicates a very significant alteration in H^+ concentration. The reason for this is that every change in one pH unit represents a tenfold change in H^+ ion concentration. Thus an alteration of pH from pH 7.4 to pH 7.3 results in a doubling of the H^+ ion concentration. In other words:

- pH 8 contains 10^{-8} mol/L or 10 nmol (nanomoles)
- pH 7 contains 10^{-7} mol/L or 100 nmol
- pH 6 contains 10^{-6} mol/L or 1000 nmol

and so on.

Homeostasis

Homeostasis is the body's attempt to maintain a stable internal environment by achieving some sort of balance. The body is normally able to achieve a relatively stable internal environment even though the external environment is constantly changing – from cold to hot, or from dry to wet, etc. The body uses various homeostatic mechanisms to monitor and maintain a dynamic state of equilibrium within the body – i.e. a balance in which the internal environment conditions can react to external environmental conditions by changing within quite narrow limits. The homeostatic mechanisms include:

- Receptors – these receptors sense external and internal environmental changes and provide information on the changes to the control centre
- Control centre – the control centre determines what a particular value (e.g. pH value or blood pressure) should be and sends out a message to the effectors

- Effectors – once they have received the information from the control centre, the effectors cause responses to take place within the body's internal environment which hopefully will produce the changes that will return the internal environment to return to normal values.

Organic and inorganic substances

All substances are classed either as organic or inorganic depending upon their molecules.

Organic molecules:

- Contain carbon (C) and hydrogen (H)
- Are usually larger than inorganic molecules
- Dissolve in water and organic liquids
- As a group include carbohydrates (sugars), proteins, lipids (fats) and nucleic acids (part of DNA).

Inorganic molecules:

- Do not generally contain carbon (C)
- Are usually smaller than organic molecules
- Usually dissolve in water or they react with water and release ions
- As a group, include water (H_2O) carbon dioxide (CO_2) and inorganic salts.

Examples of organic substances

Carbohydrates

Monosaccharides (one of the group of sugars known as carbohydrates) provide energy to cells as well as supplying the materials that allow for the building of the various structures of the cell (see Chapter 2). They contain carbon (C), hydrogen (H) and oxygen (O) and their structure can be depicted by the chemical formula $C_6H_{12}O_6$. There are three types of carbohydrates:

- Monosaccharides – glucose and fructose
- Disaccharides – sucrose, lactose
- Polysaccharides – glycogen, cellulose.

Fats (lipids)

Fats are lipids (known as triglycerides) and are soluble in organic solvents. They are mainly used to provide energy. Like carbohydrates, they consist of carbon (C), hydrogen (H) and oxygen (O), but because the numbers and proportions of these molecules are different from the carbohydrates, they have different properties. The chemical formula for stearin (one type of lipid) is $C_{57}H_{110}O_6$. Lipids can be either saturated or unsaturated. One important group of lipids is the steroid group which is used to synthesise (produce/construct) hormones. Cholesterol is an important member of the steroid group of lipids.

Proteins

Proteins are built up from amino acids – this will be discussed in Chapter 17, Genetics. Proteins are very important as they provide the structural material for the body as well as being an energy source. They also help to form many other substances, including hormones, receptors, enzymes and antibodies.

Examples of inorganic substances

Water (H_2O)

As mentioned above, water is the most abundant compound found in all living material and is a major component of all body fluids. It has an important role to play in most metabolic reactions as well as transporting chemicals around the body. Water can both absorb and transport heat, so it plays a crucial role in maintaining body temperature.

Oxygen (O_2)

Oxygen is necessary for survival. It is used by the organelles of the nucleus to release energy from nutrients (see Chapter 2, Cells).

Units of measurement

To conclude this chapter, which introduces certain bioscientific concepts and prepares the reader for the remaining chapters, just some brief notes about units of measurement. This is an important section because the ability to identify and understand units of measurement will enhance the understanding of the complex organism known as man.

A unit is a standardised, descriptive word which specifies the dimension of a number. Traditionally there have been seven properties of matter that have been measured independently of each other, namely:

- Time – measures the duration that something occurs
- Length – measures the length of an object
- Mass – measures the mass (commonly taken to be the weight) of an object
- Current – measures the amount of electric current that passes through an object
- Temperature – measures how hot or cold an object is
- Amount – measures the amount of a substance that is present
- Luminous intensity – measures the brightness of an object.

Originally, each country/society had its own units of measurement. In the United Kingdom, for example, there were such units as furlongs, miles, poles, gallons, quarts, bushels, pecks, etc. This made it difficult for people, particularly scientists, from other countries to work with each other, so several years ago, an international system of units was agreed upon by most major countries (however a notable exception to this agreement is the United States of America). This new agreed system became known as the Système International d'Unités (or SI units for short). It is a system of units that relates present scientific knowledge to a unified system of units. Included in this chapter are several tables of SI units which will be useful as reference whilst working through this book.

Table 1.1 The fundamental SI units

Quantity	Name	Symbol
Length	metre	m
Mass	kilogram	kg
Time	second	s
Current	ampere	A
Temperature	Kelvin	K
Amount of substance	mole	mol
Luminous intensity	candela	cd

Table 1.2 Other common SI units

Physical quantity	Name	Symbol
Force	Newton	N
Energy	joule	J
Pressure	pascal	Pa
Potential difference	volt	V
Frequency	hertz	Hz
Volume	litre	L

Table 1.3(a) Multiples of SI units

Prefix	Symbol	Meaning	Scientific notation
tera	T	one million million	10^{12}
giga	G	one thousand million	10^{9}
mega	M	one million	10^{6}
kilo	k	one thousand	10^{3}
hecto	h	one hundred	10^{2}
deca	da	ten	10^{1}
deci	d	one tenth	10^{-1}
centi	c	one hundredth	10^{-2}
milli	m	one thousandth	10^{-3}

Table 1.3(b) Multiples of SI units

micro	μ	one millionth	10^{-6}
nano	n	one thousandth of a millionth	10^{-9}
pico	p	one millionth of a millionth	10^{-12}
femto	f	one thousandth of a pico	10^{-15}
atto	a	one millionth of a pico	10^{-18}

Table 1.4 Measures of weight

1 kilogram = 1000 gram
1 gram = 1000 milligram
1 milligram = 10^{-3} gram
1 microgram = 10^{-6} gram
1 pound = 0.454 kilogram/454 gram
1 ounce = 28.35 gram
25 gram = 0.9 ounce
1 ounce = 8 dram

Table 1.5 Measures of volume

1 litre = 1000 millilitre
100 millilitre = 1 decilitre
1 millilitre = 1000 microlitre
1 UK gallon = 4.5 litre
1 pint = 568 millilitre
1 fluid ounce = 28.42 millilitre
1 teaspoon = 5 millilitre
1 tablespoon = 15 millilitre

Table 1.6 Measures of length

1 metre = 10^{-3} kilometre
1 centimetre = 10^{-5} metre
1 millimetre = 10^{-6} metre
1 metre = 39.37 inches
1 mile = 1.6 kilometre
1 yard = 0.9 metre
1 foot = 0.3 metre
1 inch = 25.4 millimetre

Table 1.7 Measures of energy

1 calorie = 4.184 joules
100 calories = 1 dietary Calorie or kilocalorie
1 dietary Calorie = 4184 joules or 4.184 kilojoule
1000 Calorie = 4184 kilojoule
1 kilojoule = 0.238 Calories

Conclusion

This concludes this introduction to the very basics of the biochemistry of physiology. As you can now appreciate, biochemistry and physiology are really quite complicated – but also very interesting, and indeed exciting. After all, as you work through this book, you are learning about yourself – how your body works and functions – both in good times (when you are fit and healthy) and in bad times (when you are sick or have had an accident). Everyone is interested in how they function and what happens when they eat and drink, or exercise, or go to the toilet, and so on – not just you but also your patients, and so this is important knowledge for you to have when you are talking to patients. This first chapter is just the beginning of a journey – think of it as a map to help you to complete this journey. This journey is one of self-knowledge and awareness which will lead you to your ultimate goal – a good knowledge of the human body and its functioning – good luck.

Glossary

Acid: A chemical substance with a low pH factor. The opposite of an alkaline substance.

Acid base balance: The relationship between an acidic environment and an alkaline one. This is essential for maintaining our good health. See pH.

Alkali: A chemical substance with a high pH factor. The opposite of an acidic substance.

Anatomy: The study of the structures of the body.

Antibody: Antibodies are proteins that can recognise and attach to infectious agents in the body, and so provoke an immune response to these infectious agents.

Atomic number: Relates to the number of protons to be found in any one atom.

Atoms: The base of all life, atoms are extremely minute and consist of different numbers of protons, neutron and electrons.

Base:	Another name for an alkali substance.
Bonds:	The joining together of various substances, particularly atoms and molecules. See **chemical bonds,** covalent bonds, ionic bonds, and polar bonds.
Chemical bond:	The 'attractive' force that holds atoms together.
Chemical reaction:	A process in which chemical substances are transformed into something completely different. This is usually depicted in a chemical equation.
Compounds:	A pure substance that is made up of two or more elements that are chemically bonded together.
Covalent bonds:	Bonds between atoms caused by the sharing of electrons between the atoms.
Electrolyte:	Substances that are able to move to opposite electrically charged electrodes in fluids.
Electron:	The parts of an atom that carry a negative electrical charge. See neutrons and protons.
Elements:	A pure chemical substance which cannot be broken down into anything simpler by chemical means, e.g. iron, hydrogen, etc.
Enzymes:	Proteins produced by cells that can cause very rapid biochemical reactions in the body.
Homeostasis:	The name given to processes in which both negative and positive controls are given over variables: they usually involve negative feedback, and the aim is to maintain a stable internal environment.
Inorganic substances:	Substances that do not contain carbon molecules, e.g. water.
Ionic bonds:	Bonding that takes place when atoms lose or gain electrons. This alters the electrical charge of the atoms.
Ions:	Ions are atoms that are no longer in a stable state (i.e. the are no longer electrically neutral but are either positively or negatively electrically charged).
Mole:	The unit of measurement for the amount of a substance.
Molecules:	The smallest part of an element or compound that can exist on its own (e.g. sodium chloride).
Neutral substance:	A chemical substance that is neither acidic nor alkaline.
Neutron:	The parts of an atom that carry a neutral electrical charge, i.e. they have no electrical charge. See electrons and protons.

Organic substances:	Substances that contain carbon molecules, e.g. carbohydrates, lipids (fats) and proteins.
Organelle:	Structural and functional parts of a cell.
Osmosis:	The movement of water across a semi-permeable membrane from an area of low solute concentration to an area of high solute concentration: this allows for equilibrium of solute and water density on both sides of the semi-permeable membrane.
pH:	A measure of the acidity or alkalinity of a solution. See acid base balance.
Physiology:	The study of the way in which the body structures function.
Polar bonds:	Polar bonds occur when atoms of different electronegativities form a bond. Consequently, the molecules that are then formed also carry a weak negative electrical charge, which allows molecules to ionically bond, just like atoms. They are also known as hydrogen bonds because hydrogen molecules have to be present for polar bonding to exist. Examples of such molecules include hydrochloric acid and water.
Product (chemical reactions):	The new substance formed following a chemical reaction.
Protons:	The parts of an atom that carry a positive electrical charge. See electrons and neutrons.
Reactant (chemical reactions):	The individual substances involved in a chemical reaction.
Shell (of an atom):	The name that is given to the orbits of electrons moving around the nucleus (containing protons and neutrons) of an atom.
Valency:	A measure of the combining power of atoms.

References

Fisher, J. and Arnold, J.R.P. (2004) *Chemistry for Biologists*, 2nd edn. London: BIOS Scientific Publishers.

International Bureau of Weights and Measures (2006) *The International System of Units (SI)*, 8th edn. Paris: BIPM.

Marieb, E.N. and Hoehn, K. (2009) *Human Anatomy and Physiology*, 8th edn. Harlow: Pearson Education.

Tortora, G.J. and Derrickson, B.H. (2009) *Principles of Anatomy and Physiology*, 12th edn. Hoboken, NJ: John Wiley & Sons.

Activities

www.wiley.com/go/peate

Multiple choice questions

1. An atom consists of:

   (a) electrons, neutrons and protons
   (b) electrons and neutrons
   (c) neutrons and electrons
   (d) protons

2. Electrons are held in orbit by:

   (a) electromagnetic force
   (b) solar force
   (c) nuclear force
   (d) gravitational force

3. A molecule is:

   (a) the same as an element which exists independently
   (b) the positive charge of an atom
   (c) an ion which exists independently
   (d) the smallest particle of an element which exists independently

4. The three types of chemical bonds are:

   (a) ionic, tonic covalent
   (b) tonic, polar, equatorial
   (c) ionic, covalent, polar
   (d) tonic, equatorial, polar

5. Polar bonds only occur with molecules containing:

   (a) hydrogen
   (b) oxygen
   (c) carbon
   (d) sodium

6. The three classes of elements are:

   (a) metals, crystalloids, metalloids
   (b) metalloids, non-metals, metals
   (c) non-metals, metals, crystalloids
   (d) metals, fire, water

7. Examples of elements as metals are:

   (a) calcium, sodium, carbon
   (b) calcium, carbon, chlorine
   (c) sulphur, calcium, potassium
   (d) phosphorous, carbon, sodium

8. Which is more acidic, a substance which has a pH of:

   (a) 3.2
   (b) 13.2
   (c) 2.3
   (d) 6.2

9. Lipids:

   (a) are sugars
   (b) mainly provide energy
   (c) have the chemical formula $C_6H_{12}O_6$
   (d) provide the structural material for the body

10. A substance with a pH of 11 is:

   (a) Very acidic
   (b) Slightly acidic
   (c) Neutral
   (d) Slightly alkaline
   (e) Highly alkaline

Test your learning

1. What is the importance of respiration for the body?
2. Why is water essential for all organisms, including humans?
3. How is the atomic number of an atom calculated?
4. What is an ion, and what is its importance for us?
5. Make a list of some of the common elements found in the body.
6. Explain what is happening in the chemical reaction as depicted by this chemical equation: $C_6H_{12}O_6 + 6O_2 \rightarrow 6CO_2 + 6H_2O + ATP$ (cellular energy).
7. Discuss the importance of the pH of the blood.
8. Discuss the importance of carbohydrates to the body.

Label the diagram

From the list of words, label the diagram below:

Proton, Neutron, Paths of orbit, Nucleus, Electron

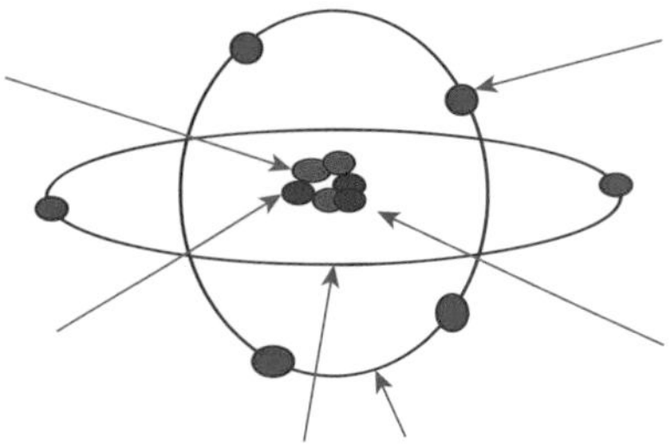

Crossword

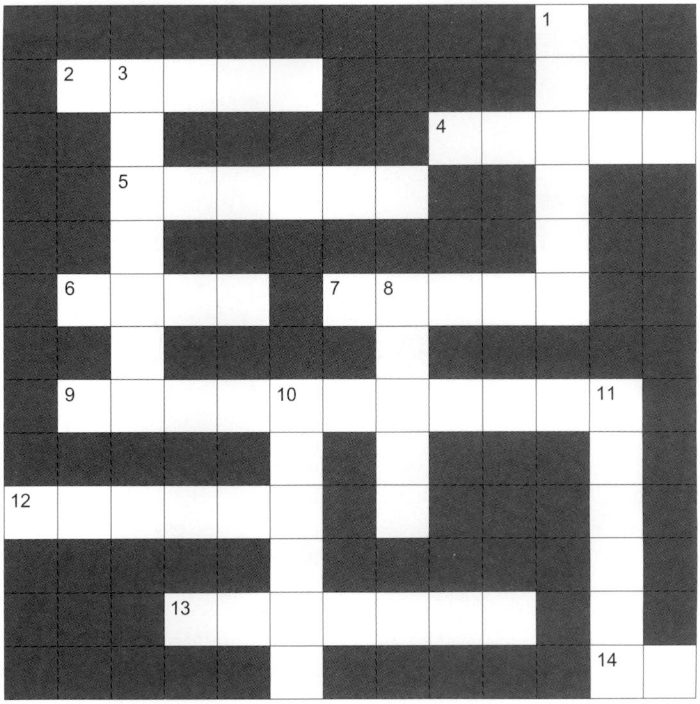
1
2 3
4
5
6
7 8
9 10 11
12
13
14

Across:

2. The symbol H_2O stands for ....? (5)
4. An ion which carries a negative charge (5).
5. What type of number represents an atom? (6)
6. The name of the process by which two atoms join together (4).
7. What bond occurs when one atom donates an electron to another atom? (5)
9. One form of pressure (11).
12. Always present following a chemical reaction (6).
13. A pure chemical substance that cannot be broken down into anything simpler by chemical means (7).
14. The chemical symbol for sodium (2).

Down:

1. An environment with a pH of 4.6 is said to be? (6)
3. The study of the structure of the body (7).
8. The rule that states that there is a maximum of 8 electrons in the second and subsequent shells of an atom, excluding the outer shell (5).
10. A gas essential for respiration (6).
11. An atom that is very important and describes the underlying make-up of the body, as in 'we are all. ...-entities' (6).

Word riddles

Answer the following riddles to find words related to basic science.

My first part begins another word for beer and wine.
My second part is an indefinite article.
My third part is neither a circle nor a square.
My whole is the opposite of acid.
What am I?

My first part is something that you agree with.
My second part is the time between being a child and being an adult.
My whole is an organic substance constructed of amino acids.
What am I?

My first part is a hairy pet.
My second part is an atom that is not in a stable state.
My whole carries a positive electrical charge.
What am I?

My first word is a musical group.
My second word is to reign.
My whole determines the number of electrons in a shell.
What am I?

My first letter is in Charley but not in barley.
My second letter is in orange but not in apple.
My third letter is in valley but not in hill.
My fourth letter is in water but not in beer.
My fifth letter is in lettuce but not in cabbage.
My sixth letter is in bent but not in straight.
My seventh letter is in newt but not in frog.
My last letter is in tea but not in coffee.
My whole is a process of bonding atoms together.
What am I?

My first letter is in cheese but not in milk.
My second letter is in farm but not in field.
My third letter is in pelt but not in fur.
My fourth letter is in raucous but not in loud.
My fifth letter is in ice cream but not in cake.
My sixth letter is in tummy but not in stomach.
My last letter is in jam but not in honey.
My whole strengthens bones.
What am I?

My first letter is in cabbage but not in onions.
My second letter is in onions but not in cabbage.
My third letter is in Timothy but not in Thomas.
My fourth letter is in Thomas but not in Timothy.
My last letter is in navy but not in army.
My whole carries a negative electrical charge.
What am I?

Answers

MCQs

1a; 2a; 3d; 4c; 5a; 6b; 7a; 8c; 9b; 10e

Crossword

Across

2. Water
4. Anion
5. Atomic
6. Bond
7. Ionic
9. Hydrostatic
12. Energy
13. Element
14. NA

Down

1. Acidic
3. Anatomy
8. Octet
10. Oxygen
11. Carbon

Word riddles

1 alkaline; 2 protein; 3 cation; 4; octet rule; 5 covalent; 6 calcium; 7; anion

2

Cells: cellular compartment, transport system, fluid movements

Muralitharan Nair

Contents

Introduction 34

Cell membrane **35**
Functions of the cell membrane 37
Transport systems 38
Active transport system 41
Endocytosis 42
Exocytosis 43
Fluid compartments 43
Composition of body fluid 46
Effects of water deficiency 47

Electrolytes **47**
Functions of electrolytes 47
Hormones that regulate fluid and electrolytes 50

Conclusion 51
Glossary 52
References 53
Activities 53

Fundamentals of Anatomy and Physiology for Student Nurses, First Edition. Edited by Ian Peate, Muralitharan Nair.

Test your knowledge

- List some of the structures of the human cell.
- What is a cytosol?
- What is the difference between active and passive transport?
- Where is most of the fluid volume found, in the intracellular or extracellular compartments?
- Define the function of body fluids and electrolytes.
- Define the terms endocytosis and exocytosis.

Learning outcomes

On completion of this section the reader will be able to:

- Outline the structure and function of the plasma membrane
- Describe the functions of the organelles
- Explain the cellular transport system
- Identify the fluid compartments of the body
- List the major electrolytes of the extracellular and intracellular compartments of the body
- Define the terms osmosis and diffusion

Introduction

Cells are the structural and functional units of all living organisms. Some organisms, such as bacteria, are unicellular, consisting of a single cell. Others, such as humans, are multicellular, indicating that humans are made up of many cells (see Figure 2.1). Cells are the smallest independent units of life with different parts (see Figure 2.2) that perform their own function (see Table 2.1) and to survive some fundamental chemical activities must occur within the cell. These activities include cellular growth, metabolism and reproduction. Each cell is an amazing unit of life; it can take in nutrients, convert these nutrients into energy, carry out specialised functions and reproduce as necessary. Most amazingly, each cell stores its own set of instructions for carrying out each of these activities.

Substances such as water, electrolytes and nutrients move in and out of a cell utilising the transport system. The cell membrane is not impermeable, it is semi-permeable to water and solutes. It regulates the movement of water, nutrients and waste products into and out of the cell. The cell consists of four basic parts:

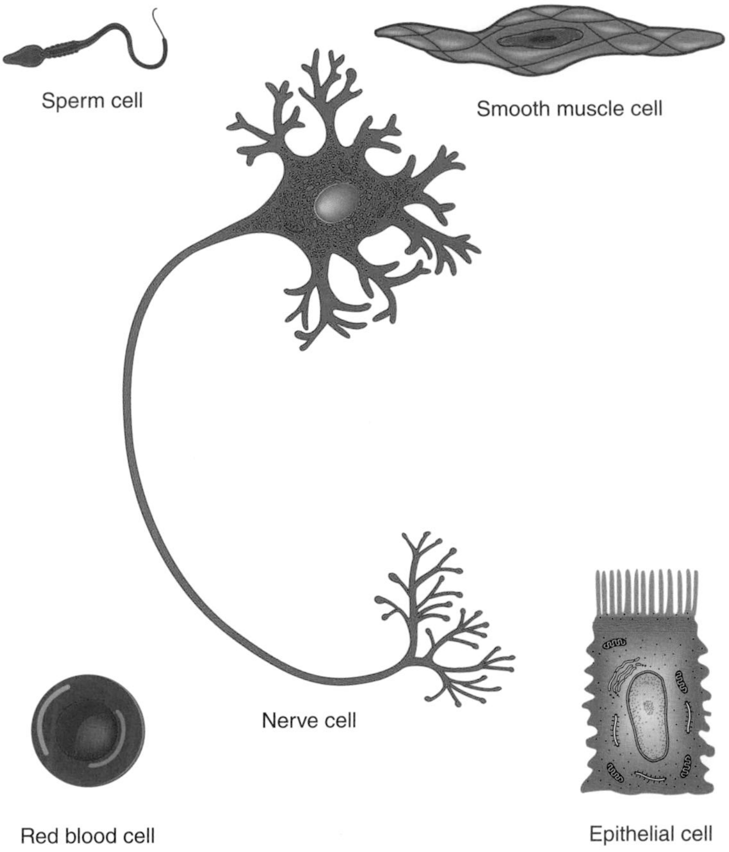
Sperm cell
Smooth muscle cell
Nerve cell
Red blood cell
Epithelial cell

Figure 2.1 Examples of some cells of the human body (Tortora and Derrickson 2009)

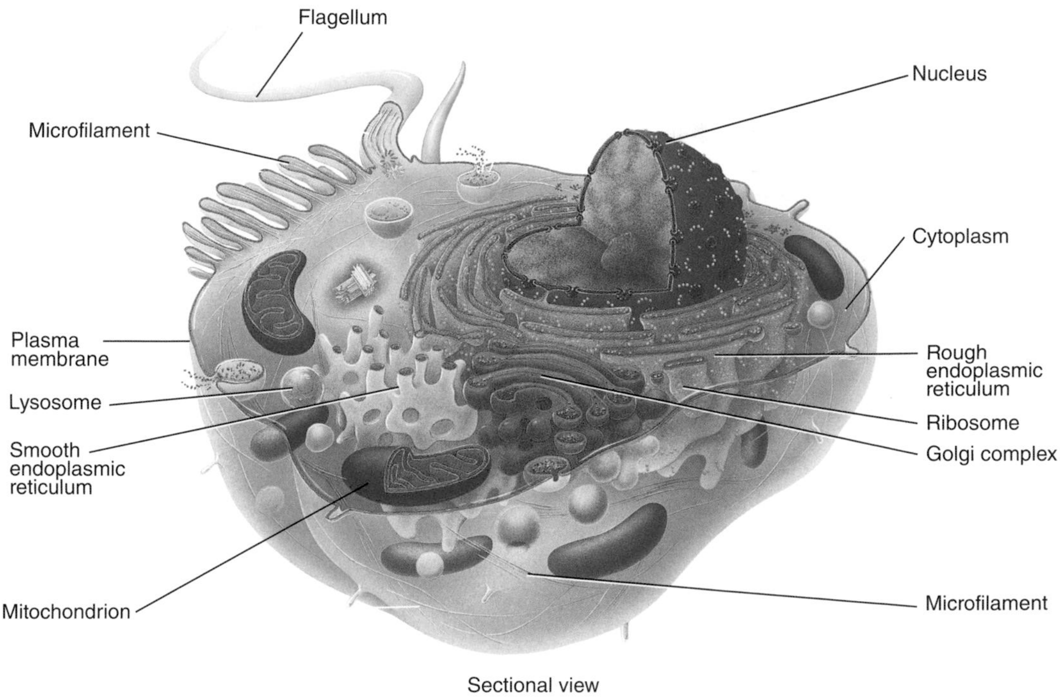
Flagellum
Nucleus
Microfilament
Cytoplasm
Plasma membrane
Rough endoplasmic reticulum
Lysosome
Ribosome
Smooth endoplasmic reticulum
Golgi complex
Mitochondrion
Microfilament
Sectional view

Figure 2.2 Structure of a cell (Nair and Peate 2009)

- The cell membrane
- Cytoplasm
- The nucleus
- Nucleoplasm.

Cell membrane

The cell membrane is thin and forms the outermost layer of a cell; it is also called the plasma membrane. This membrane ensures that the boundary and integrity of the cell and its contents are separate from the surrounding environment. The cell membrane contains a variety of biological molecules, mainly proteins and lipids which are involved in many cellular functions such as cellular communication and cellular transport. The cell membrane is made up of a double layer (bilayer) of phospholipid (fatty) molecules with protein molecules interspersed between them (see Figure 2.3). The cell membrane can vary from 7.5 nanometres (nm) to 10 nm in thickness (Vickers 2009).

The phospholipid bilayer consists of a polar 'head' end which is hydrophilic (water-loving) and fatty acid 'tails' which are hydrophobic (water-hating). The hydrophilic heads are situated on the outer and inner surface of the cell while the hydrophobic areas point into the cell membrane (see Figure 2.3). The phospholipid molecules are arranged as a bilayer with the heads facing outwards. This means that the bilayer is self-sealing. It is the central part of the plasma membrane, consisting of hydrophobic 'tails', that makes the cell membrane impermeable to water-soluble molecules,

Table 2.1 Cellular compartments and their functions

Components	Functions
Centrioles	Cellular reproduction
Chromatin	Contains genetic information
Cilia (pleural)	Moves fluid or particles over the surface of the cell
Cytoplasm	Fluid portion which supports organelles
Cytoskeleton	Provides support and site for specific enzymes
Endoplasmic reticulum (rough and smooth)	Many functions, including site for protein transportation, modification of drugs and synthesis of lipids and steroids
Glycogen granules	Stores for glycogen
Golgi complex	Packages proteins for secretion
Intermediate filament	Helps to determine the shape of the cell
Lysosomes	Break down and digest harmful substances. In normal cells, some of the synthesised proteins may be faulty – lysosymes are responsible for their removal
Microfilaments	Provide structural support and cell movement
Microtubules	Provide conducting channels through which various substances can move through the cytoplasm. Provide shape and support for cells
Microvilli	Increase cell surface; site for secretion, absorption and cellular adhesion
Mitrochondria	Energy-producing site of the cell. Mitochondria are self-replicating
Nucleolus	Site for the formation of ribosomes
Nucleus	Contains genetic information
Peroxisomes	Carry out metabolic reactions. Site for the destruction of hydrogen peroxide. Protects the cell from harmful substances such as alcohol and formaldehyde
Plasma membrane	Regulates substances in and out of a cell
Ribosomes	Sites for protein synthesis
Secretory vesicles	Secretes hormone, neurotransmitters

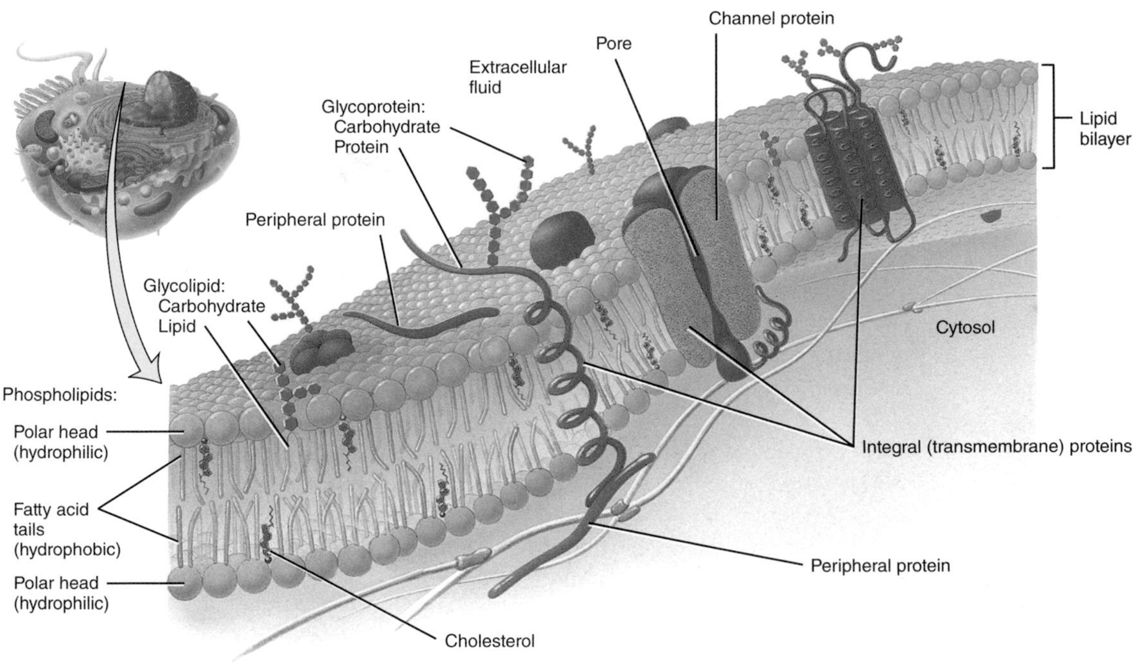
Channel protein
Pore
Extracellular fluid
Glycoprotein: Carbohydrate Protein
Lipid bilayer
Peripheral protein
Glycolipid: Carbohydrate Lipid
Cytosol
Phospholipids:
Polar head (hydrophilic)
Fatty acid tails (hydrophobic)
Polar head (hydrophilic)
Integral (transmembrane) proteins
Peripheral protein
Cholesterol

Figure 2.3 Cell membrane (Tortora and Derrickson 2009)

and so prevents the passage of these molecules into and out of the cell (Marieb and Hoehn 2007). However, for the cells to survive and function, substances need to enter and leave the cells and this is provided by special proteins, such as integral and peripheral membrane proteins (see Figure 2.3).

The integral transmembrane proteins are attached to the cell membrane and they can form channels which allow for the transportation of materials into and out of the cell. Examples of integral transmembrane proteins include voltage-gated ion channels, such as those which transport potassium ions in and out of cells, certain types of T-cell receptors, the insulin receptor and many other receptors and neurotransmitters. On the other hand, peripheral membrane proteins adhere temporarily to the cell membrane with which they are associated. Peripheral membrane proteins may interact with other proteins or directly with the lipid bilayer.

Functions of the cell membrane

Cell membranes serve several important functions. They:

- Anchor the cytoskeleton (a cellular 'skeleton' made of protein and contained in the cytoplasm) and gives shape to the cell
- Attach the cell to the extracellular matrix (non-living material that is found outside the cells), so that the cells group together to form tissues

- Transport materials needed for the functioning of the cell organelles. The cell membrane is semi-permeable and controls the in and out movements of substances. Such movement of substances may be either at the expense of cellular energy or passive, without using cellular energy
- The protein molecules in the cell membrane receive signals from other cells or the outside environment and convert the signals to messages, which are passed to the organelles inside the cell
- In some cells, the protein molecules in the cell membrane group together to form enzymes, which carry out metabolic reactions near the inner surface of the cell membrane
- The proteins in the cell membrane also help very small molecules to be transported through the cell membrane, provided the molecules are travelling from a region with lots of molecules to a region with less number of molecules.

Some of the proteins embedded in a cell membrane provide structural support to the cell, while others are enzymes where chemical reactions occur. Some membrane proteins regulate water-soluble substances through pores in the cell membrane; others are receptors where hormones and other substances such as neurotransmitters act. Other important cell membrane proteins are glycoproteins and they play an important role in cell cell recognition. One example are mucins, which are secreted in the mucus of the digestive and respiratory tracts.

Transport systems

Cells utilise two processes to move substance in and out of the cell: the passive and active transport systems. When molecules pass in and out of a cell membrane without the use of cellular energy, it is called passive transport system. This includes:

- Simple diffusion
- Facilitated diffusion
- Osmosis
- Filtration.

On the other hand, the active transport system requires energy to move substances in and out of a cell. The active transport systems include:

- Active transport with the utilisation of adenosine triphosphate (ATP)
- Endocytosis
- Exocytosis.

Simple diffusion

The term simple diffusion refers to a process whereby a substance passes through a membrane without the aid of an intermediary such as an integral membrane protein (see Figure 2.4). Water, oxygen, carbon dioxide, ethanol and urea are examples of molecules that readily cross cell membranes by simple diffusion. They pass either directly through the lipid bilayer or through pores created by certain integral membrane proteins (see Figure 2.3). Small, nonpolar substances can diffuse directly through the plasma membrane. One example of simple diffusion is the exchange of respiratory gases between the cells of the alveolar sac and the blood in the lungs. The rate of diffusion depends on several factors:

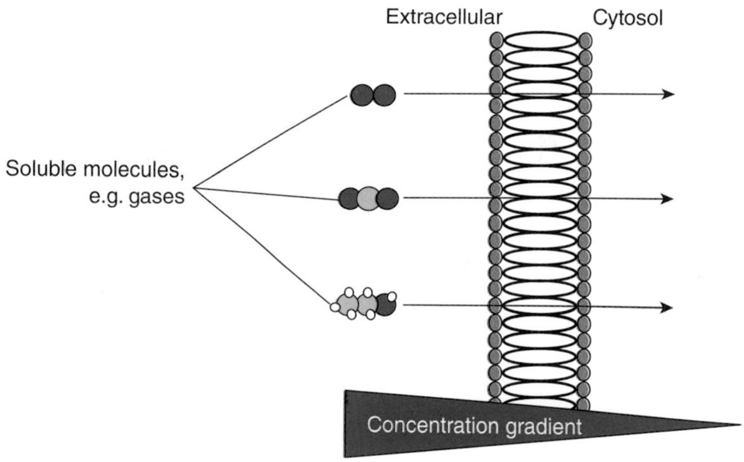
Extracellular
Cytosol
Soluble molecules, e.g. gases
Concentration gradient

Figure 2.4 Simple diffusion (Nair and Peate 2009)

- Gases diffuse rapidly and liquids diffuse more slowly
- In high temperature the rate of diffusion is much faster
- Smaller molecules such as glycerol diffuse much faster than larger molecules like fatty acids
- The surface area of the cell membrane over which the molecule can work
- The solubility of the molecule
- The concentration gradient.

Facilitated diffusion

Facilitated diffusion (facilitated transport) is a process of passive transport (diffusion) via which molecules diffuse across cell membranes, with the help of transport proteins. Small, uncharged molecules can easily diffuse across cell membranes. However, due to the hydrophobic nature of the lipids that make up cell membranes, water-soluble molecules and ions cannot do so; instead, they are helped by transport proteins. Larger molecules, such as amino acids, cannot pass the cell membrane and therefore they use a process called facilitated diffusion (see Figure 2.5). No direct cellular energy is used in this process. Glucose, sodium and chloride ions are just a few examples of molecules and ions that must efficiently get across the plasma membrane. Their transport must therefore be 'facilitated' by proteins that span the cell membrane and provide a passageway for these substances. Like simple diffusion, facilitated diffusion transports substances from an area of high concentration to an area of low concentration.

Osmosis

Osmosis is a process whereby water moves from an area of high volume to an area of low volume through a selective permeable membrane. A selective permeable membrane is one that allows the unrestricted passage of water, but not solute molecules or ions. The relative concentrations of water are determined by the amount of solutes dissolved in the water. For example, a higher

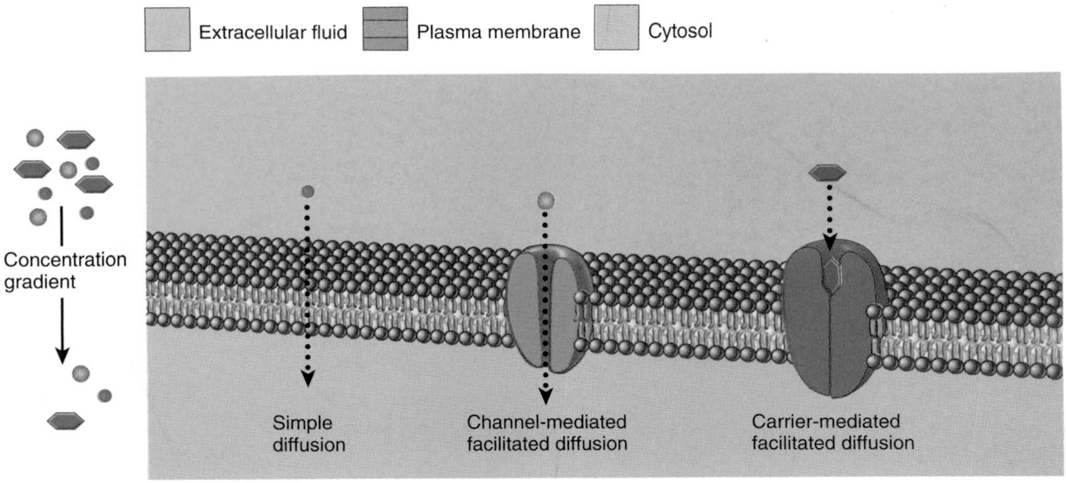
Extracellular fluid
Plasma membrane
Cytosol
Concentration gradient
Simple diffusion
Channel-mediated facilitated diffusion
Carrier-mediated facilitated diffusion

Figure 2.5 Facilitated diffusion (Tortora and Derrickson 2009)

concentration of salt on one side of the cell membrane means that there is less space for water molecules. Water then will move from the side where there is a greater number of water molecules through the cell membrane to the other side of the cell where there are fewer water molecules. This is known as osmotic pressure. The higher the concentration of the solute on one side of the membrane, the higher the osmotic pressure available for the movement of the water (Colbert *et al.* 2007).

The osmotic pressure can be sufficient to damage the cell membrane and therefore it is important for the cell to have a relatively constant pressure between the internal and external environment. If the osmotic pressure on one side of the cell is greater than that on the other side, changes to the cell could take place, resulting in cell damage. A red blood cell placed in a solution with less concentration of solute will undergo haemolysis and if placed in a fluid with high concentration of solutes the red blood cell will crenate (see Figure 2.6). On the other hand, if the red blood cell is placed in a solution with a relatively constant osmotic pressure between the internal and external environment, the red blood cell does not undergo any changes. The net movement of water in and out of the cell is minimal.

Filtration

Filtration is a process where small substances are forced through a selective permeable membrane by means of hydrostatic pressure. An example of filtration within the human body is at the capillary end of the blood vessels. With the aid of blood pressure, fluid and solutes are forced out of the single layered cells of the capillaries into the interstitial fluid space. Large molecules such as proteins and red blood cells remain in the capillaries. Another example of filtration that occurs in the human body takes place in the kidneys. Blood pressure forces water and dissolved wastes products such as urea and uric acid into the kidney tubules during the formation of urine (see Chapter 14, The renal system).

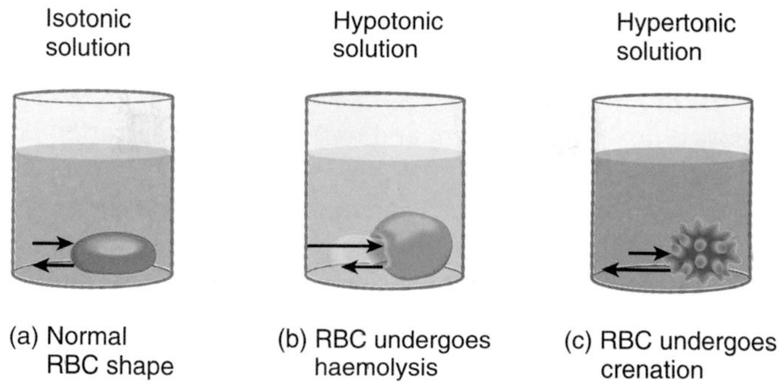

Isotonic solution
Hypotonic solution
Hypertonic solution
(a) Normal RBC shape
(b) RBC undergoes haemolysis
(c) RBC undergoes crenation

Figure 2.6 Effect of solute concentration on a red blood cell (Tortora and Derrickson 2009)

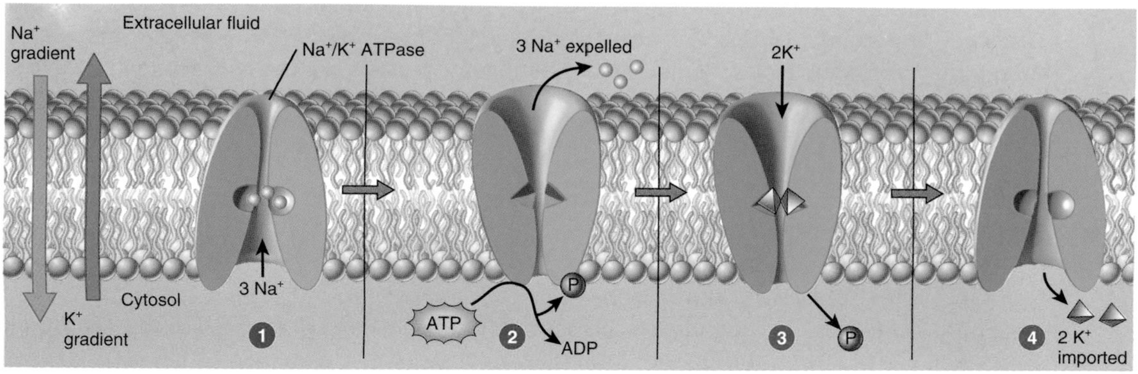

Na⁺ gradient
Extracellular fluid
Na⁺/K⁺ ATPase
3 Na⁺ expelled
2K⁺
Cytosol
K⁺ gradient
3 Na⁺
1
ATP
2
ADP
P
3
4
2 K⁺ imported

Figure 2.7 Active transport system (Tortora and Derrickson 2009)

Active transport system

The main difference between the active and passive transport systems is that the active transport system utilises cellular energy to move substances through a semipermeable membrane. The energy is obtained by splitting ATP into adenosine diphosphate (ADP) and phosphate (see Figure 2.7). Examples of active transport processes are active transport, endocytosis and exocytosis.

Active transport

An active process is one in which substances move against a concentration gradient from an area of lower to higher concentration. The cell must expend energy which is released by splitting ATP into ADP and phosphate. ATP is a compound made up of a base, a sugar and three phosphate groups (triphosphate). These phosphate groups are held together by high-energy bonds, which when broken release a high level of energy. Once one of these phosphate bonds has been broken and a phosphate group has been released, that compound now has only two phosphate groups (diphosphate) leaving a spare phosphate group, which in turn will join up with another adenosine diphosphate group, so forming another molecule of ATP (with energy stored in the phosphate bonds), and the whole process continues (Vickers 2009).

In the human body, the four main active transport systems considered when discussing cellular energy are:

- The sodium-potassium pump: sodium and potassium concentration gradients are generated to produce electrical energy
- The calcium pump: calcium ions essential for muscle contraction are transported into muscle cells
- The sodium-linked cotransporter: glucose and amino acids are actively transported into the cells and at the same time sodium moves passively via the cotransporter
- The hydrogen-linked cotransporter: glucose is actively transported into the cell and at the same time hydrogen ions move into the cell via the cotransporter.

Endocytosis

Endocytosis is the process by which cells take in molecules such as proteins from outside the cell by engulfing them with their cell membrane. It is used by all cells of the body because most substances important to them are polar and consist of big molecules, and thus cannot pass through the hydrophobic plasma membrane. During endocytosis only a small section of the cell membrane plays a part to form a fold and a new intracellular pod is formed containing the substance. There are three types endocytosis:

- Pinocytosis ('cell drinking'). In pinocytosis the molecule engulfed is relatively small (see Figure 2.8)
  - occurs in almost all cells
  - occurs continuously
- Phagocytosis ('cell eating') (see Figure 2.8)
  - results in the ingestion of particulate matter (e.g. bacteria) from the ECF
  - the endosome is so large that it is called a phagosome or vacuole
  - phagocytosis occurs only in certain specialised cells (e.g. neutrophils, macrophages)
  - occurs sporadically

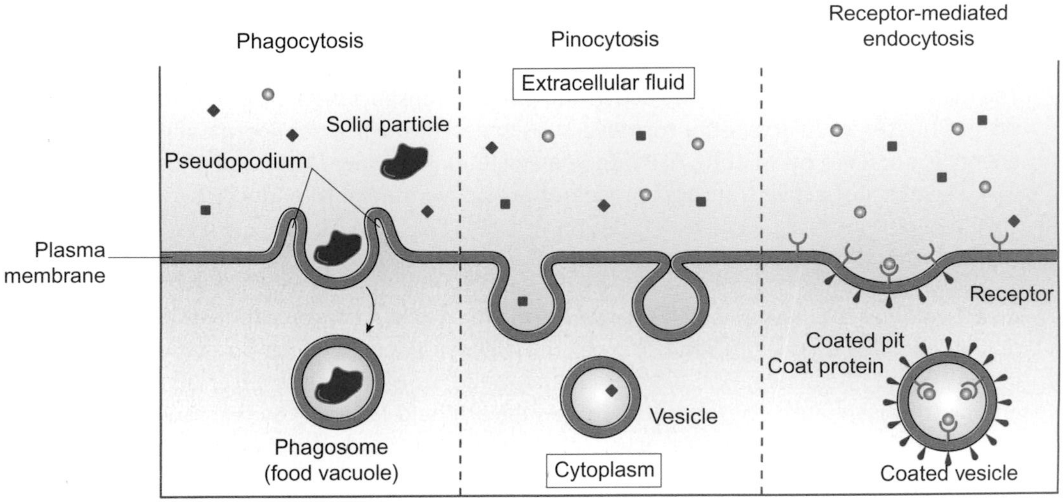
Phagocytosis
Pinocytosis
Receptor-mediated endocytosis
Extracellular fluid
Solid particle
Pseudopodium
Plasma membrane
Receptor
Coated pit
Coat protein
Vesicle
Phagosome (food vacuole)
Cytoplasm
Coated vesicle

Figure 2.8 Pinocytosis, phagocytosis and receptor-mediated endocytosis

- Receptor-mediated endocytosis (see Figure 2.8)
  - involves specific receptors that bind to large molecules in the extracellular fluid
  - the substance bound to the receptor is called a ligand.

Exocytosis

Exocytosis is a process for moving items from the cytoplasm of the cell to the outside. The intracellular vesicle with its ingested substances fuses with the cell membrane to get rid of the unwanted substance from the cell (see Figure 2.9). This process is also utilised by nerve cells to release chemical messengers into the synapse of a neurone. Gland cells release proteins by exocytosis.

Many cells in the body use exocytosis to release enzymes or other proteins that act in other areas of the body, or to release molecules that help cells communicate with one another. For instance, clusters of α- and β-cells in the islets of Langerhans in the pancreas secrete the hormones glucagon and insulin, respectively. These enzymes regulate glucose levels throughout the body. As the level of glucose rises in the blood, the β-cells are stimulated to produce and secrete more insulin by exocytosis. When insulin binds to liver or muscle, it stimulates uptake of glucose by those cells. Exocytosis from other cells in the pancreas also releases digestive enzymes into the gut.

Cells also communicate with each other, through exocytosis, more directly through the products that they secrete. For instance, a neurone cell relays an electrical pulse through the use of neurotransmitters. The neurotransmitters are stored in vesicles and lie next to the cytoplasmic face of the plasma membrane. When the appropriate signal is given, the vesicles holding the neurotransmitters must make contact with the plasma membrane and secrete their contents into the synaptic junction, the space between two neurones, for the other neurone to receive those neurotransmitters.

Fluid compartments

The two principal body fluid compartments are intracellular and extracellular. The intracellular compartment is the space inside a cell and the fluid inside the cell is called intracellular fluid (ICF). The extracellular compartment is found outside the cell and the fluid outside the cell is called

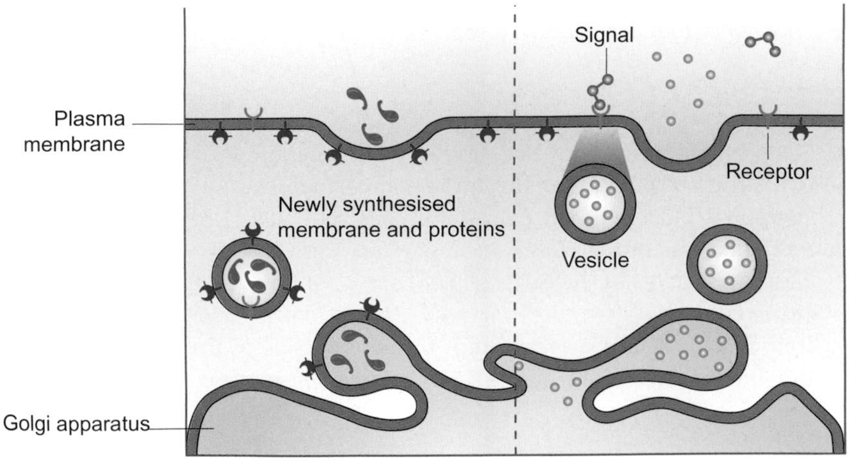
Signal
Plasma membrane
Receptor
Newly synthesised membrane and proteins
Vesicle
Golgi apparatus

Figure 2.9 Exocytosis

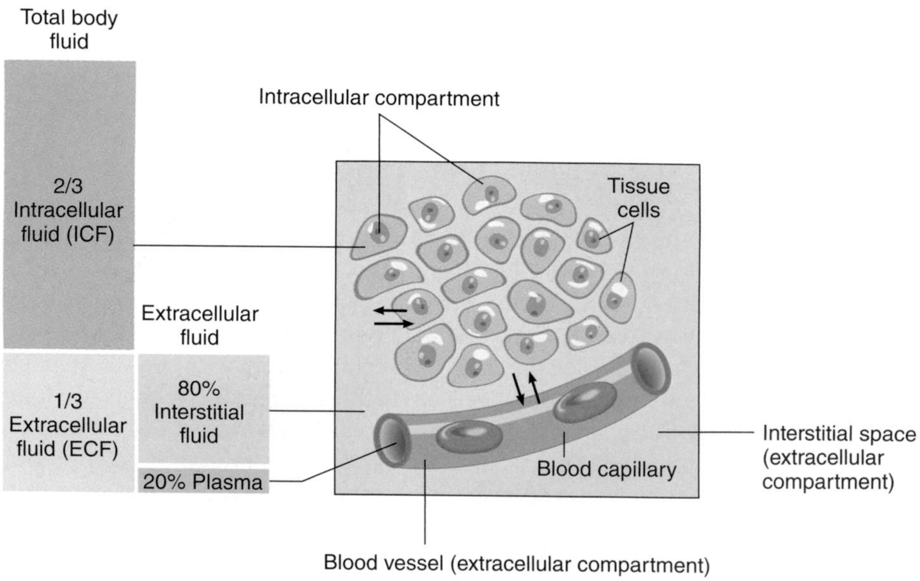
Total body fluid
2/3 Intracellular fluid (ICF)
1/3 Extracellular fluid (ECF)
Extracellular fluid
80% Interstitial fluid
20% Plasma
Intracellular compartment
Tissue cells
Interstitial space (extracellular compartment)
Blood capillary
Blood vessel (extracellular compartment)

Figure 2.10 Fluid compartments and distribution (Nair and Peate 2009)

extracellular fluid (ECF). However, the extracellular compartment is further divided into the interstitial and the intravascular compartments. Two thirds of body fluid is found inside the cell and one third outside the cell. Eighty per cent of the ECF is found in the interstitial compartment and 20% in the intravascular compartment as plasma (see Figure 2.10).

Intracellular fluid (ICF)

- The ICF is primarily a solution of potassium and organic anions, proteins, etc.
- The cell membranes and cellular metabolism control the constituents of this ICF
- ICF is not consistent in the body; it represents a collection of fluids from all the different cells.

Extracellular fluid (ECF)

- The ECF primarily consists of NaCl and $NaHCO_3$ solution.
- The ECF is further subdivided into three compartments:
  - Interstitial fluid (ISF) surrounds the cells, but does not circulate. It comprises about three quarters of the ECF
  - Plasma circulates as the extracellular component of blood. It makes up about one quarter of the ECF
  - Transcellular fluid is a set of fluids that are outside of the normal compartments. These 1–2 litres of fluid make up the CSF, digestive juices, mucus, etc.

Movement of body fluid between compartments

The movement of fluid between the intracellular and the extracellular compartments is primarily controlled by two forces:

- Hydrostatic pressure: pressure exerted by the fluid
- Osmotic pressure: the pressure that must be exerted on a solution to prevent the passage of water into it across a semipermeable membrane.

Furthermore, the movement of fluid is dependent on solutes dissolved within the fluid; changes in the concentration of solutes will affect fluid movement between compartments. Similarly, changes in fluid volume will also affect the fluid movement between compartments. An example of fluid and solute movement that occurs in the body is when blood pressure (hydrostatic pressure) forces fluid and solutes from the arterial end of the capillaries into the interstitial fluid space (see Figure 2.11). Fluid and solutes return to the capillaries at the venous end as a result of the osmotic pressure. Fluid also enters the lymphatic capillaries from the interstitial space as a result of the osmotic pressure in the lymphatic vessels.

The movement of fluid between the intracellular and extracellular compartments is the result of hydrostatic and osmotic pressures. In a normal state of health, the hydrostatic pressure in the intracellular compartment and the interstitial space is in balance and therefore the fluid movement is minimal. However, changes in the osmotic pressure, either in the intracellular or extracellular compartments, can affect fluid movement. As the capillary barrier is readily permeable to ions, the osmotic pressure within the capillary is principally determined by plasma proteins that are relatively impermeable. Therefore, instead of speaking of 'osmotic' pressure, this pressure is referred to as the 'oncotic' pressure or 'colloid osmotic' pressure because it is generated by colloids. Albumin generates about 70% of oncotic pressure. This pressure is typically 25–30 mmHg. Oncotic pressure increases along the length of the capillary, particularly in capillaries having high net filtration (e.g. in renal glomerular capillaries), because the filtering fluid leaves behind proteins, leading to an increase in protein concentration.

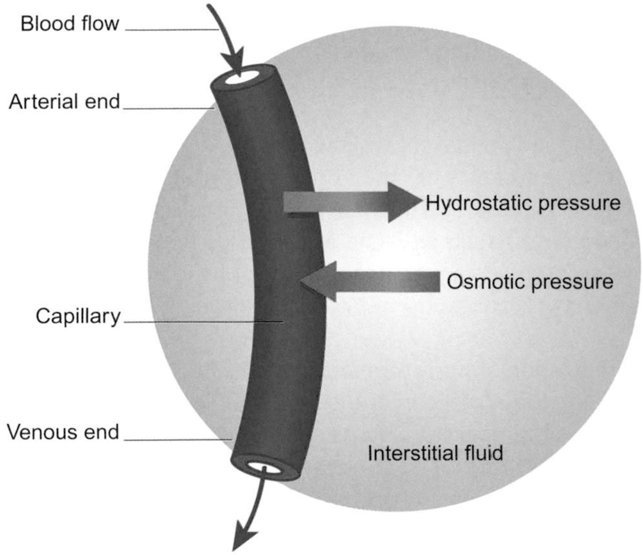
Blood flow
Arterial end
Hydrostatic pressure
Osmotic pressure
Capillary
Venous end
Interstitial fluid

Figure 2.11 Capillary hydrostatic and osmotic pressures

Clinical considerations

Intravenous infusion

Nurses are responsible for administering prescribed intravenous (IV) fluid. For a patient who is dehydrated, IV infusion is commenced for rehydration purposes. The fluid is instilled into the vascular space (extracellular compartment). Safe administration of intravenous fluid requires the nurse to understand the role of electrolytes and water in the body, the mechanism for movements between different body compartments and how fluid balance is maintained. Patients on intravenous infusion may not be able to take oral fluid as a result of their illness. The type of fluid to be administered depends on the patient's condition. Regardless of the type of intravenous fluid, nurses need to be aware that when patients are on fluid therapy, they need careful monitoring to ensure that the fluid is administered without complications, such as fluid overload.

Intravenous fluid can either be colloid or crystalloid. Colloid solutions in practice include albumin and gelfusin, and are also effective for volume replacement in major haemorrhage. Crystalloid solutions for intravascular volume replenishment are typically isotonic (e.g. 0.9% normal saline). Water freely travels outside the vasculature, so as little as 10% of isotonic fluid remains in the intravascular space. With hypotonic fluid (e.g. 0.45% normal saline), even less remains in the vasculature and thus is not ideal as fluid replacement.

Composition of body fluid

Body fluid is composed of water and dissolved substances such as electrolytes (sodium, potassium and chloride), gases (oxygen and carbon dioxide), nutrients, enzymes and hormones. Total body water constitutes 60% of total body weight and water plays an important part in cellular function (LeMone and Burke 2008). Water is essential for the body as it:

- Acts as a lubricant and so makes swallowing easy.
- Is the major component of the body's transport systems. The blood transports nutrients, oxygen, glucose and fats to various tissues and cells. Also, the waste products of cellular metabolism, such as lactic acid and carbon dioxide, are removed. Via urine, a number of waste products are transported out of the body, for example, urea, phosphates, sulphites, minerals, ketones from fat metabolism and nitrogenous waste from protein breakdown.
- Is needed for regulation of body temperature at 37°C. When body temperature starts to rise, blood vessels near the surface of the skin dilate to release some of the heat; the reverse happens when body temperature starts to drop. Also, when body temperature rises, sweat glands secrete sweat, which is 99% water. As the sweat evaporates, heat is removed from the body.
- Provides an optimum medium for the cells to function.
- There are chemical reactions in the body which require water. A synthesis reaction involves the joining of two molecules by the removal of a water molecule and a hydrolysis reaction involves a molecule being split into two smaller molecules with the addition of water.

- Breaks down food particles in the digestive system.
- Provides lubrication for the joints as it is a component of synovial fluid. It is also a component of tears which lubricate the eyes and of saliva to provide lubrication to food which aids chewing, swallowing and digestion. It also has a protective function, washing away particles that get into the eyes, providing cushioning against shock to the eyes and the spinal cord. It is also a component of amniotic fluid, which provides protection for the foetus during pregnancy.

Effects of water deficiency

Deficiency of water in the body can affect various functions and in severe conditions may lead to death. Some of the problems associated with water deficiency include:

- Low blood pressure
- Problem with clotting of blood
- Kidney dysfunction leading to renal failure
- Severe constipation
- Multisystem failure
- Proneness to infection
- Electrolyte imbalance.

Electrolytes

Chemically, electrolytes are substances that become ions in solution and acquire the capacity to conduct electricity. Electrolytes are present in the human body, and the balance of the electrolytes in our bodies is essential for normal function of our cells and our organs.

Fluid balance is linked to electrolyte balance. Electrolytes are chemical compounds that dissociate in water to form charged particles called ions (Lemone and Burke 2008). They include potassium (K), sodium (Na), chloride (Cl), magnesium (Mg) and phosphate (HPO_4). Electrolytes are either positively or negatively charged. Positively charged ions are called cations (for example, Na^+ and K^+) and negatively charged ions are called anions (for example, Cl^- and HCO_3^-). Remember that an anion and a cation will combine to form a compound, for example, potassium (K^+) and chloride (Cl^-) combine to form potassium chloride (KCl). The composition of electrolytes differs between the intracellular and the extracellular compartments (see Figure 2.12).

Functions of electrolytes

Electrolytes are compounds that dissociate into ions when placed in liquid, thus enabling the liquid to conduct an electric current. The positive ions are called cations and the negative ions are called anions. An electrolyte is a compound that does not form ions in solution. Electrolytes have numerous functions in the body. They:

- Regulate fluid movement between compartment
- Regulate hydrogen-ion concentration for normal cellular function

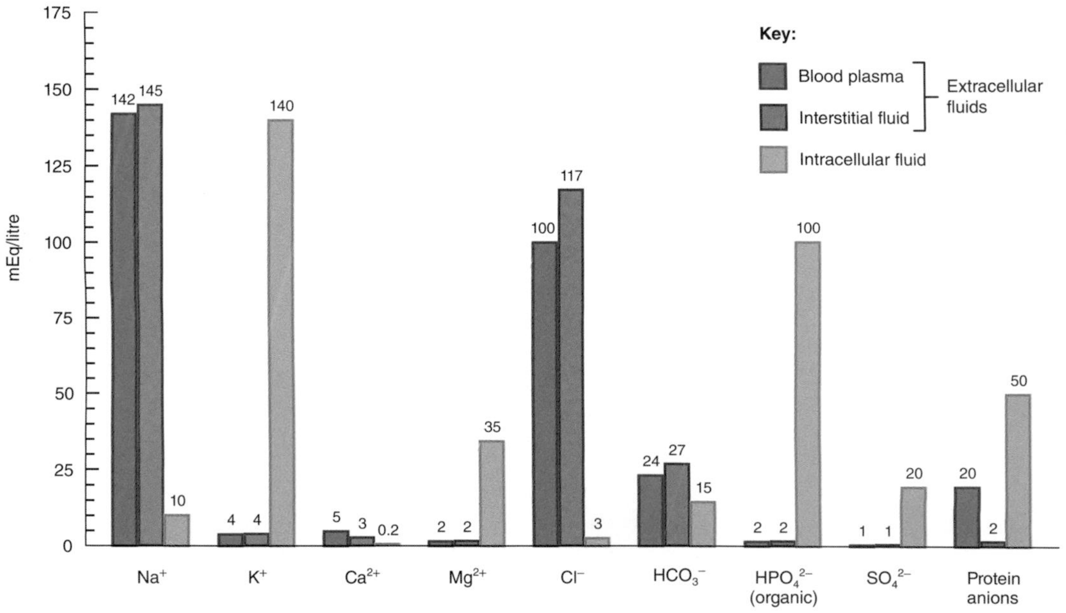
175
150
125
100
75
50
25
0
mEq/litre
Key:
Blood plasma
Interstitial fluid
Intracellular fluid
Extracellular fluids
142
145
10
4
4
140
5
3
0.2
2
2
35
100
117
3
24
27
15
2
2
100
1
1
20
20
2
50
Na+
K+
Ca2+
Mg2+
Cl−
HCO3−
HPO42− (organic)
SO42−
Protein anions

Figure 2.12 Electrolytes of intracellular and extracellular compartments (Nair and Peate 2009)

- Play a vital role in membrane potentials and action potentials
- Are essential for neuronal function.

To function normally, the body must be able to maintain the levels of electrolytes within very narrow limits. These limits are controlled by hormones. The body maintains the levels of electrolytes in each compartment (cells, tissues, organs) by moving electrolytes into, or out of, cells based upon the signals provided by the hormones. If the balance of electrolytes is disturbed, disorders can develop. An imbalance of electrolytes can occur if a person:

- Uses certain drugs, especially long-term use of laxatives and/or diuretics
- Becomes dehydrated as a result of profuse sweating, vomiting, chronic diarrhoea, very poor nutrition, etc.
- Has certain heart, liver or kidney disorders
- Is given intravenous fluids in inappropriate amounts.

Loss of electrolytes can have serious consequences for the body. In severe dehydration, the loss of electrolytes can result in circulatory problems, such as tachycardia (rapid heartbeat), and problems with the nervous system, such as loss of consciousness or shock. See Table 2.2 for a summary of electrolytes and their functions.

..2 Principal electrolytes and their functions

Electrolytes	Normal values in extracellular fluid	Function	Main distribution
Sodium (Na^+)	135–145 mmol/L	Important cation in generation of action potentials. Plays an important role in fluid and electrolyte balance. Increases plasma membrane permeability. Helps promote skeletal muscle function. Stimulates conduction of nerve impulses. Maintains blood volume	Main cation of the extracellular fluid
Potassium (K^+)	3.5–5 mmol/L	Important cation in establishing resting membrane potential. Regulates acid-base balance. Maintains intracellular fluid volume. Helps promote skeletal muscle function. Helps promote the transmission of nerve impulses	Main cation of the intracellular fluid
Calcium (Ca^{2+})	2.1–2.6 mmol/L	Important clotting factor. Plays a part in neurotransmitter release in neurones. Maintains muscle tone and excitability of nervous and muscle tissue. Promotes transmission of nerve impulses. Assists in the absorption of vitamin B_{12}	Mainly found in the extracellular fluid
Magnesium (Mg^{2+})	0.5–1.0 mmol/L	Helps to maintain normal nerve and muscle function; maintains regular heart rate, regulates blood glucose and blood pressure. Essential for protein synthesis	Mainly distributed in the intracellular fluid
Chloride (Cl^-)	98–117 mmol/L	Maintains a balance of anions in different fluid compartments. Combines with hydrogen in gastric mucosal glands to form hydrochloric acid. Helps to maintain fluid balance by regulating osmotic pressure	Main anion of the extracellular fluid
Hydro carbons (HCO_3^-)	24–31 mmol/L	Main buffer of hydrogen ions in plasma. Maintains a balance between cations and anions of intracellular and extracellular fluids	Mainly distributed in the extracellular fluid
Phosphate – organic (HCO_4^{2-})	0.8–1.1 mmol/L	Essential for the digestion of proteins, carbohydrates and fats and absorption of calcium. Essential for bone formation	Mainly found in the intracellular fluid
Sulphate (SO_4^{2-})	0.5 mmol/L	Involved in detoxification of phenols, alcohols and amines	Mainly found in the intracellular fluid

Hormones that regulate fluid and electrolytes

The three principal hormones that regulate fluid and electrolyte balance are antidiuretic hormone (ADH), aldosterone and atrial natriuretic peptide (Thibodeau and Patton 2007).

Antidiuretic hormone

Antidiuretic hormone (ADH) is a peptide and its main role is to regulate fluid balance in the body. This hormone is produced in the hypothalamus by neurones called osmoreceptors and it is stored in the posterior pituitary gland. Osmoreceptors are sensitive to plasma osmolality and a decrease in blood volume. The target organs for ADH are the kidneys. ADH acts on the distal convoluted tubule and the collecting ducts which make the tubules more permeable to water, thus increasing reabsorption of water. This occurs through insertion of additional water channels (Aquaporin-2s) into the apical membrane of the tubules and collecting duct epithelial cells. The aquaporins allow water to pass out of the nephron (at the distal convoluted tubules and the conducting tubules) and into the cells, increasing the amount of water reabsorbed from the filtrate. Therefore, when a person is lacking fluid, as in dehydration, more ADH is released, thus increasing water reabsorption resulting in less fluid loss. The secretion of ADH is decreased by a drop in plasma osmotic pressure, increased extracellular fluid volume and increased alcohol intake. ADH is also known as vasopressin because it causes constriction of arterioles, thus raising blood pressure.

Aldosterone

Aldosterone is a steroid hormone produced by the adrenal glands which are situated on top of each kidney. The adrenal gland is divided into the cortex and medulla. The cortex produces aldosterone. Aldosterone regulates electrolyte and fluid balance by increasing the reabsorption of sodium and water and the release of potassium in the kidneys. This increases blood volume and therefore increases blood pressure. Aldosterone stimulates H^+ secretion by intercalated cells in the collecting duct, regulating plasma bicarbonate (HCO_3^-) levels thus maintaining the acid base and electrolyte balance. The main target areas for aldosterone are the kidney tubules and the collecting duct epithelial cells.

Atrial natriuretic peptide

Atrial natriuretic peptide (ANP), atrial natriuretic factor (ANF), atrial natriuretic hormone (ANH), or atriopeptin, is a powerful vasodilator and a polypeptide hormone secreted by heart muscle cells (myocytes). The myocytes produce, store and release ANP in response to atrial stretch. It is involved in the homeostatic control of body water, sodium, potassium and fat (adipose tissue). It is released by muscle cells in the upper chambers (atria) of the heart (atrial myocytes), in response to high blood pressure. ANP acts to reduce the water, sodium and adipose loads on the circulatory system, thereby reducing blood pressure. ANP stimulates vasodilation, increased glomerular filtration and salt and water excretion, and blocks the release and/or actions of several hormones, including angiotensin II, aldosterone and vasopressin. ANP levels are commonly elevated in situations of excessive fluid volume or hypertension, and the hormone plays an important role in regulating fluid/electrolyte balance.

Clinical considerations

Hyponatraemia

Hyponatraemia is the commonest electrolyte imbalance encountered in clinical practice. In healthy individuals, the normal range for serum sodium is 135–147 mmol/l. In hyponatraemic patients, serum sodium levels fall below 135 mmol/l. Hyponatraemia can be fatal; in less severe cases it can significantly impede the patient's recovery. Common symptoms include weakness, agitation, confusion, nausea and vomiting. Hyponatraemia may occur when there is an excessive consumption of water, which dilutes electrolytes in the body, and/or excessive sweating or electrolyte loss as a result of vomiting and/or diarrhoea.

Causes of hyponatraemia include:

- Burns
- Congestive heart failure
- Diarrhoea
- Use of medications called diuretics, which increase urine output
- Kidney diseases
- Liver cirrhosis
- Syndrome of inappropriate antidiuretic hormone secretion (SIADH)
- Sweating
- Vomiting.

Mild chronic hyponatraemia may not require treatment other than adjustments in diet, lifestyle or medications. For severe or acute hyponatraemia, treatment typically involves the intravenous administration of fluids and electrolytes. In this case medications are often needed to treat the underlying cause of the hyponatraemia as well as medications to manage the symptoms.

Conclusion

Cells are the basic living structures of the body and they contain special proteins that perform specific functions to maintain homeostasis within the cell. All cells have four basic parts: cytoplasm, plasma membrane, nucleus and nucleolus. Although the cell membrane is in a constant state of flux, it allows substances in and out of the cell. The nucleus is the place where genetic information is stored. Cells utilise various transport systems to move nutrients, oxygen, electrolytes, water and hormones into the cell and waste products of cellular metabolism, such as carbon dioxide, urea and uric acid, out of the cell. Electrolytes and hormones play a vital role in maintaining homeostasis. Many hormones, such as antidiuretic hormone, aldosterone and atrial natriuretic hormone, help to regulate fluid balance and maintain homeostasis.

Body fluids consist of water and substances dissolved in it. Water is the main component of the human body and, in any individual, the body water content stays remarkably constant from day to day. There is constant movement of fluid between compartments. There are two main body fluid compartments: inside and outside the cells (intracellular and extracellular).

The extracellular compartment is divisible into (a) the plasma, which is extracellular fluid within the blood vessels; (b) the interstitial fluid, which is extracellular fluid outside the blood vessels and separated from plasma by the walls of the capillaries; and (c) transcellular fluids, which are fluids with specialised functions. They include synovial fluid (which lubricates joints), cerebrospinal fluid (which cushions and nurtures the brain) and the aqueous and vitreous humours of the eyes (which maintain the shape of the eyeball and the integrity of structures within it). The transcellular fluids are separated from the plasma by a cellular membrane, which takes part in their formation, in addition to the capillary wall.

Glossary

Active transport:	The process in which substances move against a concentration gradient by utilising cellular energy.
Adenosine diphosphate:	ADP is the end-product that results when ATP loses one of its phosphate groups located at the end of the molecule.
Adenosine triphosphate:	Compound that is necessary for cellular energy.
Chemical reactions:	Reactions that involve molecules, in which they are formed, changed, or broken down.
Compartments:	Spaces.
Cytoplasm:	Fluid found inside the cell.
Diffusion:	The most common form of passive transport of materials, it is the ability of gases, liquids and solutes to disperse randomly and to occupy any space available, so that there is an equal distribution.
Electrolytes:	Substances that dissociate in water to form ions.
Endocytosis:	Processes by which cells ingest foodstuffs and infectious micro-organisms.
Extracellular:	Space found outside the cell.
Exocytosis:	The system of transporting material out of cells.
Facilitated diffusion:	Diffusion with the aid of a transport protein.
Hydrophilic:	Water-loving.
Hydrophobic:	Water-hating.
Hypertonic:	Solution that has large amount of solutes dissolved in it.
Hypotonic:	Solution that has low concentration of solutes.

Interstitial: Space between cells.

Intracellular: Space inside the cell.

Organelles: Structural and functional parts of a cell.

Osmosis: Movement of water through a selectively permeable membrane so that concentrations of substances in water are the same on either side of the membrane.

Osmotic pressure: The pressure that must be exerted on a solution.

Passive transport: The process by which substances move on their own down a concentration gradient without utilising cellular energy.

Plasma membrane: Outer layer of the cell.

Transport protein: Small molecules that help in the movement of ions across a cell membrane.

References

Colbert, B.J., Ankney, J. and Lee, K.T. (2007) *Anatomy and Physiology for Health Professionals: An Interactive Journey*. Upper Saddle River, NJ: Pearson Prentice Hall.

LeMone, P. and Burke, K. (2008) *Medical–Surgical Nursing: Critical Thinking in Client Care*, 4th edn. Upper Saddle River, NJ: Pearson Education.

Marieb, E.N. and Hoehn, K. (2007) *Human Anatomy and Physiology*, 7th edn. San Francisco: Pearson Benjamin Cummings.

Nair, M. and Peate, I. (2009) *Fundamentals of Applied Pathophysiology: An Essential Guide for Nursing Students*. Oxford: Wiley-Blackwell.

Thibodeau, G.A. and Patton, K.T. (2007) *Anatomy and Physiology*, 6th edn. St Louis, MO: Elsevier Mosby.

Tortora, G.J. and Derrickson, B.H. (2009) *Principles of Anatomy and Physiology*, 12th edn. Hoboken, NJ: John Wiley & Sons.

Vickers, P.S. (2009) Cell and body tissue physiology. In: Nair, M. and Peate, I. (eds) *Fundamentals of Pathophysiology*. Chichester: John Wiley & Sons.

Activities

www.wiley.com/go/peate

Multiple choice questions

1. Which of the following is not made of microtubules?

   (a) centrioles
   (b) microvilli
   (c) cilia
   (d) cytoskeleton

2. The plasma membrane does not contain:

   (a) protein
   (b) nucleic acid
   (c) cholesterol
   (d) glycolipid

3. The movement of water through a semipermeable membrane is called:

   (a) facilitated diffusion
   (b) active transport
   (c) simple diffusion
   (d) osmosis

4. The nucleolus:

   (a) has a surrounding membrane
   (b) contains ATP
   (c) is the site for ribosomal RNA synthesis
   (d) is the site for enzyme action

5. Mitochondria produce:

   (a) ATP
   (b) CO_2
   (c) DNA
   (d) RNA

6. In the capillaries albumin produces 70% of the:

   (a) energy
   (b) oncotic pressure
   (c) cholesterol
   (d) lipids

7. Which of the following is an example of an active transport system?

   (a) pinocytosis
   (b) osmosis
   (c) diffusion
   (d) facilitated diffusion

8. A red blood cell placed in hypotonic solution will:
   (a) crenate
   (b) swell and burst
   (c) remain stable
   (d) divide

9. Lysosomes:
   (a) will produce cellular energy
   (b) will provide structural support for a cell
   (c) will digest foreign material
   (d) will store cellular material

10. The three types of endocytosis are:
   (a) phagocytosis , pinocytosis, exocytosis
   (b) phagocytosis, exocytosis, cytolysis
   (c) cytolysis, receptor-mediated endocytosis, pinocytosis
   (d) pinocytosis, receptor-mediated endocytosis, phagocytosis

Test your learning

1. What are the components of a cell?
2. Describe the structure of the cell membrane.
3. List the differences between active and passive transport systems.
4. Discuss the functions of mitochondria.
5. What is a semipermeable membrane?
6. What are organelles?
7. Discuss the role of electrolytes.
8. What are the differences between endocytosis and exocytosis?

Label the diagram

From the ...s of words, label the diagrams below:

...icrofilament, Plasma membrane, Lysosome, Smooth endoplasmic reticulum, Flagellu...drion, Sectional view, Nucleus, Cytoplasm, Rough endoplasmic reticulum, Ribosome, Mit...complex, Microfilament

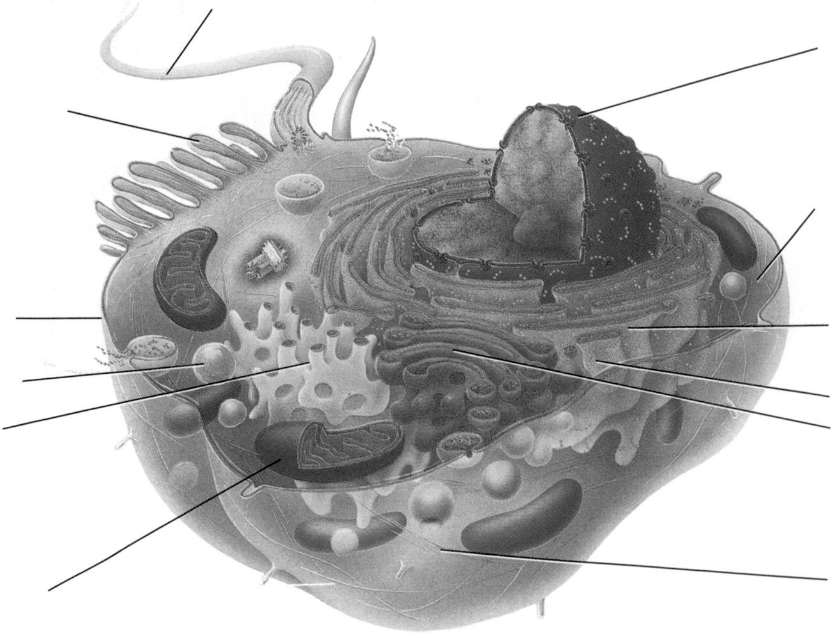

From the list of words, label the diagram below:

Phagocytosis, Solid particle, Pseudopodium, Phagosome (food vacuole), Pinocytosis, Vesicle, Receptor-mediated endocytosis, Coated pit, Receptor, Coat protein, Coated vesicle, Plasma membrane, Extracellular fluid, Cytoplasm

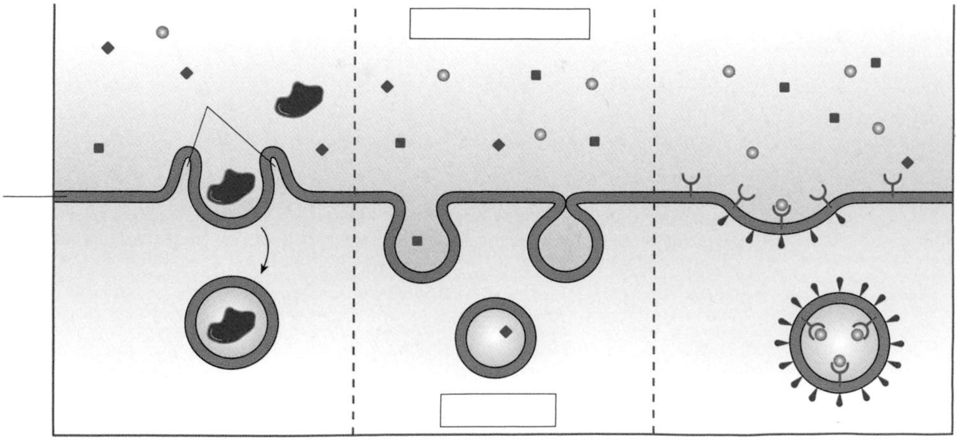

Relating to cellular organelles, circle the word or term that does not belong in the following groups

1.	Centrioles	Lysosomes	Peroxisomes	Enzymatic breakdown
2.	Centrioles	Cilia	Mitochondria	Flagella
3.	Nucleus	Nucleolus	Lysosomes	DNA
4.	Ribosomes	Rough ER	Protein synthesis	Smooth ER
5.	Microtubules	Cilia	Intermediate filaments	Cytoskeleton

Word search

In the grid below there are 20 words that you will have seen in this chapter. Can you find them all?

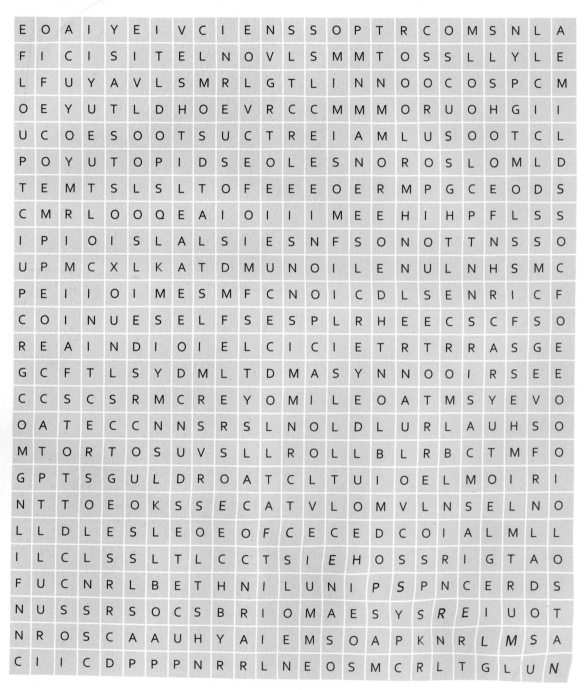

E	O	A	I	Y	E	I	V	C	I	E	N	S	S	O	P	T	R	C	O	M	S	N	L	A
F	I	C	I	S	I	T	E	L	N	O	V	L	S	M	M	T	O	S	S	L	L	Y	L	E
L	F	U	Y	A	V	L	S	M	R	L	G	T	L	I	N	N	O	O	C	O	S	P	C	M
O	E	Y	U	T	L	D	H	O	E	V	R	C	C	M	M	M	O	R	U	O	H	G	I	I
U	C	O	E	S	O	O	T	S	U	C	T	R	E	I	A	M	L	U	S	O	O	T	C	L
P	O	Y	U	T	O	P	I	D	S	E	O	L	E	S	N	O	R	O	S	L	O	M	L	D
T	E	M	T	S	L	S	L	T	O	F	E	E	E	O	E	R	M	P	G	C	E	O	D	S
C	M	R	L	O	O	Q	E	A	I	O	I	I	I	M	E	E	H	I	H	P	F	L	S	S
I	P	I	O	I	S	L	A	L	S	I	E	S	N	F	S	O	N	O	T	T	N	S	S	O
U	P	M	C	X	L	K	A	T	D	M	U	N	O	I	L	E	N	U	L	N	H	S	M	C
P	E	I	I	O	I	M	E	S	M	F	C	N	O	I	C	D	L	S	E	N	R	I	C	F
C	O	I	N	U	E	S	E	L	F	S	E	S	P	L	R	H	E	E	C	S	C	F	S	O
R	E	A	I	N	D	I	O	I	E	L	C	I	C	I	E	T	R	T	R	R	A	S	G	E
G	C	F	T	L	S	Y	D	M	L	T	D	M	A	S	Y	N	N	O	O	I	R	S	E	E
C	C	S	C	S	R	M	C	R	E	Y	O	M	I	L	E	O	A	T	M	S	Y	E	V	O
O	A	T	E	C	C	N	N	S	R	S	L	N	O	L	D	L	U	R	L	A	U	H	S	O
M	T	O	R	T	O	S	U	V	S	L	L	R	O	L	L	B	L	R	B	C	T	M	F	O
G	P	T	S	G	U	L	D	R	O	A	T	C	L	T	U	I	O	E	L	M	O	I	R	I
N	T	T	O	E	O	K	S	S	E	C	A	T	V	L	O	M	V	L	N	S	E	L	N	O
L	L	D	L	E	S	L	E	O	E	O	F	C	E	C	E	D	C	O	I	A	L	M	L	L
I	L	C	L	S	S	L	T	L	C	C	T	S	I	E	H	O	S	S	R	I	G	T	A	O
F	U	C	N	R	L	B	E	T	H	N	I	L	U	N	I	P	S	P	N	C	E	R	D	S
N	U	S	S	R	S	O	C	S	B	R	I	O	M	A	E	S	Y	S	R	E	I	U	O	T
N	R	O	S	C	A	A	U	H	Y	A	I	E	M	S	O	A	P	K	N	R	L	M	S	A
C	I	I	C	D	P	P	P	N	R	R	L	N	E	O	S	M	C	R	L	T	G	L	U	N

For the following electrolytes write the correct chemical symbols

Potassium __________
Sodium __________
Bicarbonate __________
Chloride __________
Organic phosphate __________
Sulphate __________
Calcium __________

Conditions

Below is a list of conditions that are associated with the subjects discussed in this cha[illegible] some time and write notes about each of the conditions. You may make the notes take[illegible] text books or other resources, for example, people you work with in a clinical area, or yo[illegible] make the notes as a result of people you have cared for. If you are making notes about pe[illegible] you have cared for you must ensure that you adhere to the rules of confidentiality.

Sarcoma	
Oedema	
Neoplasms	
Apoptosis	
Melanoma	
Hyponatraemia	
Hyperkalaemia	
Hypokalaemia	

Answers

MCQs

1b; 2b; 3d; 4c; 5a; 6b; 7a[illegible]; 9c; 10d

Rela[illegible]g to cellular organelles, circle the word or term that does n[illegible] [illegible]elong in the following groups

1a; 2c; 3c; 9d

Wordsearch

E	O	A	I	Y	E	I	V	C	I	E	N	S	S	O	P	T	R	C	O	M	S	N	L	A
F	I	C	I	S	I	T	E	L	N	O	V	L	S	M	M	T	O	S	S	L	L	Y	L	E
L	F	U	Y	A	V	L	S	M	R	L	G	T	L	I	N	N	O	O	C	O	S	P	C	M
O	E	Y	U	T	L	D	H	O	E	V	R	C	C	M	M	M	O	R	U	O	H	G	I	I
U	C	O	E	S	O	O	T	S	U	C	T	R	E	I	A	M	L	U	S	O	O	T	C	L
P	O	Y	U	T	O	P	I	D	S	E	O	L	E	S	N	O	R	O	S	L	O	M	L	D
T	E	M	T	S	L	S	L	T	O	F	E	E	E	O	E	R	M	P	G	C	E	O	D	S
C	M	R	L	O	O	Q	E	A	I	O	I	I	I	M	E	E	H	I	H	P	F	L	S	S
I	P	I	O	I	S	L	A	L	S	I	E	S	N	F	S	O	N	O	T	T	N	S	S	O
U	P	M	C	X	L	K	A	T	D	M	U	N	O	I	L	E	N	U	L	N	H	S	M	C
P	E	I	I	O	I	M	E	S	M	F	C	N	O	I	C	D	L	S	E	N	R	I	C	F
C	O	I	N	U	E	S	E	L	F	S	E	S	P	L	R	H	E	E	C	S	C	F	S	O
R	E	A	I	N	D	I	O	I	E	L	C	I	C	I	E	T	R	T	R	R	A	S	G	E
G	C	F	T	L	S	Y	D	M	L	T	D	M	A	S	Y	N	N	O	O	I	R	S	E	E
C	C	S	C	S	R	M	C	R	E	Y	O	M	I	L	E	O	A	T	M	S	Y	E	V	O
O	A	T	E	C	C	N	N	S	R	S	L	N	O	L	D	L	U	R	L	A	U	H	S	O
M	T	O	R	T	O	S	U	V	S	L	L	R	O	L	L	B	L	R	B	C	T	M	F	O
G	P	T	S	G	U	L	D	R	O	A	T	C	L	T	U	I	O	E	L	M	O	I	R	I
N	T	T	O	E	O	K	S	S	E	C	A	T	V	L	O	M	V	L	N	S	E	L	N	O
L	L	D	L	E	S	L	E	O	E	O	F	C	E	C	E	D	C	O	I	A	L	M	L	L
I	L	C	L	S	S	L	T	L	C	C	T	S	I	E	H	O	S	S	R	I	G	T	A	O
F	U	C	N	R	L	B	E	T	H	N	I	L	U	N	I	P	S	P	N	C	E	R	D	S
N	U	S	S	R	S	O	C	S	B	R	I	O	M	A	E	S	Y	S	R	E	I	U	O	T
N	R	O	S	C	A	A	U	H	Y	A	I	E	M	S	O	A	P	K	N	R	L	M	S	A
C	I	I	C	D	P	P	P	N	R	R	L	N	E	O	S	M	C	R	L	T	G	L	U	N

For the following electrolytes write the correct chemical symbols

Potassium	K
Sodium	Na
Bicarbonate	HCO_3
Chloride	Cl
Organic phosphate	PO_4
Sulphate	SO_4
Calcium	Ca

3 The immune system

Peter S Vickers

Contents

Introduction 64

Blood cell development 64

Organs of the immune system 67
The thymus 67

The lymphatic system 68
Lymph nodes 70
Lymphoid tissue 70
The spleen 71

Types of immunity 72
The innate immune system 72
Physical barriers 72
Mechanical barriers 73
Chemical barriers 73
Blood cells 73
Blood cells of the immune system 73
Phagocytosis 74
Cytotoxicity 76
Inflammation 76

The acquired immune system 79
Cell-meditated immunity (T-cell lymphocytes) 79
Humoral immunity (B-cell lymphocytes) 80

Immunoglobulins (antibodies) 83

Types of immunoglobulins 83
Immunoglobulin G 83
Immunoglobulin A 83
Immunoglobulin M 84
Immunoglobulin E 84
Immunoglobulin D 84
Role of immunoglobulins 84
Natural killer cells 86

Primary and secondary response to infection 86
Primary immune response 86
Secondary immune response 88

Immunisations 89
Passive immunisation 89
Active immunity 90

Conclusion 91
Glossary 92
References 95
Activities 96

Test your knowledge

- Name the blood cells involved in the immune system.
- What are the four classic signs of inflammation?
- List the chemical barriers that protect us against infection.
- What is the main role of antibodies (immunoglobulins)?

Fundamentals of Anatomy and Physiology for Student Nurses, First Edition. Edited by Ian Peate, Muralitharan Nair.

Learning outcomes

On completion of this chapter the reader will be able to:

- Describe and discuss the development of white blood cells and their roles in immunity
- Explain how the immune system works to protect us from infections
- List all the various physical, mechanical and chemical barriers that the human body possesses to prevent infectious organisms from entering the body
- Explain the process of phagocytosis
- Understand how inflammation works to protect us once the body has been damaged in some way or has been infected
- Describe and discuss cellular immunity
- Describe and discuss humoral immunity
- Explain the body's response to infection and the rationale for immunisations

Body map

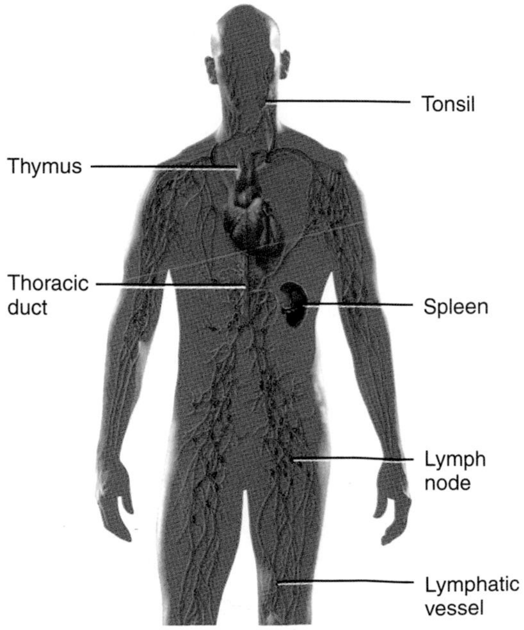
Tonsil
Thymus
Thoracic duct
Spleen
Lymph node
Lymphatic vessel

Introduction

The body is constantly under attack from organisms out to destroy it. This may sound dramatic, but it is true. Infectious micro-organisms, toxins and pollutants are some of the harmful substances from which it has to defend itself. Fortunately, the body has evolved and developed many defences to repel and destroy these harmful substances.

Immunology – the study of the **immune system** – is a relatively new branch of bioscience and medicine. Although some of the mechanisms and components of immunity, such as antibodies and blood cells, have been known for some time, it is only recently that so much research has been undertaken into the immune system.

Without a doubt, the onset of HIV and AIDS in the 1980s was the trigger for much of this research, and it is now accepted that the immune system is a complicated and wonderful system which underpins so much of the understanding of disease and disease process, and not only those diseases caused by infectious micro-organisms.

This chapter will show what the body's acquired and innate immune defences consist of and how they work together to give the body a good chance of surviving the continuous and continuing assaults by micro-organisms, toxins and other pollutants, to which it is subjected.

Blood cell development

All our blood cells are descended from a particular type of cell known as the multipotent stem cell. This **multipotent stem cell** has the ability to switch to different types of cells, and initially they, or rather their descendants, form one of two major branches of white cells.

One descendant stem cell will lead to the development of the **myeloid** family of cells, which include the white blood cells such as neutrophils and monocytes, whilst the other descendant stem cell will lead to the development of the **lymphoid** family of cells, which is made up of cells known as lymphocytes.

Figure 3.1 shows the development of the white blood cells from the initial multipotent stem cell.

It can be seen from the family tree of blood cells below that the end results from the myeloid side include the macrophages (consisting of monocytes and tissue macrophages) and granulocytes (consisting of neutrophils, eosinophils and basophils). The lymphoid branch of white blood cells ends up with T-lymphocytes and B-lymphocytes (with many of the B-lymphocytes developing into plasma cells). It can also be seen that the stem cell that develops into the myeloid branch can also provide megakaryocytes (leading to platelets) and erythroid cells, which develop into a regional sides (i.e. red blood cells).

As it is the white blood cells that make up the immune systems, in this chapter we are not interested in red blood cells, although they are important to the immune system in which they carry oxygen to the other cells of the immune system, such as the skin cells.

Similarly, although platelets do play a very important role in the defence of the body in terms of blocking any breaks in the skin and, by doing so, preventing any more infectious organisms getting into the body, this group of blood cells will only be discussed in terms of the process of inflammation.

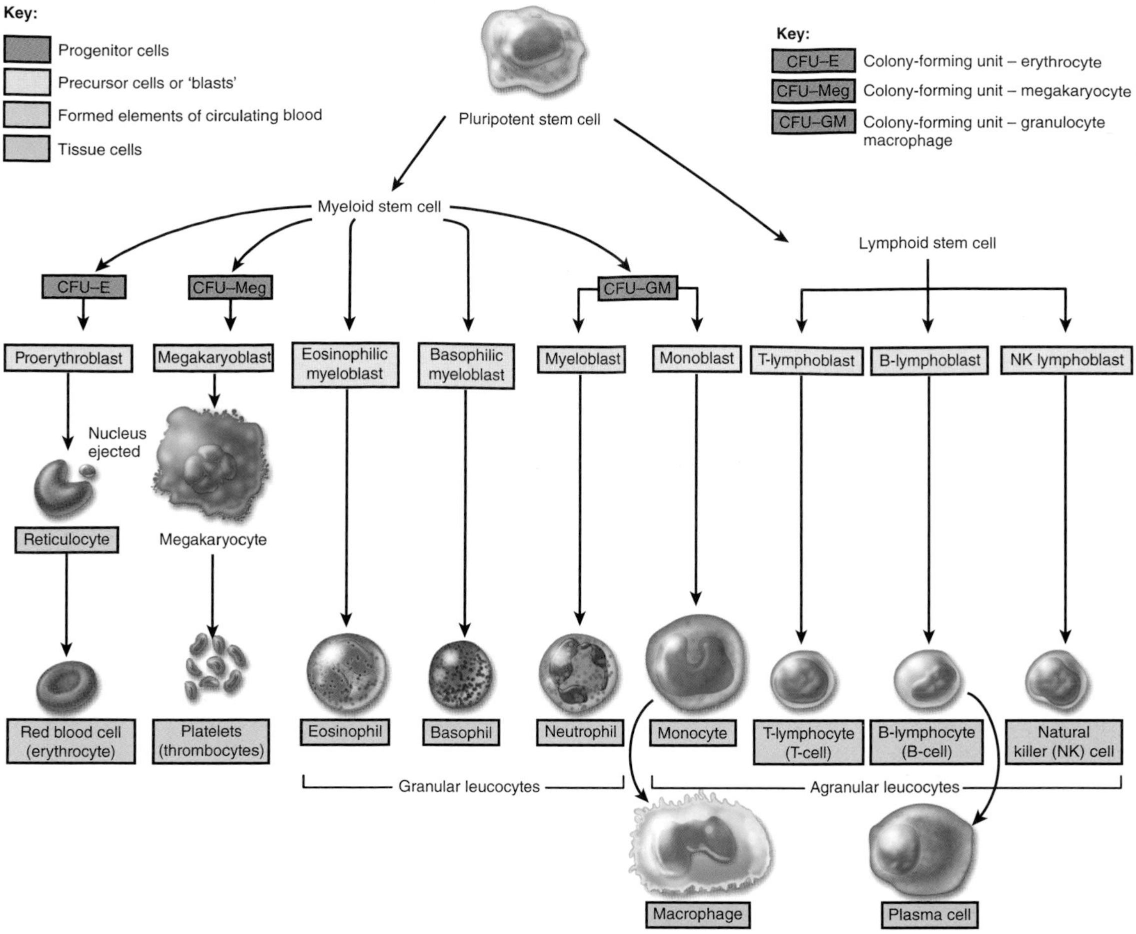
Key:
Progenitor cells
Precursor cells or 'blasts'
Formed elements of circulating blood
Tissue cells
Pluripotent stem cell
Key:
CFU–E Colony-forming unit – erythrocyte
CFU–Meg Colony-forming unit – megakaryocyte
CFU–GM Colony-forming unit – granulocyte macrophage
Myeloid stem cell
Lymphoid stem cell
CFU–E
CFU–Meg
CFU–GM
Proerythroblast
Megakaryoblast
Eosinophilic myeloblast
Basophilic myeloblast
Myeloblast
Monoblast
T-lymphoblast
B-lymphoblast
NK lymphoblast
Nucleus ejected
Reticulocyte
Megakaryocyte
Red blood cell (erythrocyte)
Platelets (thrombocytes)
Eosinophil
Basophil
Neutrophil
Monocyte
T-lymphocyte (T-cell)
B-lymphocyte (B-cell)
Natural killer (NK) cell
Granular leucocytes
Agranular leucocytes
Macrophage
Plasma cell

Figure 3.1 The development of blood cells (Tortora and Derrickson 2009)

All these blood cells start life in the bone marrow as stem cells, but as they slowly mature through various stages, they eventually find themselves at different places around the body, including:

- The blood and lymph circulation
- The thymus
- The spleen
- The tonsils and other lymph nodes.

They also are found in all the mucosal membranes, such as the lining of the mouth and the gastrointestinal tract.

Blood cells: a brief glossary

B-lymphocytes:	These lymphocytes arise in the bone marrow and differentiate into plasma cells, which in turn produce **immunoglobulins** – also known as antibodies.
Bone marrow:	The site in the body where most of the cells of the immune system are produced as immature (stem) cells.
Immunoglobulins:	Immunoglobulins are highly specialised protein molecules. They are also known as antibodies and their job is to connect with, and hold on to, foreign **antigens**, so that they cannot escape destruction by other cells of the immune system.
Monocytes:	These white blood cells are also **phagocytes** and are found in the blood. However, they have the ability to migrate into tissues, and there they are known as macrophages.
Plasma cells:	These cells develop from B-lymphocytes, and are responsible for producing **the immunoglobulins**.
Platelets:	Blood cells which have an important role to play in the clotting of blood.
Polymorphonuclear leucocytes:	These white blood cells are known as **phagocytes**, and are found in the blood.
Red blood cells:	These are the cells in the blood which carry oxygen from the lungs to the tissues.
Stem cells:	These cells have the potential to differentiate and mature into the different cells of the immune system.
Thymus:	An organ located in the chest which instructs immature T-lymphocytes to become mature T-lymphocytes.
T-effector lymphocytes:	Also known as **T-cytotoxic** lymphocytes. These lymphocytes have the ability to produce chemicals that can kill foreign cells and micro-organisms, as well as helping in the process of inflammation.
T-helper lymphocytes:	During their time in the thymus, these specialised lymphocytes develop the ability to help other lymphocytes (both T- and B-lymphocytes) to mount an immune response.
T-lymphocytes:	These lymphocytes arise in the bone marrow but migrate to the thymus where they mature into T-lymphocytes, and also learn to differentiate between 'self' and 'non-self' matter.
T-suppressor lymphocytes:	These are specialised lymphocytes which during their time in the thymus are so differentiated that they can suppress the helper T lymphocytes and help to turn off the immune system response.

(Vickers 2007: 9)

Organs of the immune system

The main organs of the immune system are concerned with the lymphatic system. These organs of the immune system consist of the:

- Thymus
- Spleen
- Lymph nodes
- Lymphoid tissues scattered throughout the gastrointestinal, respiratory and urinary tracts.

The thymus

The **thymus** is situated in the chest (Figure 3.2), and in babies it is a large organ (relative to size). It shrinks with age (atrophies).

Within the thymus, certain blood stem cells mature and differentiate into their various **T-cell lymphocyte** subclasses. In addition, they also acquire the ability to recognise and differentiate 'self' cells from 'non-self' cells.

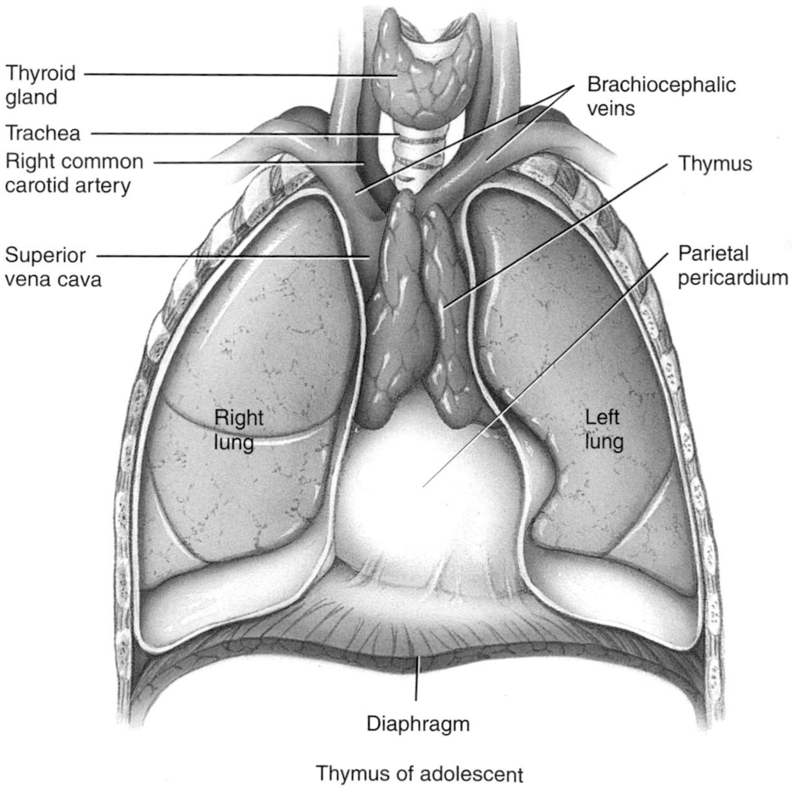

Thyroid gland
Trachea
Right common carotid artery
Superior vena cava
Brachiocephalic veins
Thymus
Parietal pericardium
Right lung
Left lung
Diaphragm
Thymus of adolescent

Figure 3.2 Position of the thymus (Tortora and Derrickson 2009)

'Self' cells are cells which originate and belong to the individual with that thymus, whilst 'non-self' cells are cells which come from outside of the individual, so think of the thymus as a school for T-cell lymphocytes in which the cells take part in learning experiences as they mature and in which they also are guided to different careers for when they leave the 'school'.

Even though the thymus starts to degenerate (atrophy) at puberty, T-cells continue to develop in the thymus throughout an individual's life (Delves and Roitt 2000; Vickers 2005).

The lymphatic system

The lymphatic system is a specialised system of **lymph vessels** (similar to blood vessels) and **lymph nodes**. The lymphatic vessels contain a fluid called **'lymph'**, which drains into the organs of the lymph system from nearby organs. This lymph originates from plasma leaking from the blood capillaries.

Lymphocytes migrate from the blood system by passing through the walls of the smallest venous capillaries in the lymph node. What may be of surprise is that lymphocytes spend only a few minutes in the blood stream during each circuit of the body, but spend several hours in the lymphoid system.

The lymphatic system can be thought of as a parallel system to the blood circulatory system, but it does not have a pump, like the heart, which pumps blood around the body. Instead, the lymph is agitated around the body by a combination of the smooth muscular walls of the lymph vessels and the flexing and relaxing of striated muscle as an individual moves around.

The peripheral lymphatic system (Figure 3.3) is made up of lymphatic vessels and lymphatic capillaries, as well as encapsulated organs (i.e. organs which are situated within their own 'capsule').

These include:

- Spleen
- Tonsils
- Lymph nodes.

In addition, the lymphatic system includes unencapsulated (not bound by a capsule, but more diffuse) **lymphoid tissue** in the gastro intestinal tract, the urogenital tract and the lungs.

The lymph vessels and capillaries form a network throughout the body which connects the tissues of the body to the lymphoid organs, such as the **spleen,** and the lymph nodes.

Lymphatic capillaries have some anatomical similarities to blood capillaries in that their walls consist of a layer of **endothelial cells**. However, lymphatic capillary walls do not have a basement membrane. This lack of a basement membrane allows substances of relatively large molecular weight, such as plasma proteins, to enter the lymphatic capillaries between the cells of the capillary walls.

Lymph flows through the vessels by means of:

- Muscle contraction in the limbs (arms and legs)
- The pulsing of arteries (caused by the beating of the heart)
- Negative intrathoracic pressure (which draws up the lymph, as from a vacuum).
- The rhythmic contraction of the lymphatic vessels themselves.

The lymph eventually flows into two large lymph ducts. One of them is called the thoracic duct and this receives lymph from the

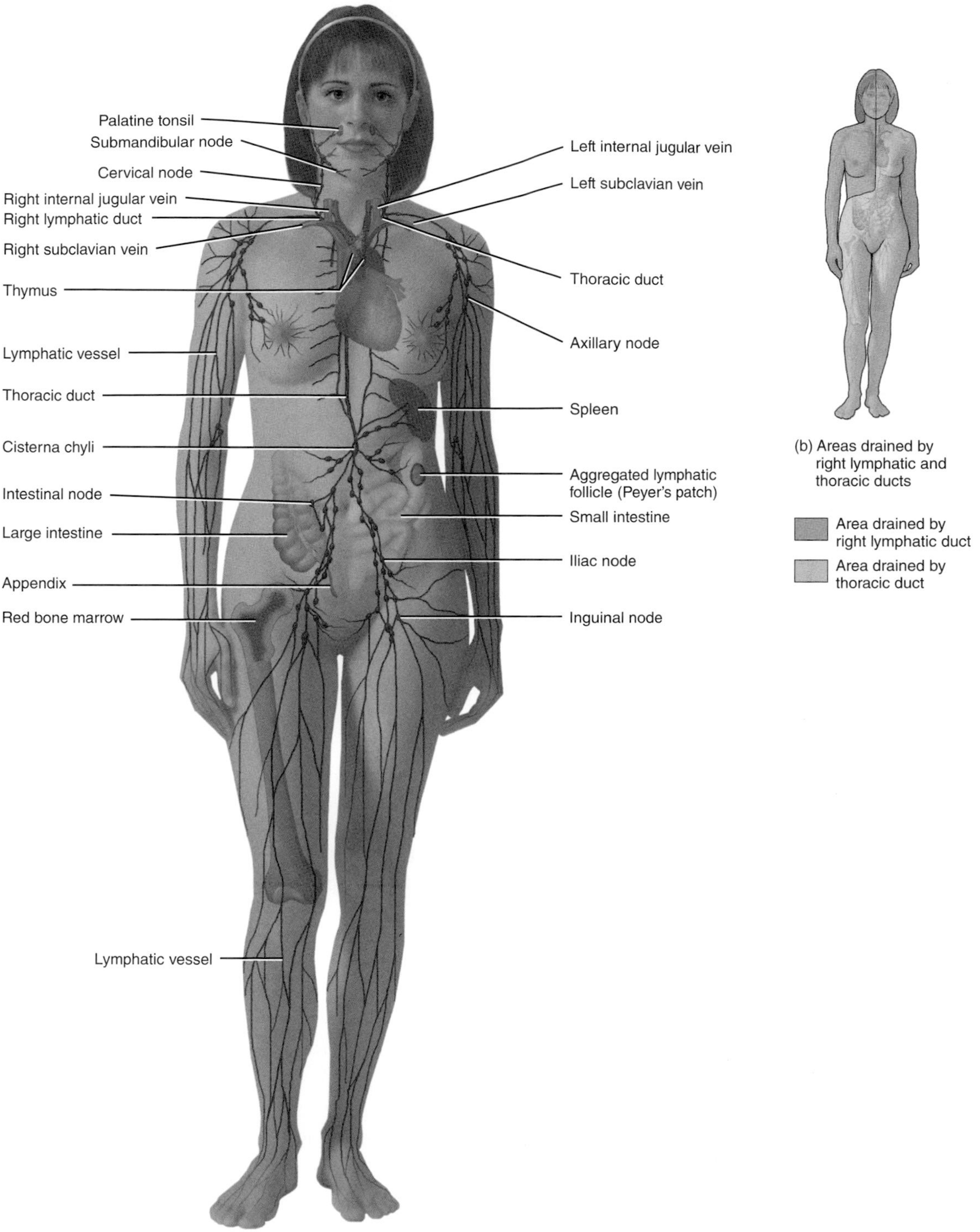
Palatine tonsil
Submandibular node
Cervical node
Right internal jugular vein
Right lymphatic duct
Right subclavian vein
Thymus
Lymphatic vessel
Thoracic duct
Cisterna chyli
Intestinal node
Large intestine
Appendix
Red bone marrow
Lymphatic vessel
Left internal jugular vein
Left subclavian vein
Thoracic duct
Axillary node
Spleen
Aggregated lymphatic follicle (Peyer's patch)
Small intestine
Iliac node
Inguinal node
(b) Areas drained by right lymphatic and thoracic ducts
Area drained by right lymphatic duct
Area drained by thoracic duct

Figure 3.3 Principal components of the lymphatic system (Tortora and Derrickson 2009)

- Lower limbs
- Digestive tract
- Left arm
- Left side of the thorax, head and neck.

The other large lymph vessel, the right lymphatic duct, receives lymph from the

- Right arm
- Right side of the head, neck and thorax.

The two lymph ducts then empty into the great veins in the neck, thus restoring fluid and proteins to the venous circulation.

Lymph nodes

Lymph enters the lymph nodes from the afferent lymphatic vessels and from there goes to the **trabeculae**. Afferent means 'leading towards', therefore, afferent vessels in the case of lymph nodes are those vessels that lead towards the lymph node.

The lymph node is made up of a mesh of cells – just like a net. The lymph at this stage contains **antigens** from infected cells and tissues. This lymph passes through this mesh in the lymph node and the antigens are trapped – like fish in fishing nets (Figure 3.4).

Antigens entering the body at any point are rapidly swept along the lymph vessels towards a lymphoid organ or lymph node.

Within the lymph node, **B-cell lymphocytes** are located in the primary lymphoid follicles as well as the secondary lymphoid follicles (which contain the germinal centres), and it is inside these germinal centres that the B-cells proliferate after encountering their specific antigen and its co-operating T-cell. The B-cells that are found at the centre of the secondary lymphoid follicles are actively dividing, whilst those at the periphery are antibody-forming.

In addition, large numbers of **phagocytic macrophages** and plasma cells producing antibodies are found in the **medulla** of the gland. Macrophages and other antigen-presenting cells spend most of their lives migrating through the tissues until they encounter antigens. These are then **phagocytosed** (engulfed by phagocytes and 'eaten') and transported to the nearest lymph node.

Macrophages in the lymph node also encounter trapped antigens within the meshwork of reticular cells, and they phagocytose the dead cells and bacteria. The lymph which has destroyed the antigens in the lymph nodes then leaves through the efferent lymphatic vessel. Efferent means 'to lead away from', therefore the efferent lymph vessels lead away from the lymph nodes.

Lymphoid tissue

As well as lymphatic vessels, the lymphatic system contains lymphoid tissue. This consists of lymph glands, called lymph nodes, which are approximately the size and shape of a broad bean, and lymphoid tissue, and which is found in specific organs, particularly the

- Spleen
- Bone marrow
- Lungs

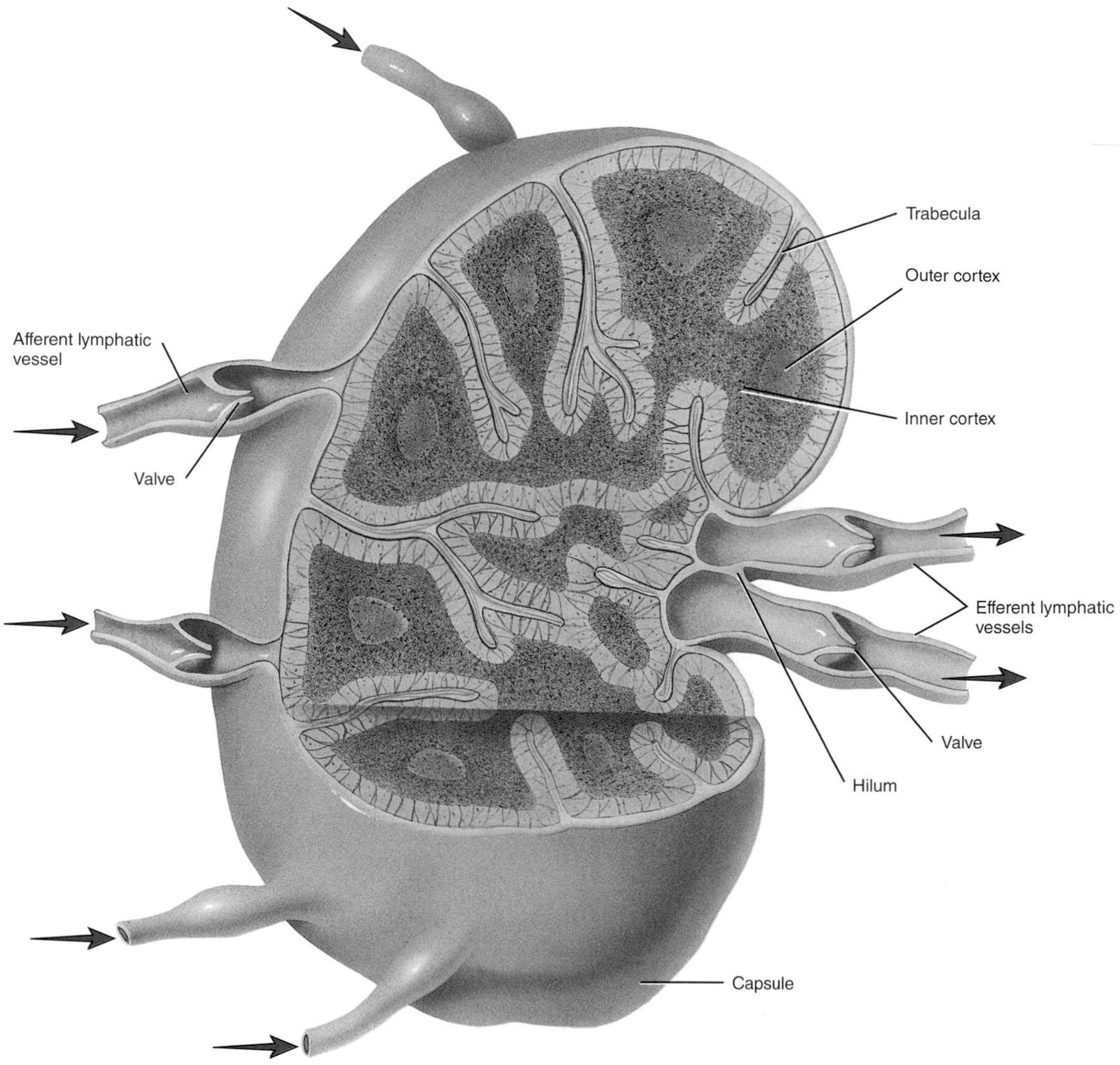
Trabecula
Outer cortex
Afferent lymphatic vessel
Inner cortex
Valve
Efferent lymphatic vessels
Valve
Hilum
Capsule

Figure 3.4 Simplified drawing of a lymph node (Nair and Peate 2009)

- Liver
- Other lymphoid tissue.

The spleen

The spleen is situated just behind the stomach and is about the size of a fist. It collects antigen from the blood for presentation to phagocytes and lymphocytes, and also collects, and disposes of, dead red blood cells.

To sum up the lymph system:

- The lymphoid system enables lymphocytes to protect the tissues and vessels of the body from infectious micro-organisms.
- It holds them in antigen 'traps' in the lymph nodes and other lymphoid organs, and it brings them into close proximity with other immune cells.
- This is essential for the cell-to-cell communication that is necessary to recruit, direct and regulate a coordinated immune response.
- Lymph glands are the major centres for lymphocyte proliferation and antibody production as well as for filtering the lymph.

(Vickers 2005)

Types of immunity

There are two major types of immunity in humans – the **innate** and the **acquired**.

Innate immunity is the immunity we possess at birth, so it is innate in all of us. On the other hand, **acquired immunity** is not present at birth; rather, it is something that we acquire as we go through life. Innate immunity is the oldest type of immunity and is present in all creatures, whereas the second type of immunity, acquired immunity, is only found in more developed organisms, such as humans and other mammals.

Another name for innate immunity is **non-specific immunity**. This means that these defences come into action no matter what infectious or non-self organism is trying to attack us, therefore they are non-specific. Similarly, acquired immunity is also known as **specific immunity** because it responds to known specific organisms.

The innate immune system

Many parts of the body, as well as the white blood cells, combine to make up the innate immune system.

It is possible to categorise the innate immune system into four groups:

- Physical barriers
- Mechanical barriers
- Chemical barriers
- Blood cells.

Physical barriers

Within the category of physical barriers can be placed skin and mucosal membranes.

The skin acts as a physical barrier to prevent infectious organisms and other matter from getting to the more delicate and undefended organs within our body. However, not only is it a physical barrier, it is also a chemical barrier in that sweat produced from the skin is **bactericidal** (dangerous for bacteria). However, skin also has weak spots, namely the various orifices that connect the internal body to the outside. These include the mouth, nose, urethral opening and anus.

Mechanical barriers

In this category are included cilia, coughing, sneezing and tears.

- **Cilia** are the tiny hairs found in the nose. They are constantly moving and they waft dirt, micro-organisms and mucus away to the adenoids (made of lymphatic tissue) where they can be dealt with.
- **Sneezing and coughing** work quite simply by expelling any micro-organisms or irritants out of the body and into the external atmosphere. So if someone has a cold or a cough and sneezes or coughs, millions of viruses are expelled into the atmosphere, which means that there are fewer viruses in that person's body to cause even worse problems. This is very effective for the infected person, but means that there are all these viruses in tiny droplets suspended in the air, just waiting for someone else to come along and breathe them in, thereby becoming infected themselves.
- **Tears** are also a mechanical barrier. When someone cries, the tears wash any dirt particles or micro-organisms away from their eyes (like a windscreen washer in a car). Tears are also a chemical barrier because they contain a bactericidal enzyme known as lysozyme. Lysozyme will crop up quite a lot in the section on the innate immune system.

Chemical barriers

Chemical barriers include **tears**, **breast milk**, **sweat**, **saliva**, **acidic secretions**, including **stomach acid**, and **semen**.

Most of these secretions contain either bactericidal enzymes, such as lysozyme, or antibodies. In addition, bacteria cannot survive in acidic secretions.

Blood cells

As well as the previously mentioned defences, the innate system includes certain blood cells, namely **leucocytes** (white cells) and **thrombocytes** (platelets).

The white cells involved in the innate immune system are known as

- **Neutrophils**, which make up 60% of the leucocytes in the body
- **Monocytes and tissue macrophages**, which make up a total of 3% of leucocytes
- **Eosinophils**, which only make up 1% of leucocytes
- **Basophils**, which also make up only 1% of leucocytes.

The neutrophils, eosinophils and basophils are known as **granulocytes**, because when seen through a powerful microscope these cells appear to be full of little granules (or grains). In fact these granules are vacuoles, or empty spaces, within the cells, and are very important when looking at a function of these white cells, which is known as **phagocytosis**.

Blood cells of the immune system

These are white blood cells which have been mentioned earlier in this chapter. The main activities of the white blood cells can be divided into three:

- **Phagocytosis** – this is the destruction of infectious organisms/non-self matter by engulfing them and then ingesting them. This will be explained a little later in this chapter.

- **Cytotoxity – cyto** means cell and **toxicity** means poisonous or, in immunological terms, 'lethal to'. So cytotoxicity is the action that some types of white cell take in killing infectious organisms by damaging their cell membranes (see also complement system).
- **Inflammation** – white cells are very much involved in the response of body tissue to infection and injury.

There are many other roles that white cells take within the immune system, and these will be discussed throughout this chapter, but for now we will concentrate on the three roles above.

Phagocytosis

The cells that make up the innate immunity have two major functions – they are either **phagocytes** or **mediator cells**.

The phagocytes are cells that actually devour the infectious organisms that have managed to get through the other innate immune defences mentioned above.

There are two types of phagocytes: **mononuclear phagocytes** and **polymorphonuclear phagocytes**.

Mononuclear phagocytes are another name for the monocytes and macrophages. They are called **mononuclear** because the nuclei of the cells are a single blob (or sphere) when looked at through a microscope; in other words, they have a clearly defined, single nucleus; **neutrophils**, on the other hand, make up the polymorphonuclear phagocytes.

When looked at through a microscope, the nuclei of neutrophils are seen as a blob which can take many shapes, hence **poly** (many) **morpho** (shape) **nuclearcyte** (cell nucleus) – in other words, polymorphonuclearcyte.

The role of a phagocytic cell is to **phagocytose**, or consume, any infectious organism or non-self matter that overcomes the external barriers. This process is known as **phagocytosis**, and works like this:

Figure 3.5: Phagocytosis (stage 1)

Stage 1. A bacterium approaches a phagocyte – in this case a neutrophil. It is held in place by **opsonins** such as **complement factors** or **antibodies** (**immunoglobulins**). Opsonins prepare the bacterium for being digested by the phagocyte by firmly holding the bacterium to the phagocyte so that it cannot escape.

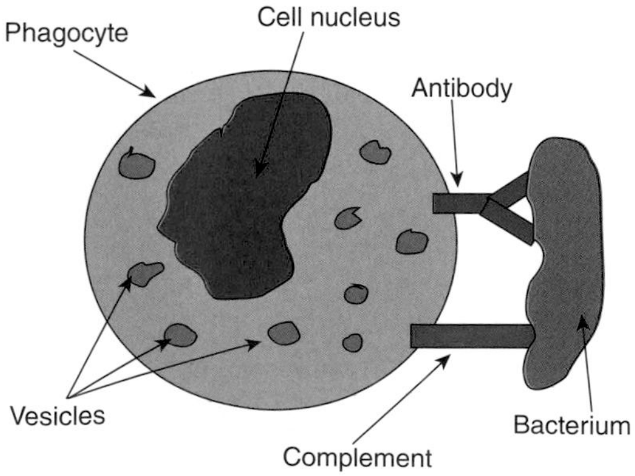
Phagocyte
Cell nucleus
Antibody
Vesicles
Complement
Bacterium

Figure 3.5 Phagocytosis (stage 1)

Figure 3.6: Phagocytosis (stage 2)

Stage 2. As the bacterium approaches the neutrophil, the neutrophil recognises that it is non-self matter and it sends out **pseudopodia** (false arms) and starts to surround the bacterium.

Stage 3. Once surrounded by the phagocyte, the bacterium comes into contact with the vacuoles (as mentioned above). A vacuole completely surrounds the bacterium and kills it, and then breaks it up by means of bactericidal enzymes such as lysozyme. The phagocyte then uses what it can from the bacterium for its own functions – growth, nutrition, etc. – and then ejects the parts that it cannot use. This is the process of phagocytosis (Figure 3.7).

As well as bacteria, phagocytes also remove pus and other infected matter, as well as any other non-self matter which has found its way into the body.

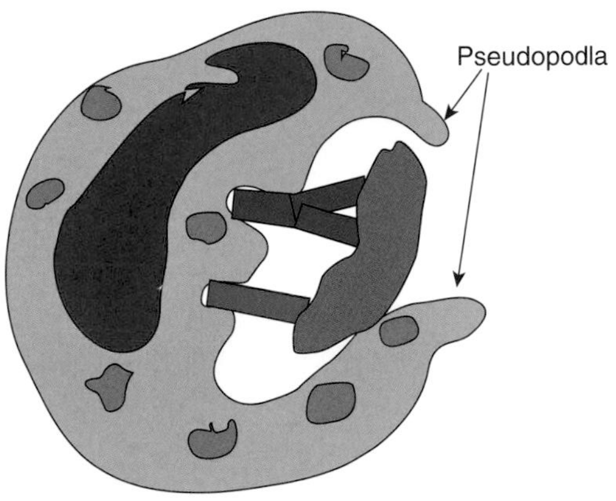
Pseudopodla

Figure 3.6 Phagocytosis (stage 2)

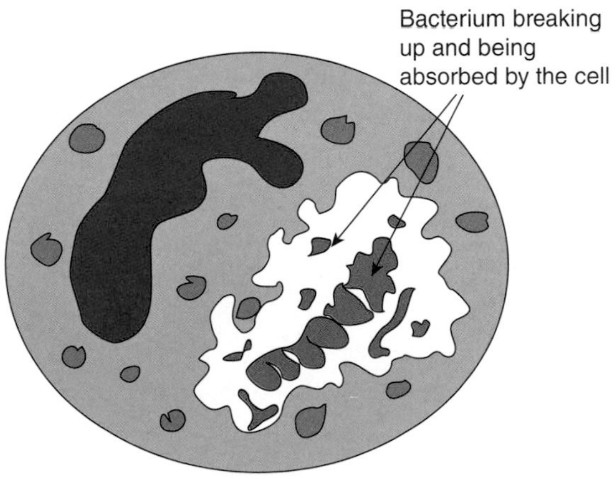
Bacterium breaking up and being absorbed by the cell

Figure 3.7 Phagocytosis (stage 3)

Cytotoxicity

Cytotoxicity is the process of damage to or death of cells. Many substances are toxic to cells, including certain chemicals, components of the immune system, viruses and bacteria, and some types of venom (e.g. from certain snakes).

With regards to the immune system, T-cells that can kill other cells are known as cytotoxic T-cells, and produce proteins that can play a role in the destruction of target cells. Cytotoxic T-cells (Tc cells) work by programming their target cells (often cells that have been infected by viruses, or even cancerous/pre-cancerous cells) to undergo apoptosis – otherwise known as cell suicide.

Inflammation

Inflammation is the body's immediate reaction to tissue injury or damage. This can be caused by:

- Physical trauma
- Intense heat
- Irritating chemicals
- Infection by viruses, fungi or bacteria (Marieb 2006).

The inflammatory process involves the movement of white cells, complement and other plasma proteins into a site of infection or injury (Roitt and Rabson 2000).

There are four **cardinal signs and symptoms of inflammation**:

- Swelling (also known as oedema)
- Pain
- Heat
- Redness

at the site of the injury. There may also have been:

- Nausea
- Sweating
- Raised pulse
- Lowered blood pressure
- Possibly loss of consciousness.

These last symptoms and signs are the body's response to pain and shock, but in terms of immunology, the first four signs and symptoms are the important ones, and that is why they are known as the four cardinal signs of inflammation.

Although inflammation does cause pain and other problems, it actually has beneficial properties and effects. These are:

- The prevention of the spread to nearby tissues of infectious micro-organisms and other damaging agents
- The disposal of killed pathogens and cell debris
- Preparation for repair of the damage (Marieb 2006).

According to Nairn and Helbert (2007), inflammation can be defined clinically as the presence of swelling, redness and pain.

Following injury or other damage to the body, three processes occur at the same time:

- **Mast cell degranulation**. Mast cells are tissue cells which contain granules in their cytoplasm. These granules contain, amongst other substances, **serotonin** and **histamine** which, during the process of degranulation, are released into the tissues. These substances cause some of the signs and symptoms of inflammation, but they also work with the other two processes to provide the complete inflammatory signs and symptoms.
- **The activation of four plasma protein systems**. These systems are: the complement system, the clotting system, the kinin system and immunoglobulins. The complement system consists of more than 30 proteins, which are found in blood plasma and on cell surfaces and it works very closely with antibodies, and indeed is so called because the proteins in the system are seen to 'complement' antibodies in the destruction of bacteria (Walport 2001). The complement system activates and assists the inflammatory and immune processes, and plays a major role in the destruction of bacteria. The clotting system traps bacteria that have entered the wound and also interacts with platelets to stop any bleeding. The kinin system helps to control vascular permeability, whilst immunoglobulins help in the destruction of bacteria.
- **The movement of phagocytic cells** to the area in order to phagocytose bacteria or any other non-self debris in the wound (Figure 3.8).

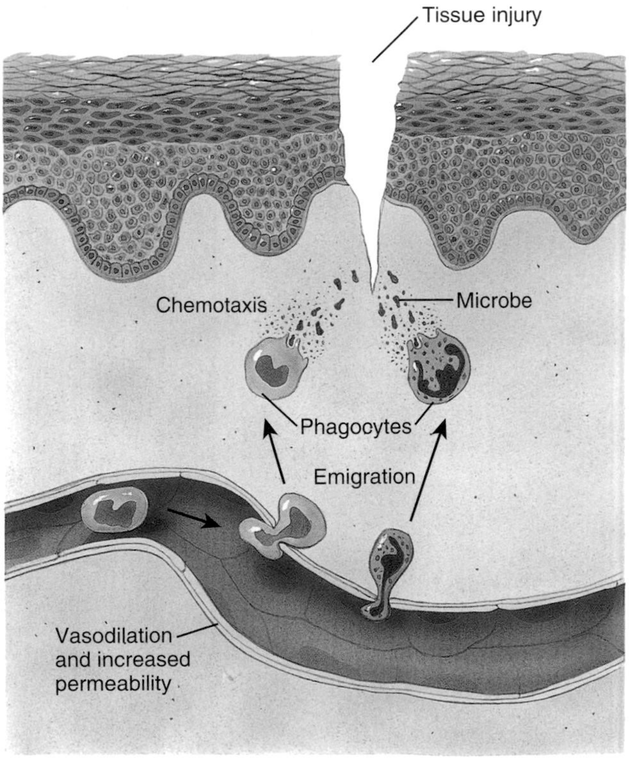
Tissue injury
Chemotaxis
Microbe
Phagocytes
Emigration
Vasodilation and increased permeability

Figure 3.8 Phagocytes migrate from blood to the site of tissue injury (Tortora and Derrickson 2009)

Complement factors stimulate the mast cells to release histamine and other chemicals, which in turn can increase the permeability of blood vessels (Tortora *et al.* 2004).

Other factors involved in vascular permeability are: **cytokines** (cell messengers), which promote inflammation and also attract white blood cells to the affected area (Marieb 2006); **kinins** and **prostaglandins**, which are also chemical messengers which are released from damaged and stressed tissue cells, phagocytes and lymphocytes.

All these factors – histamine, complement, cytokines and kinins – as well as having their own specific individual inflammatory roles, cause the small blood vessels in the area that has been damaged to dilate so that more blood is able to flow into the region surrounding the damaged area. This causes the redness and heat associated with inflammation (Marieb 2006).

These chemicals also increase the permeability of the capillary walls, which allows blood cells and protein-rich fluid to seep into the surrounding tissues, which leads to **oedema** – the third of the classic signs of inflammation. This performs three functions that are important to the healing of damaged tissue, namely:

- The dilution of harmful substances in the area to make them less concentrated
- The movement into the area of large quantities of oxygen as well as the nutrients necessary for the repair of any damage
- The entry of clotting proteins to help seal off the damage (Marieb 2006).

That leaves **pain** as the remaining classic sign of inflammation. Pain is caused partly by the pressure on the nerve endings as a result of the oedema in the tissues and partly by the release of bacterial toxins (Marieb 2006).

So to sum up inflammation:

The timetable of a typical inflammatory response to tissue in injury is:

- Arterioles near the injury site constrict briefly.
- This vasoconstriction is followed by vasodilation which increases blood flow to the site of the injury (redness and heat).
- Dilation of the arterioles at the injury site increases the pressure in the circulation.
- This increases the exudation of both plasma proteins and blood cells into the tissues in the area.
- Exudation then causes oedema and **swelling**.
- The nerve endings in the area are stimulated, partly by pressure **(pain)**.
- The clotting and kinin systems, along with platelets, move into the area and block any tissue damage by commencing the clotting process.
- White blood cells – phagocytes and lymphocytes – move into the area and start to destroy any infectious organisms in the vicinity of the trauma.
- These phagocytes and protein cells, along with the substances they produce, kill any bacteria or other micro-organisms in the vicinity, and remove the debris which results from the battle between the micro-organisms and the immune system – this includes exudates and dead cells (pus).
- All these parts of the immune and blood systems remain in the area until tissue regeneration (repair) takes place – this is known as resolution.

The acquired immune system

Acquired immunity is the immunity that we acquire as we go through life – the acquired immune system is barely functioning when we are born. Another name for the acquired immune system is the specific immune system because it is aimed at specific infectious organisms. It is very much based upon the white blood cells known as lymphocytes.

There are two types of acquired immunity: cell-mediated immunity and humoral immunity.

Cell-mediated immunity (T-cell lymphocytes)

This type of immunity is known as cell-mediated immunity because the cells themselves destroy any invading antigens.

T-cell lymphocytes originate in the bone marrow, but they do not remain there. At a certain stage in their development they leave the bone marrow as immature lymphocytes. These immature lymphocytes find their way to the thymus where they develop. In addition, they learn to recognise our own cells and so do not destroy them, only invading cells, e.g. bacteria and viruses (see Figure 3.11). The thymus is situated in the chest, and in babies it is a large organ (relative to size), but atrophies (shrinks) with age.

T-cell lymphocytes have different functions to perform within the acquired immune system, and the functions that they perform are dependent upon the differentiation they undergo within the thymus (Figure 3.9). Different types of T-cells carry different receptors on their surfaces, and these are known as clusters of definition (CDs) – so called because the way in which these receptors are organised on the cell surface defines their role and function.

There are four classes of T-lymphocyte cells:

- T-cytotoxic lymphocytes
- T-helper lymphocytes
- T-suppressor lymphocytes
- T-memory lymphocytes.

The major functions performed by the T-cell lymphocytes are:

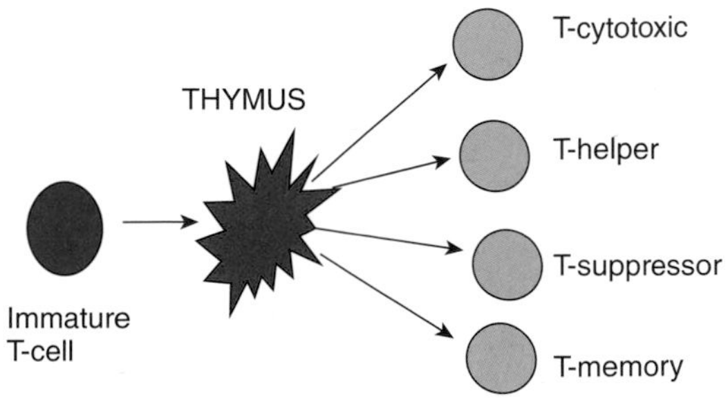
T-cytotoxic
THYMUS
T-helper
T-suppressor
Immature
T-cell
T-memory

Figure 3.9 Development and types of T-lymphocytes

Cytotoxicity (cell destruction)

This function is performed by the T-cytotoxic lymphocytes that possess CD8 glycoprotein on their membrane. These cells mediate the direct cellular killing of target cells (Rote and Crippes Trask 2006). The target cells may be virally infected cells, tumours or 'non-self' grafts, such as kidney transplants.

The T-cytotoxic lymphocytes bind to the target cell and release toxic substances into the target cell, which are capable of destroying it. If the target cell is a virally infected cell, that cell is destroyed, as are the viruses that have infected it. In this way the viruses are unable to go on to invade other cells.

Control of the immune system

This is a task undertaken by the T-helper and T-suppressor lymphocytes.

T-helper cells are coated with CD4 proteins and they stimulate the immune system – both the acquired immune system and many parts of the innate immune system – to proliferate in response to infectious organisms (or other antigens) present in the body. There are two types of T-helper cell: type 1 T-helper cells and type 2 T-helper cells.

The body is usually very efficient at stimulating immune activity in response to an invasion by antigens, but there is a need for balances and checks to prevent the overstimulation of immunological activity, and this function is performed by the T-suppressor cells.

Many studies have identified T-suppressor cells, but there appears to be no unique receptor marker for T-suppressor cells, and so immune suppression may actually be a task performed by a combination of T-helper and T-cytotoxic cells by means of a negative feedback mechanism (Male 2006).

Memory

A special quality that the acquired immune system possesses is the ability to remember antigen receptors which have been previously detected by the immune system, and so produce a group of lymphocytes which can stimulate the parts of the immune system that are able to counter these antigens immediately if that antigen is detected in future infections. T-memory lymphocytes are responsible for a rapid response to further attacks by specific infectious micro-organisms (Rote and Crippes Trask 2006). This process is known as the secondary immune response and will be explained towards the end of this chapter (Figure 3.10 and Figure 3.11).

Memory cells are long-lived and also, regardless of cell division, there is always a constant number of T-memory cells for a given antigen in circulation (Janeway *et al.* 2005).

Humoral immunity (B-cell lymphocytes)

This second type of acquired immunity is known as humoral immunity because the components effective in the immune system are soluble in fluids (and so is called humoral immunity from the old English term 'humours').

B-cell lymphocytes originate in the bone marrow where they also mature.

As with the T-cell lymphocytes, the B-cells need to undergo a maturation process in which they have to survive a negative selection process. This is an attempt to ensure that the antigen receptors on their surface membrane do not display self-reactivity (i.e. do not react against our own cells) (Nairn and Helbert 2007).

During this process, those B-cell lymphocytes that are auto-reactive to the host cells and tissues are destroyed, leaving only non-auto-reactive naïve lymphocytes behind which will then be able

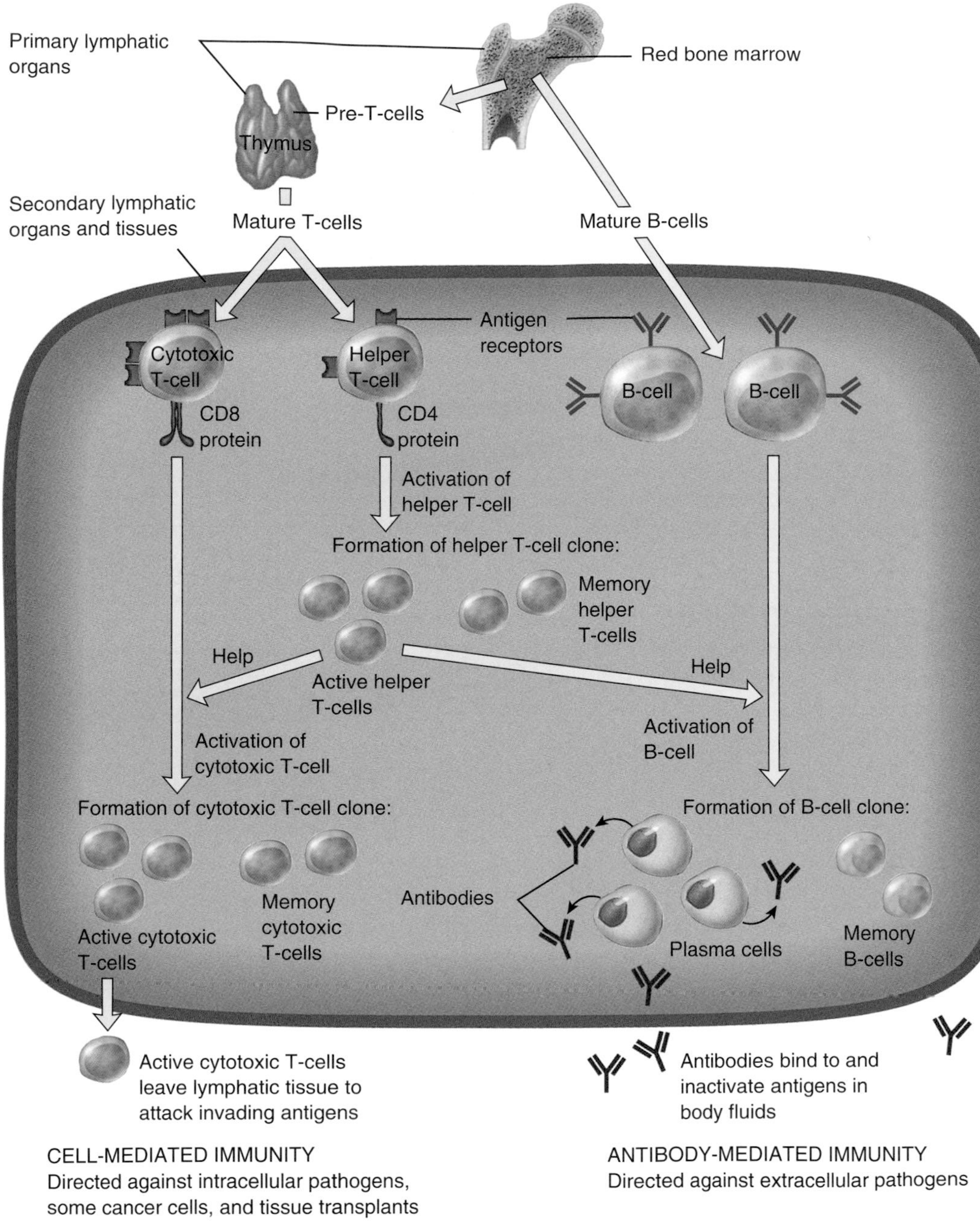

Primary lymphatic organs
Red bone marrow
Pre-T-cells
Thymus
Secondary lymphatic organs and tissues
Mature T-cells
Mature B-cells
Antigen receptors
Cytotoxic T-cell
Helper T-cell
B-cell
B-cell
CD8 protein
CD4 protein
Activation of helper T-cell
Formation of helper T-cell clone:
Memory helper T-cells
Help
Active helper T-cells
Help
Activation of B-cell
Activation of cytotoxic T-cell
Formation of cytotoxic T-cell clone:
Formation of B-cell clone:
Antibodies
Memory cytotoxic T-cells
Active cytotoxic T-cells
Plasma cells
Memory B-cells
Active cytotoxic T-cells leave lymphatic tissue to attack invading antigens
Antibodies bind to and inactivate antigens in body fluids
CELL-MEDIATED IMMUNITY
Directed against intracellular pathogens, some cancer cells, and tissue transplants
ANTIBODY-MEDIATED IMMUNITY
Directed against extracellular pathogens

Figure 3.10 Cellular and humoral immune responses (Tortora and Derrickson 2009)

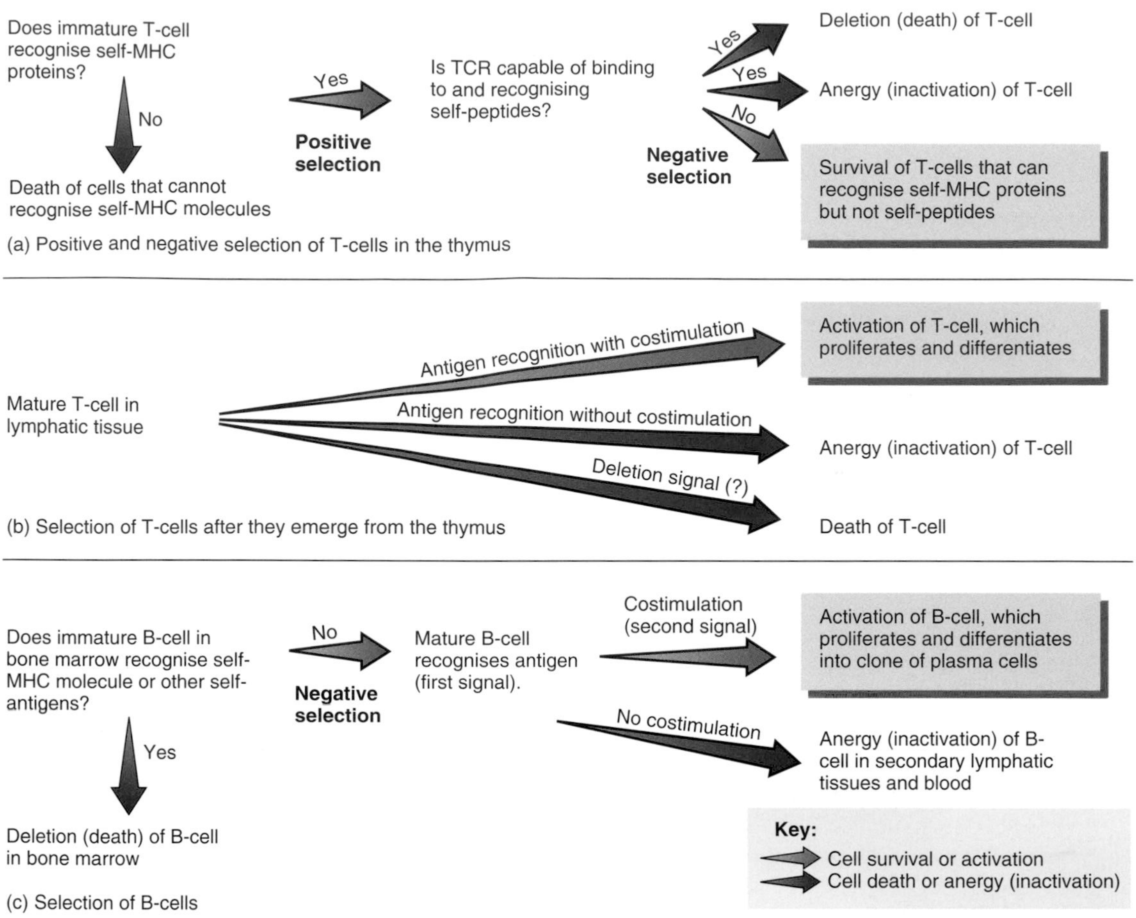
Does immature T-cell recognise self-MHC proteins?
No
Death of cells that cannot recognise self-MHC molecules
Yes
Positive selection
Is TCR capable of binding to and recognising self-peptides?
Yes
Yes
No
Negative selection
Deletion (death) of T-cell
Anergy (inactivation) of T-cell
Survival of T-cells that can recognise self-MHC proteins but not self-peptides
(a) Positive and negative selection of T-cells in the thymus
Mature T-cell in lymphatic tissue
Antigen recognition with costimulation
Antigen recognition without costimulation
Deletion signal (?)
Activation of T-cell, which proliferates and differentiates
Anergy (inactivation) of T-cell
Death of T-cell
(b) Selection of T-cells after they emerge from the thymus
Does immature B-cell in bone marrow recognise self-MHC molecule or other self-antigens?
Yes
Deletion (death) of B-cell in bone marrow
No
Negative selection
Mature B-cell recognises antigen (first signal).
Costimulation (second signal)
No costimulation
Activation of B-cell, which proliferates and differentiates into clone of plasma cells
Anergy (inactivation) of B-cell in secondary lymphatic tissues and blood
Key:
Cell survival or activation
Cell death or anergy (inactivation)
(c) Selection of B-cells

Figure 3.11 Process of teaching T-cells and B-cells to recognise pathogens (infectious organisms) (Tortora and Derrickson 2009)

to go on to the next stage of maturation and selection (Figure 3.10). This is a very important process because if there should be any self-reactivity of the B-cells, as with T-cell self-reactivity, then autoimmunity may be the result.

The actual mechanism of the B-cell negative selection process within the bone marrow is similar to that process which is undergone by T-cells during their maturation and differentiation within the thymus (Figure 3.11). However, in addition, B-cells undergo a positive selection process in which those lymphocytes that are able to respond to non-self antigens are preserved, whilst those that are not are left to die. The B-cells that have survived this negative selection find their way to the peripheral lymphoid organs where they may encounter actual non-self antigens for which they have specificity. It is thought that more than 10^8 (100,000,000) different antigens may be recognised by the B-cell lymphocytes.

Mature B-cells are of two types: B-memory cells (with a similar role to play as the T-memory cells) and antibody-secreting plasma cells.

Immunoglobulins (antibodies)

The antibodies secreted by the plasma cells are also known as **immunoglobulins** (Igs), and their role is to act as mediators in the destruction of non-self antigens. These immunoglobulins are not responsible for the actual killing. Instead, they assist other components of the immune system in destroying non-self antigens.

There are five classes of immunoglobulin, which are known as:

- IgG
- IgA
- IgM
- IgE
- IgD.

Types of immunoglobulins

Immunoglobulin G

This is the most important class of immunoglobulin involved in the secondary immune response. It makes up about 75% of total serum immunoglobulin (Seymour *et al.* 1995), and it divides into four subclasses, namely IgG1, IgG2, IgG3 and IgG4.

Because it has a low molecular weight, IgG is found within both the intravascular and extravascular areas of the body. This means that it can reach all parts of the body, and therefore its effects are far reaching. In particular, it plays a major role against blood-borne infective organisms as well as those invading the tissues.

The low molecular weight also means that IgG can cross the placental barrier to give a high degree of temporary passive immunity to the newborn child. This is important because although maternal IgG disappears by the age of 9 months, by then hopefully, the infant is producing its own IgG.

IgG helps the immune system in several ways

- It is important for activating the complement system
- It can bind to macrophages and so enhance phagocytosis
- It binds to the T cytotoxic cells and helps them in destroying infected cells
- It binds to platelets and helps with the inflammatory response.

(Seymour *et al.* 1995; Vickers 2005; Nairn and Helbert 2007; Roitt 2007)

Immunoglobulin A

There are two types of IgA: 'serum' and 'secretory'. Serum IgA has similar roles to IgG.

Secretory IgA is most important because it is the major immunoglobulin found in external body secretions, such as saliva, breast milk, colostrum, tears, nasal secretions, sweat and the secretions of the respiratory tract and gastrointestinal tract.

Secretory IgA has a molecule of a secretory component, which allows for the easy transfer of secretory IgA across the epithelial cells into various bodily secretions. It also helps to protect the IgA from the proteolytic (destruction of protein) attack mounted by enzymes which are themselves secreted by bacteria.

The main function of secretory IgA (sIgA) is to prevent antigens crossing the epithelium. In addition, sIgA can activate the complement system.

Secretory IgA plays an important role in the protection of the host's body against respiratory, urinary and bowel infections. Also, because it is present is such large quantities in colostrum and breast milk, it performs a vital role in the prevention of neonatal gut infections – this is one of the reasons why breast-feeding is so heavily promoted (Seymour *et al.* 1995; Vickers 2005; Nairn and Helbert 2007; Roitt 2007).

Immunoglobulin M

IgM is the predominant antibody involved in the primary immune response (see below), as well as being involved in the early stages of the secondary immune response.

It is very effective at activating the classic pathway of the complement system.

Because of its large size, IgM is restricted almost entirely to the intravascular (within blood vessels) spaces, and it is also often involved with any response by the immune system to complex, blood-borne infectious micro-organisms (Seymour *et al.* 1995; Vickers 2005; Nairn and Helbert 2007; Roitt 2007).

Immunoglobulin E

IgE is found only sparingly in the body – in normal circumstances it makes up less than 0.01% of the total serum immunoglobulins, but is also found on the surfaces of mast cells and basophils. It has a very high avidity (binding potential) to tissue mast cells and circulatory basophils, and it is the binding of IgE to receptors on these cells in the presence of antigen that can trigger an allergic reaction.

This allergic reaction consists of the:

- Activation of the mast cell
- Degranulation of the cell
- Release of mediators such as histamine.

Degranulation of the mast cell and release of histamine helps to cause an acute inflammatory response, which leads to the classic signs of allergic reactions such as those seen in hay fever and asthma. Immunoglobulin E is also responsible for sensitising cells on mucosal surfaces, such as the conjunctival, nasal and bronchial mucosa. This gives rise to other symptoms of an allergy, including rhinitis and conjunctivitis.

Immunoglobulin D

The first thing to say is that little is known about the functions of IgD. However, we do know that it is chiefly found on B-cell surface membranes and that it acts as a receptor molecule, but work is ongoing in trying to decipher and understand this particular immunoglobulin.

Role of immunoglobulins

According to Roitt (2007), the primary function of an antibody is to bind antigen by attaching to **epitopes** (or receptors) on the surface of the antigen (Figures 3.12 and 3.13), thus the main functions of antibodies are to protect the host by:

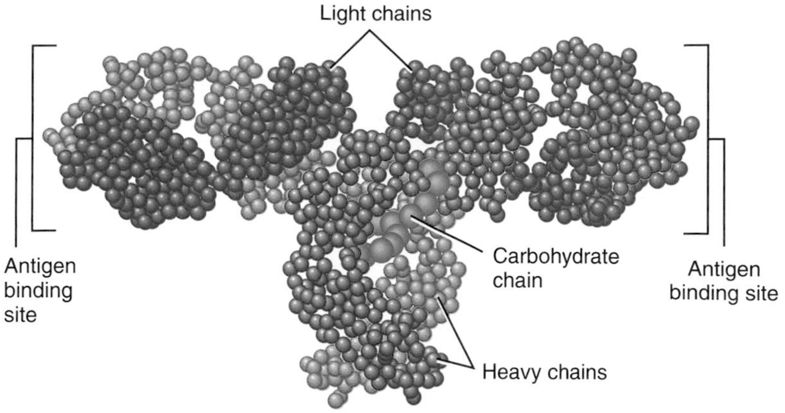
Light chains
Antigen binding site
Carbohydrate chain
Antigen binding site
Heavy chains

Figure 3.12 Model of an antibody (IgG) (Tortora and Derrickson 2009)

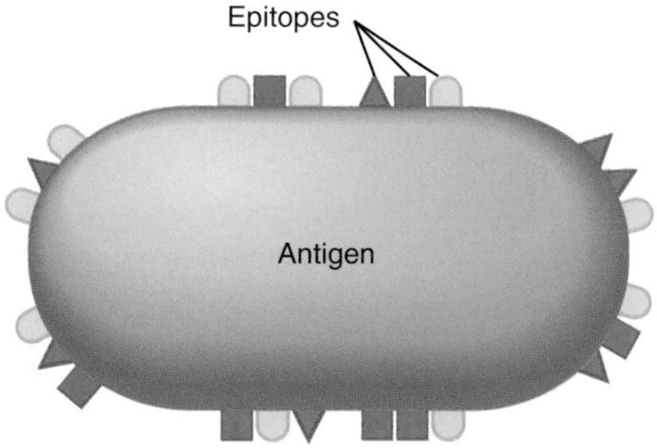
Epitopes
Antigen

Figure 3.13 Model of an antigen showing the epitopes (receptors) (Tortora and Derrickson 2009)

- Neutralising bacterial toxins
- Neutralising viruses
- Opsonising bacteria – opsonins are molecules that bind to non-self matter and to receptors on phagocytes, in this way acting as a bridge between the two and holding the non-self matter bound to the phagocytes (Male 2006)
- Activating components of the inflammatory response.

(Rote and Crippes Trask 2006)

Antibodies rarely act in isolation. Instead, they join with other components of the immune system to destroy the infecting organisms.

A second role of the immunoglobulin is the neutralisation of bacterial toxins. These toxins are produced by the bacteria and make them more pathogenic (harmful), thus causing more harm to the host. When this happens, the immunoglobulins function as antitoxins.

Similarly, the immunoglobulins neutralise viruses by binding to the viral surface receptors, so preventing them from binding to the host's cells, allowing the viruses then to be phagocytosed and so preventing the viruses from infecting cells of the body.

Immunoglobulins also activate components of the inflammatory response.

Natural killer cells

There is a further type of lymphocyte, which appears to express only the earliest markers of T-cell differentiation. These are known as **null cells** or **NK (natural killer) cells**. The NK cells do not bind antigen, nor are they induced to proliferate by contact with an antigen. Rather, they bind to chemical changes on the surfaces of virally infected cells or malignant cells, rather than antigen receptors (Rote and Crippes Trask 2006).

Although they are lymphocytes, these cells are usually classified within the innate immune system.

Primary and secondary response to infection

Finally, we will examine the immune system's response to infections. The one thing that really marks out the acquired immune system as special is its ability to 'remember' previous encounters with an antigen. Without this ability, each time an individual came into contact with a particular antigen, there would be a risk of a serious, possibly fatal, illness. This immune memory is crucial because it allows the body to mount an immediate immune response to an antigen, without waiting for the immune system to work out a way of destroying that antigen each time it infects us.

How does the immune system gain this memory of a specific antigen? There are two immune responses – the primary and secondary responses. The primary response occurs when the immune system first comes into contact with a new antigen (infectious organism), and the secondary response occurs with all subsequent encounters with that same antigen.

Primary immune response

Clinical considerations

Rheumatoid disease

Rheumatoid disease is caused by an autoimmune reaction (the body's immune system attacking the body's own cells). It is one of the commonest chronic inflammatory conditions in developed countries. Some inflammatory cytokines have a major role to play in the pathogenesis of this disease. Rheumatoid arthritis is a common cause of disability, with one-third of patients likely to be severely disabled. The joint changes, which almost certainly represent an autoimmune reaction, consist of:

- Inflammation
- Erosion of cartilage and bone.

Autoimmune diseases

Specific examples of autoimmune diseases include such diverse conditions as rheumatoid arthritis, type 1 diabetes mellitus, multiple sclerosis and systemic lupus erythromatosus (lupus).

Autoimmune diseases affect 3% of the Western population, and are found to be more common in people living in the more northerly latitudes. Almost all autoimmune diseases are more common in women and they are rare in childhood, with the onset usually occurring between puberty and retirement. In addition, there tend to be clusters in families – not necessarily of the same disease but of a tendency to an autoimmune disease.

Drug treatment

The drugs most frequently used in rheumatoid disease are disease-modifying anti-rheumatoid drugs (DMARDS) as well as non-steroidal anti-inflammatory drugs (NSAIDS). These drugs reduce the symptoms of rheumatoid disease, but do not prevent the progress of the disease. Other drugs that are used with this disease include:

- Some immunosuppressants (drugs that suppress the immune system to try to prevent it attacking the body's own cells)
- Steroids
- Anticytokine drugs – these are newer drugs and they have more specific action against the disease processes of rheumatoid disease.

Included within the category of DMARDs is a variety of drugs with different chemical structures and mechanisms of action. They can improve symptoms and reduce disease activity in rheumatoid arthritis. This can be measured by a reduction in:

- The number of swollen and tender joints
- The pain score
- The disability score.

There are, however, doubts as to whether or not they halt the long-term progress of the disease.

With the primary immune response, there is always a long time period before a response can be made. This is known as the 'lag' phase because the response lags some way behind the encounter with the antigen (Figure 3.14). During this time there are no detectable antibodies produced by the mature B-cell lymphocytes, but the immune system is working out how to destroy the antigen.

In the case of the primary immune response, the lag phase can take anything from 5 to 10 days before there has been sufficient production of antibodies to make a difference. During this period, the host can become very sick and may even die!

The major immunoglobulin class produced at this stage is IgM, and only small amounts of IgG are produced but hopefully enough to destroy the antigen.

At the same time as the antigen is being destroyed, the memory cells are retaining a memory of this specific antigen and how to defeat it, and this memory will stay with the host for a long time. Each time the host is infected by that same antigen, the memory cells are reinforced.

Clinical considerations

Hand washing

Hand washing is the single most important measure in preventing cross-infection. The technique employed involves thoroughly cleaning, rinsing and drying both hands. Hand are the principal route by which cross-infection occurs.

There have been many concerted efforts to enforce stricter hand washing policies in all health and social care settings; effective hand washing remains an essential public health initiative. Hand washing is an essential aspect of any caregivers repertoire of skills and these skills must be mastered in order to provide all people with a safe environment. Those people with immunological deficiencies are at particular at risk of infection and as such attention to scrupulous hand washing techniques must be carried out at all times.

All healthcare providers should strive to make hand washing an automatic behaviour that is performed by all in homes, schools and other environments. Families and carers who come into contact will those people with an immunological deficiency must adhere to effective hand washing. The key aim of effective hand washing is to prevent the spread of micro-organisms between people or between other living things and people. Inanimate objects and surfaces such as contaminated cutlery or clinical equipment may put the health and wellbeing of an immunologically compromised person at risk.

Using the correct hand washing technique not only saves lives but can also save money. Poor hand washing practices can lead to urinary tract infections, bloodstream infections, respiratory infections and infection of incisional wounds. These infections are caused by the transfer of micro-organisms from staff and families to vulnerable people, which could be prevented by using the correct hand washing procedures.

In all healthcare environments hand washing is mandatory and must be carried out using established policies and procedures. There are a number of practices associated with hand hygiene – for example, using alcohol hand rubs and the act of physically washing the hands. The consequences of failing to use the correct procedure are many; the impact this can have on the health and wellbeing of the person you are caring for can be devastating.

Secondary immune response

If, at a later date, the same antigen infects the body again, because of the memory T-cell lymphocytes, the body is capable of mounting a secondary immune response which is much quicker. Because the memory cells are carrying their memory of this antigen, production of antibodies can take place very quickly, so that there is a very short lag phase.

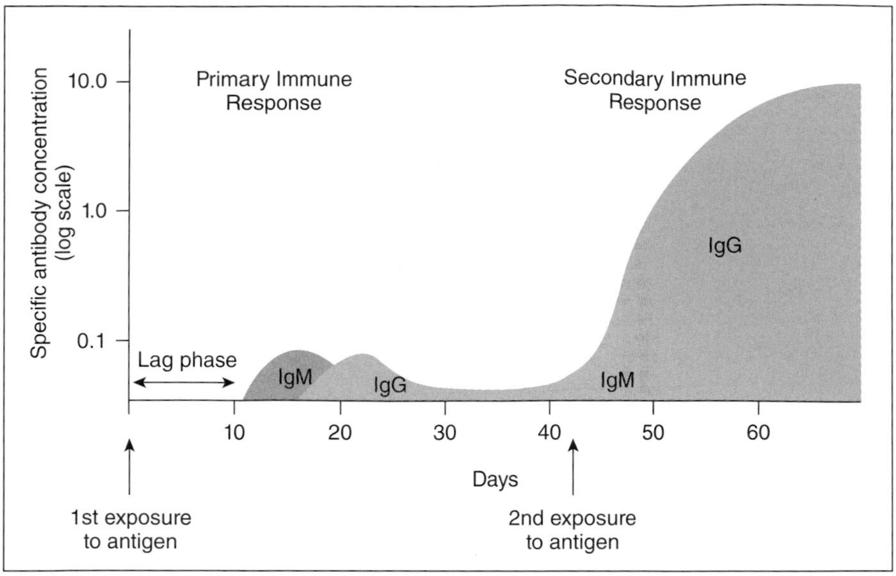

Specific antibody concentration (log scale)
10.0
1.0
0.1
Primary Immune Response
Secondary Immune Response
Lag phase
IgM
IgG
IgM
IgG
10
20
30
40
50
60
Days
1st exposure to antigen
2nd exposure to antigen

Figure 3.14 Responses to infection

In a secondary immune response, the major antibody class produced is IgG, although occasionally IgA or IgE may be produced depending upon the nature of the antigen and its route of entry (Nairn and Helbert 2007). IgG is produced in huge quantities very quickly, and therefore the response is very rapid and effective – often the antigen is destroyed before any signs and symptoms appear.

Immunisations

Immunisation, or vaccination, is either the process of transferring antibodies to an individual who is lacking them (passive immunisation) or the process of inducing an immune reaction in an individual (active immunisation). Immunisations induce the primary response by exposing the immune system to a vaccine that includes an infectious organism which is either inactivated (killed) or attenuated (weakened) so that it is no longer infectious, but still possesses the receptors that can stimulate the immune system.

Passive immunisation

In passive immunisation, the individual is actually injected with the antibodies. There are two types of passive immunisation which are natural and very common:

- The mother transfers IgG antibodies across the placenta to the foetus. Whatever organisms the mother is immune to, the newborn baby will also be immune to them.
- During breastfeeding, when the mother passes IgA antibodies to the baby in her colostrum and milk.

Passive immunisation is also short lived and lasts only as long as it takes for these antibodies to be cleared from the body. This type of immunisation will not normally provoke an immune response in the recipient, and therefore there will be no immunological cover for subsequent exposure to that particular antigen.

Active immunity

Active immunity is the process of presenting antigen to the immune system to induce an immune response to it. This is the type of immunity that takes advantage of the primary and secondary responses to immunity and is the basis for all the immunisations/vaccinations that we have throughout our lives.

A vaccine has to be able to stimulate both T- and B-cell lymphocytes to provide an immune response. If a vaccine is effective, it provides common immunity to a population.

Clinical considerations

Secondary immunodeficiencies

Secondary immunodeficiencies are those disorders that, due to another illness, age, injury, environmental poisons or treatment result in an increased susceptibility to infection. Indeed, almost all serious illnesses are associated with some impairment of one or more components of the immune system.

Most people are aware of one particular secondary immunodeficiency, namely acquired immunodeficiency syndrome (AIDS) caused by the human immunodeficiency virus (HIV), but there are many other causes of secondary immunodeficiencies.

One of the major causes of immunodeficiency globally is protein deficiency due to malnutrition or to such disorders as Kwashiorkor disease. In developed countries, apart from HIV, the major causes of secondary immunodeficiencies are iatrogenic, i.e. caused by medical personnel/treatment. These particularly include immunodeficiencies that occur following steroid or cytotoxic drug therapy for various diseases.

Someone with a secondary immunodeficiency will have a susceptibility to opportunistic infections, anorexia, diarrhoea and an increased risk of cancer.

Secondary immunodeficiencies are associated with a multitude of factors, of which we only have time to look at a very few, including:

- Infections, including HIV, hepatitis, measles, mumps, TB, congenital rubella, cytomegalovirus (CMV) and infectious mononucleosis (glandular fever)
- Medications, including steroids, cytotoxic drugs and immunosuppressive drugs, and even antibiotics, as well as so-called recreational drugs, such as alcohol, cocaine and heroin

- Stress, including psychological and physical stress
- Malnutrition
- Cancers
- Autoimmune diseases
- Ageing
- Environmental chemicals, such as polychlorinated biphenyls (PBCs) and dioxin
- Burns and other traumas
- Pregnancy
- Anaesthesia and surgery (stress)
- Radiation.

The treatment of secondary immunodeficiencies consists of removing or treating the cause (if at all possible) and supportive therapy. For example, if an infection is the cause, then the relevant antimicrobial drugs need to be given. If there is an iatrogenic cause such as drugs or surgery, once these are stopped and recovery is underway, the immune system will usually right itself. Similarly, if other diseases are causing the immunodeficiency, then they have to be tackled. If malnutrition is the cause, then the solving of the problem leading to malnutrition needs to take place.

Along with the elimination of the cause, supportive therapy is required to help to boost the immune system and to prevent infections. Drugs and nutrition, changes of lifestyle, occasionally isolation, may be necessary.

Secondary immunodeficiencies are often transient, and supportive therapy is usually only necessary until the cause has been dealt with and the immune system starts to recover. Unfortunately, however, there are some secondary immunodeficiencies to which this does not apply. The best known of these is AIDS, although if a cure were ever found for it, then it in turn would become a transient immunodeficiency.

Conclusion

This completes the chapter on the immune system. As you have learned, it is a very complex system with each of the many components interacting with others to provide us with the protection that we need to survive in this very dangerous world. But, above all, hopefully you will be amazed and awe-struck at its ability to fulfil its major role – that of keeping us safe from infections and other potential harm that could befall us.

What you must remember is that immunology is a dynamic subject. Research in the specialty is continually bringing us new knowledge, not only of the anatomy and physiology of the immune system, but also of disorders affected by it and of new therapies.

There is now so much progress being made in immunology that it is impossible to predict the future. But then, this is what makes immunology such an exciting specialty with which to be involved.

Glossary

Acquired immunity:	Immunity that is acquired throughout life by coming into contact with many different infectious agents.
Active immunity:	Immunity developed inside the body as a result of encountering infectious agents.
Antibodies:	Also known as **immunoglobulins**, antibodies can recognise and attach to infectious agents and so provoke an immune response to these infectious agents. They are also **opsonins**.
Antigens:	Anything that provokes an antibody response.
Atopy:	A type of hypersensitivity that is linked to **immunoglobulin** E.
Bactericidal:	The ability to kill bacteria.
Basophils:	White blood cells which take part in the process of phagocytosis. Also involved in allergic/atopic reactions.
B-cell lymphocytes:	Blood cells from which antibodies (immunoglobulins) develop. Part of the humoral immune system.
Cell-mediated immunity:	The type of acquired immunity generated by the T-cell **lymphocytes**.
Complement factors:	A group of proteins that are involved in many of the immune processes, e.g. phagocytosis and inflammation. They are also **opsonins**.
Clotting system:	The clotting of blood to reduce blood loss. Also involving **thrombocytes** (platelets). See Chapter 12, The circulatory system.
Cytokines:	Chemical messengers that affect the behaviour of other cells, including cells of the immune system.
Cytotoxicity:	The process by which infectious micro-organisms are killed or damaged (cyto = cell; toxicity = dangerous to).
Eosinophils:	White blood cells involved in the destruction of parasitic worms, but also linked to hypersensitivity.
Epitopes:	The parts of a cell that can bind to other cells (i.e. cell receptors).
Granulocytes:	White blood cells which take part in the process of phagocytosis.
Humoral immunity:	Another name for antibody immunity. This is the part of the **acquired immune** system that relies upon antibodies to help in the destruction of infectious agents.

Hypersensitivity: A heightened immune response that can cause allergies and atopic diseases.

Immunisation: The process of either transferring antibodies to someone (i.e. passive immunisation) or inducing an immune reaction naturally but safely (i.e. active immunity).

Immunity: The body's response to infection, damage or other diseases.

Immunoglobulins: Also known as antibodies.

Inflammation: The body's immediate reaction to tissue injury or damage.

Innate immunity: The immunity with which we are born.

Kinins: A specialist group of plasma proteins (i.e. proteins that circulate within blood plasma) and have a role to play in the process of inflammation.

Kinin system: The system in which kinins operate in order to activate and help inflammatory cells, such as neutrophils, to function properly as well as being involved in making the blood vessels more permeable to allow cells of the immune system to get to the area of inflammation or damage.

Leucocyte: Another term for a white blood cell (leuco = white, cyte = cell).

Lymph: A colourless liquid derived from blood.

Lymphatic system: This shadows the blood system, but is vey much involved in immunity and consists of lymph vessels that contain **lymph** which transports antigens and antibodies, and also lymph nodes and other lymphatic tissues, such as the tonsils and the spleen.

Lymph nodes: Nodules within the lymphatic system which contain mesh traps which are able to trap antigens in order for them to be destroyed by antibodies and other components of the immune system.

Lymphocyte: The major white blood cell of the acquired immune system.

Lymph vessels: These are similar to blood vessels, but they carry lymph, antigens (e.g. bacteria), antibodies and other components of the immune system, from the site of infection towards **lymph nodes**.

Macrophage: Also known as a tissue macrophage, it is white blood cell which takes part in the process of phagocytosis within the tissues as opposed to within the blood circulation.

Mast cells: Cells of connective tissue that are involved in the activation of the inflammatory response (inflammation).

Medulla: The central part of an organ.

Monocyte: A type of phagocytic white blood cell (known as a tissue macrophage once it migrates into the tissues).

Neutrophils: White blood cells which take part in the process of phagocytosis.

NK cells: Natural killer cells are a class of lymphocytes that are not specific to certain infectious agents and so are often classed with innate immunity as opposed to acquired immunity.

Null cells: Another name for the NK cells.

Oedema: A scientific term for swelling.

Opsonins: Substances that bind antigens to phagocytic cells, and so enhance the process of phagocytosis, e.g. complement factors and antibodies.

Passive immunity: The process of transferring **antibodies** to someone who is vulnerable to infections and cannot make their own active immunity.

Phagocyte: White blood cells that are able to ingest and destroy infectious micro-organisms and other non-self matter, and include, amongst others, neutrophils and macrophages.

Phagocytosis: The ingestion and destruction of infectious micro-organisms and other non-self matter by specialised cells (phagocytes).

Plasma cells: Cells that develop from B-cell **lymphocytes** and that produce antibodies.

Platelet: See thrombocyte.

Primary response: The immune response that occurs when we first come into contact with a new infectious agent.

Prostaglandins: Fatty acids that function as part of the inflammatory process (inflammation).

Pseudopodia: (literal meaning = 'false arms'). These are finger-like projections that emerge from cells and, within immunity, they are very important in the process of phagocytosis.

Secondary response: The immune response that, following a successful primary immune response to a specific infectious agent, occurs every time we encounter that same specific infectious agent.

Spleen: Part of the lymphatic system, it functions to fight infections and to filter and clean blood. In addition it serves as a blood reservoir.

T-cell lymphocytes: White blood cells that have many functions, including control of the acquired immune system and killing viruses. The major component of the cell-mediated immune system.

Thrombocyte: Another name for a platelet, it is important in the **clotting** process (see Chapter 12, The circulatory system).

Thymus: The organ of the body where T-cell lymphocytes mature, distinguish between self and non-self cells and differentiate into various types of T-cells which each have different functions within the acquired immune system.

Tonsils: Lymph tissue that is situated within the oral region (the mouth) and helps to protect the respiratory and gastrointestinal tracts from infections.

Trabeculae: Connective tissue strands that help to form part of the framework of organs, so giving them rigidity.

References

Delves, P.J. and Roitt, I.M. (2000) The immune system: part 1. *New England Journal of Medicine* 343:137–149.

Janeway, C.A., Travers. P., Walport, M., *et al.* (2005) *Immunobiology*, 6th edn. New York: Garland Publishing.

Male, D. (2006) *Immunology: An Illustrated Outline*, 7th edn. London: Gower Medical Publishing.

Marieb, E.N. (2006) *Human Anatomy and Physiology*, 6th edn. San Francisco: Pearson Benjamin Cummings.

Nair, M. and Peate, I. (2009) *Fundamentals of Applied Pathophysiology: An Essential Guide for Nursing Students*. Oxford: Wiley-Blackwell.

Nairn, R. and Helbert, M. (2007) *Immunology for Medical Students*, 2nd edn. St Louis, MO: Mosby.

Roitt, I.M. (2007) *Roitt's Essential Immunology*, 11th edn. Oxford: Blackwell Science.

Roitt, I.M. and Rabson, A. (2000) *Really Essential Medical Immunology*. Oxford: Blackwell Science.

Rote, N.S. and Crippes Trask, B. (2006) Adaptive immunity. In: McCance, K.L. and Huether, S.E. (eds) *Pathophysiology: The Biologic Basis for Disease in Adults and Children*, 5th edn. St Louis: Mosby, pp. 211–248.

Seymour, G.J., Savage, N.W. and Walsh, L.J. (1995) *Immunology: An Introduction for the Health Sciences*. Roseville, Australia: McGraw-Hill.

Tortora, G.J. and Derrickson, B.H. (2009) *Principles of Anatomy and Physiology*, 12th edn. Hoboken, NJ: John Wiley & Sons.

Tortora, G.J., Funke, B.R. and Case, C.L. (2004) *Microbiology: An Introduction*, 8th edn. San Francisco: Pearson Benjamin Cummings.

Vickers, P.S. (2005) Acquired defences. In: Montague, S. Watson, R. and Herbert, R.A. (eds) *Physiology for Nursing Practice*. Edinburgh: Elsevier, pp. 685–724.

Vickers, P.S. (2007) Section 1: Anatomy and physiology of the immune system. In: *Immunology/ Immunodeficiencies – Antibody Deficiency*. CD Rom, Baxter (pp. 3–51).

Walport, M.J. (2001) Complement: part 1. *New England Journal of Medicine* 344:14; 1058–1066.

Activities

www.wiley.com/go/peate

Multiple choice questions

1. Which of the following are blood cells of the immune system? [2 answers]
   (a) lymphocytes
   (b) monocytes
   (c) red blood cells
   (d) antigens

2. Which of the following blood cells are phagocytes? [2 answers]
   (a) lymphocytes
   (b) platelets
   (c) monocytes
   (d) eosinophils

3. Where do T-cells mature?
   (a) spleen
   (b) bone marrow
   (c) thymus
   (d) liver

4. What are the functions of the lymph nodes?
   (a) to trap and destroy infectious organisms
   (b) to produce antibodies
   (c) to mature B-cells
   (d) to mature and differentiate macrophages

5. Which of the following is/are chemical barriers to infection? [3 answers]
   (a) breast milk
   (b) skin
   (c) basophil enzyme
   (d) saliva

6. Which of the following is/are a sign of inflammation? [2 answers]

   (a) pallor
   (b) pain
   (c) oedema
   (d) shivering

7. Which class of T-lymphocyte is involved in killing infected body cells?

   (a) T-helper
   (b) T-cytotoxic
   (c) T-memory
   (d) T-natural killer

8. Other names for antibody are: [2 answers]

   (a) immunoglobulin
   (b) gammaglobulin
   (c) omegaglobulin
   (d) proglobulin

9. Antibodies are produced on which cell?

   (a) T-cytotoxic
   (b) B-memory
   (c) plasma
   (d) natural killer

10. Which is the main immunoglobulin involved in the secondary response to infection?

    (a) IgM
    (b) IgD
    (c) IgG
    (d) IgE

Label the diagram

From the list of words, label the diagram below:

Afferent lymphatic vessel, Valve, Trabecula, Outer cortex, Inner cortex, Efferent lymphatic vessels, Valve, Hilum, Capsule

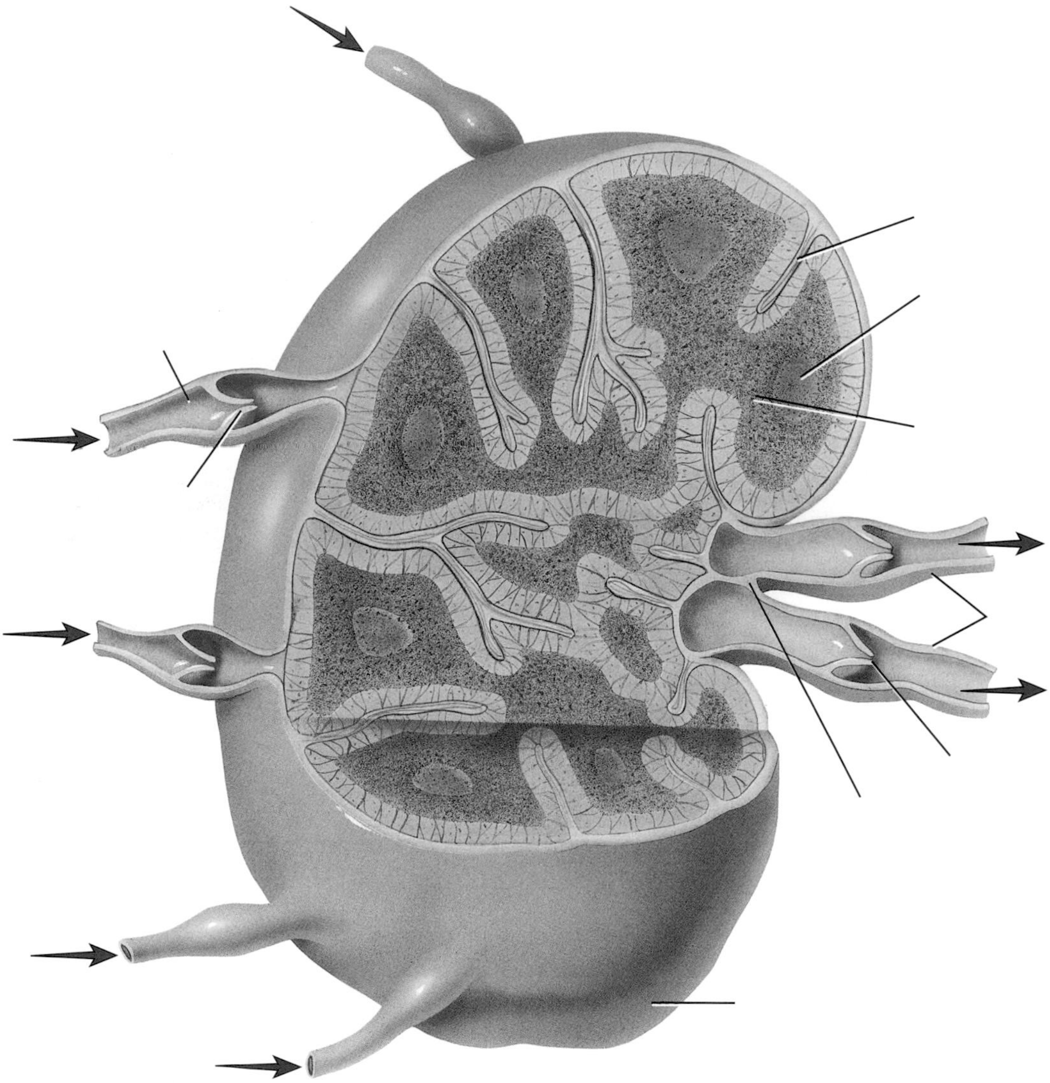

Crossword

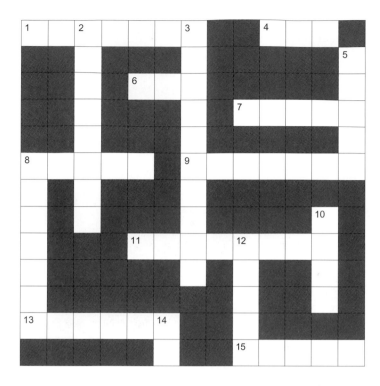
1
2
3
4
5
6
7
8
9
10
11
12
13
14
15

Across:

1. The part of the immune system that contains B-cell lymphocytes (7).
4. The most numerous antibody in the body (3).
6. The first antibody to be produced following an infection by a new organism (3).
7. Substance often produced by a bacterium as it is being destroyed by the immune system (5).
8. The cell involved in cell-mediated immunity (1, 4).
9. Prepares an infectious organism for phagocytosis (7).
11. An opsonin produced by plasma cells (8).
13. An organ of the lymphatic system (6).
15. The material in which are to be found most of the lymphocytes (5).

Down:

2. Cells that contain histamine and are involved in allergic reactions (4, 4).
3. The major blood cell of the acquired immune system (10).
5. One of the plasma protein systems involved in inflammation (5).
8. A lymphoid organ that we often lose as children (7).
10. Another scientific name for a 'cell' (4).
12. A major component of the humoral immune system (1, 4).
14. A lymphocyte that is not really part of the acquired immune system (abbreviation) (2).

Words

Find the words linked to immunology that are hidden in each of these sentences:

e.g. Tell Sal I've a pen for her (saliva)

1. Auntie Jenny invited us to stay with her.
2. The family Robinson acquired some new friends whilst working in France.
3. The student forgot to cite 'O'Kine' in his essay.
4. Jean did so well with her assignment that the teacher felt that he had to compliment her on it.
5. I have had lots of fun giving you these puzzles.
6. I have no memory of what you said.
7. Alice went to the theatre to listen to some classical music.
8. When Jenny's mother broke her leg, Jenny visited her in hospital and her first words were 'Oh dear Ma, what have you done?'.
9. When I was two years old I first started to go to the primary school.

Conditions

Below is a list of conditions that are associated with the immune system. Take some time and write notes about each of the conditions. You may make the notes taken from text books or other resources, for example, people you work with in a clinical area, or you may make the notes as a result of people you have cared for. If you are making notes about people you have cared for you must ensure that you adhere to the rules of confidentiality.

Rheumatoid arthritis	
Systemic lupus erythematosus (SLE/lupus)	
Common variable immune deficiency (CVID)	
Insulin-dependent diabetes	
Anaphylaxis	
Asthma	
AIDS	
Malaria	

Answers

Multiple choice questions

1a+b; 2c+d; 3c; 4a; 5a+b+d; 6b+c; 7b; 8a+b; 9c; 10c

Crossword

Across		Down	
1.	Humoral	**2.**	Mast cell
4.	IGG	**3.**	Lymphocyte
6.	IGM	**5.**	Kinin
7.	Toxin	**8.**	Tonsils
8.	T Cell	**10.**	Cyte
9.	Opsonin	**12.**	B Cell
11.	Antibody	**14.**	NK
13.	Spleen		
15.	Lymph		

Words

1 antigen; 2 acquired; 3 cytokine; 4 complement; 5 fungi; 6 memory (as in T memory cells); 7 classical (as in classical pathway of complement); 8 oedema; 9 primary (as in primary response to infection)

4

Tissue

Anthony Wheeldon

Contents

Introduction 104

Epithelial tissue 104
Simple epithelia 105
Stratified epithelia 108
Glandular epithelia 110

Connective tissue 110
Connective tissue proper 113
Loose connective tissue 113
Dense connective tissue 113
Cartilage 114

Bone 115

Liquid connective tissue 115

Membranes 115
Cutaneous membrane 115
Mucous membranes 115
Serous membranes 117
Synovial membranes 118

Muscle tissue 118

Nervous tissue 118

Tissue repair 119

Conclusion 121
Glossary 122
References 123
Activities 124

Fundamentals of Anatomy and Physiology for Student Nurses, First Edition. Edited by Ian Peate, Muralitharan Nair.

Test your knowledge

- List the four main types of body tissue.
- What are the main functions of epithelial tissue?
- Which types of muscle are involuntary?
- What are the main steps of tissue repair?

Learning outcomes

On completion of this section the reader will be able to:

- Describe the characteristics of epithelial tissue
- List the classifications of epithelial tissue
- Discuss the functions of connective tissue
- List the classifications of muscle tissue
- Describe the process of tissue repair

Introduction

The human body consists of around 50–106 trillion individual structural working units called cells (Marieb and Hoehn 2008). Cells work together to ensure that homeostasis is maintained. Cells come in many different shapes, sizes and life spans, however they can be categorised depending on their structure and functions. A group of cells that have a similar structure and function are called tissue and within the human body there are four distinct types of tissue. Cells that provide a covering for organs and structures, for example, are referred to as epithelial tissue, whereas cells that provide support for structures are called connective tissue. Cells that govern body movement are muscle tissue and cells that help control homeostasis are nervous tissue. Most organs of the body contain a selection of all four tissue types. The heart, for example, contains muscle tissue, is controlled by nervous tissue, lined by epithelial tissue and supported by connective tissue. Tissue also has the capacity to repair itself. This chapter examines all four types of tissue and the process of tissue repair.

Epithelial tissue

Epithelial tissue is essentially a sheet of cells which cover an area of the body. Epithelial tissue covers or lines body surfaces, i.e. skin, or it lines the walls and the organs within body cavities. The major role of epithelial tissue is as an interface; indeed, nearly all the substances absorbed or secreted by the body must pass through epithelial tissue. Broadly speaking, epithelial tissue has six main functions:

- Absorption
- Protection
- Excretion
- Secretion
- Filtration
- Sensory reception.

Not all epithelial tissue carries out all six functions. In many areas of the body epithelial tissue specialises in just one or two functions. Epithelial tissue in the digestive system, for example, specialises in absorption of nutrients, whereas epithelial tissue within skin provides a protective layer.

Epithelial tissue cells are closely bonded together in continuous sheets, which have an apical and basal surface. The apical surface faces outwards, towards the exterior of the organ it is lining. Apical surfaces can be smooth, but most have hair-like extensions called micro-villi. Micro-villi dramatically increase the surface area of the epithelial tissue and therefore increase its ability for absorption and secretion. Some areas, within the respiratory tract for example, possess larger hair-like extensions called cilia, which are capable of propelling substances. Lying close to the basal surface is a thin sheet of glycoproteins which acts as a selective filter, governing which substances can enter epithelial tissue. Epithelial tissue is innervated by nerves, however it has no blood supply as such. Rather than containing capillaries, epithelial tissue receives its nutrients from nearby blood vessels. Due to their protective role they have to endure a great deal of abrasion and environmental damage. Nevertheless epithelial cells are very hardy and tough. This is due to their ability to divide and regenerate rapidly, which results in damaged epithelial cells being quickly replaced. However, this regenerative capacity is reliant upon a plentiful supply of nutrients.

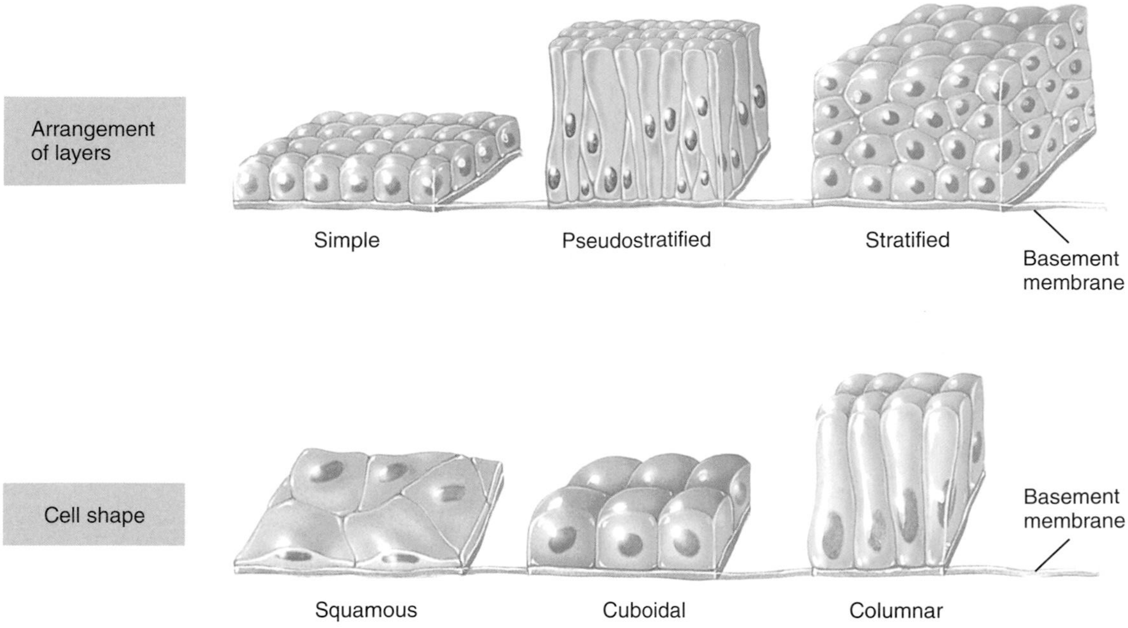
Arrangement of layers
Simple
Pseudostratified
Stratified
Basement membrane
Cell shape
Squamous
Cuboidal
Columnar
Basement membrane

Figure 4.1 Epithelial tissue classified by shape and depth (Tortora and Derrickson 2009)

The varying types of epithelial tissue are named after the shape and number of cells bound in the continuous sheet. Narrow epithelial tissue consisting of one layer of cells is referred to as simple epithelium, whereas stratified epithelium is thicker with numerous layers of cells. All epithelial cells have six sides, indeed a cross-section of epithelial tissue looks like a honeycomb. However epithelial cells can be subdivided into three different six-sided shapes. As their name suggests cuboidal and columnar epithelial cells are square and tall respectively, whereas squamous epithelial cells are rather flat and scaly (see Figure 4.1). When examining the many different types of epithelial cell it is easy to work out its size and shape by its name. For instance, simple squamous epithelium is thin, flat and scale-like.

Simple epithelia

Because simple epithelia consist of a single cellular layer and specialise in absorption, secretion and filtration rather than protection. **Simple squamous epithelium** is quite often very permeable and is found where the diffusion of nutrients is essential. The alveoli, for example, are lined with simple squamous epithelium, allowing the diffusion of oxygen and carbon dioxide to occur. Simple squamous epithelium found within hollow organs, such as the alveoli, is called endothelium. Endothelium is also found in the kidneys and blood vessels, especially capillaries, providing the perfect conditions for the diffusion of nutrients between the blood stream and cells (see Figure 4.2).

Simple cuboidal epithelium specialises in secretion as well as absorption. Simple cuboidal epithelium is found in the lining of the ovaries, the kidney tubules and the ducts of smaller glands. It also forms part of the secretory portions of glands such as the thyroid and pancreas (see Figure 4.3).

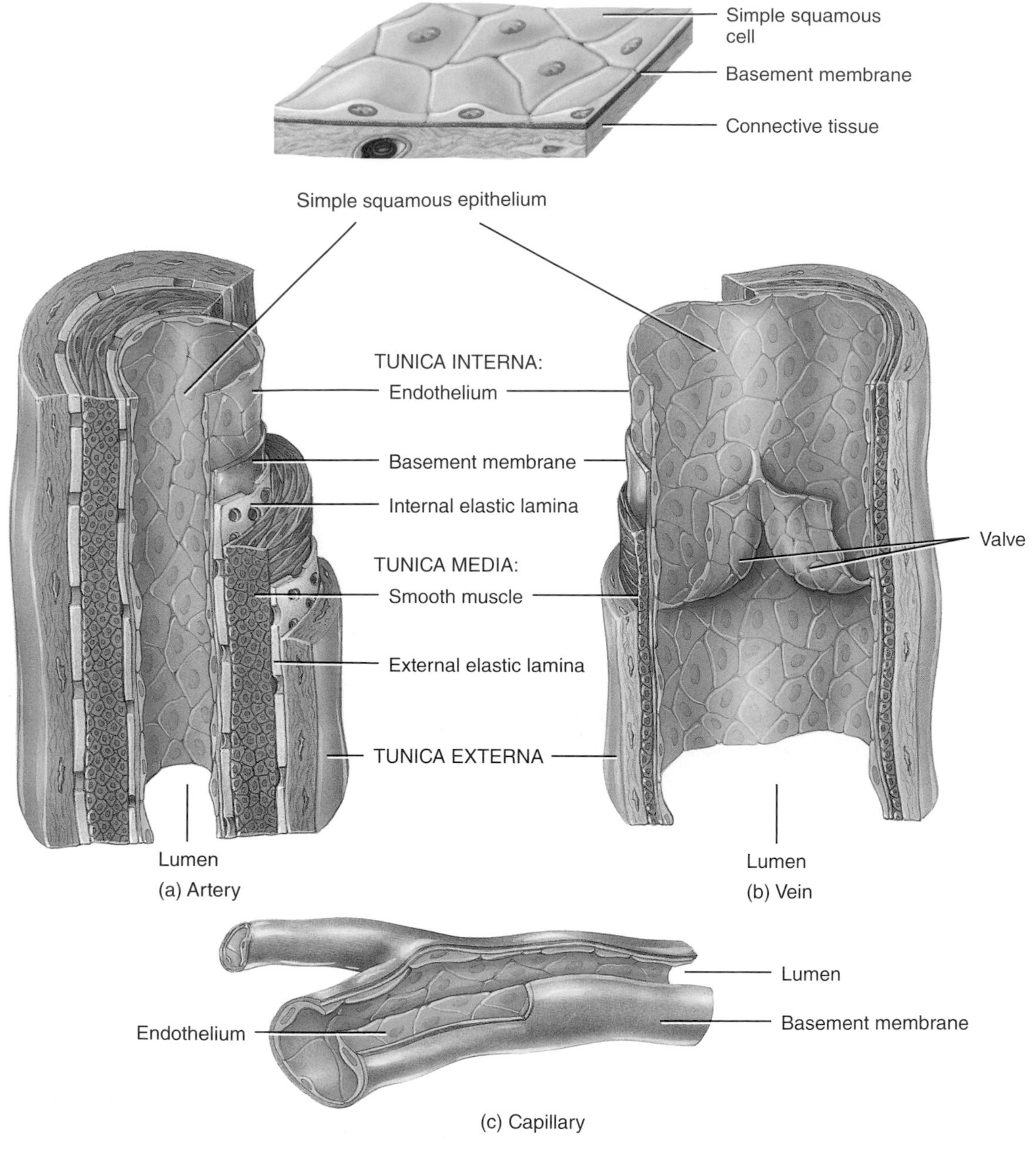
Simple squamous cell
Basement membrane
Connective tissue
Simple squamous epithelium
TUNICA INTERNA:
Endothelium
Basement membrane
Internal elastic lamina
TUNICA MEDIA:
Smooth muscle
External elastic lamina
TUNICA EXTERNA
Valve
Lumen
(a) Artery
Lumen
(b) Vein
Lumen
Basement membrane
Endothelium
(c) Capillary

Figure 4.2 Simple squamous epithelium forms the endothelial layer of blood vessels (Tortora and Derrickson 2009)

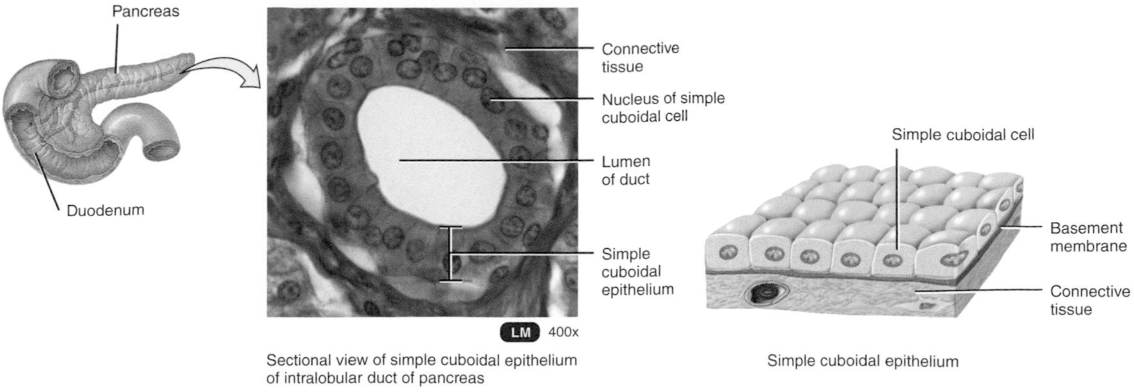
Pancreas
Duodenum
Connective tissue
Nucleus of simple cuboidal cell
Lumen of duct
Simple cuboidal epithelium
LM 400x
Sectional view of simple cuboidal epithelium of intralobular duct of pancreas
Simple cuboidal cell
Basement membrane
Connective tissue
Simple cuboidal epithelium

Figure 4.3 Simple cuboid epithelium forms part of the secretory portion of the pancreas (Tortora and Derrickson 2009)

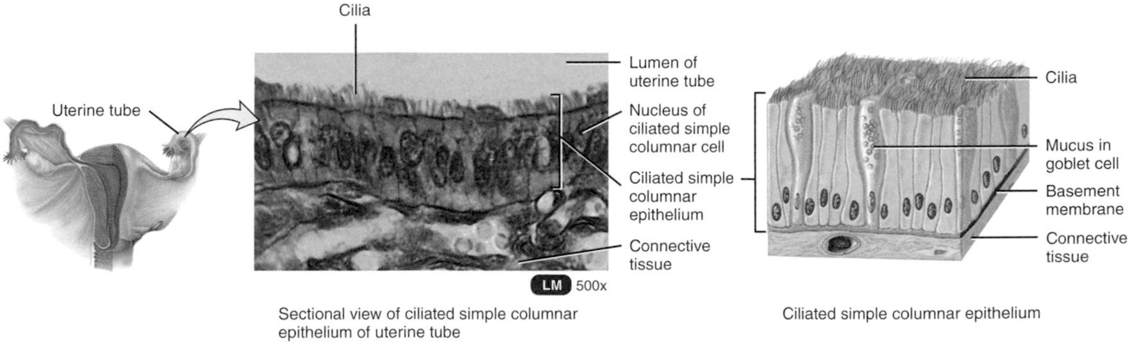
Cilia
Uterine tube
Lumen of uterine tube
Nucleus of ciliated simple columnar cell
Ciliated simple columnar epithelium
Connective tissue
LM 500x
Sectional view of ciliated simple columnar epithelium of uterine tube
Cilia
Mucus in goblet cell
Basement membrane
Connective tissue
Ciliated simple columnar epithelium

Figure 4.4 Ciliated simple columnar epithelium lines the fallopian tubes (Tortora and Derrickson 2009)

Simple columnar epithelium can be ciliated or non-ciliated. As its name suggests, ciliated simple columnar epithelium has cilia on its apical surface. It is found in areas of the body where movement of fluids, mucus or other substances is required. Ciliated simple columnar epithelial cells line the passageways of the central nervous system and help propel cerebrospinal fluid. They also line the fallopian tubes and help move oocytes recently expelled from the ovaries (see Figure 4.4). A common location for non-ciliated simple columnar epithelium is the lining of the digestive tract from the stomach to the rectum (see Figure 4.5). Non-ciliated simple columnar epithelium performs two broad functions. Some possess micro-villi, greatly increasing their surface area for absorption, others specialise in the secretion of mucus. Such cells are referred to as goblet cells owing to their cup shape.

Simple columnar epithelial cells are generally of equal size. However, in some instances simple columnar epithelial cells vary in height with only the tallest reaching the apical surface. This gives the illusion that the tissue has many layers, like stratified epithelium. Such examples of columnar epithelial tissue are called **pseudostratified columnar epithelium**. Pseudostratified columnar

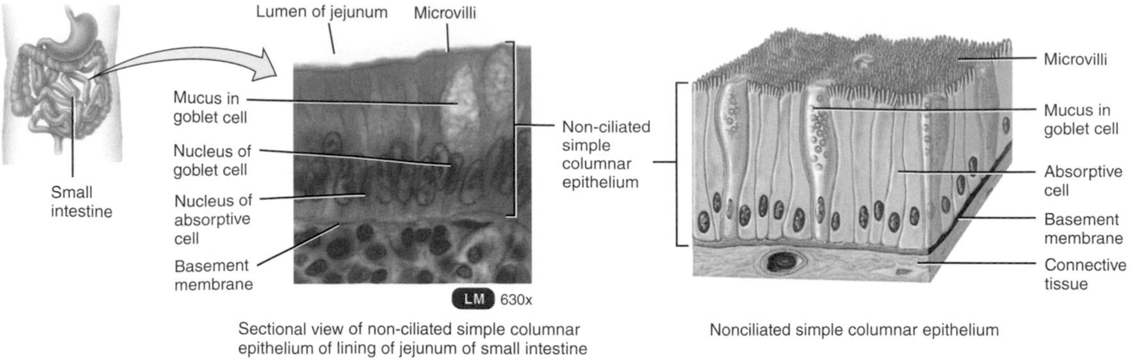
Small intestine
Lumen of jejunum
Microvilli
Mucus in goblet cell
Nucleus of goblet cell
Nucleus of absorptive cell
Basement membrane
Non-ciliated simple columnar epithelium
LM 630x
Sectional view of non-ciliated simple columnar epithelium of lining of jejunum of small intestine
Microvilli
Mucus in goblet cell
Absorptive cell
Basement membrane
Connective tissue
Nonciliated simple columnar epithelium

Figure 4.5 Non-ciliated columnar epithelium lines the digestive tract (Tortora and Derrickson 2009)

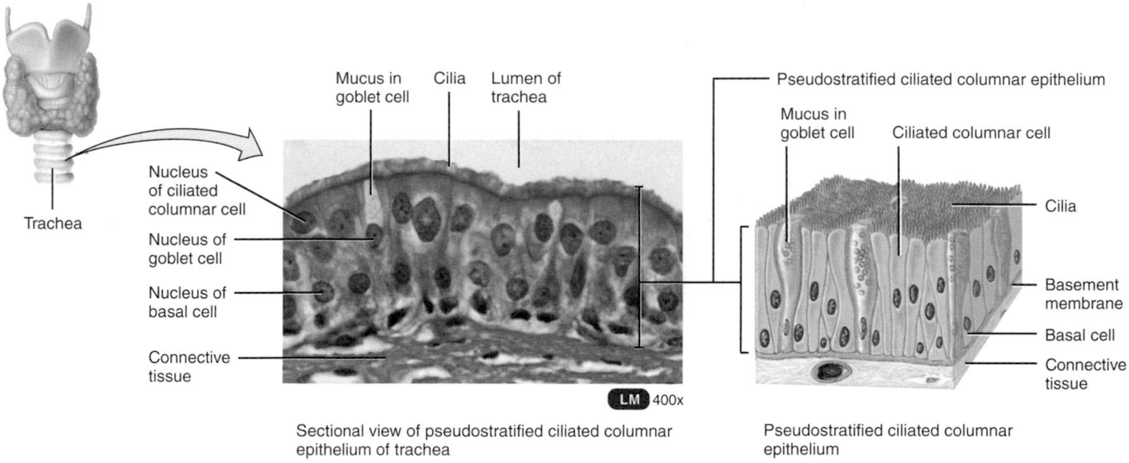
Trachea
Mucus in goblet cell
Cilia
Lumen of trachea
Nucleus of ciliated columnar cell
Nucleus of goblet cell
Nucleus of basal cell
Connective tissue
LM 400x
Sectional view of pseudostratified ciliated columnar epithelium of trachea
Pseudostratified ciliated columnar epithelium
Mucus in goblet cell
Ciliated columnar cell
Cilia
Basement membrane
Basal cell
Connective tissue
Pseudostratified ciliated columnar epithelium

Figure 4.6 Pseudostratified ciliated columnar epithelium lines the trachea (Tortora and Derrickson 2009)

epithelium is found within the lining of the male reproductive system, however the most common location is the lining of the respiratory tract (see Figure 4.6).

Stratified epithelia

Unlike simple epithelia, stratified epithelia have many layers. The cells regenerate from below, with new cells dividing on the basal layer pushing the older cells towards the surface. As stratified epithelium is thicker its principal function is protection. **Stratified squamous epithelium** is the most common stratified epithelium and forms the external part of skin (see Chapter 5, The skin). Skin stratified squamous epithelial tissue is keratinised, toughened by the presence of keratin, a special tough fibrous protein. Non-keratinised stratified squamous epithelial tissue lines wet areas of the body, the mouth, the tongue and the vagina for example (see Figure 4.7). Only the outer layers of stratified squamous epithelium are actually squamous in shape, the basal layers may be cuboidal or columnar. **Stratified cuboidal epithelium** is found in the oesophagus, sweat glands and in the male urethra (see Figure 4.8). **Stratified columnar epithelium** however is quite rare. Small amounts can be found in the male urethra and in the ducts of some glands. Another common example of stratified epithelium is **transitional epithelium**, which may have both squamous and cuboidal cells in its apical surface. The basal surface may contain both cuboidal and columnar cells. Transitional epithelium can withstand a great deal of stretch and is found in organs such as the bladder, which is subject to considerable distension (see Figure 4.9).

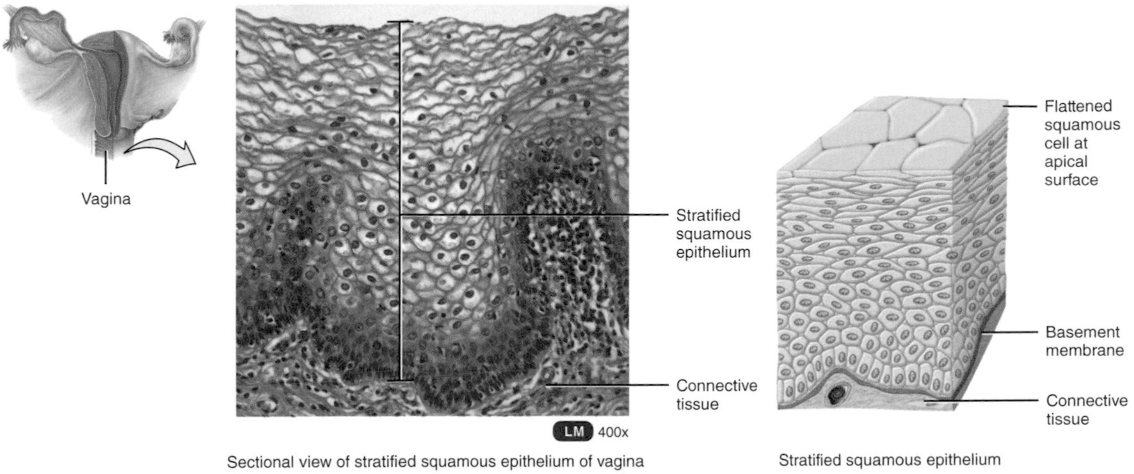
Vagina
Stratified squamous epithelium
Connective tissue
LM 400x
Sectional view of stratified squamous epithelium of vagina
Flattened squamous cell at apical surface
Basement membrane
Connective tissue
Stratified squamous epithelium

Figure 4.7 Non-keratinised stratified squamous epithelial tissue lines the vagina (Tortora and Derrickson 2009)

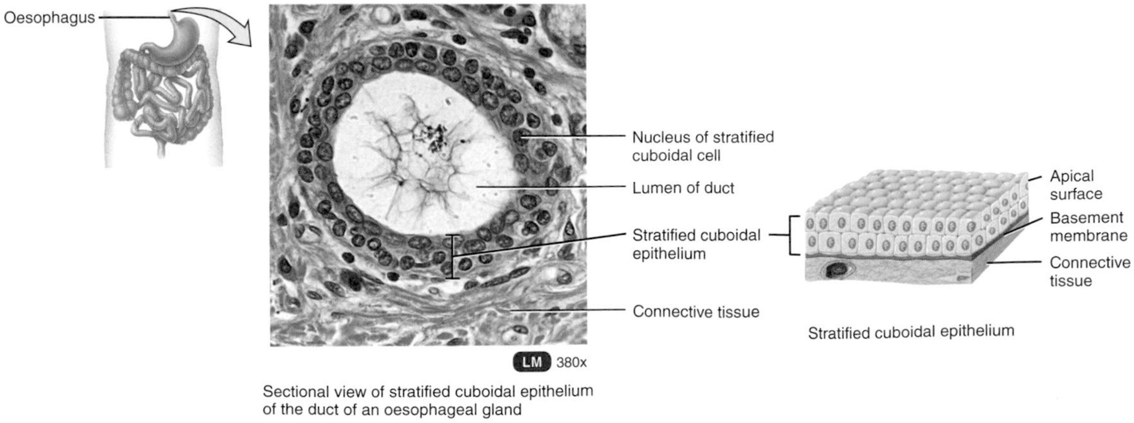
Oesophagus
Nucleus of stratified cuboidal cell
Lumen of duct
Stratified cuboidal epithelium
Connective tissue
LM 380x
Sectional view of stratified cuboidal epithelium of the duct of an oesophageal gland
Apical surface
Basement membrane
Connective tissue
Stratified cuboidal epithelium

Figure 4.8 Cuboidal epithelial tissue is found in the oesophagus (Tortora and Derrickson 2009)

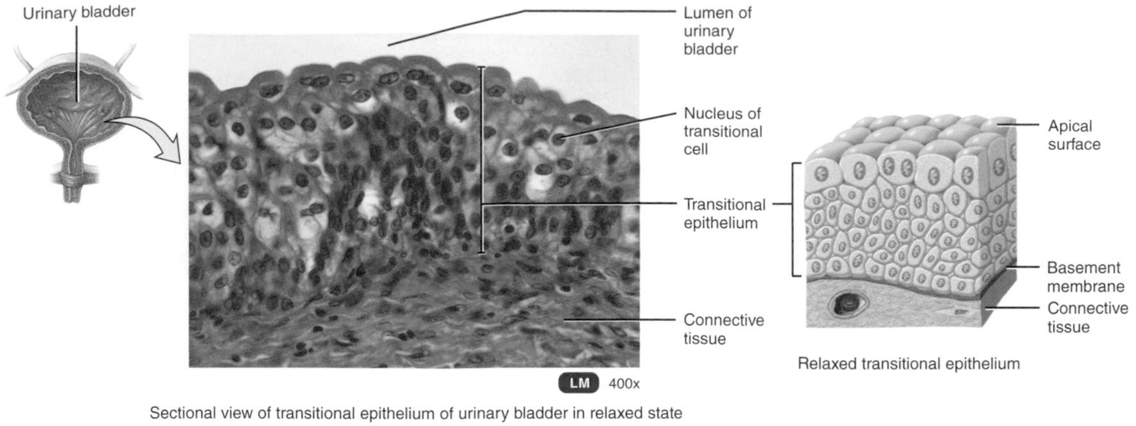
Urinary bladder
Lumen of urinary bladder
Nucleus of transitional cell
Transitional epithelium
Connective tissue
LM 400x
Sectional view of transitional epithelium of urinary bladder in relaxed state
Apical surface
Basement membrane
Connective tissue
Relaxed transitional epithelium

Figure 4.9 Transitional epithelium lines the bladder and allows for distension (Tortora and Derrickson 2009)

Glandular epithelia

The glands of the body are formed by glandular epithelia. All glands are classified as endocrine or exocrine. Glands which secrete their products internally are called endocrine glands. Endocrine glands release hormones, regulatory chemicals for use elsewhere in the body (see Chapter 7, The endocrine system). Exocrine glands release their products onto the surface of epithelial tissue. Exocrine glands are either unicellular or multicellular. Unicellular exocrine glands consist of a single cell type and the main example is the goblet cell which releases a glycoprotein called mucin. Once dissolved in water mucin forms mucus, which lubricates and protects surfaces. Multicellular exocrine glands are far more complex, coming in several shapes and sizes. Some exocrine glands are simple and consist of a single branched duct, others are more complex with multi-branched ducts (see Figure 4.10). However, they all contain two distinct areas, an epithelial duct and secretory cells (acinus). Exocrine glands that are tubular in shape can be found within the digestive system and stomach. Other exocrine glands are spherical and referred to as alveolar or acinar. The oil glands within skin and mammary glands are just two examples. Glands which are both tubular and acinar are referred to as tubulacinar, salivary glands, for example.

Connective tissue

Connective tissue is the most abundant tissue in the human body. Its main functions are to bind tissues together, reinforcement, insulation, protection and support. All epithelial tissue is reinforced by the connective tissue base it rests upon (see Figure 4.11). There are four types of connective tissue: **connective tissue proper, cartilage, bone** and **blood**. Connective tissue is not present on body surfaces and, unlike epithelial tissue, is highly vascular and receives a rich blood supply.

Several types of cell are present in connective tissue, macrophages, plasma cells, mast cells, adipocytes, white blood cells and primary blast cells. Macrophages, plasma cells and white blood cells form part of the body's immune system.

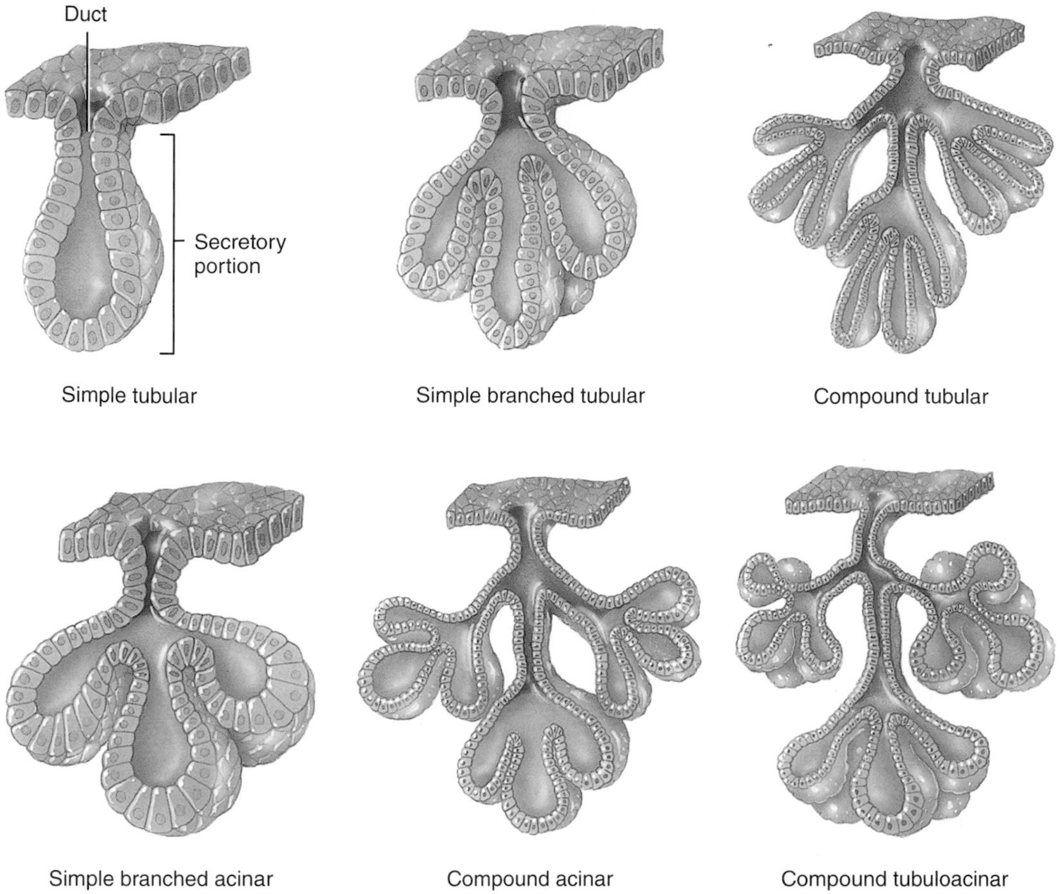
Duct
Secretory portion
Simple tubular
Simple branched tubular
Compound tubular
Simple branched acinar
Compound acinar
Compound tubuloacinar

Figure 4.10 Exocrine glands classified by shape, with examples of location (Tortora and Derrickson 2009)

- Macrophages engulf invading substances and plasma cells produce antibodies
- White blood cells are not normally found in significant numbers within connective tissue; however, they do migrate into connective tissue during inflammation
- Mast cells produce histamine, which promotes vasodilation during the body's inflammatory response
- Adipocytes are fat cells. Within connective tissue adipocytes store triglycerides (fats)
- Primary blast cells continually secret ground substance and produce mature connective tissue cells. Each type of connective tissue contains its own unique primary blast cells (see Table 4.1).

Connective tissue cells are surrounded by a collection of substances referred to as the extracellular matrix. The function of the extracellular matrix is to ensure that connective tissue can bear weight and withstand tension, abuse and abrasion. As a result connective tissue can cope with

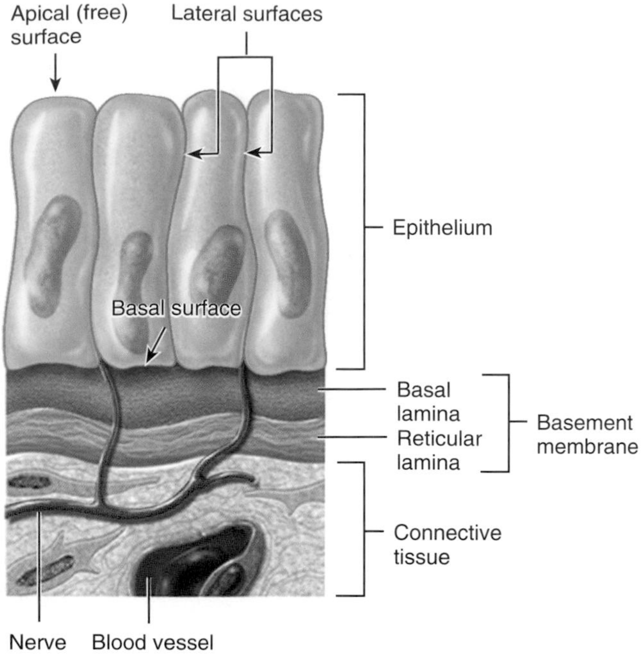
Apical (free) surface
Lateral surfaces
Epithelium
Basal surface
Basal lamina
Reticular lamina
Basement membrane
Connective tissue
Nerve
Blood vessel

Figure 4.11 Connective tissue reinforces epithelial tissue (Tortora and Derrickson 2009)

Table 4.1 The major primary blast cells and their connective tissue type

Connective tissue type	Primary blast cell	Connective tissue cell
Connective tissue proper	Fibroblast	Fibrocyte
Cartilage	Chondroblast	Chondrocyte
Bone	Osteoclast	Osteocyte

stresses and strains other tissues wouldn't be able to tolerate. The two main elements of extracellular matrix are **ground substance** and **fibres** (see Figure 4.12). Ground substance consists of interstitial fluid, cell adhesion proteins and glycoaminoglycans (GAGs). Cell adhesion proteins act as connective glue, keeping the tissue cells together. GAGs trap water, making ground substance jelly like. The higher the amount of GAGs the harder the ground substance will be.

There are three types of fibre found within extracellular matrix: **collagen, elastic** and **reticular**.

- The most abundant are collagen fibres, which are essentially the protein collagen. Collagen is very tough; indeed, collagen fibres are stronger than similar-sized steel fibres (Marieb and Hoehn 2008)
- Reticular fibres are much thinner but also contain bundles of collagen. They provide support and strength and are found in greater numbers in soft organs, spleen and lymph nodes, for example

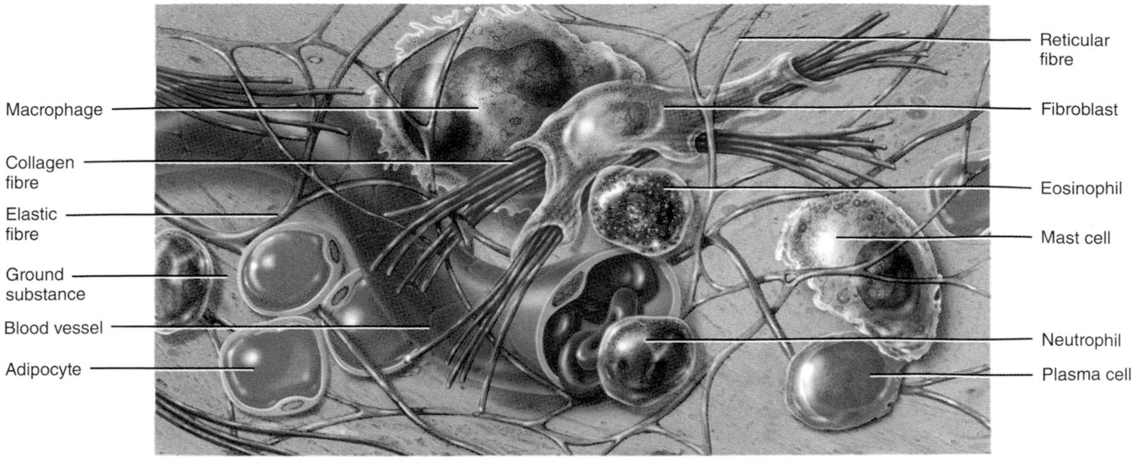
Macrophage
Collagen fibre
Elastic fibre
Ground substance
Blood vessel
Adipocyte
Reticular fibre
Fibroblast
Eosinophil
Mast cell
Neutrophil
Plasma cell

Figure 4.12 Constituents of connective tissue (Tortora and Derrickson 2009)

- Elastic fibres contain the rubber-like protein called elastin, which facilitates stretch and recoil. Elastic fibres are found in greater numbers in tissue that has to endure stretch, skin and blood vessel walls for example.

Connective tissue proper

Aside from cartilage, bone and blood all connective tissue belongs to this class. Connective tissue proper is subdivided further into **loose connective** and **dense connective** tissue (see Table 4.2). Loose connective tissue contains fewer fibres than dense connective tissue.

Loose connective tissue

There are three types of loose connective tissue: **areolar, adipose** and **reticular**.

- Areolar is the most abundant connective tissue. It contains all three fibres (collagen, elastic and reticular) and its primary function is support, elasticity and strength. Areolar tissue is combined with adipose tissue to form the subcutaneous layer, which connects skin with other tissues and organs.
- Adipose tissue contains adipocytes, whose primary function is to store triglycerides (fat). The primary functions of adipose tissue are to provide insulation, protection and an energy store.
- As its name suggests, reticular tissue only contains reticular fibres. Its main function is to form a protective framework or stroma which surrounds the liver, spleen and lymph nodes. Within the spleen reticular connective tissue can also filter blood, assisting with the removal of old blood cells.

Dense connective tissue

Dense connective tissue contains more collagen or elastic fibres. Dense connective tissue that is made primarily from collagen is said to be either **regular** or **irregular** depending on the organisation of the collagen fibres. Dense regular connective tissue contains collagen fibres, which are arranged

Table 4.2 Types of connective tissue proper, their main constituents, functions and locations

Connective tissue	Main constituent	Functions	Main locations
Loose areolar	Collagen, elastic, reticular fibres	Strength Elasticity Support	Subcutaneous layer beneath skin
Loose adipose	Adipocytes	Insulation Protection Energy store	Subcutaneous layer beneath skin Tissue surrounding heart and kidneys Padding around joints
Loose reticular	Reticular fibres Reticular cells	Support Filtration	Liver Spleen Lymph nodes
Dense regular	Collagen fibres in parallel	Strength Support	Tendons Ligaments
Dense irregular	Collagen fibres arranged randomly	Strength	Skin Heart Tissue surrounding bone Tissue surrounding cartilage
Dense elastic	Elastic fibres	Stretch	Lung tissue Arteries

in parallel rows. It has a silvery appearance and is both tough and pliable. Dense, irregular connective tissue is found in ligaments and tendons. Its collagen fibres are randomly arranged but closely knitted together. Dense irregular tissue can withstand pressure and pulling forces and is found in skin and the heart as well as the membranes that surround cartilage and bone. Dense elastic connective tissue consists of elastic fibres. Dense elastic connective tissue is found in areas of the body that have to withstand great amounts of stretch, such as arteries and lung tissue.

Cartilage

Cartilage contains a compact network of collagen fibres and is stronger than both loose and dense connective tissue. It has the ability to return to its original shape after stress and movement. Its strength and resilience are provided by a gel-like substance called **chondroitin sulphate**, which is found in cartilage ground substance. Cartilage is surrounded by a layer of dense irregular tissue called **perichondrium**. Perichondrium is the only area of cartilage that is served by blood and nervous tissue. There are three types of cartilage: **hyaline, fibrocartilage** and **elastic**.

- Hyaline cartilage is the most common cartilage in the human body. It mainly comprises collagen fibres with cartilage cells, chondrocytes accounting for around 10% of its volume. The collagen fibres are so fine they are almost invisible, giving hyaline cartilage a bluish appearance. Because hyaline cartilage is both strong and flexible it can act as a shock absorber reducing friction around joints. Hyaline cartilage is also found in the rib cage and airways

- Elastic cartilage is almost identical to hyaline cartilage. Its major difference is the greater presence of elastic fibres. Elastic cartilage can withstand greater movement and bending than hyaline cartilage and is found in areas of the body where stretchability is required, i.e. the outer ear
- Fibrocartilage is the strongest of the three cartilages. Its strength is provided by rows of chondrocytes and collagen. Because it can withstand great pressure it is found where hyaline cartilage meets tendons or ligaments, between the discs of the vertebrae for example (see Figure 4.13).

Bone

Along with cartilage, bones make up the human skeletal frame. Bone is similar to cartilage but contains even greater amounts of collagen. For this reason bone is harder and more rigid, facilitating greater protection and support for body structures. However, unlike cartilage, bone receives a rich supply of blood. Bone also stores fat and plays an important role in the production of blood cells. A more detailed examination of bones can be found in Chapter 8, The skeletal system.

Liquid connective tissue

Connective tissue that has a liquid extracellular matrix includes **blood** and **lymph**. Blood and lymph are said to be atypical connective tissues because, strictly speaking, they do not connect tissues or provide mechanical support. The extracellular matrix of blood is plasma. Blood cells include erythrocytes, leucocytes and platelets. Blood and plasma perform many important functions. For a detailed explanation of blood see Chapter 12, The circulatory system. Lymph has a clear extracellular matrix very similar to plasma. The primary function of lymph is defence against invading pathogens. A more detailed exploration of lymph can be found in Chapter 3, The immune system.

Membranes

Membranes are sheets of tissue, which cover or line areas of the human body. Membranes contain both epithelial and connective tissue. Structurally, membranes consist of an epithelial tissue layer that is bound to a basement layer of connective tissue. There are four major types of membrane: **cutaneous, mucous, serous** and **synovial**.

Cutaneous membrane

The principal example of a cutaneous membrane is skin. It consists of an outer stratified squamous epithelial layer, which sits on top of a thick layer of dense irregular connective tissue. Chapter 5, The skin, is dedicated to the functions and structure of skin.

Mucous membranes

Mucous membranes line the external surfaces of body cavities. Examples include hollow organs of the digestive tract, the respiratory system and the renal system. All mucous membranes are wet or moist, but not all secrete lubricating mucus. The mucous membranes of the renal system, for example, are wet due to the presence of urine. Most mucous membranes contain stratified

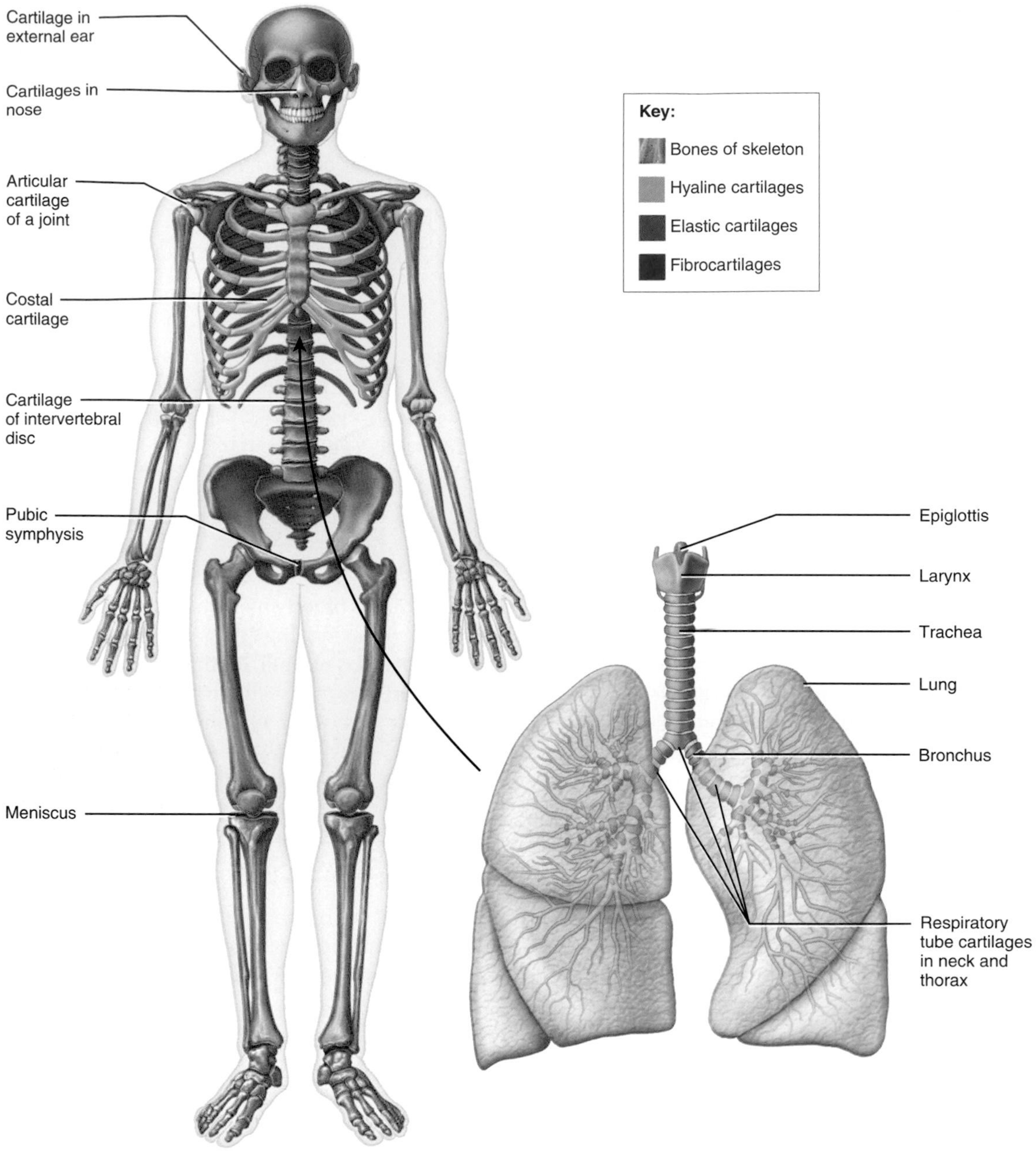
Cartilage in external ear
Cartilages in nose
Articular cartilage of a joint
Costal cartilage
Cartilage of intervertebral disc
Pubic symphysis
Meniscus
Key:
Bones of skeleton
Hyaline cartilages
Elastic cartilages
Fibrocartilages
Epiglottis
Larynx
Trachea
Lung
Bronchus
Respiratory tube cartilages in neck and thorax

Figure 4.13 Where cartilage is found within the body (Jenkins *et al.* 2007)

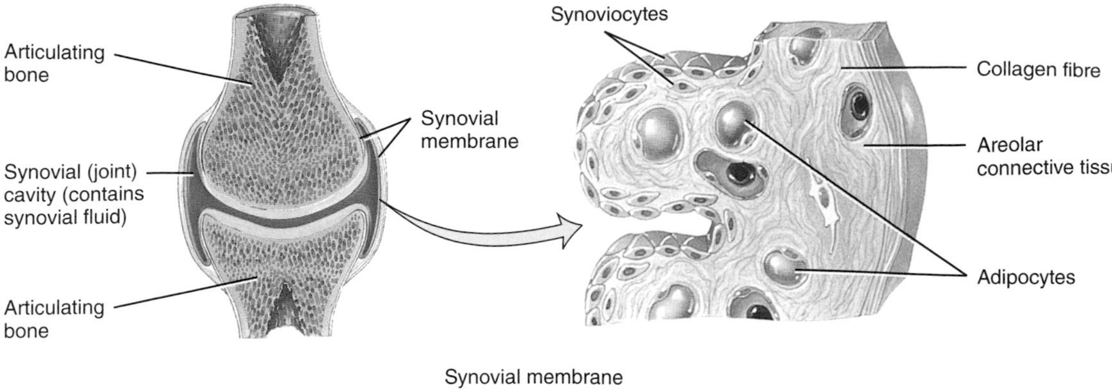
Articulating bone
Synovial (joint) cavity (contains synovial fluid)
Articulating bone
Synovial membrane
Synoviocytes
Collagen fibre
Areolar connective tissue
Adipocytes
Synovial membrane

Figure 4.14 Synovial membranes fill joint cavities (Tortora and Derrickson 2009)

squamous or simple columnar epithelium supported by a layer of connective tissue referred to as **lamina propria**.

Serous membranes

Serous membranes or a *serosa* cover internal body cavities. They consist of areolar connective tissue which is covered by a special kind of simple squamous epithelium called **mesothelium**. Mesothelium secretes a watery substance referred to as serous fluid, which allows organs to slide against one another with ease. Serous membranes consist of an outer or **parietal** layer and an inner or **visceral** layer. The largest example is the peritoneum, which lines the organs of the abdominopelvic cavity. The protective lining of the lungs, the parietal and visceral pleura, provides another example of an important serous membrane. The parietal and visceral pleura glide over one another when the thorax expands on inspiration.

Clinical considerations

Peritonitis

Peritonitis is the inflammation of the peritoneum, the serous membrane that lines both the digestive organs and the wall of the abdominopelvic cavity. The causes of peritonitis are either **chemical** or **bacterial**. Chemical peritonitis results from damage to neighbouring structures, i.e. a piercing wound or ulcer which leaks digestive juices into the peritoneum. Bacterial peritonitis results from the direct contamination of the peritoneum, i.e. a burst appendix or perforated bowel. If left unaddressed chemical peritonitis will lead to bacterial peritonitis.

Peritonitis is an acute medical emergency, which is associated with high mortality. Survival rates have improved since the use of prophylactic antibiotics.

(Lawrence *et al.* 2003; Gould 2006)

Clinical considerations

Pneumothorax

A pneumothorax or collapsed lung occurs when air accumulates in the pleural cavity, the small space between the visceral and parietal pleura. It most often occurs as the result of trauma but can also occur in chronic lung disease. In a small number of cases the pleura separate spontaneously due to a congenital defect. In small pneumothoraces the lungs will reinflate over time but large pneumothoraces are potentially life-threatening. Chest drains are often inserted to remove the air from the pleura and allow the lung to reinflate.

(Allibone 2003; Ryan 2005)

Synovial membranes

Unlike serous, mucous and cutaneous membranes, synovial membranes do not contain any epithelial tissue. Synovial membranes are mainly found in moving joints and consist of areolar connective tissue, adipocytes and elastic and collagen fibres. They secrete synovial fluid which bathes, nourishes and lubricates the joints. Synovial fluid also contains macrophages which destroy invading microbes and debris from the joint cavity. Synovial membranes are also found in cushion-like sacs in the hands and feet that ease the movement of tendons (see Figure 4.14).

Muscle tissue

Muscle tissue contains long muscle fibres whose primary function is to generate force. Muscle tissue is found where there is a need for movement and maintenance of posture. Muscle is classified in three ways: **skeletal, smooth** and **cardiac** (see Figure 4.15).

- Skeletal muscle is found adjacent to the skeleton and its function is twofold: the movement of the skeleton and the maintenance of body posture. The structure of the muscle fibres within skeletal muscle gives a striped or **striated** appearance. Skeletal muscle is also voluntary, meaning its movement can be controlled by conscious control.
- Smooth muscle, on the other hand, is both involuntary and **non-striated**. Smooth muscle is found in hollow internal structures where fluid or solid substances need to be propelled from one area to another. Smooth muscle is found in blood vessels where blood is propelled through the vascular system and the gastrointestinal tract where chyme is moved from the stomach through the intestines towards the rectum.
- Cardiac muscle is striated, but it is also involuntary. As its name suggests cardiac muscle is only found in the heart and provides the driving force of contraction. A more detailed examination of muscle can be found in Chapter 9, The muscular system.

Nervous tissue

Nervous tissue is found within the nervous system (See Chapter 6, The nervous system). There are two types of nervoues tissue cells: neurones and neuroglia (see Figure 4.16). Neurones are the functioning unit of the nervous system. They consist of three basic parts: **the cell body, an axon** and

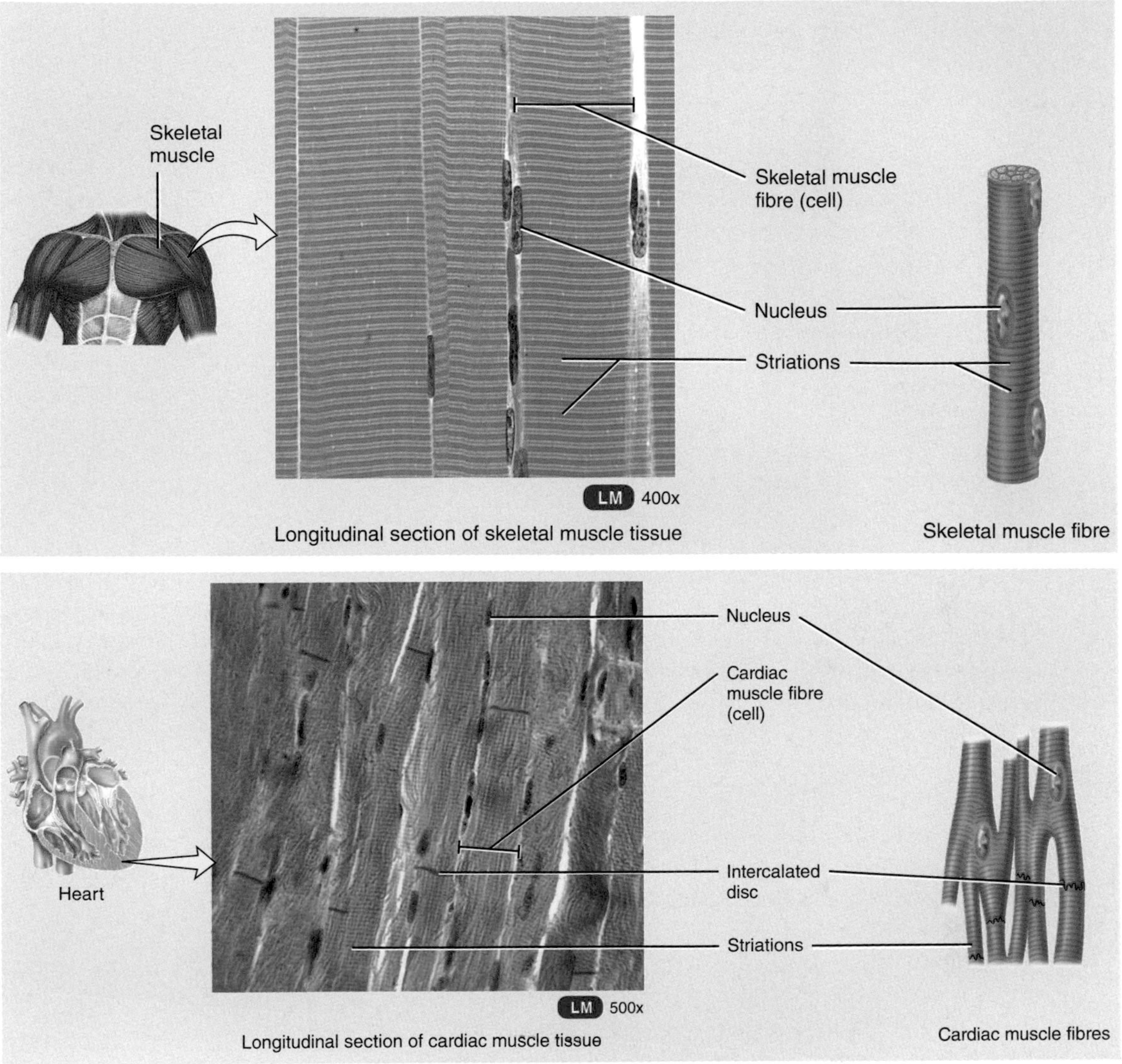

Skeletal muscle
Skeletal muscle fibre (cell)
Nucleus
Striations
LM 400x
Longitudinal section of skeletal muscle tissue
Skeletal muscle fibre
Heart
Nucleus
Cardiac muscle fibre (cell)
Intercalated disc
Striations
LM 500x
Longitudinal section of cardiac muscle tissue
Cardiac muscle fibres

Figure 4.15 The major muscle types with examples of their location (Tortora and Derrickson 2009)

dendrites. There primary function is the propagation of nerve signals within the central and peripheral nervous systems. Neuroglia do not propagate nerve signals; rather, they nourish, protect and support neurones.

Tissue repair

Tissue repair occurs in order to replace cells that are damaged, worn out or dead. Each of the four tissue types has the capacity to regenerate and replace cells injured by trauma, disease or

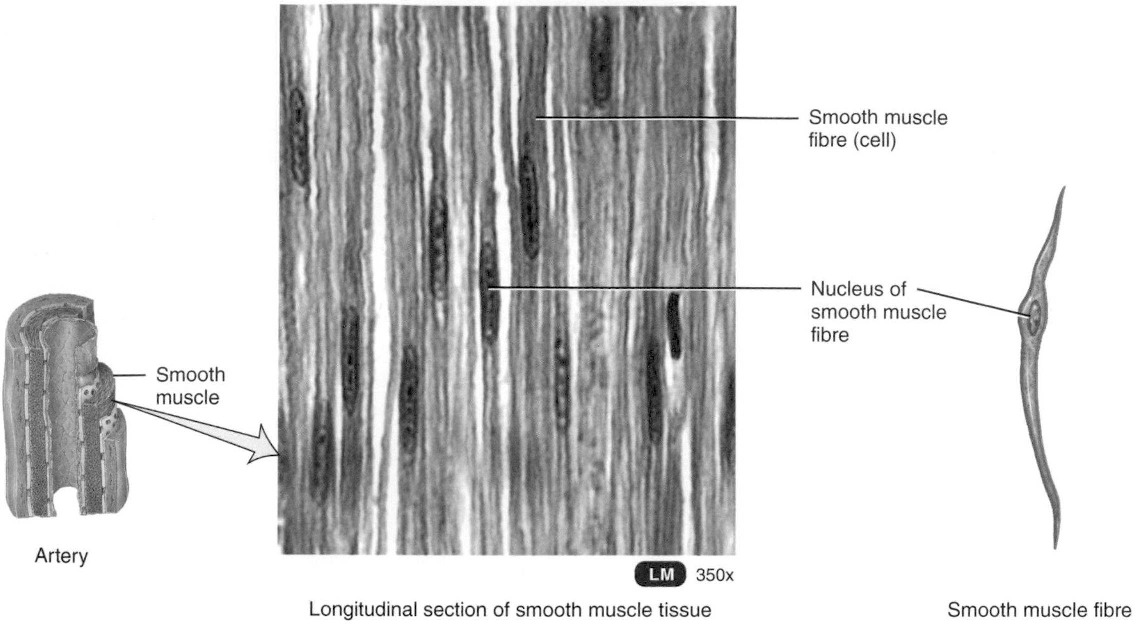
Smooth muscle fibre (cell)
Nucleus of smooth muscle fibre
Smooth muscle
Artery
LM 350x
Longitudinal section of smooth muscle tissue
Smooth muscle fibre

Figure 4.15 *Continued*

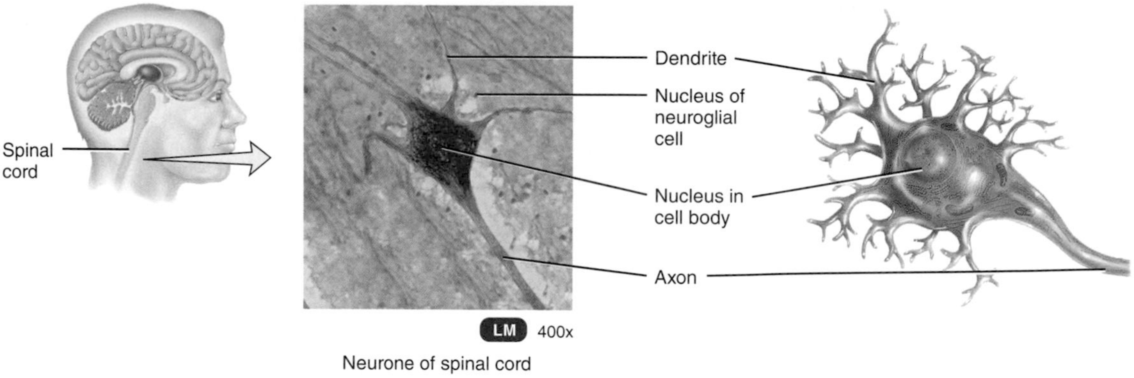
Spinal cord
Dendrite
Nucleus of neuroglial cell
Nucleus in cell body
Axon
LM 400x
Neurone of spinal cord

Figure 4.16 An example of nervous tissue (Tortora and Derrickson 2009)

other events. However, the tissue types have differing success rates. Because epithelial cells have to withstand large amounts of wear and tear they have great capacity for renewal. Epithelial tissue often contains immature cells called **stem cells**, which can divide and replace lost cells easily. Most connective tissue also has great capacity for renewal, however due to the lack of blood supply cartilage can take a long time to heal.

Muscle and nervous tissue by comparison have poor regeneration properties. Skeletal muscle and smooth muscle fibres divide very slowly and mitosis does not occur in cardiac muscle tissue.

Stem cells migrate from blood to the heart where they divide and produce a small number of new cardiac muscle fibres. Nervous tissue does not normally undergo mitosis to replace damaged neurones.

Tissue repair involves the proliferation of new cells, which stem from cell division in the parenchyma (tissue cells/organ cells) or from the stroma (supporting connective tissue). The replenishing of tissue by parenchymal and stroma cells is called **regeneration**. If parenchymal cells are solely responsible for tissue repair, then a near-perfect regeneration may occur. If fibroblasts from stroma are involved in tissue repair, new connective tissue is generated to replace the damaged tissue. This new connective tissue, primarily consisting of collagen, is referred to as **scar tissue**. The process of scar tissue generation is called **fibrosis**. Unlike cells regenerated from parenchymal cells, scar tissue cells are not designed to perform the original functions of the damaged cells. Therefore any organ or structure with scar tissue will have impaired function.

In open or large wounds **granulation** occurs. Granulation describes the formation of granulation tissue, which covers the healing tissue and secretes bacterial fluid. During this process both parenchymal and stroma cells are active in the repair. Fibroblasts provide new collagen tissue to strengthen the area and new blood capillaries sprout new buds and bring the necessary nutrients to the area.

Clinical considerations

Diabetic foot ulcers

Between 12% and 25% of diabetic patients develop leg and foot ulcers. This is because diabetes can cause macroangiopathy, which obstructs blood flow in large arteries. The slower flow of blood through the arteries in legs results in the development of leg and foot ulcers. Diabetic patients also experience lengthy recovery times from leg and foot injuries. The lack of bloodflow also reduces the tissue's ability to fight off infection. Diabetic patients are therefore at increased risk of developing gangrene and amputation.

(Cavanagh *et al.* 2005; Gould 2006)

Conclusion

All human cells can be categorised into four classifications: epithelial tissue, connective tissue, muscle tissue and nervous tissue. Epithelial tissue covers or lines structures and organs. It specialises in absorption, secretion, protection, excretion, filtration and sensory reception. Almost every substance that passes in and out of the body travels through epithelial tissue. Connective tissue not only connects tissues it also protects, supports and insulates them. Connective tissue is dense and strong; examples include cartilage and bone. Muscle tissue provides movement and posture, whereas nervous tissue forms the major part of the nervous system. Tissue has the ability to regenerate and renew itself, however epithelial and connective tissue have a greater capacity for repair than other tissues.

Glossary

Abdominopelvic cavity: Body cavity that encompasses the abdominal and pelvic cavities. The abdominal cavity contains the stomach, intestines, spleen, liver and other associated digestive organs. The pelvic cavity contains the bladder and some reproductive organs.

Apical surface: Surface of body organ that faces outwards, towards the surface.

Avascular: Structure that does not contain blood vessels.

Basal surface: Surface that forms the base of a body organ.

Cartilage: Strong form of connective tissue which contains a dense network of collagen and elastic fibres.

Chyme: A fluid substance consisting of partially digested food and digestive enzymes, which is found travelling through the digestive tract.

Connective tissue: Tissue that binds, reinforces, insulates, protects and supports structures.

Diffusion: The movement of particles from areas of high concentration to low concentration.

Endocrine gland: Glands that release hormones.

Epithelial tissue: Tissue that lines or covers body surfaces.

Exocrine glands: Glands that secrete their products externally, i.e. mucus, sweat.

Extracellular matrix: A collection of largely non-living substances that separate the living cells of connective tissue.

Gland: A structure that manufactures a product, i.e. hormones, mucus, sweat, etc.

Glycoproteins: Special proteins that contain simple sugar chains. Glycoproteins play an important role in cell-to-cell communication.

Hormones: Regulatory chemicals released by endocrine glands for use elsewhere in the body. i.e. thyroxine, insulin.

Innervated (innervate): Stimulated by nerve cells.

Interstitial fluid: The fluid which bathes cells.

Keratin: A special tough fibrous protein found in skin.

Lymph nodes: Small lymphatic structures that filter lymphatic fluid.

Macrophages:	White blood cells that specialise in the destruction and consumption of invading pathogens.
Membrane:	A sheet of tissue that covers or lines an area of the body.
Mitosis:	The division and replication of cells.
Neuroglia:	Cells of the nervous system that support and nourish neurons.
Neurone:	A nerve fibre.
Parenchyma:	The cells that constitute the function part of an organ.
Prophylactic antibiotics:	Antibiotics prescribed to prevent infection.
Oocytes:	Female reproductive cell.
Spleen:	Large lymph organ, responsible for production of lymphocytes, immune response and the cleansing of blood.
Stroma:	The internal framework of an organ.
Subcutaneous:	Underneath the skin.
Vertebrae:	The disc-shaped bones that make up the spinal column.

References

Allibone, L. (2003) Nursing management of chest drains. *Nursing Standard* 17(22):45–54.

Cavanagh, P.R., Lipsky, B.A., Bradbury, A.W. and Botek, G. (2005) Treatment for diabetic foot ulcers. *Lancet* 366:1725–1735.

Gould, B.E. (2006) *Pathophysiology for the Health Professions*, 3rd edn. Philadelphia: Saunders Elsevier.

Jenkins, G.W., Kemnitz, C.P. and Tortora, G.J. (2007) *Anatomy and Physiology from Science to Life.* Hoboken, NJ: John Wiley & Sons.

Lawrence, K.R., Adra, M. and Schwaitzberg, S.D. (2003) An overview of the pathophysiology and treatment of secondary peritonitis. *Formulary* 38:102–111.

Marieb, E. and Hoehn, K. (2008) *Human Anatomy and Physiology*, 8th edn. San Francisco: Pearson Benjamin Cummings.

Ryan, B. (2005) Pneumothorax assessment and diagnostic testing. *Journal of Cardiovascular Nursing* 20(4):251–253.

Tortora, G.J. and Derrickson, B.H. (2009) *Principles of Anatomy and Physiology*, 12th edn. Hoboken, NJ: John Wiley & Sons.

Activities

www.wiley.com/go/peate

Multiple choice questions

1. Which of the following epithelial tissue has a single layer of square-shaped cells?
   (a) pseudostratified columnar epithelium
   (b) ciliated simple columnar epithelium
   (c) simple cuboidal epithelium
   (d) stratified cuboidal epithelium

2. Which of the following is not a function of simple epithelium?
   (a) protection
   (b) secretion
   (c) absorption
   (d) filtration

3. What is the primary function of transitional epithelium?
   (a) absorption
   (b) stretch
   (c) secretion
   (d) protection

4. Which fibres ensure that connective tissue is strong and tough?
   (a) collagen fibres
   (b) reticular fibres
   (c) elastic fibres
   (d) plasma fibres

5. Which of the following connective tissues is found in heart valves?
   (a) areolar tissue
   (b) dense irregular connective tissue
   (c) dense regular connective tissue
   (d) reticular tissue

6. Which of the following statements on cartilage is true?

(a) Fibrocartilage contains the most elastic fibres
(b) Hyaline cartilage is found within the ears
(c) Elastic cartilage is the most abundant in the human body
(d) The weakest cartilage tissue is hyaline cartilage

7. Blood is an example of ____________ connective tissue.

(a) liquid
(b) loose
(c) avascular
(d) dense

8. Which of the following areas does not contain mucous membranes?

(a) the urinary tract
(b) the respiratory system
(c) the pericardium
(d) the digestive tract

9. Smooth muscle is both

(a) involuntary and striated
(b) involuntary and non-striated
(c) voluntary and striated
(d) voluntary and non-striated

10. Scar tissue is generated by

(a) fibroblasts
(b) osteoclasts
(c) stem cells
(d) parenchymal cells

Test your learning

1. What types of simple epithelial tissue are found in the lining of the following structures?
   (a) the respiratory tract
   (b) the fallopian tubes
   (c) the small intestine
   (d) the kidney tubules.
2. Explain why connective tissues such as bone and cartilage can sustain great tension.
3. Describe the structure and location of cartilage within the body.
4. List the major types of membrane and their locations.
5. Describe how connective and epithelial tissue may repair itself after surgery.

Label the diagram

From the lists of words, label the diagrams below:

Arrangement of layers, Simple, Pseudostratified, Stratified, Basement membrane, Cell shape, Squamous, Cuboidal, Colunmar, Basement membrane

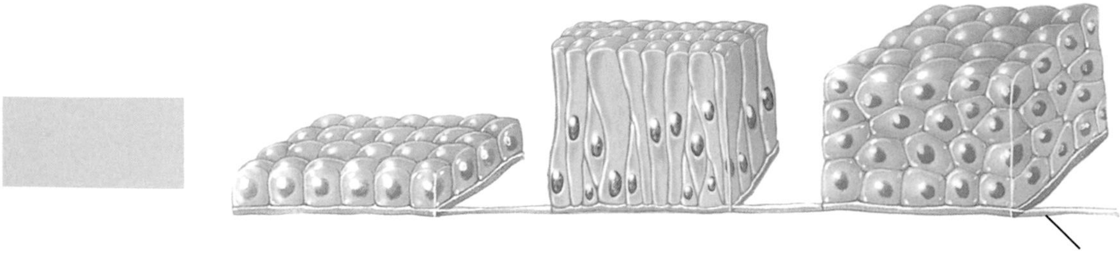

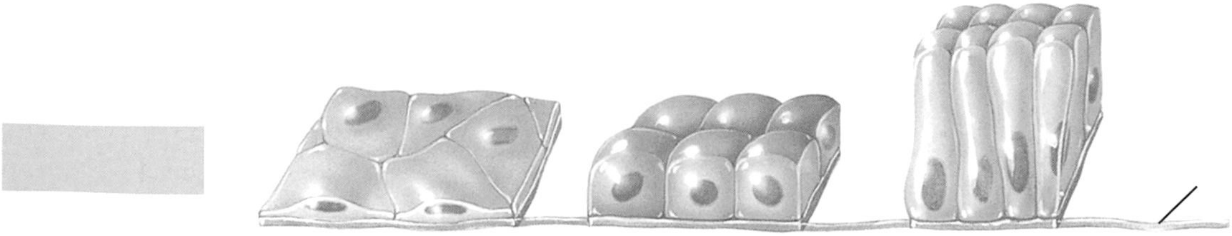

Duct, Secretory portion, Simple tubular, Simple branched tubular, Compound tubular, Simple branched acinar, Compound acinar, Compound tubuloacinar

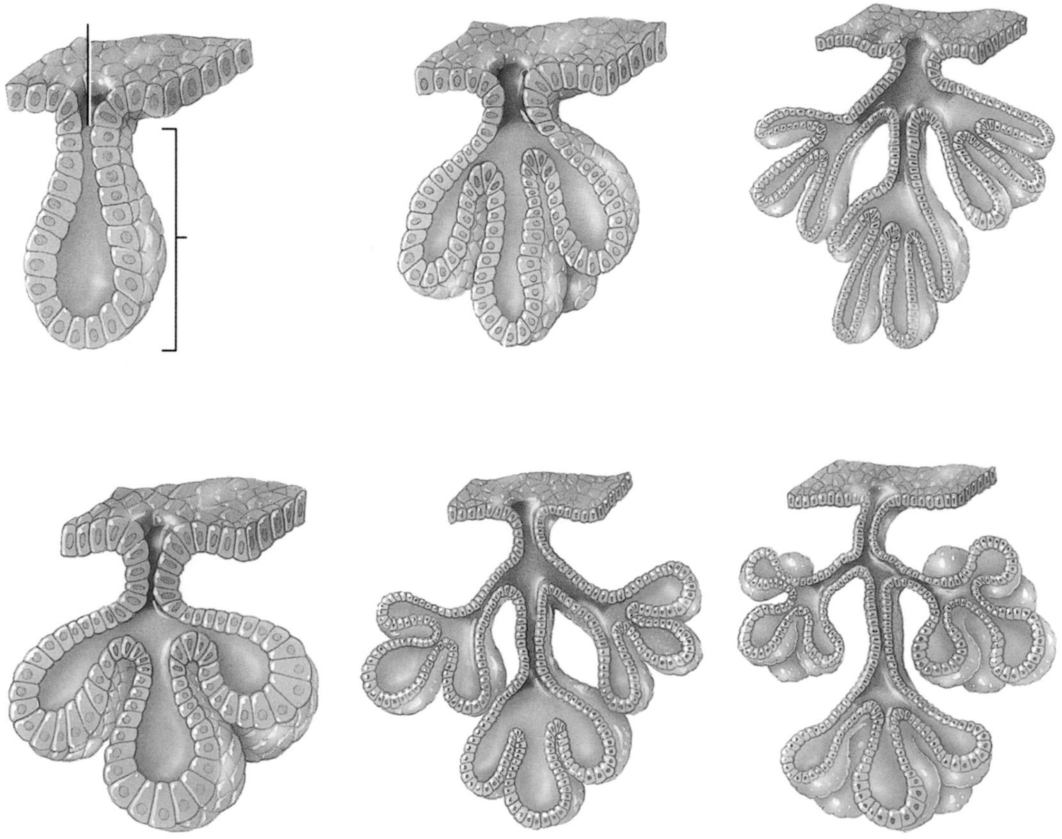

Crossword

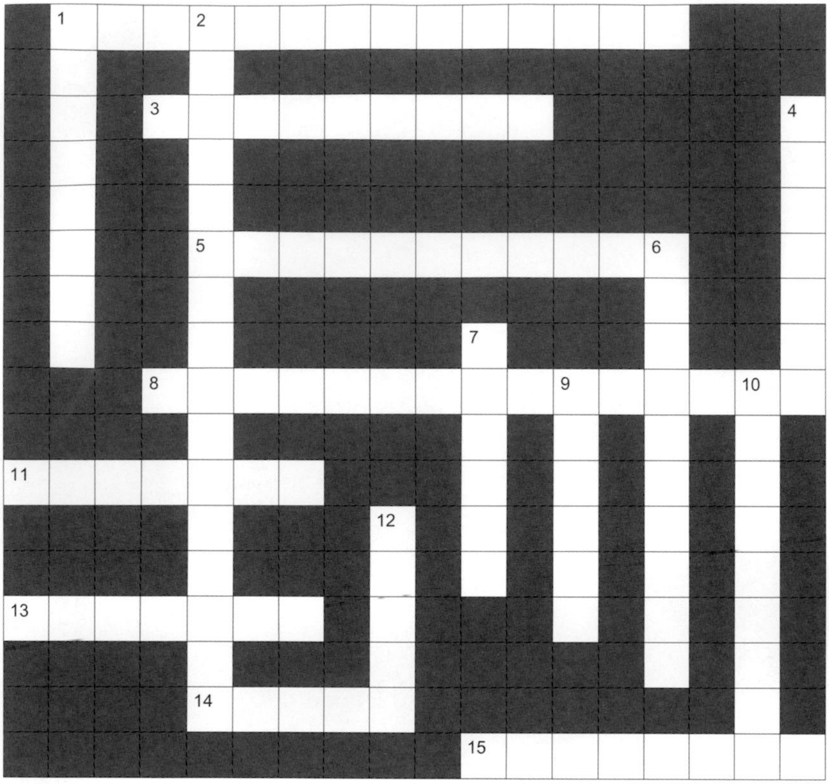
1
2
3
4
5
6
7
8
9
10
11
12
13
14
15

Across:

1. Epithelial tissue that consists of a single layer of square shaped cells (6, 8).
3. Type of loose connective tissue (9).
5. Bone cells (11).
8. Forms a substantial part of the extracellular matrix (6, 9).
11. Type of dense connective tissue (7).
13. Most abundant type of cartilage (7).
14. ______ connective tissue can be regular, or irregular (5).
15. Major constituent of bone (8).

Down:

1. Type of muscle (8).
2. Word that describes single-layered epithelial tissue that contains different shaped cells (16).
4. Fat tissue (7).
6. Word used to describe multilayered epithelial tissue (10).
7. _______ membranes have wet or moist surfaces (6).
9. _______ membranes cover organs that lie within a cavity (6).
10. Type of connective tissue that is avascular (9).
12. Areolar is an example of which type of connective tissue (5).

Answers

MCQs

1c; 2a; 3b; 4a; 5b; 6d; 7a; 8c; 9b; 10a

Crossword

Across

1. Simple cuboidal
3. Reticular
5. Osteoclasts
8. Ground Substance
11. Elastic
13. Hyaline
14. Dense
15. Collagen

Down

1. Skeletal
2. Pseudostratified
4. Adipose
6. Stratified
7. Mucous
9. Serous
10. Cartilage
12. Loose

5 The skin

Ian Peate

Contents

Introduction	*132*
The structure of skin	**132**
The epidermis	**132**
Keratinocytes	133
Melanocytes	133
Langerhans cells	133
Merkel cells	133
Stratum basale	134
Stratum spinosum	135
Stratum granulosum	135
Stratum lucidum	136
Stratum corneum	136
The dermis	**137**
The papillary and reticular aspects	138
The accessory skin structures	**139**
The hair	139
Skin glands	**140**
Eccrine glands	140
Apocrine glands	141
Nails	**141**
The functions of the skin	**142**
Sensation	143
Thermoregulation	143
Protection	143
Excretion and absorption	144
Synthesis of vitamin D	145
Conclusion	*145*
Glossary	*146*
References	*147*
Activities	*148*

Test your knowledge

- Name the layers of the skin.
- Describe the role of the skin in health.
- What are three key functions of the skin?

Fundamentals of Anatomy and Physiology for Student Nurses, First Edition. Edited by Ian Peate, Muralitharan Nair.

- How does the skin provide or help to provide the body with various defence mechanisms?
- Why is ultraviolet light sometimes harmful to the skin?
- What is the role of the skin in relation to thermoregulation?
- Discuss skin changes as the body ages.
- What is melanin?
- How does skin regenerate?
- How does pigment add to skin colour?

Learning outcomes

After reading this chapter you will be able to:

- Discuss the anatomy and physiology of the skin
- Describe the various functions of the skin
- Discuss the structure and growth of the appendages
- Explain how the skin functions as a homeostatic mechanism
- Outline the factors that determine skin colour

Body map

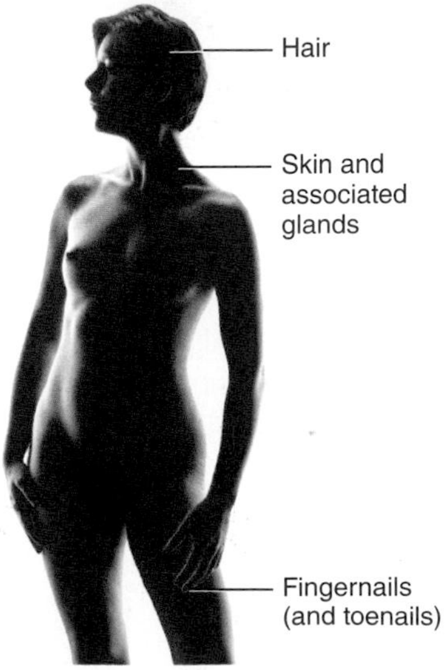
Hair
Skin and associated glands
Fingernails (and toenails)

Introduction

The skin, sometimes referred to as the integumentary system, protects the body in a number of ways; without skin and its protective mechanisms the human being would not survive. The skin is often the only organ of the body that is on show all of the time, and because of this the skin can reveal how we feel emotionally, for example, we may blush. It can also reveal how we are from a physiological perspective, for example, it can appear cyanosed. The skin is the organ that is the most commonly exposed to disease or infection. The skin is almost entirely waterproof.

The skin has a number of homeostatic elements, for example, it can regulate body temperature and is often spoken of as the skin with appendages. The appendages are modifications of the skin. LeMone and Burke (2009) suggest that the average adult has 2 m^2 of skin, which weighs approximately 4.1 kg. The skin is twice as heavy as the brain. There are about 4.5 m of blood vessels, 3.6 m of nerves, 2.6 million sweat glands, 1500 sensory receptors and over 3 million cells that are continuously dying and being replaced. The skin receives nearly one third of all blood that flows through the body (Rizzo 2006).

The skin plays a vital role in health and wellbeing. Any disturbance in skin can lead to physical and or psychological problems and this in turn has the ability to impact on a person's quality of life. Just as a house needs bricks and mortar to act as a framework, the house would be of little value if it were not waterproof. Using this analogy, the house also needs shelter from the environment and in the human this job is carried out by the skin. The skin provides a defensive barrier defending the body from the elements and safeguards against pathogens, it also offers a number of other functions. The skin is made up of a superficial epidermis and a deeper structure called the dermis. Prior to discussing the functions of the skin the next section will outline the structure of the skin.

The structure of skin

According to Shier *et al.* (2009) the skin is one of the more versatile organs of the body. The skin is composed of two distinct regions: the dermis and the epidermis. The subcutaneous facia (sometimes referred to as the hypodermis) lies under the dermis (Colbert *et al.* 2007), these masses of loose connective and adipose tissue attach to the skin and organs beneath; they are not part of the skin.

The epidermis

The superficial and thinnest aspect of the skin, the epidermis is the area of skin that can most commonly be seen. Whilst the skin covers the whole of the body there are several regional distinctions and these are associated with flexibility, distribution and type of hair, density and types of gland, pigmentation, vascularity, innervations and thickness (Jenkins *et al.* 2010). The thinnest part of the skin can be found on the eyelids; here it is just 0.5 mm in thickness whereas at the heel it is 4.0 mm thick.

The epidermis is made up epithelium, called keratinised stratified squamous epithelium, and contains four key cell types, these are:

- Keratinocytes
- Melanocytes

- Langerhans cells
- Merkel cells.

Keratinocytes

These cells are organised in four layers. They are responsible for producing a protein called keratin. Keratin is a tough, fibrous protein which aids in the protection of the skin and tissues below from the heat, micro-organisms and chemicals. The keratinocytes are also responsible for the production of the water-resistant properties of the skin, and act as a type of sealant that reduces water entry as well as water loss; they also prevent the entry of foreign matter.

Melanocytes

The developing embryo produces the pigment melanin from the melanocytes. Melanocytes are most profuse in the epidermis of the penis, nipples, the areola, face and limbs. Melanocytes have long, slender projections that extend between the keratinocytes and have the ability to transfer melanin granules. Melanocytes are cells which produce a pigment called melanin. Melanin is responsible for the natural colour of a person's skin and it helps to defend it from the damaging effects of the sun.

When skin has been exposed to a great deal of sun the melanocytes multiply the quantity of melanin in order to absorb more ultraviolet rays. This activity makes the skin darker, giving it a suntanned appearance. A suntan indicates that the skin has been harmed and is attempting to defend itself.

All people have about the same number of melanocytes, those people with brown or black skin have the same number of melanocytes but they make more of the pigment melanin; it is the amount of melanin produced and how it is distributed that results in a variation of skin colour. These people have more natural protection from the harmful ultraviolet rays of the sun. Moles (sometimes called naevi) are a group or a cluster of melanocytes that lie close together. The majority of people with white skin have approximately 10–50 moles on their skin.

Langerhans cells

These cells are part of the immune system and arise from the red bone marrow (see Chapter 8, The skeletal system, for a discussion on the red bone marrow) these cells migrate from the bone marrow to the epidermis, and make up a small part of the epidermal cells. The Langerhans cells regulate immune reactions in the skin as a defence against micro-organisms that invade it (Lewis and Roberts 2009); these cells are very fragile when exposed to the sun.

The Langerhans cells process microbial antigens (they help to stimulate lymphocytes); their role is to assist other cells of the immune system in response to and recognition of micro-organisms and destroy the invading microbes.

Merkel cells

A Merkel cell has the ability to have contact with a flattened process of a sensory neurone (a synaptic contact), this is a structure called a tactile disc (sometimes this is called a Merkel disc). The Merkel cells and the tactile discs (the least numerous of cells on the epidermis) are capable of detecting touch sensations (Tortora and Derrickson 2009).

Figures 5.1 (a), (b), (c) and (d) demonstrates the types of cells in the epidermis.

Just as there are two distinct layers of skin – the dermis and epidermis – there are also a number of distinct layers of keratinocytes. These layers are developed over time and form the epidermis. These layers are called strata and are microscopically visible (see Figure 5.2).

The superficial and deeper levels of the skin are:

- Stratum basale
- Stratum spinosum
- Stratum granulosum
- Stratum lucidum
- Stratum corneum.

Clinical considerations

Personal hygiene

One of the most important aspects of the role and function of the nurse is to help persons to wash themselves when they are unable to do so. Washing is often seen as a basic nursing task but, as Hemming (2010) points out, this is a skilled activity and requires much thought and assessment of the person being cared for.

Understanding the anatomy and physiology of the skin and the complexities associated with this body system can help you to help the people you care for. When helping a person to maintain personal hygiene you should ensure that you use soaps and other toiletries that will not damage or potentially damage skin integrity. This will include ensuring that the person is not allergic to any of the products that have been chosen to wash and cleanse the skin. As far as is possible you should always ask the person if they are allergic to any toiletries or other skin products as some people are allergic to some of the chemicals found in soaps and cleansing products. This element of care provision requires you to be able to assess an individual's needs.

You should bear in mind that when using some kinds of soap this can have the same effect on the skin as swimming in the sea, the lather worked up by the soap when it is on the skin has a higher concentration and this can then draw out water from the epidermis. The product that has been chosen to clean the skin may have a harmful effect on the person's skin and can potentially lead to the development of some skin conditions, for example, dermatitis and eczema.

Stratum basale

The stratum basale rests on the basement membrane and is the deepest layer of the epidermis; this layer provides a definite border between the dermis and epidermis. This is made up of a single row of columnar kerinocytes. The cells (stem cells or mother cells) of the epidermis originate from this deep layer. New cells are being constantly produced, they are continually dividing (the

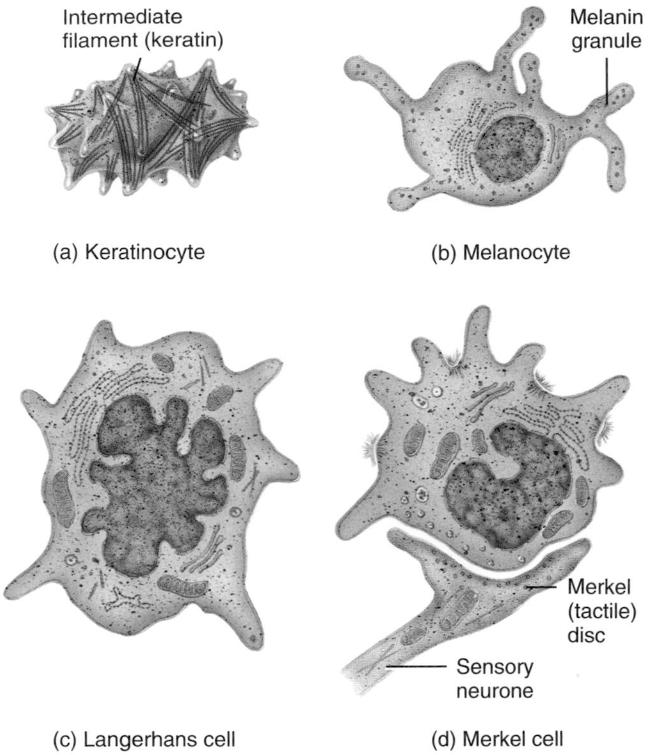
Intermediate filament (keratin)
Melanin granule
(a) Keratinocyte
(b) Melanocyte
Merkel (tactile) disc
Sensory neurone
(c) Langerhans cell
(d) Merkel cell

Figure 5.1 The types of cells in the epidermis (Tortora and Derrickson 2009)

constant regeneration of the skin), slowly pushing older cells (called daughter cells) up through the other layers of the epidermis until they reach the surface.

Stratum spinosum

Above the stratum basale lies the stratum spinosum. The keratinocytes in this layer have spine-like projections (spinosum means thorn-like or prickly). The keratinocytes are tightly packed here. This tight packing arrangement provides strength and flexibility to the skin.

Stratum granulosum

As the layers move towards the superficial level the next layer is the stratum granulosum. There are between three and five layers of flattened keratinocytes in this aspect of the skin. These cells contain granules (hence the name stratum granulosum), form a water-resistant lipid (lamellar granules), protect the body from losing excess fluid and at the same time guard against the entry of microbes. The flattening of the cells occurs as a result of pressure from below. The cells here undergo apoptosis; they lose their nucleus prior to dying, becoming compact and brittle as they

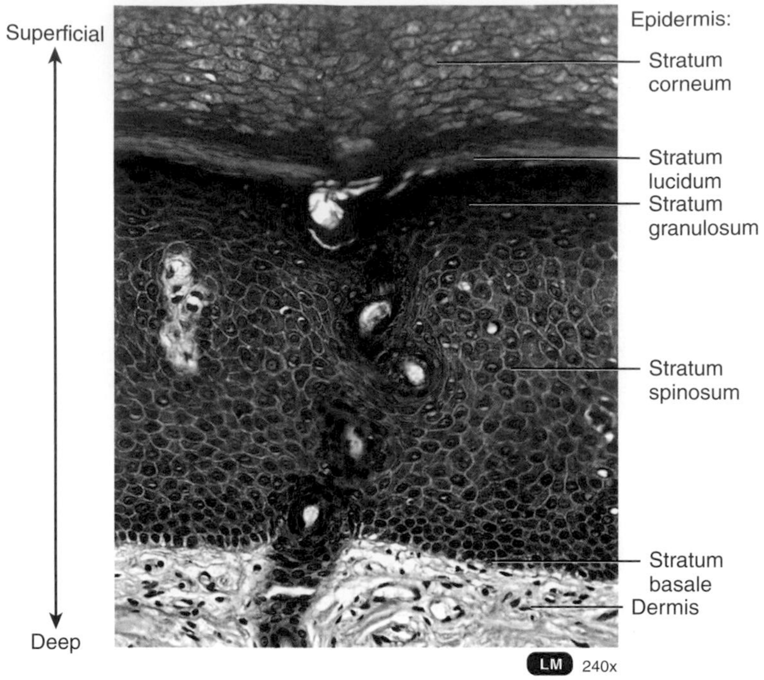
Superficial
Deep
Epidermis:
Stratum corneum
Stratum lucidum
Stratum granulosum
Stratum spinosum
Stratum basale
Dermis
LM 240x

Figure 5.2 A microscopic perspective of the skin with the various strata (Tortora and Derrickson 2009)

move slowly up towards the surface; this process is known as keratinisation. The skin is now becoming tougher and stronger, getting ready to perform its protective function. This layer lies below the stratum lucidum.

Stratum lucidum

Lying below the stratum corneum is the stratum lucidum, also known as the clear layer. There are five layers of flat dead cells here; this layer is not found on all aspects of the body, only on areas of thick skin, for example, the heels. The cells have no nucleus and are tightly packed, providing a barrier to fluid loss.

Stratum corneum

This is the outer layer of the epidermis and is made up of a number (about 25) of scale-like layers that are dead and overlap with each other; the chief component of these dead cells is keratin, most of the fluid within these cells has been lost. The cells of the lower layers are composed of approximately 70% water whereas this layer is made up of 20% fluid (Rizzo 2006). These cells are very tough and horny. The surface is covered in lipids which provide a protective barrier; this layer provides structural strength. Constant friction means that this layer is being continuously rubbed off (sloughed off).

Table 5.1 The layers of the epidermis

Layer	Location	Description
Stratum basale (sometimes called the basal cell layer)	The deepest layer	Cuboidal cells that are arranged as a single row which divide and grow. The stratum basale also contains melanocytes
Stratum spinosum	Above the stratum basale and below the stratum granulosum	These keratinocytes are tightly packed, flat and have spine-like projections
Stratum granulosum	Under the stratum corneum	Flattened cells arranged in approximately 3 to 5 layers. Protects the body from losing fluid and also protects from harm. Compact brittle cells as they lose their nucleus.
Stratum lucidum	When present, situated between the stratum corneum and the stratum granulosum	These cells are not present on the soles and palms. The cells have no nucleus and are tightly packed
Stratum corneum	The most superficial of layers	Several layers of keratinised, dead epithelial cells. These cells are flattened and have no nucleus

There are other important functions associated with this layer and these are in relation to a physical barrier to light and heat waves, micro-organisms, chemicals and injury. The stratum corneum becomes thicker when it is exposed to strong sunlight, providing a barrier to ultraviolet rays. If the ultraviolet rays do reach the dermis, they will destroy the protein content of the skin and this can lead to cancer of skin. Table 5.1 provides an overview of the layers of the epidermis.

The dermis

The deepest part of the skin is called the dermis and lies directly below the epidermis; it is predominantly composed of dense connective tissue which contains collagen and elastic fibres. Embedded within the dermis are:

- Blood vessels
- Nerves
- Lymph vessels
- Smooth muscles
- Sweat glands
- Hair follicles
- Sebaceous glands.

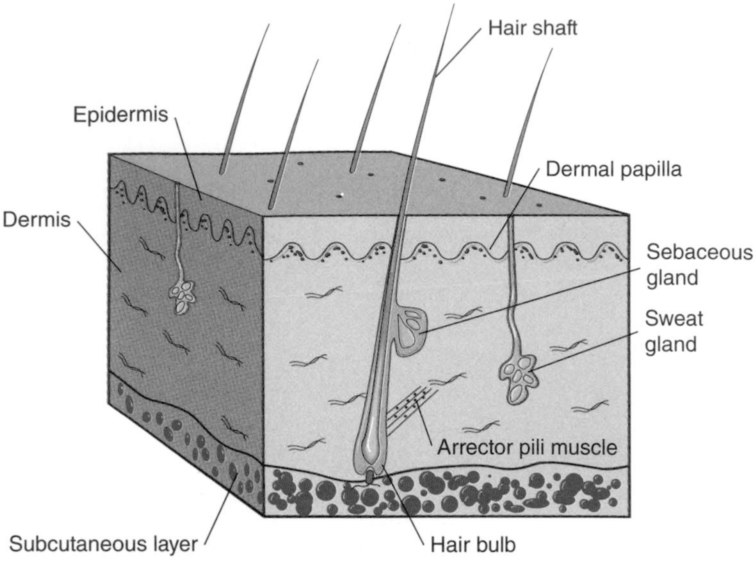
Hair shaft
Epidermis
Dermal papilla
Dermis
Sebaceous gland
Sweat gland
Arrector pili muscle
Subcutaneous layer
Hair bulb

Figure 5.3 Three layers of skin: the epidermis, the dermis and subcutaneous layer (Nair and Peate 2009)

The elastic system associated with the dermis supports the components above, as well as allowing the skin to flex with movement made and to return to its normal shape when at rest. The dermis can be divided into two layers:

- The papillary aspect
- The reticular aspect.

The surface area of the dermis is much increased as a result of the projectile-like papillary layers; the papillary layers connect the dermis to the epidermis. The fingerprints arise from this layer. The deeper aspect of the dermis is attached to the subcutaneous layer. Figure 5.3 shows the epidermis, the dermis and the subcutaneous layer.

The papillary and reticular aspects

This aspect of the dermis, according to Tortora and Derrickson (2009), accounts for one fifth of the total dermal layer, the superficial layer. The ridges caused by the papillary aspect are also known as friction ridges. These friction ridges can help the hand or foot grasp by increasing friction.

There is a capillary network within the papillary aspect. The dermal papillae also contain Meissner's corpuscles, and these are tactile receptors or touch receptors. The nerve endings here are sensitive to touch, as well as to sensations associated with warmth, coolness, pain and itching.

Attached to the subcutaneous layer are irregular, dense, connective tissues containing fibroblasts and collagen bundles, and coarse elastic fibre forms the reticular aspect. Other sensory receptors are found in this layer, for example, the Pacinian receptors for deep sensory pressure.

This layer also contains sweat glands, lymph vessels, smooth muscle and hair follicles; these are called the accessory structures and are discussed next.

The accessory skin structures

The accessory structures are also known as the appendages. The following accessory structures of the skin will be outlined in this section of the chapter:

- Hair
- Skin glands
- Nails.

The hair

Hair can be found on most surfaces of the body apart from the palms, soles and lips; the amount, its distribution, the colour and texture differ depending on location, gender, age and ethnic group. There are different types of hair and the earliest type is distinctive at approximately the fifth month of foetal development. Known as lanugo, it is a very fine, downy, non-pigmented hair and covers the body of the foetus. Just prior to birth the lanugo of the eyelashes, eyebrows and scalp is shed and this is replaced by coarse hair, longer in length and heavily pigmented.

The hair can play a part in a person's distinctive appearance. The colour of the hair is influenced by the melanocytes that are found within the hair bulb. A progressive decline in melanin results in hair that is grey in colour. Hair growth is determined by genetic and hormonal factors.

Hairs are growths of dead keratin; each hair is a thread of keratin and is formed from cells at the base of a single follicle (Timby 2005). There are a number of functions associated with hair:

- Sexual
- Social
- Thermoregulation
- Protection.

The primary role of hair is to inhibit heat loss. The whole of the skin surface has hair follicles; every pore is an opening to a follicle and these are located deep in the dermis on top of the subcutaneous layer. When heat leaves the body through the skin, it becomes trapped in the air between the hairs. Each gland has attached to it a small collection of smooth muscle known as the arrector pili. These muscles contract and become erect in response to cold, fear and emotion. The contraction of the muscle can be seen on the skin in the form of 'goose bumps'.

Hair on the head can protect the scalp from the damaging effects of the sun. The hair on the eyelashes and eyebrows guards the eyes from foreign particles entering and the hair situated in the nostrils help to protect against the inhalation of foreign material, for example, insects.

Sebaceous glands accompany the hair follicles and sebum (a liquid substance) is exuded by these glands, supplying lubrication to the skin and at the same time ensuring that the skin and hair are waterproof as well as removing waste, for example, old dead cells. Sebum is a slightly acidic substance and has antibacterial and antifungal properties (Page 2006). The distribution of the sebaceous glands differs. They are foremost on the scalp, face, upper torso and anogenital region and these glands are at their most active during puberty. Lawton (2006) and Page (2006) point out that the manufacture of sebum is influenced by sex hormone levels. Figure 5.4 shows

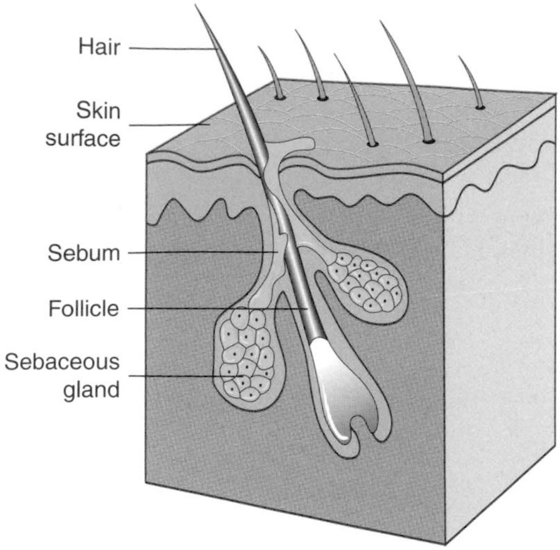
Hair
Skin surface
Sebum
Follicle
Sebaceous gland

Figure 5.4 A pilosebaceous unit (Nair and Peate 2009)

a pilosebaceous unit; this is made up of the follicle, the hair shaft, the sebaceous gland and the arrector pili. The base of the onion-shaped bulb – the follicle – contains blood vessels, providing nourishment for the developing hair.

Skin glands

There are a number of glands located within the skin; these can be thought of as mini-organs of the skin, which have a number of functions to fulfil. The sweat glands are coiled tubes composed of epithelial tissue and open out to pores that are located on the skin surface (see Figure 5.5). All of the glands have separate nerve and blood supplies; each secretes a slightly acidic fluid made up of water and salts.

There are two sorts of sweat gland: eccrine and apocrine.

Eccrine glands

Reaction to heat and fear and the production of secretions by the eccrine glands occur in response to activity of the sympathetic nervous system. These two types of gland are located all over the body; there are however sites on the body where they are more numerous, for example, the forehead, axillae, soles and palms. The primary function of the eccrine glands is associated with thermoregulation. This is accomplished through the cooling effect of the evaporation of sweat on the surface of the skin. During hot weather, stress, exercise and pyrexia these glands produce more sweat.

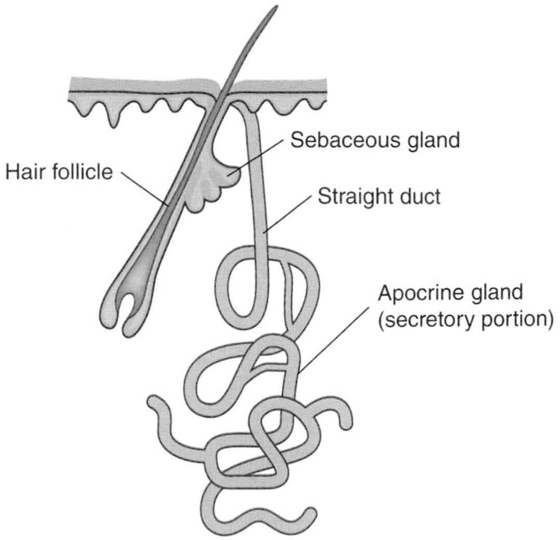
Sebaceous gland
Hair follicle
Straight duct
Apocrine gland
(secretory portion)

Figure 5.5 A sweat gland (Nair and Peate 2009)

Apocrine glands

The apocrine glands are also coiled; there are not as many of these in comparison to the eccrine glands and they are found in more localised sites, for example, the pubic and axillary areas, the nipples and perineum. The exact function of the apocrine glands is not fully understood. These glands are not fully active until the person reaches puberty; they are larger, deeper and produce thicker secretions than the eccrine glands. During periods of stress and when in a heightened emotional state these glands produce more sweat.

There are a number of modified types of apocrine glands (specialised types), for example, those that are seen on the eyelids, the cerumen-producing (ear wax) glands of the external auditory canal; and the milk-producing glands of the breasts.

The apocrine glands first develop on the soles and palms and then gradually appear all over the body. It is understood that they secrete pheromones; these are released into the external environment enabling communication through the sense of smell with other members of the species and this can provoke a number of reactions, including a sexual arousal reaction. A viscous material is excreted which results in body odour when activated by surface bacteria.

Nails

The nails provide a protective covering for the ends of the fingers and the toes. Nails are tightly packed, dead, hard, keratinised epidermal cells that form a clean, solid covering over the digits (see Figure 5.6).

The horn-like structure of the nails is a result of the concentrated amount of keratin present; there are no nerve endings in nails. Lawton (2006) notes that the nails act as a counterforce to the fingertips, the fingertips have numerous nerve endings, permitting a person to receive information about objects that are touched.

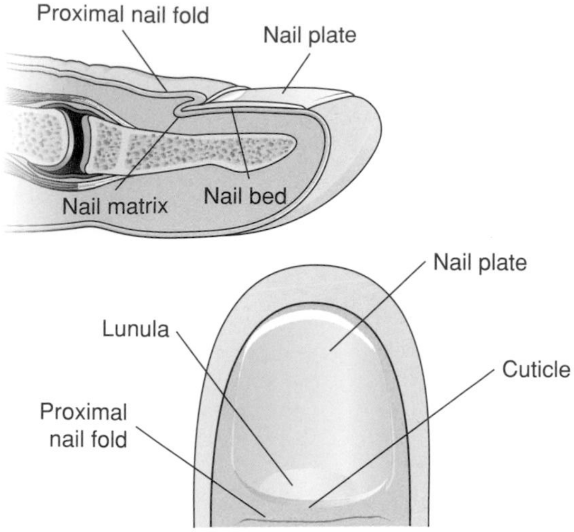
Proximal nail fold
Nail plate
Nail matrix
Nail bed
Nail plate
Lunula
Cuticle
Proximal
nail fold

Figure 5.6 The nail (Nair and Peate 2009)

The majority of the nail body is pink and this is a result of the blood capillaries lying underneath. The white crescent present at the proximal ends of the nail is known as the lunula and is formed by air mixed with keratin matrix. The size of the lunula varies with individuals. The cuticle (also called the eponychium) is stratum corneum extending over the proximal end of the nail body.

Fingernails grow faster than toenails; as a person ages the growth of nails slows. Nail growth varies, on average they grow at a rate of 00.1 cm per day (1 cm per 100 days). Four to six months is required for fingernails to regrow completely; it takes toenails between 12 and 18 months for total regrowth. There are a number of factors that will influence the growth, for example, the age of the individual, the time of year, the amount of exercise undertaken, as well as hereditary factors (Haneke 2006). The growth of nails can be delayed by trauma and inflammation; changes in the integrity of the nails can be caused by injury or infection. In some cases evidence of systemic diseases can be identified by the condition of the nails, for example, chronic cardiopulmonary disease or fungal infection (Timby 2005).

The functions of the skin

A fundamental understanding of the structure of the skin allows the reader to begin to understand the numerous functions of the skin. These functions include:

- Sensation
- Thermoregulation
- Protection
- Excretion and absorption
- Synthesis of vitamin D.

Sensation

There are several receptor sites on the skin which have the ability to sense change in the external environment in respect to temperature and pressure; these receptors throughout the skin are made up of a wide and varied range of nerve ending. The messages picked up in the skin are then usually transferred to the brain. Chapter 16 of this text considers the senses in more detail.

Sensations that arise in the skin are known as cutaneous sensations; other sensations are those associated with vibration and tickling and irritations. There are some areas of the body that have more sensory receptors than others, for example, the lips, genitalia and tips of the fingers. The sensation of pain can signify actual or potential tissue injury.

Thermoregulation

The skin has a role to play in homeostasis through thermoregulation, helping to keep the temperature of the body within narrow ranges, adapting and adjusting as a person engages in a number of different activities. Effective thermoregulation is essential for survival; temperature changes can influence alteration in enzyme function and as such can impact on the chemical makeup of cells. The skin acts as a temperature regulator through a range of complex and integrated activities.

Changes in the size of blood vessels in the skin can help to regulate temperature. As body temperature rises so the blood vessels dilate – this is known as vasodilation; this is a multifaceted bodily defence mechanism that is attempting to get hot blood from the deeper tissues beneath to the surface of the skin for cooling down: the surface of the skin is cooler, as heat radiates away from the body. As this is happening the sweat glands secrete water onto the surface of the skin. Evaporation occurs and as a result of this so too does cooling.

The opposite will occur when the person is in a cold environment. The blood vessels constrict – vasoconstriction – and blood stays closer to the core of the body preserving heat.

The hair (as previously described) plays an important part in thermoregulation. Pockets of air are trapped in the hair when the arrector pili are stimulated to contract, making the hairs stand up. The trapped air causes insulation to occur, insulating the surrounding environment on the skin from the cooler atmosphere.

Protection

There are many ways in which the skin protects the body and a number of these have already been discussed, for example, the skin's ability to protect by the production of melanin against the harmful effects of UV light. Through its ability to intensify normal cell replacement when needed and the ability to shed dead skin and cause the migration of cells, the skin maintains the integrity of the body. Wound healing is an example of the skin's protective mechanism.

By eliminating waste products through the pores on the skin (and there are over 2 million of these), the skin can help to protect the body from a buildup of poisonous substances. The skin also has the ability to prevent body fluids from escaping, preventing dehydration and helping to regulate the amount of fluid through the content and volume of sweat produced. As a waterproof barrier the skin can also ensure that harmful fluids in the environment are prevented from entering the body.

Clinical considerations

Dehydration

Many people in a number of care environments are prone to dehydration. The older person is particularly at risk and your role is to prevent and to identify dehydration and to take actions to remedy any deficits; you will be required to assess, plan, implement and evaluate care.

Performing a safe and effective assessment of needs will require you to use a number of skills: you will be required to observe, measure and ask questions (Sibson 2010). The skin can tell you much about the people you care for. You can make a diagnosis of dehydration by observing the skin of those in your care, although this is not and should not be used as the sole diagnostic tool. The classic signs of dehydration in older people include loss of skin recoil (also described as loss of skin turgor), increased thirst, reduced urinary output, tachycardia and hypotension; the person may also be confused.

The skin may lack its normal elasticity and revert to its usual position slowly when gently pinched up into a fold if lack of skin turgor is present. Normally, the skin springs right back into position in a hydrated person. Care must be taken not to harm the person when trying to make an assessment and diagnosis.

Sebum (an oily substance) secreted by the skin contains bacterial chemicals that have the ability to destroy surface bacteria. When sweat is produced the acidic pH has the potential to hamper the proliferation of bacteria. Phagocytic macrophages present in the dermis have the ability to ingest and destroy viruses and bacteria that have penetrated the surface of the skin.

Excretion and absorption

Some elements of secretion and absorption have already been mentioned in respect to the skin's function in protecting the person. The skin has the ability to excrete substances from the body, sweat is composed of water, sodium, carbon dioxide, ammonia and urea. Jenkins *et al.* (2010) point out that the body (despite its almost waterproof nature) can excrete approximately 400 ml of water daily; those who lead a less active lifestyle will lose less, and a more active person will lose more.

The skin also has the ability to absorb substances from the environment. Materials are absorbed from the external environment into the body cells and some of these substances when absorbed are toxic, for example, heavy metals such as lead and mercury. There are some therapeutic and non-therapeutic medications that can be absorbed through the skin. A number of fat-soluble vitamins – A, D, E and K – oxygen and carbon dioxide are also absorbed.

Clinical considerations

Administration of medicines

There are some medications that you may be asked to administer via the skin. These include ointments, lotions, creams and gels. The application of medicines via the skin through an adhesive patch is also used in a number of care areas. All of these medicines are subject to the same rules and regulations associated with the administration of any medicine. Medicines applied to skin are often needed to treat skin conditions and they are known as topical medications; they are administered externally onto the body as opposed to being ingested or injected.

Lotions are used to protect, soften and soothe and can provide relief from itching. Ointments are oil-based and body heat causes them to melt after application; often these medications are used to fight infection or relieve inflamed tissue. Gloves must be used when applying these medicines; they must be applied in thin, even layers unless the prescription states otherwise (Peate 2009).

Most skin medications are provided for use in tubes; one tube must only be used for one person in order to prevent cross-infection. There are some skin medicines that must be sterile for use and when this is the case after application the leftover medication must be discarded.

When you are applying the medication you must take care that you do not increase discomfort by using too much pressure or rubbing areas that are inflamed or causing the person pain.

Synthesis of vitamin D

The skin is actively involved in the production and synthesis of vitamin D. For vitamin D to synthesise effectively activation of a precursor molecule in the skin by UV rays in the sunlight (ultraviolet radiation) is required. Enzymes present in the kidneys and liver alter the molecules producing calcitriol. Calcitriol (a hormone) assists in the absorption of calcium present in food in the intestines into the blood.

Conclusion

The skin is an exceptional organ, and is also known as the integumentary system. There is a variety of diseases or injuries that can easily be observed on the surface of the skin, for example, a skin rash, the presence of jaundice or cyanosis. It is the largest organ in the body in weight and surface area. The skin has the ability to reveal how we feel and what emotional state we may be in: humans blush, sweat and tremble. No other organ in the body is as easily looked over or palpated as the skin; the skin is also more easily exposed to injury, for example, infection and trauma.

This organ is the interface between the external and internal environments. The skin contributes to the homeostasis of the body and the physical changes noted can point to homeostatic imbalance. The skin is also composed of the accessory structures, for example, the nails and a number of glands; these are sometimes called the appendages.

The skin has the ability to allow a person to experience pleasure, pain and other stimuli from the external environment.

Glossary

Absorption: Intake of fluids or other materials by cells of the skin.

Apocrine: A type of gland found in the skin, apocrine glands in the skin and eyelids are sweat glands.

Apoptosis: Death of cell as signalled by the nuclei in a normally functioning cell.

Arrector pili: A microscopic muscle attached to hair follicles.

Calcitonin: A hormone that participates in calcium metabolism.

Cerumen: Ear wax secreted by ceruminous glands.

Collagen: A protein that is the main component of connective tissue.

Cutaneous: Relating to the skin.

Cyanosis: A bluish discolouration of the skin and mucous membranes.

Dermatitis: Inflammation of the skin.

Enzyme: A substance that accelerates chemical reactions.

Erythema: Redness.

Excretion: The process of elimination of waste products from the body.

Extrinsic: Originates externally.

Fascia: A fibrous membrane covering, supporting and separating muscles.

Hair: A thread-like structure produced by the hair follicles emerging from the dermis.

Homeostasis: The ability to maintain a constant internal environment.

Hyperkeratosis: Excess keratins are produced, resulting in thickening of the skin.

Innervation: Related to the supply of nerves.

Integumentary: The external covering of the body, relating to the skin.

Intrinsic: Originates internally.

Keratin: A tough, insoluble protein found in the hair and nails and other keratinised areas of the body.

Keratinise: To convert into keratin.

Lanugo: Fine, downy hair covering the foetus.

Lunula: The moon-shaped white area at the base of nails.

Melanin: Pigment found in some parts of the body, for example, the skin and hair.

Metabolism: A set of chemical reactions in the body required to maintain life.

Nail: A hard plate that is mainly composed of keratin.

Organ: A structure that is composed of two or more kinds of tissue with a specific function and a recognised shape.

Organism: A total living form.

Pathogen: A disease-producing microbe.

Phagocytosis: The act of destroying and ingesting microbes by phagocytes.

Pheromones: A chemical that triggers an innate behavioural response in another.

Prognosis: A prediction about how a patient's disease will progress.

Proliferation: A rapid and repeated reproduction of new cells.

Pruritus: Itching.

Sebum: An oily substance made of fat and the debris of fat-producing cells produced by the sebaceous glands.

Stratum: A layer.

Tactile: Pertaining to touch.

Thermoreceptor: A sensory receptor that has the ability to detect changes in heat.

Thermoregulation: Ability to regulate temperature.

Vasoconstriction: Reduction in the diameter of blood vessels.

Vasodilation: Increase in diameter of blood vessels.

References

Colbert, B.J., Ankney, J. and Lee, K.T. (2007) *Anatomy and Physiology for Health Professionals: An Interactive Journey*. Upper Saddle River, NJ: Pearson.

Haneke, E. (2006) Surgical anatomy of the nail apparatus. *Dermatology Clinic* 24(3):291–296.

Hemming, L. (2010) Personal cleansing and dressing. In Peate, I. (ed.) *Nursing Care and the Activities of Living*, 2nd edn. Oxford: Wiley-Blackwell, pp. 171–187.

Jenkins, G.W., Kemnitz, C.P. and Tortora, G.J. (2010) *Anatomy and Physiology: From Science to Life*, 2nd edn. Hoboken, NJ: John Wiley & Sons.

Lawton, S. (2006) Anatomy and Function of the Skin. Part 4 – Appendages. *Nursing TImes* 102(34):26–27.

LeMone, P. and Burke, K. (2009) *Medical–Surgical Nursing. Critical Thinking in Client Care*, 4th edn. Upper Saddle River, NJ: Pearson.

Lewis, K. and Roberts, R. (2009) Skin integrity. In: Mallik, M., Hall, C. and Howard, D. (eds), 3rd edn. *Nursing Knowledge and Practice. Foundations for Decision Making.* Edinburgh: Baillière Tindall, pp. 337–362.

Page, B.E. (2006) Skin disorders. In: Alexander, M.F., Fawcett, J.N. and Runciman, P.J. (eds), 3rd edn. *Nursing Practice, Hospital and Home: The Adult*. Edinburgh: Churchill Livingstone, pp. 525–552.

Peate, I. (2009) Principles of medicine management. In: Lawson, L. and Peate, I. (eds) *Essential Nursing Care. Workbook for Clinical Practice.* Oxford: Wiley-Blackwell, pp. 31–78.

Rizzo D.C. (2006) *Fundamentals of Anatomy and Physiology*, 2nd edn. New York: Thomson.

Shier, D., Butler, J. and Lewis, R. (2009) *Hol\e's Anatomy and Physiology*, 12th edn. Boston, MA: McGraw-Hill.

Sibson, L. (2010) Assessing needs and the nursing process. In Peate, I. (ed.) *Nursing Care and the Activities of Living*, 2nd edn. Oxford Wiley-Blackwell, pp. 38–59.

Timby, B.K. (2005) *Fundamental Nursing Skills and Concepts*, 8th edn. Philadelphia: Lippincott.

Tortora, G.J. and Derrickson, B. (2009) *Principles of Anatomy and Physiology*, 12th edn. Hoboken, NJ: John Wiley & Sons.

Activities

www.wiley.com/go/peate

Multiple choice questions

1. How often (approximately) are the epidermal cells replaced? Every:

   (a) 30 days
   (b) 42 days
   (c) 15 days
   (d) 28 days

2. The skin is thickest on:

   (a) the lips
   (b) the earlobes
   (c) the hands
   (d) the nose

3. What is the name of the pigment that makes skin different colours?

   (a) melaena
   (b) melatonin
   (c) melonite
   (d) melanin

4. Hair follicles are made of:

   (a) sebum
   (b) sweat
   (c) keratin
   (d) muscle

5. The outermost layer of the skin is called the:

   (a) dermis
   (b) epidermis
   (c) muscularis
   (d) subcutaneous

6. The skin does all of these except:

   (a) absorb sugar
   (b) protect the body
   (c) provide the sense of touch
   (d) help to thermoregulate

7. The word used when the skin has no melanin is:

   (a) aged
   (b) exhausted
   (c) eczema
   (d) albino

8. In what aspect of the skin are the cells which divide to form new cells?

   (a) the medulla
   (b) the follicle
   (c) the basal layers of the epidermis
   (d) the sebaceous glands

9. What will eventually happen to the cells of the epidermis?

   (a) They are reabsorbed
   (b) They become scars
   (c) They become infected
   (d) They die off and flake

10. The structures in the dermis that produce oil are called the:

   (a) sebaceous glands
   (b) the Merkel cells
   (c) the Meissner corpuscle
   (d) lamellar granules

True or false

1. Skin is the largest organ of the body.
2. Total healing of body piercings takes between 2 and 4 months.
3. Nerve endings tell the body when things are too hot.
4. Blood vessels bring sweat to the skin.
5. The skin's natural oil is called serum.
6. Goose bumps are caused by the pilomotor reflex.
7. The thickest part of the skin is to be found at the heels.
8. The hypodermis is also known as the epidermis.
9. Innervation relates to blood supply.
10. The Merkel cells are the least numerous of the epidermal cells.

Label the diagram

From the lists of words, label the diagrams below:

Superficial, Deep, Epidermis, Stratum corneum, Stratum lucidum, Stratum granulosum, Stratum spinosum, Stratum basale, Dermis

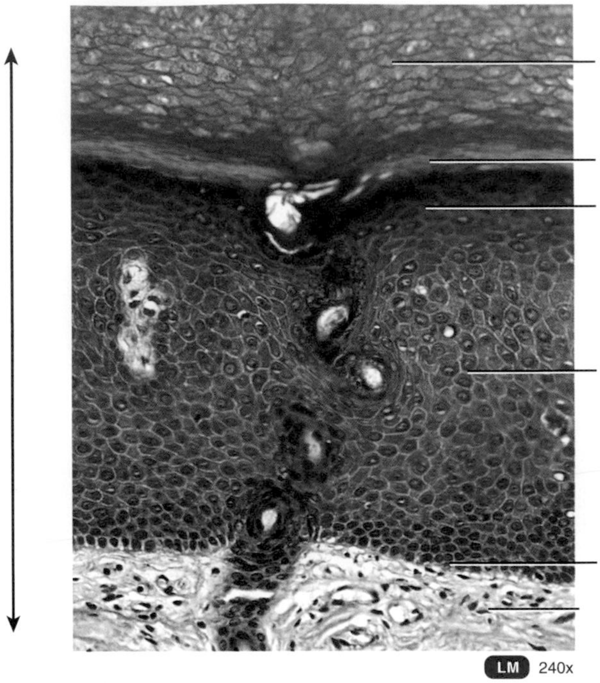
LM 240x

Hair, Skin surface, Sebum, Follicle, Sebaceous gland

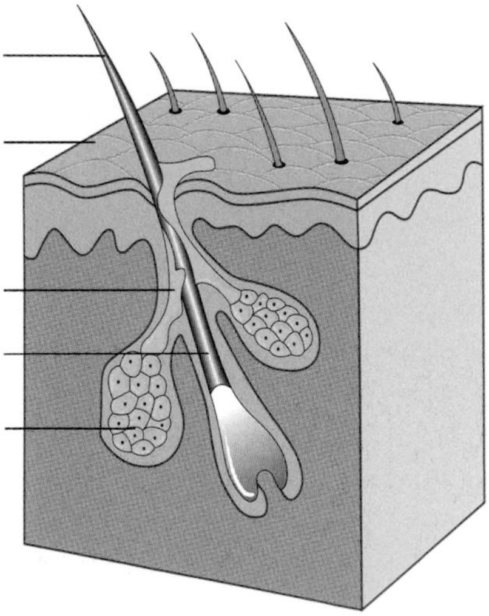

Word Search

In the grid below there are 22 words that you will have seen in this chapter. Can you find them all?

S	N	G	S	E	V	R	E	N	C	L	H	T
U	I	L	I	P	R	O	T	C	E	R	R	A
B	N	A	S	S	K	I	N	S	L	U	W	E
C	A	N	R	I	A	H	Q	I	L	O	V	W
U	L	D	E	J	M	K	C	M	T	D	P	S
T	E	B	N	E	A	R	T	R	H	O	B	O
A	M	A	O	L	L	F	E	E	I	O	L	K
N	A	S	M	C	U	P	A	D	N	W	O	C
E	L	A	R	I	N	H	C	T	I	U	O	I
O	E	L	O	T	U	D	U	C	T	P	D	H
U	M	B	H	U	L	A	Y	E	R	S	E	T
S	U	O	E	C	A	B	E	S	O	L	I	P

Fill in the blanks

The skin has ________________. The outer layer is called the ____________________ and the inner layer is the ____________________. The dermal layer contains hair ____________________, sebaceous ________________________, small blood vessels called ________________ and a pigment called ___________ that helps to protect against ____________________ light. The skin has a number of functions and one of those functions is related to heat control; this is called _______________, the skin can also protect from ____________________ invading the body. The skin is the ________________ organ of the body. When a person becomes hot the blood vessels on the ________________ of the skin ____________________. ________________ when released helps a person to _________________ down.

The epidermis is situated on the _________________ of the skin and is made from _________________ of ___________ with a basal layer. This layer drives through _______ ___________. The newly divided cells gradually ______ _______ _________ ______, this can take about _____ _________. As the cells gradually ______, they become ____________ and ___________, the outermost layer of ____________ ______________ _______ is being ______________ eroded by _____________. The keratin and _________ from the sebaceous __________ assist in making the skin ________________.

Find out more

1. What are the names of the touch receptors?
2. Where does nail growth originate?
3. Describe the anatomical and physiological changes that occur when a person experiences goose bumps.
4. Name three potential complications of body piercing.
5. What procedures can be used to remove tattoos?
6. What is needed to activate vitamin D and why?
7. What is the role and function of the arrector pili?
8. Describe what happens to the skin when vasodilation occurs.
9. Outline the processes involved as skin repairs itself after being damaged.
10. How does the skin and renal system work together to maintain homeostasis?

Conditions

Below is a list of conditions that are associated with the skin. Take some time and write notes about each of the conditions. You may make the notes taken from textbooks or other resources, for example, people you work with in a clinical area, or you may make the notes as a result of people you have cared for. If you are making notes about people you have cared for you must ensure that you adhere to the rules of confidentiality.

Allergy	
Skin cancer • Malignant melanoma • Basal cell carcinoma (BCC) • Squamous cell carcinoma (SCC)	
Eczema	
Psoriasis	
Burns • First degree • Second degree • Full thickness	
Pressure sores	

Answers

MCQs

1d; 2c; 3d; 4c; 5b; 6a; 7d; 8c; 9d; 10a

True or false

1T; 2F; 3T; 4F; 5F; 6T; 7T; 8F; 9F; 10T

Word search

S	N	G	S	E	V	R	E	N	C	L	H	T
U	I	L	I	P	R	O	T	C	E	R	R	A
B	N	A	S	S	K	I	N	S	L	U	W	E
C	A	N	R	I	A	H	Q	I	L	O	V	W
U	L	D	E	J	M	K	C	M	T	D	P	S
T	E	B	N	E	A	R	T	R	H	O	B	O
A	M	A	O	L	L	F	E	E	I	O	L	K
N	A	S	M	C	U	P	A	D	N	W	O	C
E	L	A	R	I	N	H	C	T	I	U	O	I
O	E	L	O	T	U	D	U	C	T	R	D	H
U	M	B	H	U	L	A	Y	E	R	S	E	T
S	U	O	E	C	A	B	E	S	O	L	I	P

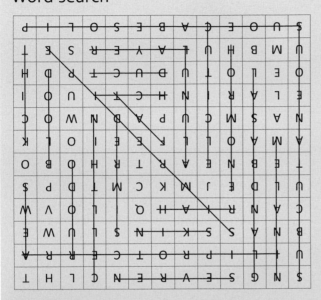

Fill in the blanks

The skin has **two layers**. The outer layer is called the **epidermis** and the inner layer is the **dermis**. The dermal layer contains hair **follicles**, sebaceous **glands**, small blood vessels called **capillaries** and a pigment called **melanin** that helps to protect against **ultraviolet** light. The skin has a number of functions and one of those functions is related to heat control this is called **thermoregulation**, the skin can also protect from **micro-organisms** invading the body. The skin is the **largest** organ of the body. When a person becomes hot the blood vessels on the **surface** of the skin **dilate**. **Sweat** when released helps a person to **cool** down.

The epidermis is situated on the **outside** of the skin and is made from **layers** of **cells** with a basal layer. This layer drives through **cell division**. The newly divided cells gradually **move towards the surface**, this can take about **1–2 months**. As the cells gradually **die**, they become **flattened** and **keratin** the outermost layer of **flat dead cells** is being **continually** eroded by **friction**. The keratin and **oil** from the sebaceous **glands** assist in making the skin **waterproof**.

6

The nervous system

Louise McErlean and Janet G Migliozzi

Contents

Introduction 156

Organisation of the nervous system 156

Sensory division of the peripheral nervous system 157

Central nervous system 157

Motor division of the peripheral nervous system 157
- Somatic nervous system 157
- Autonomic nervous system 157
- Neurones 157
- Dendrites 158
- Cell body 158
- Axons 158
- Myelin sheath 158
- Sensory (afferent) nerves 160
- Motor (efferent) nerves 160
- The action potential 160
- Simple propagation of nerve impulses 161
- Saltatory conduction 161
- The refractory period 161

Neurotransmitters 161

Neuroglia 163

The meninges 163

Cerebrospinal fluid (CSF) 164

The brain 166

The peripheral nervous system 170
- Cranial nerves 170

The spinal cord 170
- Functions of the spinal cord 172
- Spinal nerves 173

The autonomic nervous system 176
- Sympathetic division (fight or flight) 176
- Parasympathetic division (rest and digest) 178

Conclusion 178

Glossary 180

References 182

Activities 183

Fundamentals of Anatomy and Physiology for Student Nurses, First Edition. Edited by Ian Peate, Muralitharan Nair.

Test your knowledge

- Which other system does the nervous system work closely with?
- List the structures of the central nervous system.
- How many pairs of cranial nerves are there?
- Name the two divisions of the autonomic nervous system.

Learning outcomes

On completion of this chapter the reader will be able to:

- Describe the structures of the nervous system
- Describe some of the functions of each of these structures
- Describe conduction of nerve impulses
- List the functions of the neuroglial cells
- Identify the function of different areas of the brain
- Understand the structure and function of the spinal cord
- Differentiate between the sympathetic and parasympathetic nervous systems

Body map

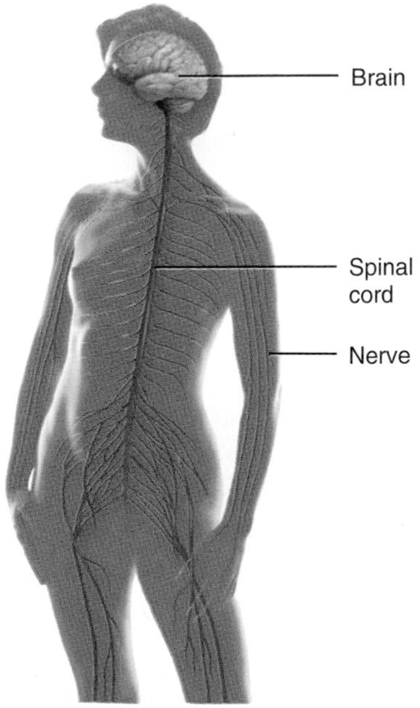
Brain
Spinal cord
Nerve

Introduction

The nervous system is a major communicating and control system within the body. It works with the endocrine system to control many body functions. The nervous system provides a rapid and short acting response and the endocrine system provides a slower but often more sustained response. The two systems work together to maintain homeostasis.

The nervous system interacts with all of the systems of the body. This system is large and complex. In order to facilitate understanding of the nervous system it has to be divided into smaller functional and anatomical parts. This chapter outlines the divisions of the nervous system; it discusses the structure and function of the nervous system and how it influences other structures of the body. Having such an important role in maintaining homeostasis, the nervous system possesses additional protection and that too will be investigated.

Organisation of the nervous system

The nervous system can be divided into two parts: the central nervous system and the peripheral nervous system. The central nervous system consists of the brain and spinal cord and is the control and integration centre for many body functions.

The peripheral nervous system carries sensory information to the central nervous system and motor information out of the central nervous system. The direction of information flow to and from the nervous system is important and is shown in Figure 6.1.

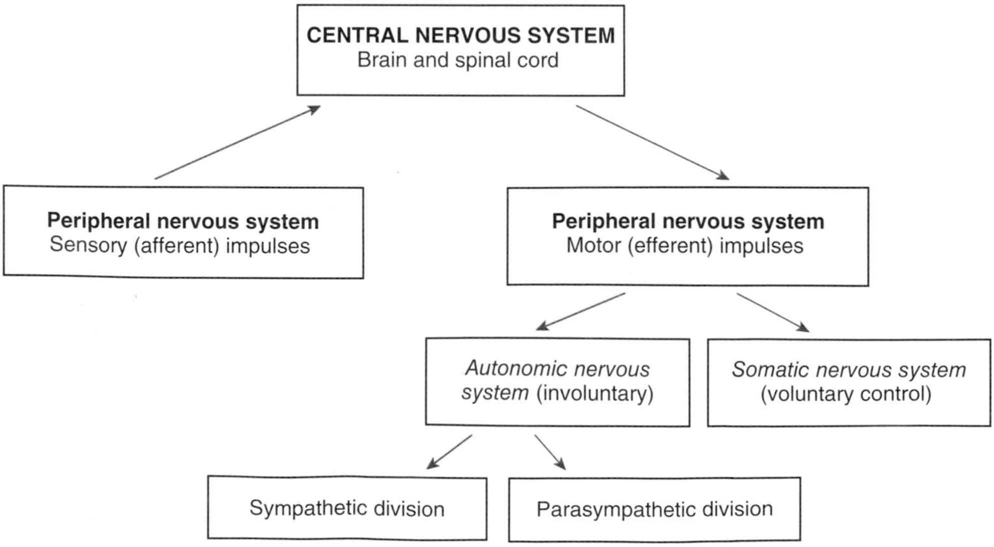
CENTRAL NERVOUS SYSTEM
Brain and spinal cord
Peripheral nervous system
Sensory (afferent) impulses
Peripheral nervous system
Motor (efferent) impulses
Autonomic nervous system (involuntary)
Somatic nervous system (voluntary control)
Sympathetic division
Parasympathetic division

Figure 6.1 Organisation of the nervous system

Sensory division of the peripheral nervous system

Sensory information is gathered from both inside and outside of the body. This sensory input is delivered to the central nervous system via the peripheral nerves. Sensory nerve fibres are also called afferent fibres. Sensory information always travels from the peripheral nervous system towards the central nervous system. An example of sensory information is temperature. Temperature receptors in the skin called thermoreceptors detect changes in temperature and this information is relayed to the central nervous system.

Central nervous system

The central nervous system consists of the brain and spinal cord. The central nervous system processes and integrates sensory information. The received information can be stored to be dealt with later or it can be acted upon immediately with one or more motor responses. The central nervous system can also be divided into functional areas. One such functional area is the hypothalamus. The sensation of temperature change would be received and interpreted by the hypothalamus and an appropriate action would be initiated.

Motor division of the peripheral nervous system

Somatic nervous system

Motor information always travels away from the central nervous system. Motor nerve fibres are also called efferent fibres. The response to sensory information may be to activate the somatic nervous system eliciting a voluntary response involving skeletal muscle movement. So from the example of temperature, if an increase in temperature is detected, then it might require the removal of a coat or the opening of a window – this is the motor response that involves the somatic nervous system.

Autonomic nervous system

The response to sensory information may require an involuntary action. The autonomic nervous system is responsible for involuntary motor responses. In the example of increased temperature, the involuntary response is to lose heat through the skin – so warm blood is directed to the skin when peripheral blood vessels vasodilate. Vasodilatation is an example of an involuntary autonomic nervous system response.

The autonomic nervous system is further divided into the sympathetic (fight or flight) and the parasympathetic (rest and digest) divisions. The autonomic nervous system will be discussed later in the chapter. A fine balance between both of these divisions is required for the maintenance of homeostasis.

Neurones

The functional unit of the nervous system is the neurone or nerve cell. It has many features in common with other cells, including a nucleus and mitochondria, but because of its vital role it is well protected and has some specialist modifications. Two specialist characteristics of neurones are:

- Irritability, in response to a stimulus – the ability to initiate a nerve impulse
- Conductivity – the ability to conduct an impulse.

Neurones consist of an axon, dendrites and a cell body. Their function is to transmit nerve impulses. Nerve impulses only travel in one direction: from the receptive area – the dendrites, to the cell body, and down the length of the axon (see Figure 6.2).

Axons bundled together are called *nerves*. Neurones rely on a constant supply of oxygen and glucose. Once the neurones of the brain and spinal cord have matured after birth they will not be replaced or regenerate if they become damaged. Peripheral neurones can regenerate if the cell body is not damaged and the alignment of the neurone is not disrupted.

Dendrites

Dendrites are short branching processes that receive information. Their branching processes provide a large surface area for this function. In sensory neurones the dendrites may form the part of the sensory receptors and in motor neurones they can form part of the synapse between one neurone and the next.

Cell body

Most of the neurone cell bodies are located inside the central nervous system and form the grey matter. When clusters of cell bodies are grouped together in the central nervous system they are called nuclei. Cell bodies located in the peripheral nervous system are called ganglia.

Axons

Each neurone has only one axon, but the axon can branch to form an axon collateral (see Figure 6.2). The axon will also branch at its terminal into many axon terminals. The axon length can vary quite significantly from very short to 100 cm long (Marieb and Hoehn 2007).

Myelin sheath

Peripheral nerve axons and long or large axons are covered in a myelin sheath. Myelin is a fatty material and its purpose is to protect the neurone and to electrically insulate it, speeding up impulse transmission. Within the peripheral nervous system Schwann cells wrapped in layers around the neurone form the myelin sheath. The outermost part of the Schwann cell is its plasma membrane and this is called the neurilemma. There is a regular gap (about 1 mm) between adjacent Schwann cells. The gaps are called the nodes of Ranvier. Collateral axons can occur at the node (see Figure 6.2). Some nerve fibres are unmyelinated and this makes nerve impulse transmission significantly slower.

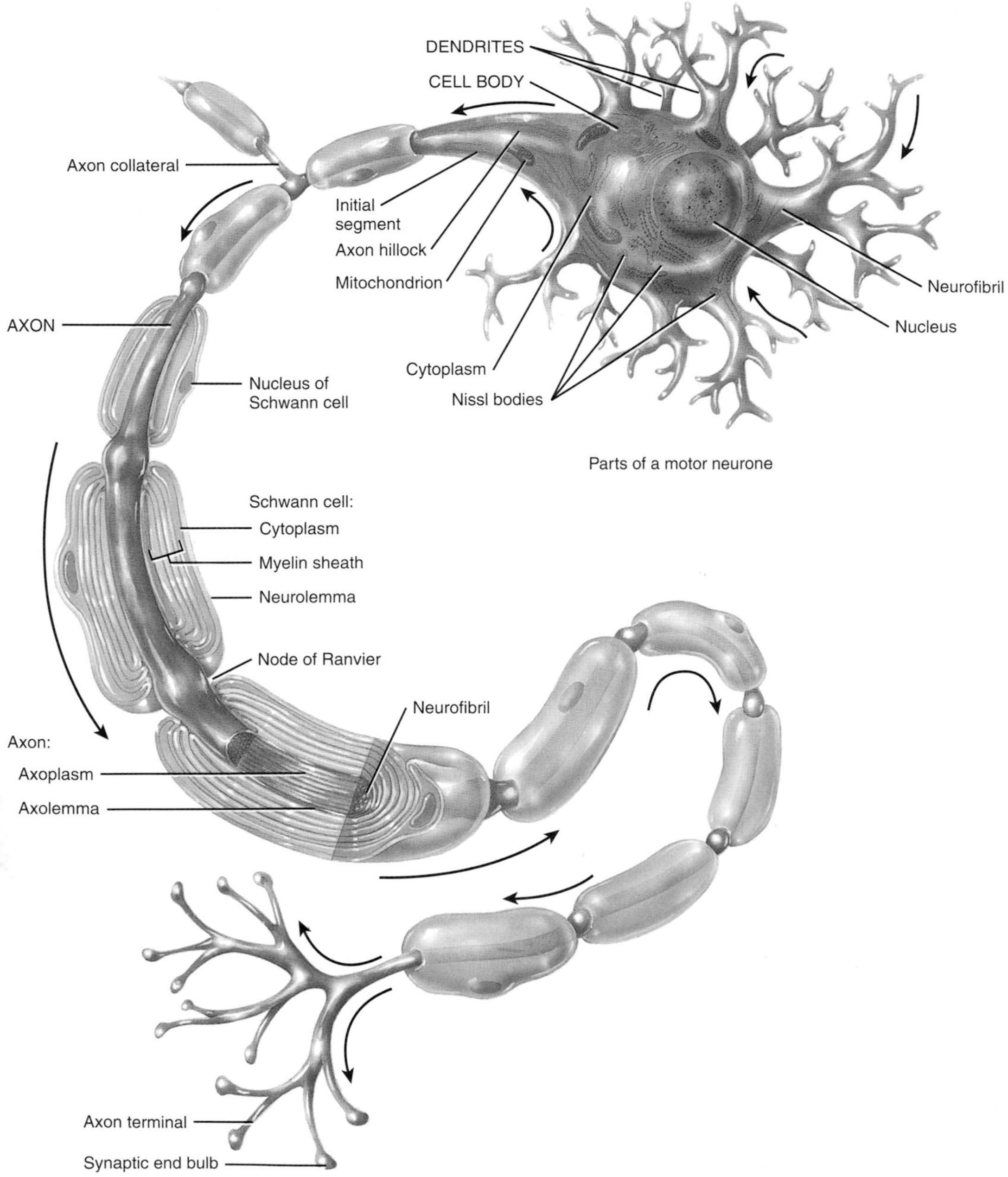
DENDRITES
CELL BODY
Axon collateral
Initial segment
Axon hillock
Mitochondrion
Neurofibril
Nucleus
AXON
Nucleus of Schwann cell
Cytoplasm
Nissl bodies
Parts of a motor neurone
Schwann cell:
Cytoplasm
Myelin sheath
Neurolemma
Node of Ranvier
Neurofibril
Axon:
Axoplasm
Axolemma
Axon terminal
Synaptic end bulb

Figure 6.2 Motor neurone (Tortora and Derrickson 2009)

Clinical considerations

Multiple sclerosis

Multiple sclerosis is a disease where areas of demyelination of the white matter (myelinated fibres form white matter) can occur. Areas of demyelination are called plaques. Multiple sclerosis affects the 20–40 year age range and is most frequently seen in temperate climates. The cause is unknown but it is suspected that there may be a genetic link; viral infection has also been implicated. Neuronal damage caused by the demyelination leads to:

- Skeletal muscle weakness, often progressing to paralysis
- Visual disturbances
- Uncoordinated movements
- Burning or tingling sensations.

Multiple sclerosis can be a chronic disease characterised by periods of remission or the disease can progress rapidly, leading to death.

Sensory (afferent) nerves

The dendrites of sensory neurones are often sensory receptors and when they are stimulated the impulse generated travels towards the spinal cord and brain. There are different types of sensory receptors:

- Special senses (as discussed in Chapter 16)
- Somatic sensory receptors located in the skin, such as touch, temperature and pain
- Autonomic nervous system receptors located throughout the body, such as baroreceptors monitoring blood pressure, chemoreceptors monitoring blood pH and visceral pain receptors
- Propioceptors monitoring muscle movement, stretch and pain.

Motor (efferent) nerves

Information from the central nervous system is delivered to the peripheral nervous system via the motor nerves. Information transmitted through a voluntary somatic nerve may result in skeletal muscle contraction or the information may be autonomic in nature, not under voluntary control, and may lead to smooth muscle contraction or the release of the products of a gland.

The action potential

The nervous system is a vast communicating network sending information from the internal and external environment to the central nervous system and from the central nervous system to the muscles and glands. The way that the functional unit, the neurone, achieves this is by the generation and conduction of impulses or action potentials.

Generation of the action potential occurs due to the movement of ions into and out of the neurone and the electrical charge associated with this movement.

Two principal ions are involved:

- Sodium – normally found outside of the cell (principal extracellular cation)
- Potassium – normally found inside the cell (principal intracellular cation).

Simple propagation of nerve impulses

When there is no impulse being transmitted the cell is said to be in its resting state – the nerve cell membrane is said to be *polarised.* When stimulated by an impulse, the cell membrane changes its permeability and the extracellular sodium ions move into the cell – this is called depolarisation. The movement of these ions changes the electrical charge on either side of the cell membrane from more positive extracellularly to more negative extracellularly as the impulse travels the length of the axon. This activity creates the action potential. This process happens in a wave along the length of the neurone from the active part of the neurone to the resting part of the neurone, always in one direction. At the same time potassium ions move out of the neurone into the extra-cellular space returning the electrical charge associated with the polarised neurone back to more positive outside the cell and more negative inside. This is the repolarising phase. The sodium potassium pump is activated to return sodium to the extracellular space in exchange for potassium (see Figure 6.3).

Saltatory conduction

Saltatory conduction occurs in myelinated neurones as the electrical charge associated with the nerve impulse jumps between one node of Ranvier and the next. This occurs much faster than simple propagation. Conduction is also faster when the neurone has a larger diameter.

The refractory period

When the action potential is stimulated the neurone cannot accept another impulse or generate another action potential no matter how strong the impulse is. This is known as the refractory period.

Neurotransmitters

Neurones do not come into contact with one another. Where one neurone ends and another begins, there is a space called the synapse. In order for communication to occur between neurones or between the neurone and a muscle or gland, a chemical messenger called a *neurotransmitter* is secreted by the neurone into the extracellular space at the synapse. Those effector cells or neurones in close proximity to the neurotransmitter will either be stimulated or inhibited by the neurotransmitter depending upon which neurotransmitter is secreted. The action of the neurotransmitter is short lived and any neurotransmitter not used is absorbed by the neurone to be recycled and used again or deactivated by enzymes.

Some examples of neurotransmitters are:

- Acetylcholine released within the central nervous system and also at the neuromuscular junction
- Norepinephrine released within the central nervous system and also at autonomic nervous system synapses

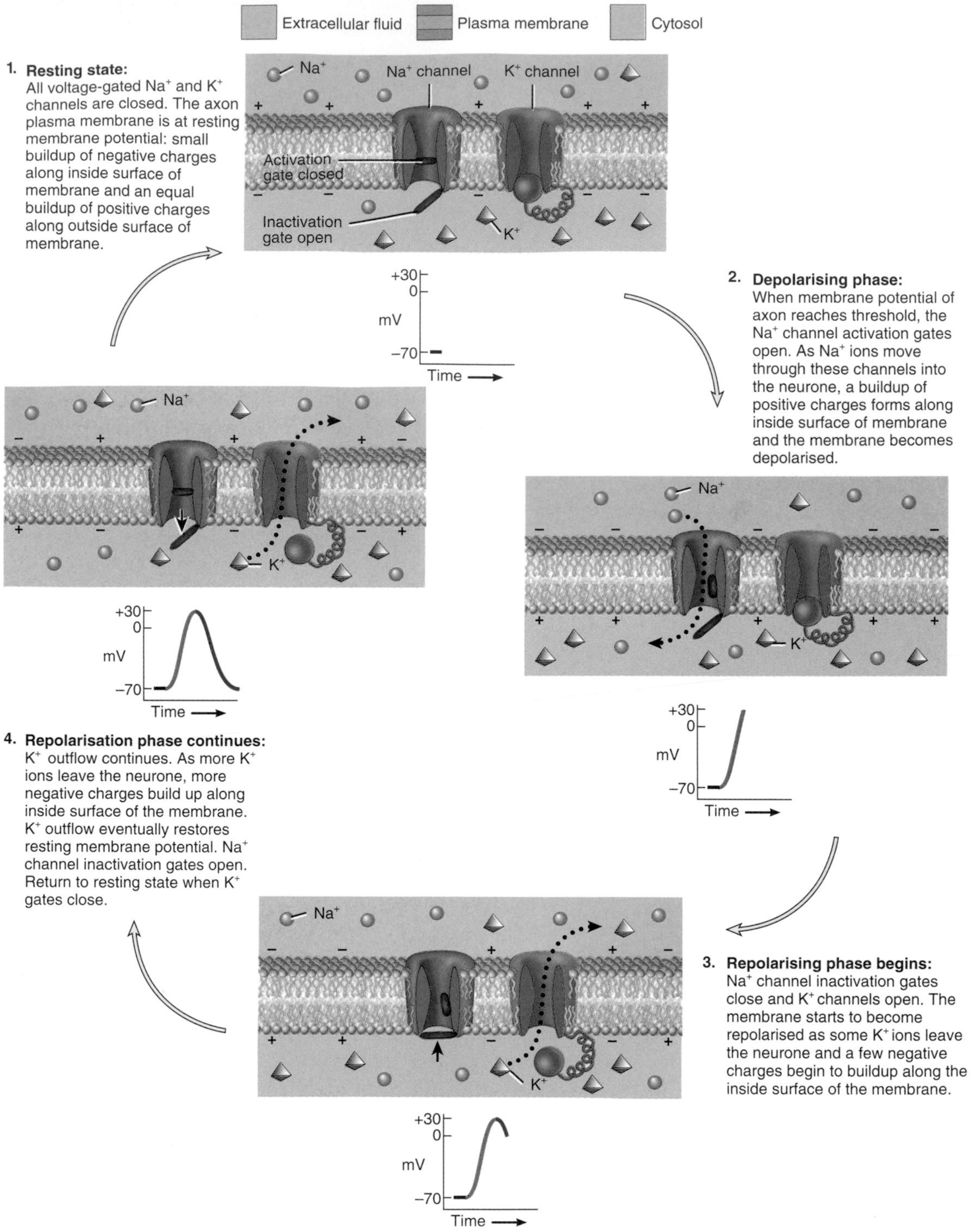

Extracellular fluid
Plasma membrane
Cytosol
1. Resting state:
All voltage-gated Na+ and K+ channels are closed. The axon plasma membrane is at resting membrane potential: small buildup of negative charges along inside surface of membrane and an equal buildup of positive charges along outside surface of membrane.
Na+
Na+ channel
K+ channel
Activation gate closed
Inactivation gate open
K+
+30
0
mV
–70
Time
2. Depolarising phase:
When membrane potential of axon reaches threshold, the Na+ channel activation gates open. As Na+ ions move through these channels into the neurone, a buildup of positive charges forms along inside surface of membrane and the membrane becomes depolarised.
3. Repolarising phase begins:
Na+ channel inactivation gates close and K+ channels open. The membrane starts to become repolarised as some K+ ions leave the neurone and a few negative charges begin to buildup along the inside surface of the membrane.
4. Repolarisation phase continues:
K+ outflow continues. As more K+ ions leave the neurone, more negative charges build up along inside surface of the membrane. K+ outflow eventually restores resting membrane potential. Na+ channel inactivation gates open. Return to resting state when K+ gates close.

Figure 6.3 Action potential (Tortora and Derrickson 2009)

- Dopamine released within the central nervous system and also at autonomic nervous system synapses.

Neuroglia

Neuroglia (see Figure 6.4) are cells that support neurones. They are more numerous than neurones. Within the central nervous system the neuroglial cells account for more than half of the weight of the brain (Marieb and Hoeh 2007). Within the peripheral nervous system two types of neuroglia have been identified:

- Schwann cells, responsible for forming the myelin sheath
- Satellite cells, whose function is not known.

Within the central nervous system four type of neuroglial cell have been identified:

- Astrocytes are star-shaped cells which occur in large quantities between neurones and blood vessels, supporting and anchoring them to each other. They help form the *blood – brain barrier* which gives the neurones an extra layer of protection from any toxic substances within the blood
- Microglia lie close to neurones and can move closer if they need to fulfil their function as nervous system macrophages. They phagocytose pathogens or cell debris
- Oligodendrocytes are found close to myelinated neurones. They help to form and maintain the myelin sheath
- Ependymal cells are often ciliated and are found lining cavities, such as the spinal cord or the ventricles of the brain. Their role is to circulate cerebrospinal fluid (Waugh and Grant 2001).

The meninges

Nervous tissue is easily damaged by pressure and therefore needs to be protected. The hair, skin and bone offer an outer layer of protection. Adjacent to the nervous tissue are the meninges (see Figure 6.5). The meninges cover the delicate nervous tissue, providing further protection. They also protect the blood vessels that serve nervous tissue and contain cerebrospinal fluid.

The meninges consist of three connective tissue layers:

- Dura mater – this layer lies closest to the bone of the skull and is a double layer of tough, fibrous, connective tissue. The outer layer is called the periosteal layer (the spinal cord lacks this layer) and the meningeal layer lies closest to the brain.
- Arachnoid mater – between the dura mater and the arachnoid mater there is a space called the subdural space. The arachnoid mater is a delicate serous membrane (Seeley *et al.* 2006). The subarachnoid space is below the arachnoid mater and above the pia mater. The subarachnoid space contains cerebrospinal fluid and is also home to some of the larger blood vessels serving the brain.
- Pia mater – this is a delicate connective tissue layer that clings tightly to the brain. It contains many tiny blood vessels that serve the brain.

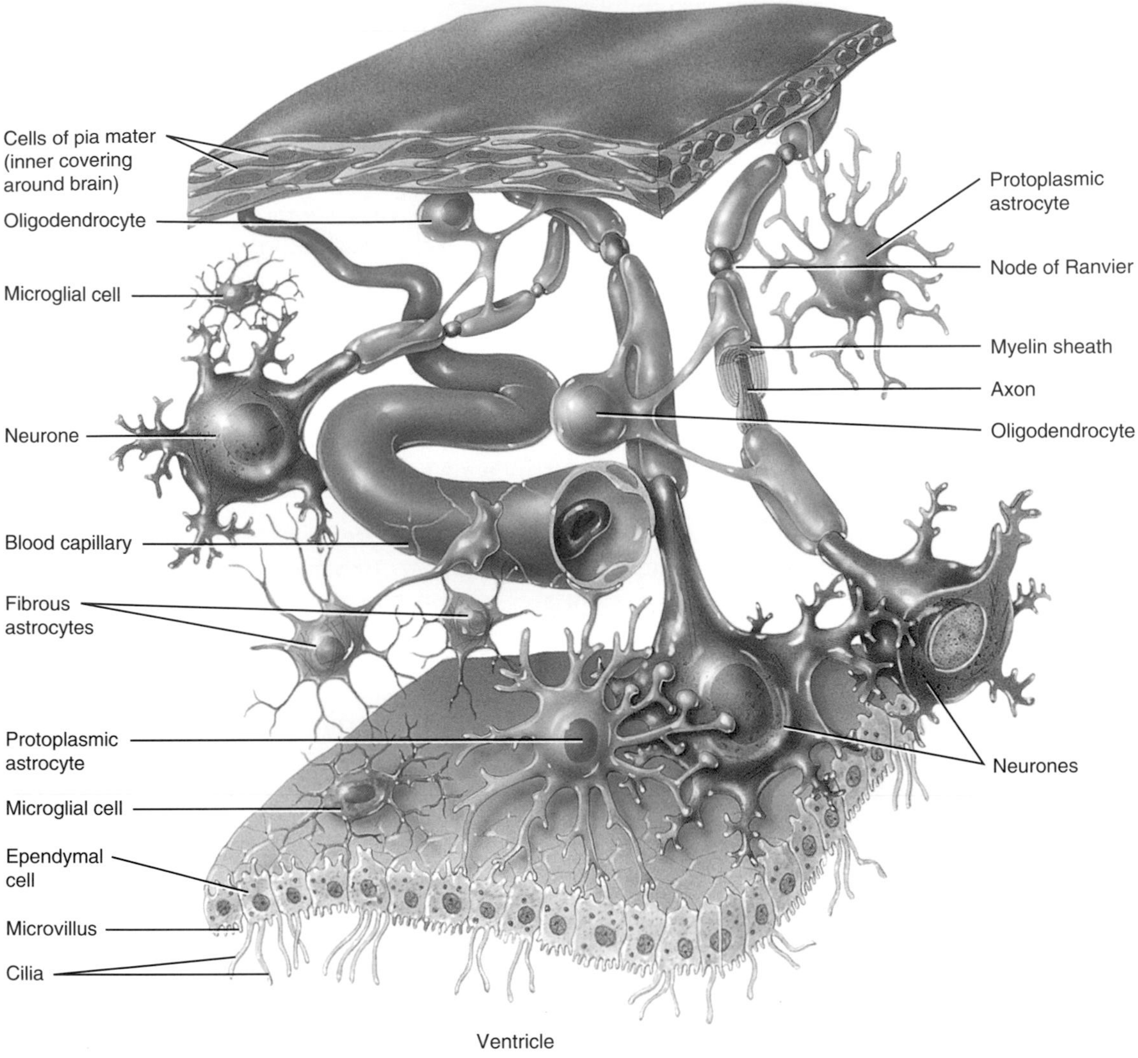
Cells of pia mater (inner covering around brain)
Oligodendrocyte
Microglial cell
Neurone
Blood capillary
Fibrous astrocytes
Protoplasmic astrocyte
Microglial cell
Ependymal cell
Microvillus
Cilia
Ventricle
Protoplasmic astrocyte
Node of Ranvier
Myelin sheath
Axon
Oligodendrocyte
Neurones

Figure 6.4 Neuroglia (Tortora and Derrickson 2010)

Cerebrospinal fluid (CSF)

Cerebrospinal fluid is produced by the *choroid plexus* in the ventricles of the brain (see Figure 6.6). There is approximately 150 ml of CSF circulating around the brain, in the ventricles and around the spinal cord. The CSF is replaced every eight hours (Marieb and Hoehn 2007). It is a thin fluid similar to plasma and has several important functions:

- It acts as a cushion supporting the weight of the brain and protecting it from damage
- It helps to maintain a uniform pressure around the brain and spinal cord
- There is a limited exchange of nutrients and waste products between neurones and CSF.

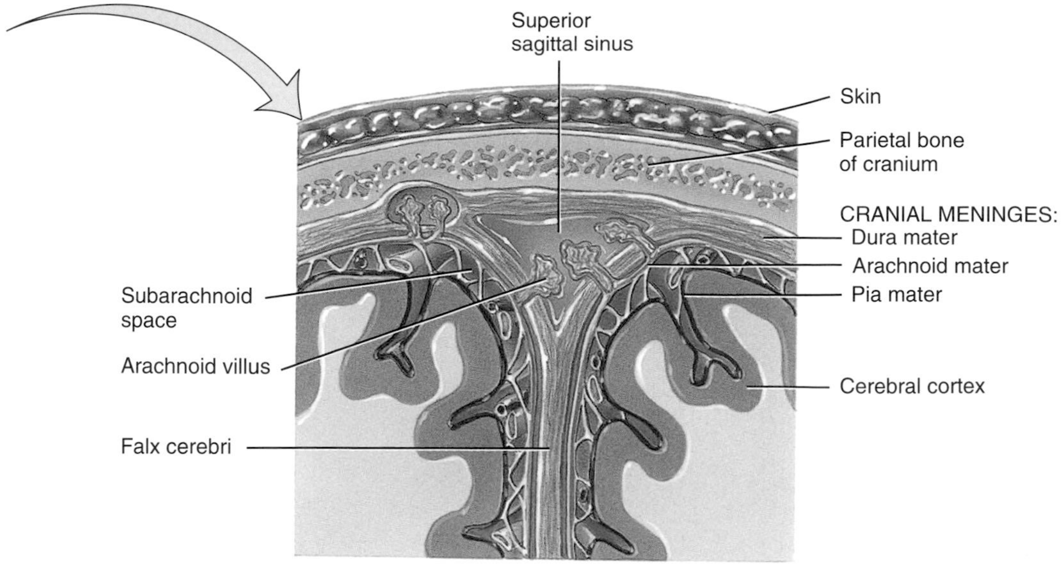
Superior
sagittal sinus
Skin
Parietal bone
of cranium
CRANIAL MENINGES:
Dura mater
Arachnoid mater
Pia mater
Subarachnoid
space
Arachnoid villus
Cerebral cortex
Falx cerebri

Figure 6.5 The meninges (Tortora and Derrickson 2009)

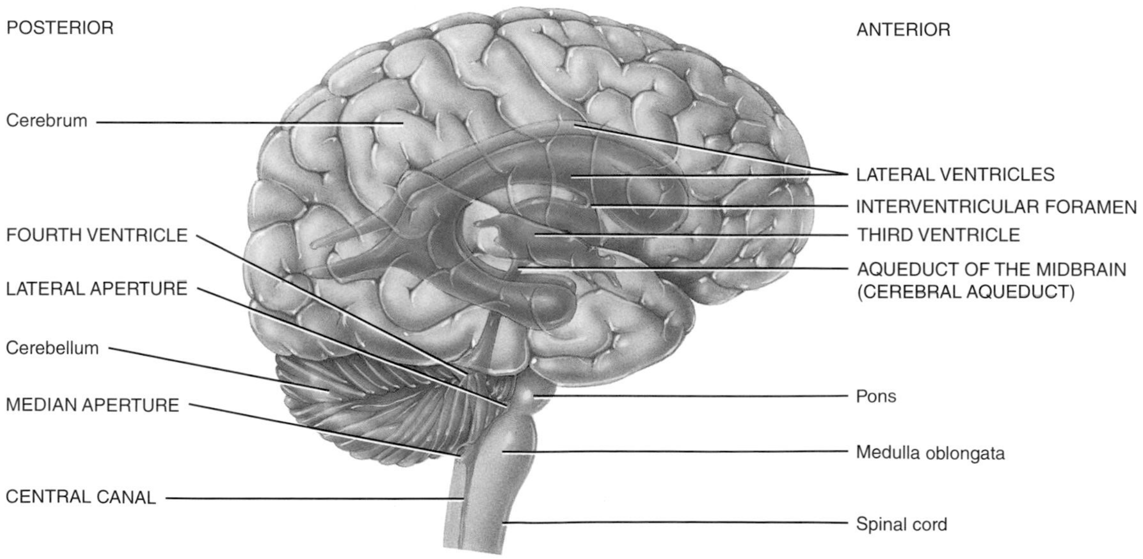
POSTERIOR
ANTERIOR
Cerebrum
LATERAL VENTRICLES
INTERVENTRICULAR FORAMEN
FOURTH VENTRICLE
THIRD VENTRICLE
LATERAL APERTURE
AQUEDUCT OF THE MIDBRAIN
(CEREBRAL AQUEDUCT)
Cerebellum
MEDIAN APERTURE
Pons
Medulla oblongata
CENTRAL CANAL
Spinal cord

Figure 6.6 The ventricles [right lateral view of the brain] (Tortora and Derrickson 2009)

There are four ventricles in the brain. The paired lateral ventricles – one in each cerebral hemisphere, the third ventricle situated below this and the fourth ventricle located inferior to the third. The third and fourth ventricles communicate via the central canal and cerbrospinal fluid circulates through the central canal and into the spinal cord.

Any additional pressure applied to the brain caused by swelling (cerebral oedema), tumour or haemorrhage (through trauma) can lead to a reduced volume of CSF being produced.

Clinical considerations

Meningitis

Meningitis is inflammation of the meninges caused by either bacteria or viruses. It can be diagnosed through symptoms which include photophobia, headache, nausea and vomiting and also by a procedure called a lumbar puncture. In lumbar puncture a small amount of CSF is removed and examined in the lab for the presence of microbes. A lack of prompt treatment can have fatal consequences.

The brain

The brain lies in the cranial cavity and weighs between 1450 g and1600 g (Marieb and Hoehn 2007). It receives 15% of the cardiac output and has a system of *autoregulation* ensuring the blood supply is constant despite positional changes. The arrangement of the arteries serving the brain is unique and they are connected to each other by a structure called the circle of Willis (see Figure 6.7). This arrangement ensures that blood pressure remains equal in both halves of the brain. Should one of the arteries serving the brain become narrowed by arterial disease or thrombus

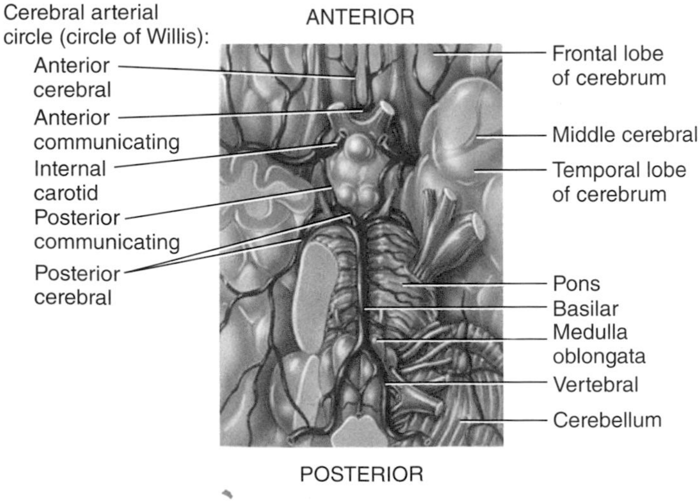

Cerebral arterial circle (circle of Willis):
Anterior cerebral
Anterior communicating
Internal carotid
Posterior communicating
Posterior cerebral
ANTERIOR
POSTERIOR
Frontal lobe of cerebrum
Middle cerebral
Temporal lobe of cerebrum
Pons
Basilar
Medulla oblongata
Vertebral
Cerebellum

Figure 6.7 Circle of Willis (Tortora and Derrickson 2009)

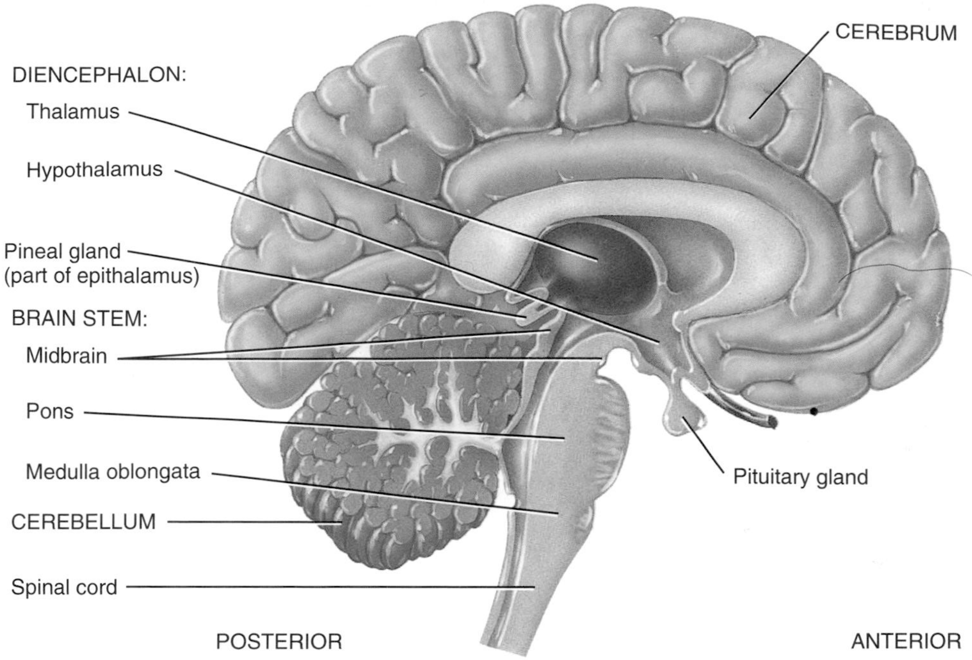
CEREBRUM
DIENCEPHALON:
Thalamus
Hypothalamus
Pineal gland
(part of epithalamus)
BRAIN STEM:
Midbrain
Pons
Medulla oblongata
CEREBELLUM
Spinal cord
Pituitary gland
POSTERIOR
ANTERIOR

Figure 6.8 The structures of the brain (Tortora and Derrickson 2009)

then there will be an alternative route available, maintaining the essential supply of oxygen and glucose required by the brain.

The brain can be divided into four anatomical regions. Each region contains one or more structures (see Figure 6.8):

- Cerebrum
  - Cerebral hemispheres
- Diencephalon
  - Thalamus
  - Hypothalamus
  - Epithalamus
- Brain stem
  - Midbrain
  - Pons
  - Medulla oblongata
  - Reticular formation
- Cerebellum.

Cerebrum

This is the largest brain structure. It is divided into the left and right hemispheres by the *longitudinal cerebral fissure.* Each hemisphere can be divided into lobes – occipital, frontal, parietal and

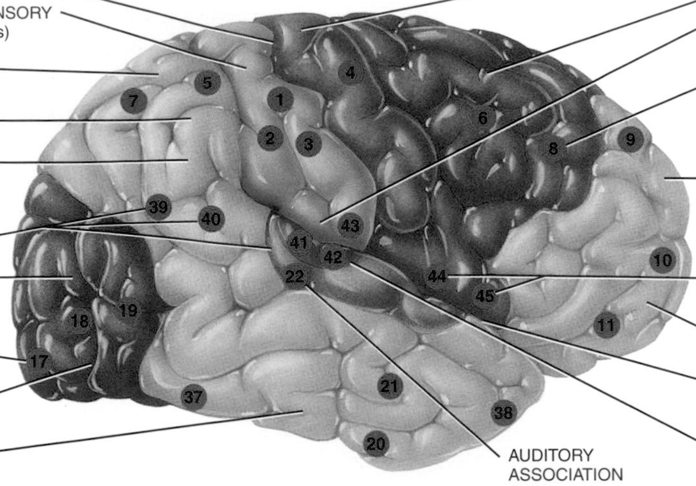

Central sulcus
PRIMARY SOMATOSENSORY AREA (postcentral gyrus)
SOMATOSENSORY ASSOCIATION AREA
Parietal lobe
COMMON INTEGRATIVE AREA
WERNICKE'S AREA
VISUAL ASSOCIATION AREA
PRIMARY VISUAL AREA
Occipital lobe
Temporal lobe
POSTERIOR
PRIMARY MOTOR AREA (precentral gyrus)
PREMOTOR AREA
PRIMARY GUSTATORY AREA
FRONTAL EYE FIELD AREA
Frontal lobe
BROCA'S SPEECH AREA
PREFRONTAL CORTEX
Lateral cerebral sulcus
PRIMARY AUDITORY AREA
AUDITORY ASSOCIATION AREA
ANTERIOR
1
2
3
4
5
6
7
8
9
10
11
17
18
19
20
21
22
37
38
39
40
41
42
43
44
45

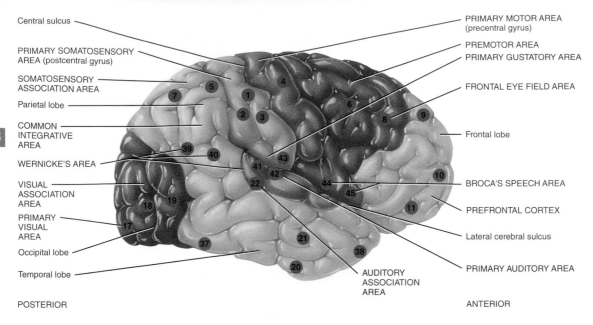

Figure 6.9 Right cerebral hemisphere showing Brodmann's area (Tortora and Derrickson 2009)

temporal. The outer layer of the cerebrum is called the cerebral cortex and is made of grey matter (nerve cell bodies). The layers below this are white matter (nerve fibres). The cerebral cortex is responsible for our conscious mind and consists of interneurones (the neurones that lie between sensory and motor neurones). The cerebral cortex can be divided into functional areas which were mapped by K Brodmann in 1906 (see Figure 6.9). The circled numbers on the diagram represent important areas on Brodmann's map. While functional and structural areas of the brain have been identified, it is important to remember that the areas do not function independently from one another and damage to one structure may have consequences for another.

The first of the functional areas is the motor area and it is subdivided as follows:

- The primary motor area: responsible for contraction of skeletal muscles
- The premotor area: involved in fine skeletal muscle movement creating the manual dexterity associated with repetitive or learned motor movement (e.g. tying a shoelace, learning to paint, etc.)
- Broca's area is responsible for the motor movement required to produce speech
- The frontal eye field area controls voluntary movement of the eyes.

The second functional area is the sensory area responsible for awareness of sensation. It can be divided as follows:

- The primary somatosensory area receives sensory information from the skin and also from proprioreceptors in skeletal muscles
- The somatosensory association area integrates the sensory information being relayed to the primary somatosensory area and provides information about size, texture, previous experience

- The visual areas – the primary visual area receives information from the eye and the visual association area helps to connect this information with past visual experiences
- The auditory areas are associated with the interpretation of sounds
- The olfactory area interprets smell information received from the nose via the olfactory nerves
- The gustatory area interprets taste information.

There are many other association areas within the cerebrum which act as communication areas between different functional regions in the cerebrum such as Wernicke's area which is responsible for understanding written and spoken language and is closely associated with Broca's speech area.

Diencephalon

This part of the brain is surrounded by the cerebrum and contains three paired structures:

- Thalamus – acts as a relay station for sensory impulses going to the cerebral cortex for integration and motor impulses entering and leaving the cerebral hemispheres. It also has a role in memory
- Hypothalamus – is closely associated with the pituitary gland and produces two hormones: antidiuretic hormone (ADH) and oxytocin. It is also the chief autonomic integration centre and is part of the *limbic system* which is the *emotional brain*
- Epithalamus – this structure is linked to the pineal gland which secretes the hormone melatonin responsible for sleep-wake cycles.

Brain stem

The structures that form the brain stem are involved in many activities that are essential for life. The brain stem is associated with the cranial nerves.

- Midbrain – conduction pathway that connects the cerebrum with the lower brain structures and spinal cord
- Pons – also a conduction pathway communicating with the cerebellum. The pons works with the medulla oblongata to control depth and rate of respiration.
- Medulla oblongata – relay station for sensory nerves going to the cerebrum. The medulla contains autonomic centres such as the cardiac centre, the respiratory centre, the vasomotor centre and the coughing, sneezing and vomiting centre. The medulla is also the site of decussation of the pyramidal tracts – this means that the right side of the body is controlled by the left cerebral hemisphere and vice versa.

Cerebellum

The cerebellum coordinates voluntary muscle movement, balance and posture. It ensures that muscle movements are smooth, coordinated and precise.

The limbic system and the reticular formation

The limbic system and the reticular formation are more functional than anatomical systems as they consist of networks of neurones that can be located close to many anatomical structures.

The limbic system is located close to the cerebrum and the diencephalon. It is known as the emotional brain and is responsible for the interpretation of facial expression helping identify fear and danger.

The reticular formation is a functional system located in the core of the brain stem and consists of a collection of neurones that have several functions:

- Contains reticular activating system that is responsible for alertness
- Filters or blocks repetitive stimuli such as background noise
- Regulates skeletal and muscle activity
- Coordinates visceral activity controlled by the autonomic nervous system.

The brain is a well-protected control and integration centre which receives information from the peripheral sensory nervous system and sends motor information to the peripheral nervous system through a comprehensive network of pathways via the spinal cord.

The peripheral nervous system

The peripheral nervous system (PNS) includes all the tissues that lie outside of the CNS and includes:

- Cranial nerves
- Spinal nerves
- Spinal cord
- Autonomic nervous system (ANS).

The PNS is subdivided into the efferent or motor system and the afferent or sensory system. The somatic sensory system serves the skeletal muscles, joints, tendons and the skin and includes the senses of vision, hearing, smell and taste (Logenbaker 2008). The internal organs of the body are supplied by the visceral sensory system. Both the somatic and visceral sensory systems take information from peripheral sensory receptors towards the CNS.

Commands from the CNS to the skeletal muscles are carried by the somatic motor system. The autonomic motor system predominantly regulates the activity of smooth and cardiac muscles and glands (Logenbaker 2008).

Cranial nerves

The human body contains 12 pairs of cranial nerves which emerge from the brain and supply various structures most of which are associated with the head and neck. Figure 6.10 provides an overview of the location and function of the cranial nerves.

The 12 pairs of cranial nerves, differ in their functions – some are **sensory nerves**, i.e. contain sensory fibres, some are **motor nerves**, i.e. contain only motor fibres, and some are **mixed nerves**, i.e. contain both sensory and motor nerves.

Table 6.1 provides a summary of the cranial nerves, their different components and function.

The spinal cord

The average adult spinal cord (see Figure 6.11) is between 42 and 45 cm long and extends from the medulla oblongata (lower part of the brain) to the upper part of the second lumbar vertebra. The

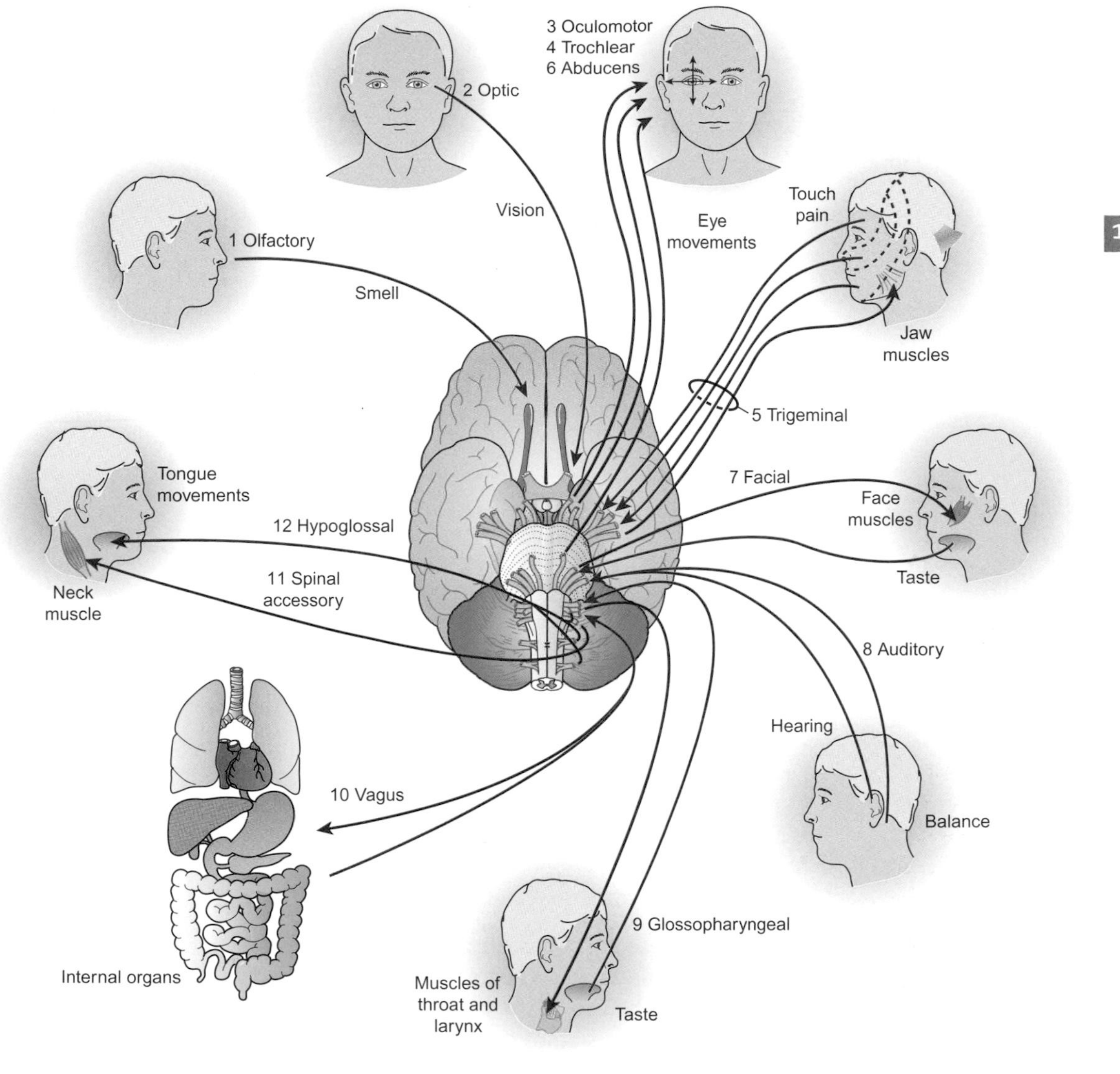
3 Oculomotor
4 Trochlear
6 Abducens
2 Optic
Vision
Eye movements
Touch pain
1 Olfactory
Smell
Jaw muscles
5 Trigeminal
Tongue movements
7 Facial
Face muscles
12 Hypoglossal
Taste
11 Spinal accessory
Neck muscle
8 Auditory
Hearing
10 Vagus
Balance
9 Glossopharyngeal
Internal organs
Muscles of throat and larynx
Taste

Figure 6.10 Functions of the cranial nerves

spinal cord is enclosed within the vertebral canal which forms a protective ring of bone around the cord. Other protective coverings include the spinal meninges, which are three layers of connective tissue coverings which extend around the spinal cord. The spinal meninges consist of:

- **Pia mater** – the innermost layer
- **Arachnoid mater** – the middle layer
- **Dura mater** – the outermost layer, which consists of a dense, irregular connective tissue.

The spinal cord consists of a central canal and grey and white matter. The central canal and the spinal meninges contain cerebrospinal fluid. The grey matter consists mostly of cell bodies and

Table 6.1 The cranial nerves

Number	Name	Components	Location/Function
I	Olfactory	Sensory	Olfactory receptors for sense of smell
II	Optic	Sensory	Retina (sight)
III	Oculomotor	Motor	Eye muscles (including eyelids and lens, pupil)
IV	Trochlear	Motor	Eye muscles
V	Trigeminal	Sensory and motor	Teeth, eyes, skin, tongue for sensation of touch, pain and temperature
VI	Abducens	Motor	Jaw muscles (chewing) Eye muscles
VII	Facial	Sensory and motor	Taste buds Facial muscles, tear and salivary glands
VIII	Vestibulocochlear	Sensory	Inner ear (hearing and balance)
IX	Glossopharyngeal	Sensory and motor	Pharyngeal muscles (swallowing)
X	Vagus	Sensory and motor	Internal organs
XI	Spinal accessory	Motor	Neck and back muscles
XII	Hypoglossal	Motor	Tongue muscles

their dendrites and the whiter areas consist of the axons of neurones which carry signals up and down the cord via ascending and descending tracts. These tracts cross as they enter and exit the brain and this explains why the right side of the brain controls the left side of the body and the left side of the brain controls the right side of the body.

The spinal cord is divided into the right and left halves by the deep **anterior median fissure** and the shallow **posterior median sulcus** (Torotora and Derrickson 2010).

Functions of the spinal cord

The spinal cord provides a means of communication between the brain and the peripheral nerves that leave the spinal cord (Logenbaker 2008) and has two major functions in maintaining homeostasis:

- The tracts of the white matter of the spinal cord carry sensory impulses to the brain and motor impulses from the brain to the skeletal muscles and other effector muscles
- The grey matter of the spinal cord is a site for integration of reflexes which is a rapid, involuntary action in relation to a particular stimulus.

(Tortora and Derrickson 2010)

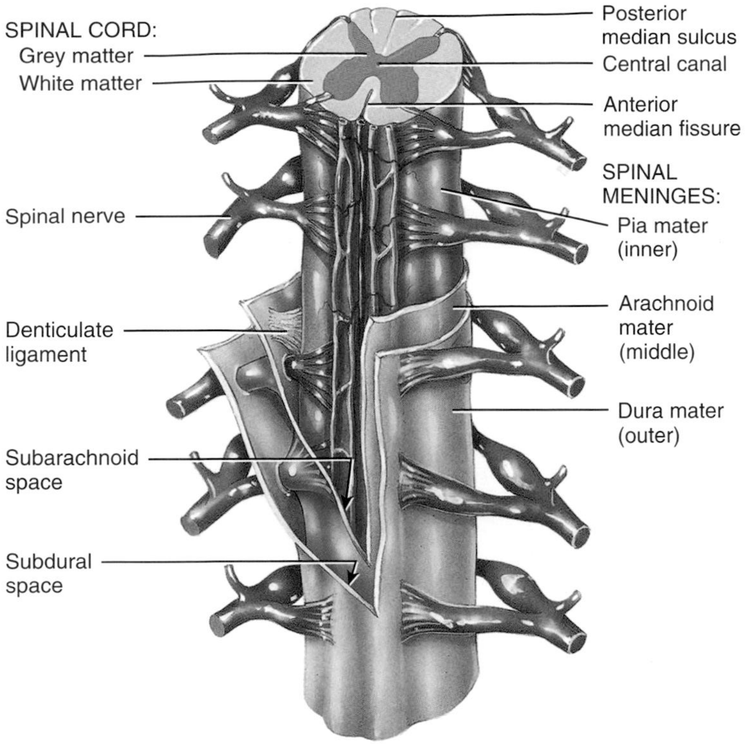
SPINAL CORD:
Grey matter
White matter
Spinal nerve
Denticulate ligament
Subarachnoid space
Subdural space
Posterior median sulcus
Central canal
Anterior median fissure
SPINAL MENINGES:
Pia mater (inner)
Arachnoid mater (middle)
Dura mater (outer)

Figure 6.11 The spinal cord (Tortora and Derrickson 2009)

Spinal nerves

There are 31 pairs of spinal nerves attached to the spinal cord within the human body which are named and numbered according to the region and level of the vertebral column from which they emerge (Figure 6.12).

Each nerve innervates a group of muscles (myotome) and an area of skin (dermatome) and most also innervate some of the thoracic and abdominal organs (Figure 6.13).

The spinal nerves provide the paths of communication between the spinal cord and specific regions of the body as they connect the CNS to sensory receptors, muscles and glands in all the parts of the body. A typical spinal nerve (Figure 6.14) has two connections to the spinal cord: a posterior root and an anterior root, which unite to form a spinal nerve at the **intervertebral foramen**. A spinal nerve is an example of a mixed nerve as it contains both sensory (posterior root) and motor (anterior root) nerves.

Clinical considerations

Acute spinal cord compression is a neurological emergency that requires rapid diagnosis and treatment if permanent loss of function is to be avoided. Common causes of spinal cord compression include:

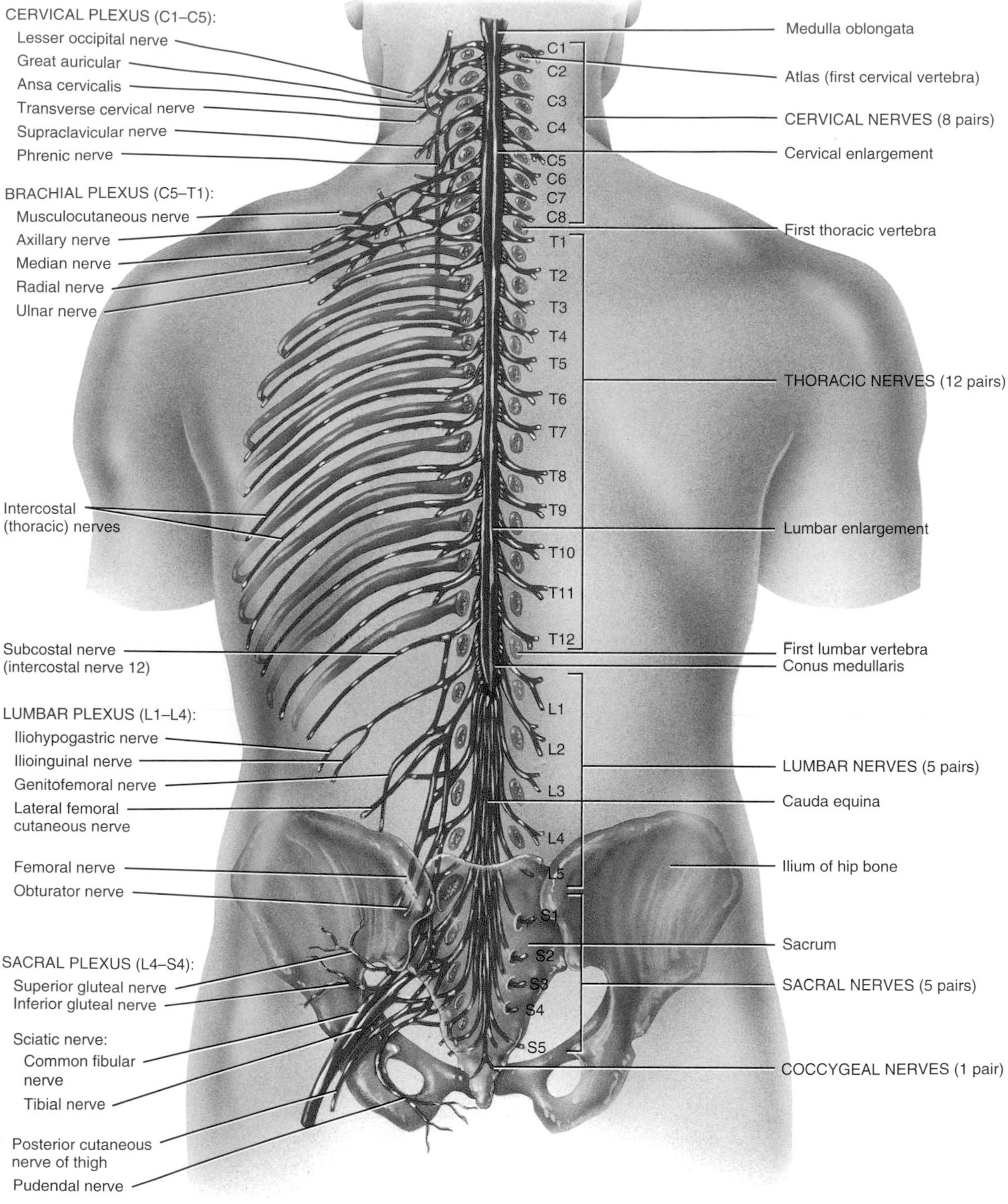
CERVICAL PLEXUS (C1–C5):
Lesser occipital nerve
Great auricular
Ansa cervicalis
Transverse cervical nerve
Supraclavicular nerve
Phrenic nerve
BRACHIAL PLEXUS (C5–T1):
Musculocutaneous nerve
Axillary nerve
Median nerve
Radial nerve
Ulnar nerve
Intercostal (thoracic) nerves
Subcostal nerve (intercostal nerve 12)
LUMBAR PLEXUS (L1–L4):
Iliohypogastric nerve
Ilioinguinal nerve
Genitofemoral nerve
Lateral femoral cutaneous nerve
Femoral nerve
Obturator nerve
SACRAL PLEXUS (L4–S4):
Superior gluteal nerve
Inferior gluteal nerve
Sciatic nerve:
Common fibular nerve
Tibial nerve
Posterior cutaneous nerve of thigh
Pudendal nerve
C1
C2
C3
C4
C5
C6
C7
C8
T1
T2
T3
T4
T5
T6
T7
T8
T9
T10
T11
T12
L1
L2
L3
L4
L5
S1
S2
S3
S4
S5
Medulla oblongata
Atlas (first cervical vertebra)
CERVICAL NERVES (8 pairs)
Cervical enlargement
First thoracic vertebra
THORACIC NERVES (12 pairs)
Lumbar enlargement
First lumbar vertebra
Conus medullaris
LUMBAR NERVES (5 pairs)
Cauda equina
Ilium of hip bone
Sacrum
SACRAL NERVES (5 pairs)
COCCYGEAL NERVES (1 pair)

Posterior view of entire spinal cord and portions of spinal nerves

Figure 6.12 The spinal cord and spinal nerves (Tortora and Derrickson 2009)

- Trauma (car accidents, sports injury and falls)
- Tumours, both benign and malignant
- A prolapsed intervertebral disc (L4-L5 and L5-S1 are the most common levels of disc prolapse)
- An epidural or subdural haemorrhage
- Inflammatory disease, e.g. rheumatoid arthritis
- Infection.

Signs and symptoms include sensory loss, paraesthesia, disturbance of gait, loss of power or paralysis.

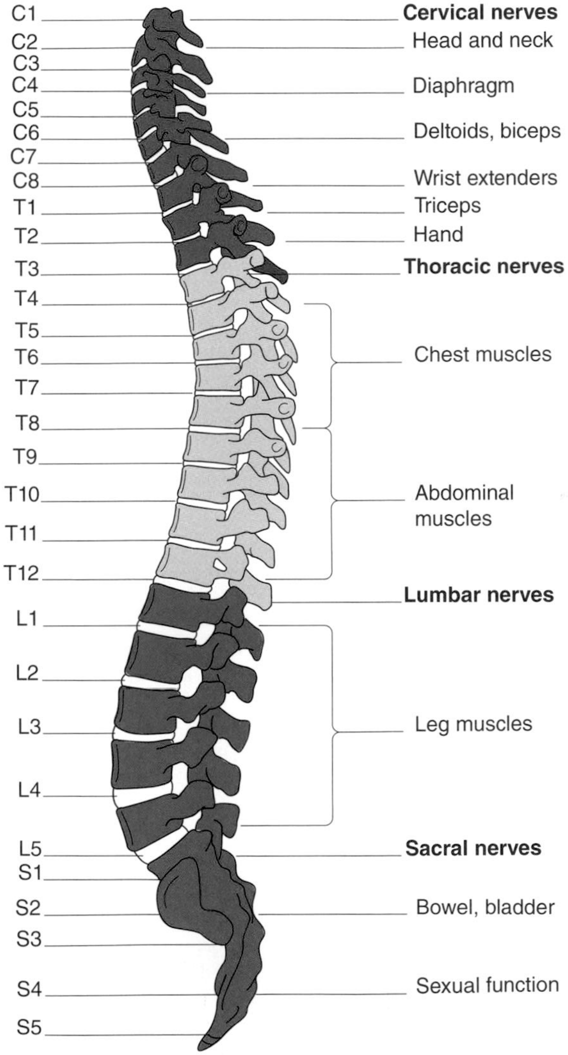
C1
C2
C3
C4
C5
C6
C7
C8
T1
T2
T3
T4
T5
T6
T7
T8
T9
T10
T11
T12
L1
L2
L3
L4
L5
S1
S2
S3
S4
S5
Cervical nerves
Head and neck
Diaphragm
Deltoids, biceps
Wrist extenders
Triceps
Hand
Thoracic nerves
Chest muscles
Abdominal muscles
Lumbar nerves
Leg muscles
Sacral nerves
Bowel, bladder
Sexual function

Figure 6.13 The spinal nerves and their areas of innervations

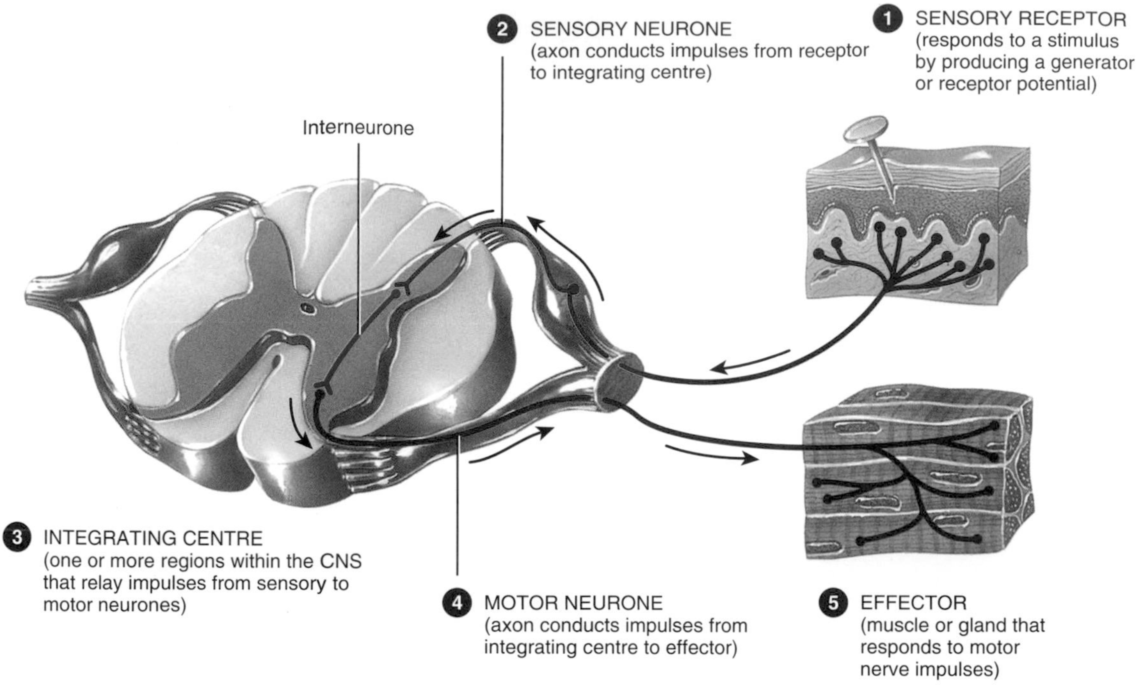

2 SENSORY NEURONE
(axon conducts impulses from receptor to integrating centre)
1 SENSORY RECEPTOR
(responds to a stimulus by producing a generator or receptor potential)
Interneurone
3 INTEGRATING CENTRE
(one or more regions within the CNS that relay impulses from sensory to motor neurones)
4 MOTOR NEURONE
(axon conducts impulses from integrating centre to effector)
5 EFFECTOR
(muscle or gland that responds to motor nerve impulses)

Figure 6.14 A typical spinal nerve (Tortora and Derrickson 2009)

The autonomic nervous system

The autonomic nervous system (ANS) plays a major role in the maintenance of homeostasis by regulating the body's automatic, involuntary functions and, in common with the rest of the nervous system, consists of **neurones**, **neuroglia** and other connective tissue. However, its structure is unique in that it is divided into two, namely the **sympathetic division** and the **parasympathetic division**. These two divisions have several common features:

- They innervate all internal organs
- They utilise two motor neurones and one ganglion to transmit an action potential
- They function automatically and usually in an involuntary manner.

(Logenbaker 2008)

Sympathetic division (fight or flight)

The sympathetic division (see Figure 6.15) includes nerve fibres that arise from the 12 thoracic and first two lumbar segments of the spinal, hence it is also referred to as the **thoracicolumbar** division. The sympathetic division takes control of many internal organs when a stressful situation occurs. This can take the form of physical stress if undertaking strenuous exercise or emotional stress at times of anger or anxiety. In emergency situations, the sympathetic nervous system releases **norepinephrine** which assists in the 'fight or flight' response (Migliozzi 2009).

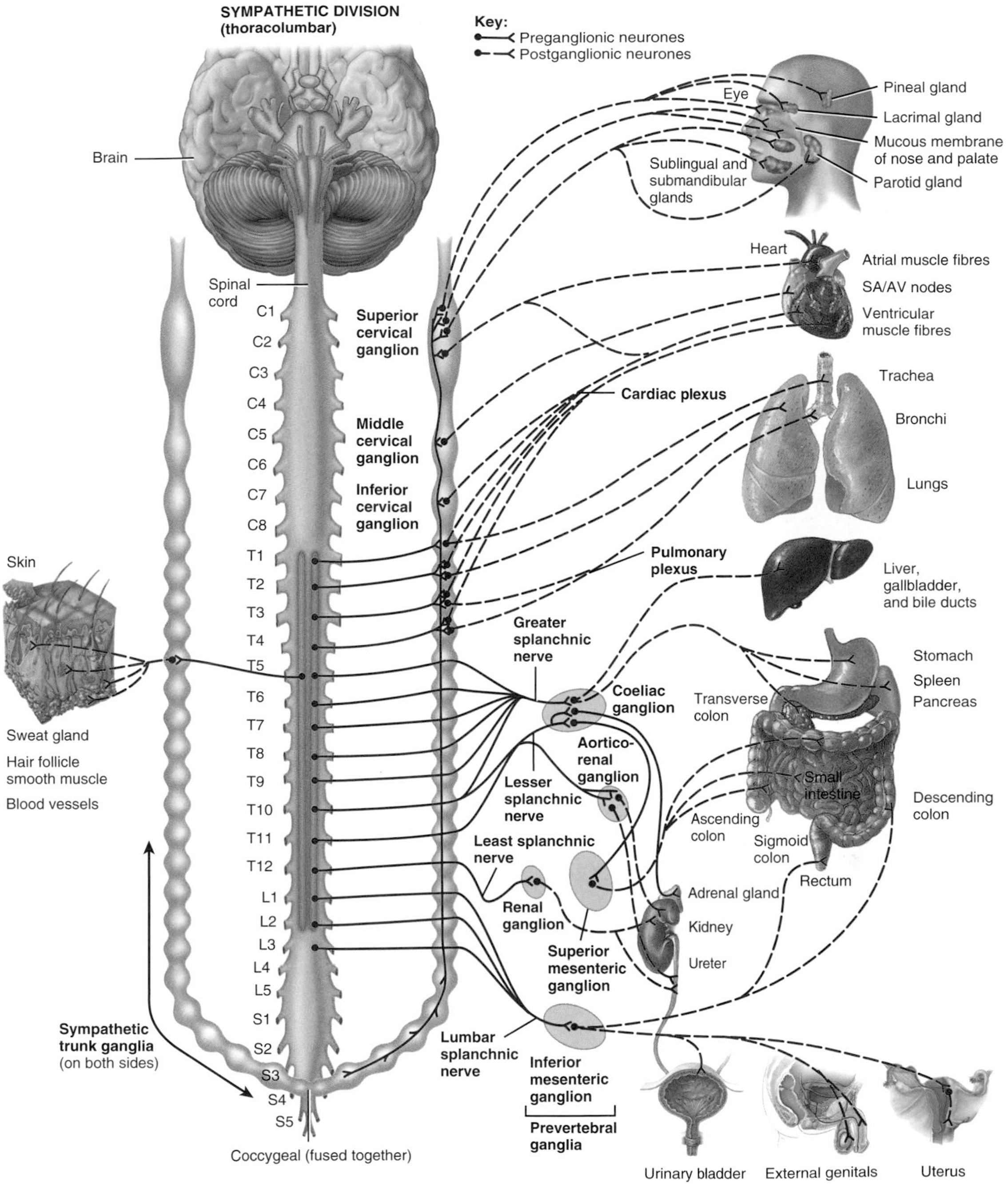
SYMPATHETIC DIVISION
(thoracolumbar)
Key:
Preganglionic neurones
Postganglionic neurones
Brain
Spinal cord
C1
C2
C3
C4
C5
C6
C7
C8
T1
T2
T3
T4
T5
T6
T7
T8
T9
T10
T11
T12
L1
L2
L3
L4
L5
S1
S2
S3
S4
S5
Coccygeal (fused together)
Superior cervical ganglion
Middle cervical ganglion
Inferior cervical ganglion
Eye
Pineal gland
Lacrimal gland
Mucous membrane of nose and palate
Sublingual and submandibular glands
Parotid gland
Heart
Atrial muscle fibres
SA/AV nodes
Ventricular muscle fibres
Cardiac plexus
Trachea
Bronchi
Lungs
Skin
Sweat gland
Hair follicle smooth muscle
Blood vessels
Pulmonary plexus
Liver, gallbladder, and bile ducts
Greater splanchnic nerve
Coeliac ganglion
Stomach
Spleen
Pancreas
Transverse colon
Aortico-renal ganglion
Lesser splanchnic nerve
Small intestine
Descending colon
Ascending colon
Sigmoid colon
Least splanchnic nerve
Rectum
Adrenal gland
Renal ganglion
Kidney
Superior mesenteric ganglion
Ureter
Sympathetic trunk ganglia (on both sides)
Lumbar splanchnic nerve
Inferior mesenteric ganglion
Prevertebral ganglia
Urinary bladder
External genitals
Uterus

Figure 6.15 Sympathetic nervous system (Tortora and Derrickson 2009)

Table 6.2 Effects of the parasympathetic and sympathetic divisions of the autonomic nervous system

Organ/System	Sympathetic effects	Parasympathetic effects
Cell metabolism	Increases metabolic rate, stimulates fat breakdown and increases blood sugar levels	No effect
Blood vessels	Constricts blood vessels in viscera and skin Dilates blood vessels in the heart and skeletal muscle	No effect
Eye	Dilates pupils	Constricts pupils
Heart	Increases rate and force of contraction	Decreases rate
Lungs	Dilates bronchioles	Constricts bronchioles
Kidneys	Decreases urine output	No effect
Liver	Causes the release of glucose	No effect
Digestive system	Decreases peristalsis and constricts digestive system sphincters	Increases peristalsis and dilates digestive system sphincters
Adrenal medulla	Stimulates cells to secrete epinephrine and norepinephrine	No effect
Lacrimal glands	Inhibits the production of tears	Increases the production of tears
Salivary glands	Inhibits the production of saliva	Increases the production of saliva
Sweat glands	Stimulates to produce perspiration	No effect

Parasympathetic division (rest and digest)

The parasympathetic division includes fibres that arise from the lower end of the spinal cord and includes several cranial nerves – hence it is often referred to as the **craniosacral** division. The parasympathetic division is most active when the body is at rest and utilises **acetylcholine** to control all the internal responses associated with a state of relaxation (Figure 6.16) and therefore has many opposite effects on the body to the sympathetic nervous system (Migliozzi 2009).

Table 6.2 provides a summary of the physiological effects of the sympathetic and parasympathetic divisions of the nervous system.

Conclusion

In conclusion, the human nervous system is a highly organised network of cells and structures that include the brain and cranial nerves and the spinal cord and spinal nerves which play a major role

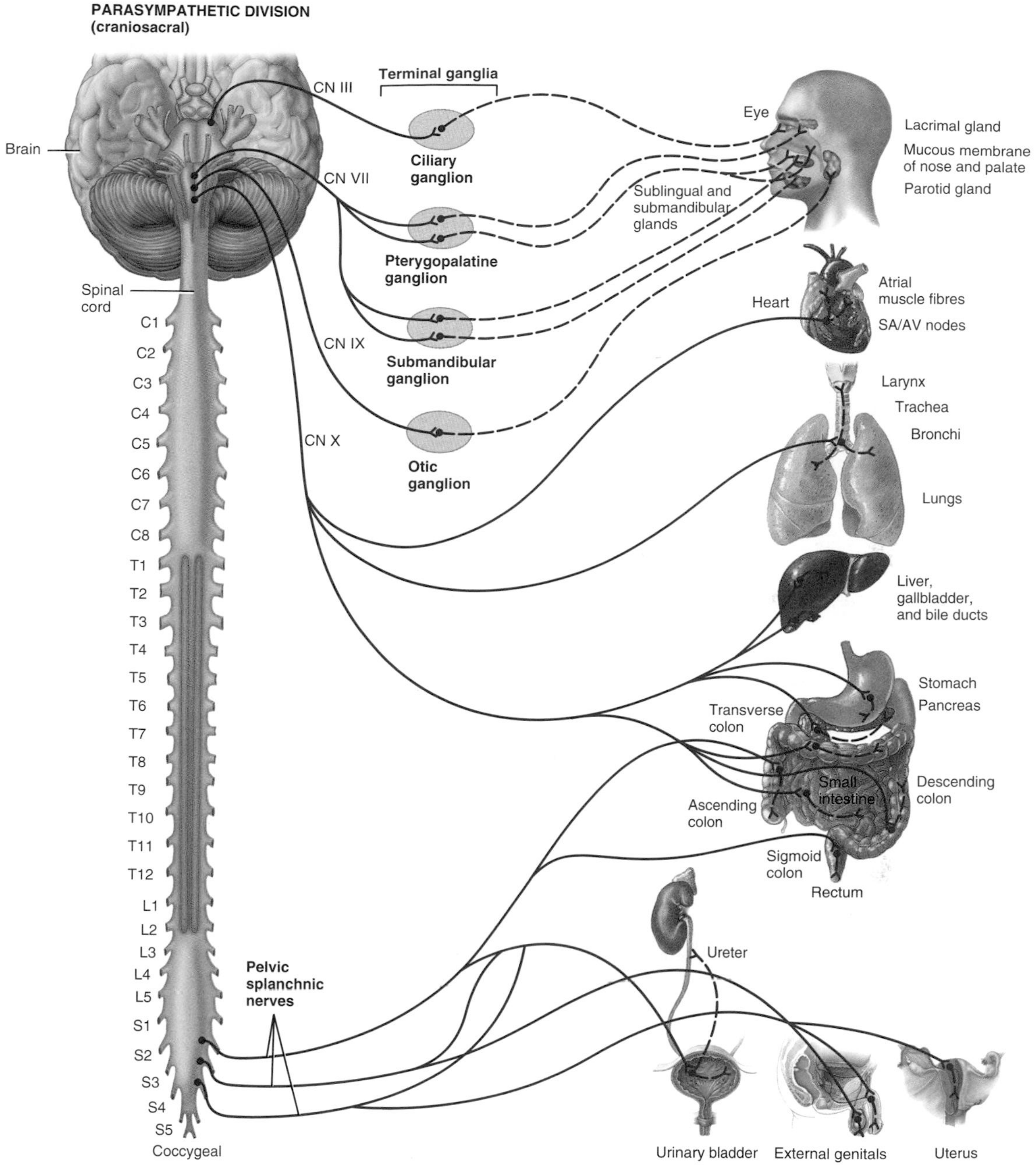
PARASYMPATHETIC DIVISION
(craniosacral)
Brain
Terminal ganglia
CN III
Ciliary ganglion
CN VII
Pterygopalatine ganglion
Submandibular ganglion
CN IX
CN X
Otic ganglion
Eye
Lacrimal gland
Mucous membrane of nose and palate
Parotid gland
Sublingual and submandibular glands
Heart
Atrial muscle fibres
SA/AV nodes
Larynx
Trachea
Bronchi
Lungs
Liver, gallbladder, and bile ducts
Stomach
Pancreas
Transverse colon
Small intestine
Descending colon
Ascending colon
Sigmoid colon
Rectum
Ureter
Spinal cord
C1
C2
C3
C4
C5
C6
C7
C8
T1
T2
T3
T4
T5
T6
T7
T8
T9
T10
T11
T12
L1
L2
L3
L4
L5
S1
S2
S3
S4
S5
Coccygeal
Pelvic splanchnic nerves
Urinary bladder
External genitals
Uterus

Figure 6.16 Parasympathetic nervous system (Tortora and Derrickson 2009)

in maintaining homeostasis. The nervous system responds to external and internal stimuli through three basic functions: the sensory, integrative and motor functions which generate responses and creates changes in bodily functions as required. Conditions affecting the nervous system can have a devastating effect on the quality of life and the functions essential for survival.

Glossary

Action potential: Conduction along a nerve or muscle cell membrane caused by a large, transient depolarisation.

Antidiuretic hormone (ADH): Hormone that acts on the kidneys to reabsorb more water, thus reducing urine output.

Afferent fibres: Carry nerve impulses towards the central nervous system.

Arachnoid mater: Middle layer of the meninges.

Astrocyte: Neuroglial cell that helps for the blood–brain barrier.

Autonomic nervous system: Involuntary motor division of the motor nervous system.

Axon: Process of a neurone that carries impulses away from the cell body.

Brain stem: Collective name given to the pons, medulla and midbrain.

Cation: An ion with a positive charge.

Central nervous system: Brain and spinal cord.

Cerebellum: Anatomical region of the brain responsible for coordinated and smooth skeletal muscle movements.

Cerebral hemispheres: Division of the cerebrum.

Cerebrospinal fluid: Fluid that surrounds the central nervous system.

Cerebrum: Large anatomical region of the brain which is divided into the cerebral hemispheres.

Circle of Willis: Part of arterial blood supply to the brain.

Cranial nerves: Twelve pairs of nerves that leave the brain and supply sensory and motor neurones to the head, neck, part of the trunk and the viscera of the thorax and abdomen.

Dendrite: Part of neurone that transmits impulses towards the cell body

Diencephalon Anatomical region of the brain consisting of the thalamus, hypothalamus and epithalamus.

Dura mater: Tough outer layer of the meninges.

Effector: Muscle, gland or organ stimulated by the nervous system.

Efferent fibres: Carry nerve impulses away from the central nervous system.

Ependymal cells: Neuroglial cells that line the cavities of the central nervous system.

Epinephrine: Hormone produced by the adrenal medulla that is also a neurotransmitter.

Epithalamus: Part of the brain that forms the diencephalon.

Ganglia: A group of neuronal cell bodies lying outside the central nervous system.

Hypothalamus: Part of the diencephalon with many functions.

Limbic system: Part of the brain involved in emotional responses.

Lobe: A clear anatomical division or boundary within a structure.

Medulla oblongata: Part of the brain stem.

Meninges: Three layers of tissue that cover and protect the central nervous system (dura, arachnoid and pia maters).

Midbrain: Part of the brain stem that links the brain stem to the diencephalon.

Microglia: Neuroglia that has the ability to phagocytose material.

Motor area: Area located in the cerebral cortex that controls voluntary motor function.

Motor nerves: Neurones that conduct impulses to effectors which may be either muscle or glands.

Myelin sheath: Fatty insulating layer that surrounds nerve fibres responsible for speeding up impulse conduction.

Neuroglia: Cells of the nervous system that protect and support the functional unit – the neurone.

Neuromuscular junction: Region where skeletal muscle comes into contact with a neurone.

Neurone: Functional unit of the nervous system responsible for generating and conducting nerve impulses.

Nuclei: Cluster of cell bodies within the central nervous system.

Oligodendrocytes: Glial cell that helps produce the myelin sheath.

Peripheral nervous system: All nerves located outside of the brain and spinal cord (the central nervous system).

Pia mater: Innermost layer of the meninges.

Pineal gland: Part of the diencephalon that has an endocrine function.

Pituitary gland: An endocrine gland located next to the hypothalamus that produces many hormones.

Receptor: Sensory nerve ending or cell that responds to stimuli.

Refractory period: The period immediately after a neurone has fired when it cannot receive another impulse.

Reticular formation: Area located throughout the brain stem that is responsible for arousal, regulation of sensory input to the cerebrum and control of motor output.

Saltatory conduction: Transmission of an impulse down a mylelinated nerve fibre where the impulse moves from node of Ranvier to node.

Sensory area: Area of the cerebrum responsible for sensation.

Sensory nerves: Neurones that carry sensory information from cranial and spinal nerves into the brain and spinal cord.

Somatic nervous system: Voluntary motor division of the peripheral nervous system.

Spinal nerves: Thirty-one pairs of nerves that originate on the spinal cord.

Synapse: Junction between two neurones or neurones and effector site.

Thalamus: Part of the diencephalon.

Ventricle: Cavity in the brain.

White matter: Myelinated nerve fibres.

References

Logenbaker, S.N. (2008) *Mader's Understanding Human Anatomy and Physiology*, 6th edn. London: McGraw-Hill.

Marieb, E.N. and Hoehn, K. (2007) *Human Anatomy and Physiology*, 7th edn. San Francisco: Pearson Benjamin Cummings.

Migliozzi, J.G. (2009) The nervous system and associated disorders. In: Nair, M. and Peate, I. (2009) *Fundamentals of Applied Pathophysiology: An Essential Guide for Nursing Students*. Oxford: Wiley-Blackwell.

Seeley, R.R., Stephens T.D. and Tate, P. (2006) *Anatomy and Physiology*, 7th edn. New York: McGraw-Hill.

Tortora, G.J. and Derrickson, T. (2009) *Principles of Anatomy and Physiology*, 12th edn. Hoboken, NJ: John Wiley & Sons.

Tortora, G.J. and Derrickson, B. (2010) *Essentials of Anatomy and Physiology*, 8th edn. New York: John Wiley & Sons.

Waugh, A. and Grant, A. (2001) *Ross and Wilson Anatomy and Physiology in Health and Illness*, 9th edn. Edinburgh: Elsevier Churchill Livingstone.

Activities

www.wiley.com/go/peate

Multiple choice questions

1. Which part of the brain is responsible for thinking, reasoning and intelligence?
   (a) cerebellum
   (b) hypothalamus
   (c) cerebrum
   (d) epithalamus
2. Which structures are involved in the control of respiration?
   (a) pons and medulla
   (b) thalamus and epithalamus
   (c) somatic and sensory nervous system
   (d) cerebellum and cerebrum
3. Which neuroglial cell acts as a macrophage?
   (a) oligodendrocyte
   (b) astrocyte
   (c) microglia
   (d) Schwann cell
4. Which layer of the meninges is closest to the skull bone?
   (a) dura mater
   (b) arachnoid mater
   (c) pia mater
   (d) subarachnoid space
5. Which neurotransmitter is associated with the neuromuscular junction?
   (a) dopamine
   (b) norepinephrine
   (c) acetylcholine
   (d) CSF
6. Which part of the brain is closely associated with the pituitary gland?
   (a) thalamus
   (b) epithalamus
   (c) hypothalamus
   (d) pons

7. Which is true of the autonomic nervous system?
   (a) it has two divisions – the somatic and voluntary divisions
   (b) it is housed in the cerebrum
   (c) it helps regulate heart rate and blood pressure
   (d) it does not influence any other system of the body

8. Nerves that carry impulses towards the central nervous system are:
   (a) afferent nerves
   (b) efferent nerves
   (c) motor nerves
   (d) mixed nerves

9. Sympathetic stimulation of the nervous system would lead to all but which of the following responses:
   (a) bronchioles dilate
   (b) urine output increases
   (c) heart rate increases
   (d) epinephrine (adrenaline) is released

10. Nerves that carry impulses away from the central nervous system are:
   (a) afferent nerves
   (b) efferent nerves
   (c) motor nerves
   (d) mixed nerves

True or false

1. The hypothalamus produces oxytocin.
2. Voluntary muscle movement is controlled by the afferent nervous system.
3. Ependymal cells help to circulate CSF.
4. The cranial nerves are all motor nerves.
5. There are eight thoracic nerves.

Test your learning

- Name the two major divisions of the nervous system.
- Differentiate between the parasympathetic nervous system and the sympathetic nervous system.
- Identify the functions of the neuroglia.
- Describe the action potential.
- Identify the functions of the different regions of the brain.

Label the diagram

From the lists of words, label the diagrams below:

Axon collateral, AXON, Axon, Axoplasm, Axolemma, Axon terminal, Synaptic end bulb, Nucleus of Schwann cell, Schwann cell:, Cytoplasm, Myelin sheath, Neurolemma, Node of Ranvier, Neurofibril, Initial segment, Axon hillock, Mitochondrion, Cytoplasm, Nissl bodies, DENDRITES, CELL BODY, Neurofibril, Nucleus, Dendrite, Neuroglial cell, Cell body, Axon

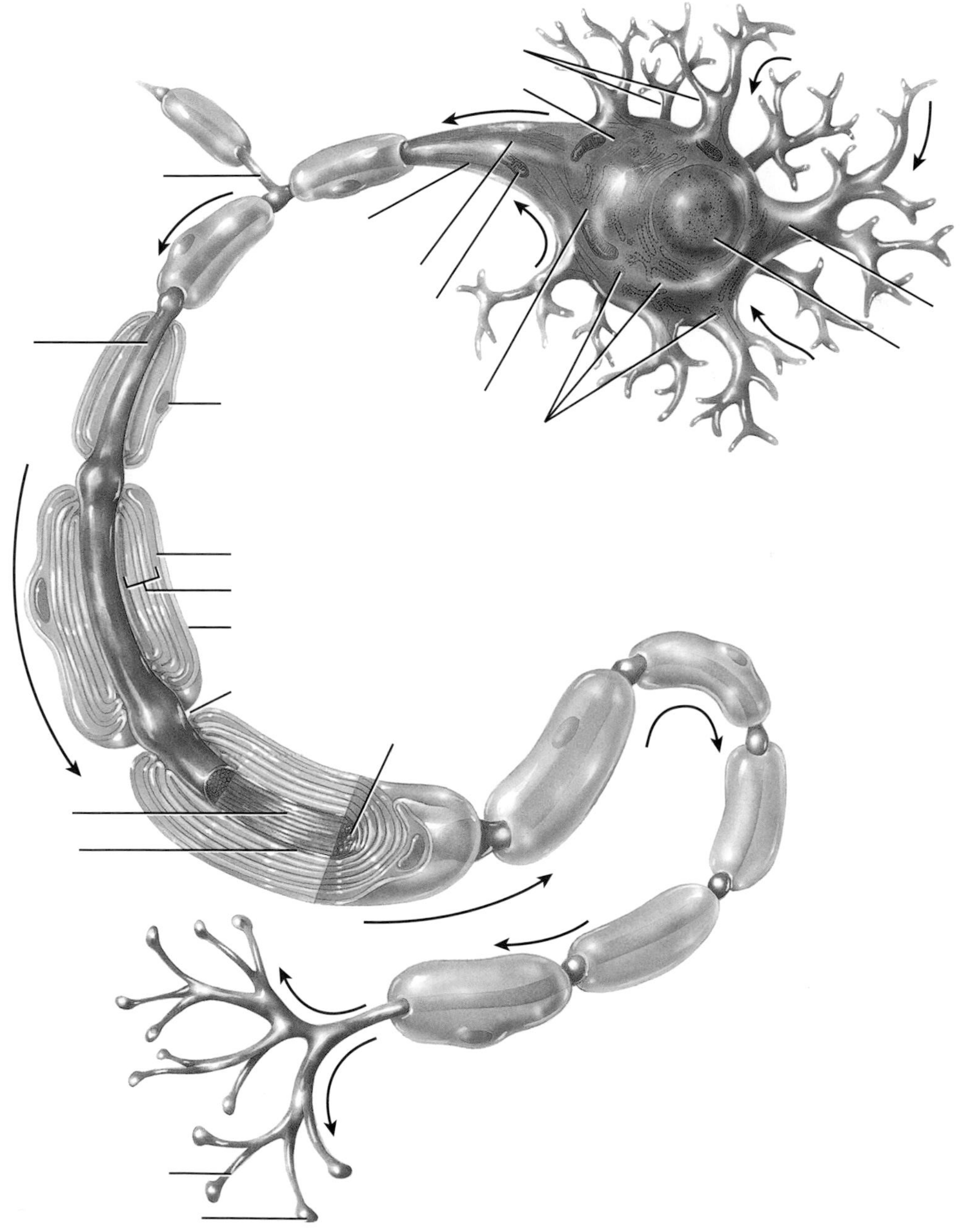

DIENCEPHALON:, Thalamus, Hypothalamus, Pineal gland (part of epithalamus), BRAIN STEM:, Midbrain, Pons, Medulla oblongata, CEREBELLUM, Spinal cord, POSTERIOR, CEREBRUM, Pituitary gland, ANTERIOR

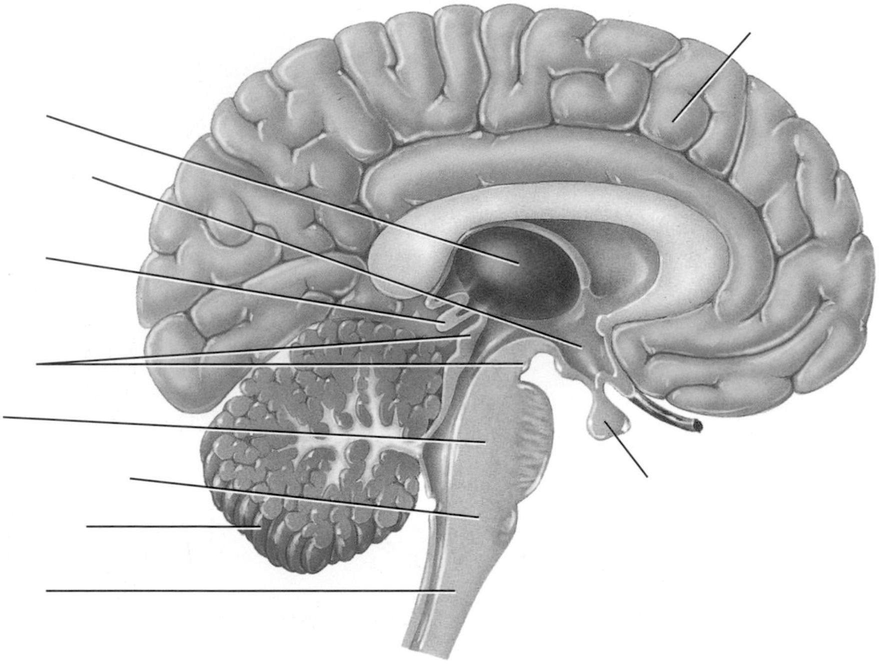

Crossword

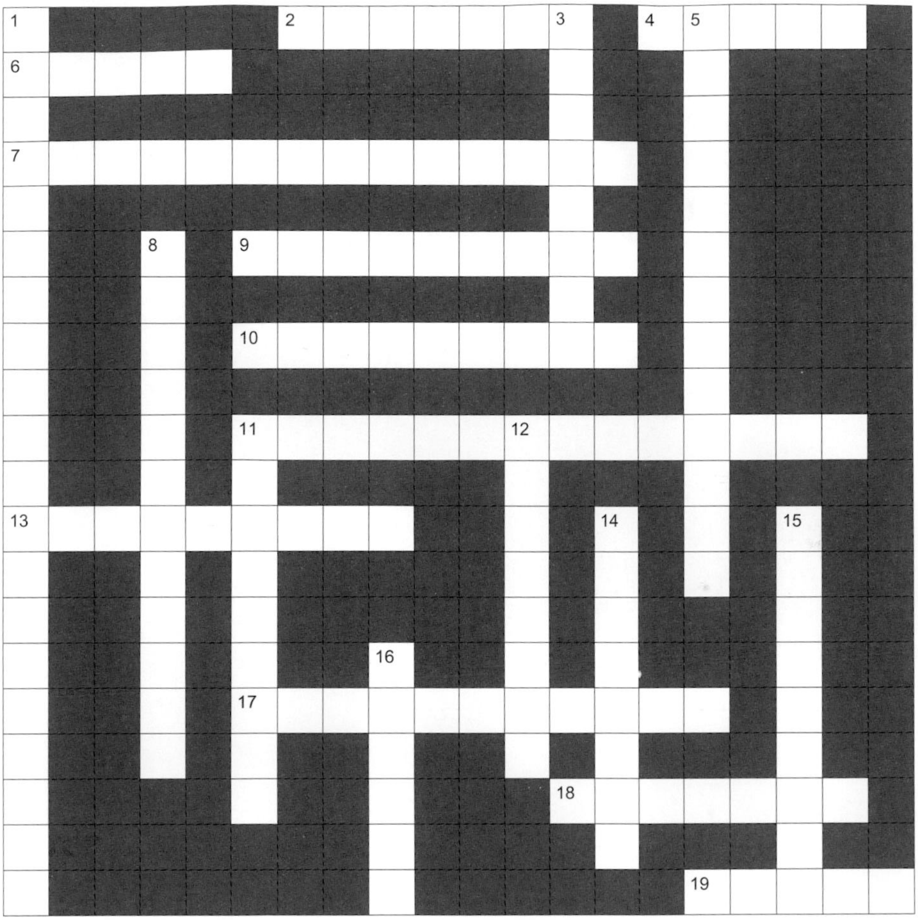

Across:

2. Cell of the nervous system (7).
4. Cranial nerve X (5).
6. Cranial nerve II (5).
7. Middle layer of the meninges (9, 5).
9. Outer layer of the meninges – closest to the skull (4, 5).
10. Star-shaped microglia (9).
11. A structure of the endocrine system that is located next to the hypothalamus (9, 5).
13. Cranial nerve I (9).
17. Describes the autonomic nervous system control (11).
18. Part of the brain that has a role in respiratory and heart rate (7).
19. One half of the central nervous system (5).

Down:

1. Voluntary part of the peripheral nervous system (7, 7, 6).
3. Name given to a nerve delivering the impulse away from the central nervous system (8).
5. Neuromuscular junction neurotransmitter (13).
8. Brain structure responsible for the autonomic nervous system (12).
11. Principal intracellular cation involved in the action potential (9).
12. Name given to a nerve delivering the impulse towards the central nervous system (8).
14. Layer of the meninges that is in contact with the brain (3, 5).
15. Nervous system phagocyte (9).
16. Principal extracellular cation involved in the action potential (6).

Conditions

Below is a list of conditions that are associated with the nervous system. Take some time and write notes about each of the conditions. You may make the notes taken from text books or other resources, for example, people you work with in a clinical area, or you may make the notes as a result of people you have cared for. If you are making notes about people you have cared for you must ensure that you adhere to the rules of confidentiality.

Multiple sclerosis	
Botulism	
Fibromyalgia	
Parkinson's disease	
Epilepsy	
Raised intracranial pressure	
Alzheimer's disease	

Answers

Crossword

Across:

2. Neurone

4. Vagus

6. Optic

7. Arachnoid mater

9. Dura mater

10. Astrocyte

11. Pituitary gland

13. Olfactory

17. Involuntary

18. Medulla

19. Brain

Down:

1. Somatic nervous system

3. Efferent

5. Acetylcholine

8. Hypothalamus

11. Potassium

12. Afferent

14. Pia mater

15. Microglia

16. Sodium

7 The endocrine system

Carl Clare

Contents

Introduction *192*

The endocrine organs **193**

Hormones **194**
Effects of hormones 196
Destruction and removal of hormones 197
Control of hormone release 197

The physiology of the endocrine organs **198**
The hypothalamus and the pituitary gland 198
Hormones released by the anterior pituitary gland 199
Growth hormone 200
Prolactin 200
Follicle stimulating hormone and luteinising hormone (gonadotrophins) 201
Thyroid stimulating hormone (TSH) 201
Adrenocorticotrophic hormone (ACTH) 201

The thyroid gland **202**

The parathyroid glands **205**

The adrenal glands **205**
Adrenal medulla 206
Adrenal cortex 207

Mineralocorticoids **208**

Glucocorticoids **208**

Pancreas **211**

Insulin **211**

Glucagon **212**

Somatostatin **213**

Conclusion *213*
Glossary *214*
References *216*
Activities *216*

Fundamentals of Anatomy and Physiology for Student Nurses, First Edition. Edited by Ian Peate, Muralitharan Nair.

Test your knowledge

- Name one hormone released by the pituitary gland.
- Where in the body is the thyroid gland found?
- What stimulates the release of insulin?

Learning outcomes

By the end of this chapter the reader will be able to:

- Name the endocrine glands in the body and the hormones they secrete
- Discuss the different forms of stimulus for the release of hormones
- Explain the control of hormone release by the hypothalamus
- Discuss the hormonal responses to stress

Body map

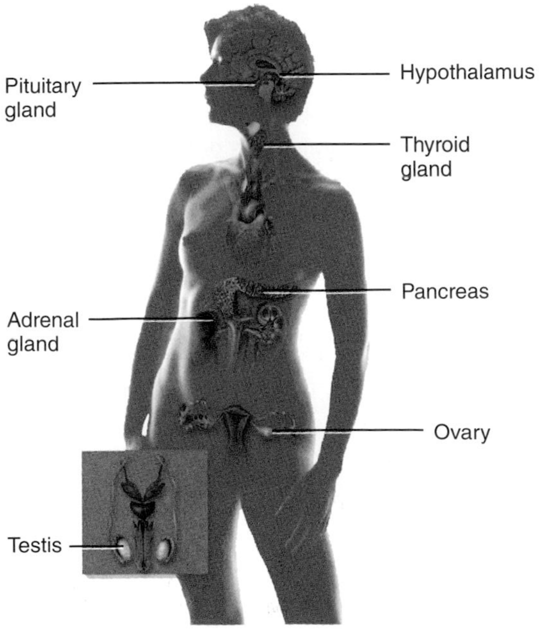
Pituitary gland
Hypothalamus
Thyroid gland
Pancreas
Adrenal gland
Ovary
Testis

Introduction

Homeostasis (from the Greek homoios, 'similar'; and histēmi, 'standing still') refers to the process of maintaining a stable internal environment. In other words, homeostasis refers to the maintenance of normal physiological balance and functioning within the body. There are two major systems in the body for maintaining homeostasis: the nervous system and the endocrine system. Table 7.1 shows the differences between these two systems.

The nervous system reacts rapidly to stimuli and effects its changes over a period of seconds or minutes, thus it is involved in the immediate and short-term maintenance of homeostasis. Due to its rapid onset of action the nervous system is responsible for the control of rapid bodily processes such as breathing and movement. The endocrine system is often responsible for the regulation of longer-term processes. The major functions it coordinates are:

- Homeostasis – maintains the internal body environment
- Storage and utilisation of energy substrates (carbohydrates, proteins and fats)
- Regulation of growth and reproduction
- Control of the body's responses to external stimuli (particularly stress).

It should be noted, however, that though these two systems are separate they often act together and complement each other in the maintenance of homeostasis.

The endocrine system is made up of a collection of small organs that are scattered throughout the body, each of which releases hormones into the blood supply ('endo' = within, 'crine' = to secrete). These hormone-releasing organs can be split into three main categories (Jenkins *et al.* 2007):

- Endocrine glands, organs whose only function is the production and release of hormones. These include:
  - pituitary gland
  - thyroid gland
  - parathyroid gland
  - adrenal gland
- Organs that are not pure glands (as they have other functions as well as the production of hormones) but contain relatively large areas of hormone producing tissue. These include:
  - hypothalamus
  - pancreas

Table 7.1 Nervous system versus endocrine system

	Nervous System	Endocrine System
Speed of action	Seconds	Minutes to hours (even days)
Duration of action	Seconds to minutes	Minutes to days
Method of transmitting messages	Electrical	Chemical
Transport method	Neurones	Hormones

- other tissues and organs also produce hormones – areas of hormone-producing cells are found in the wall of the small intestine and the stomach.

There are no cell types, organs or processes that are not influenced by the endocrine system in some way and whilst there are many hormones that we know of there are probably many more that are yet to be discovered.

The endocrine organs

See Figure 7.1 for the endocrine organs and their position within the body.

Each of these organs will typically have a rich blood supply delivered by numerous blood vessels. The hormone-producing cells within the organ are arranged into branching networks around this

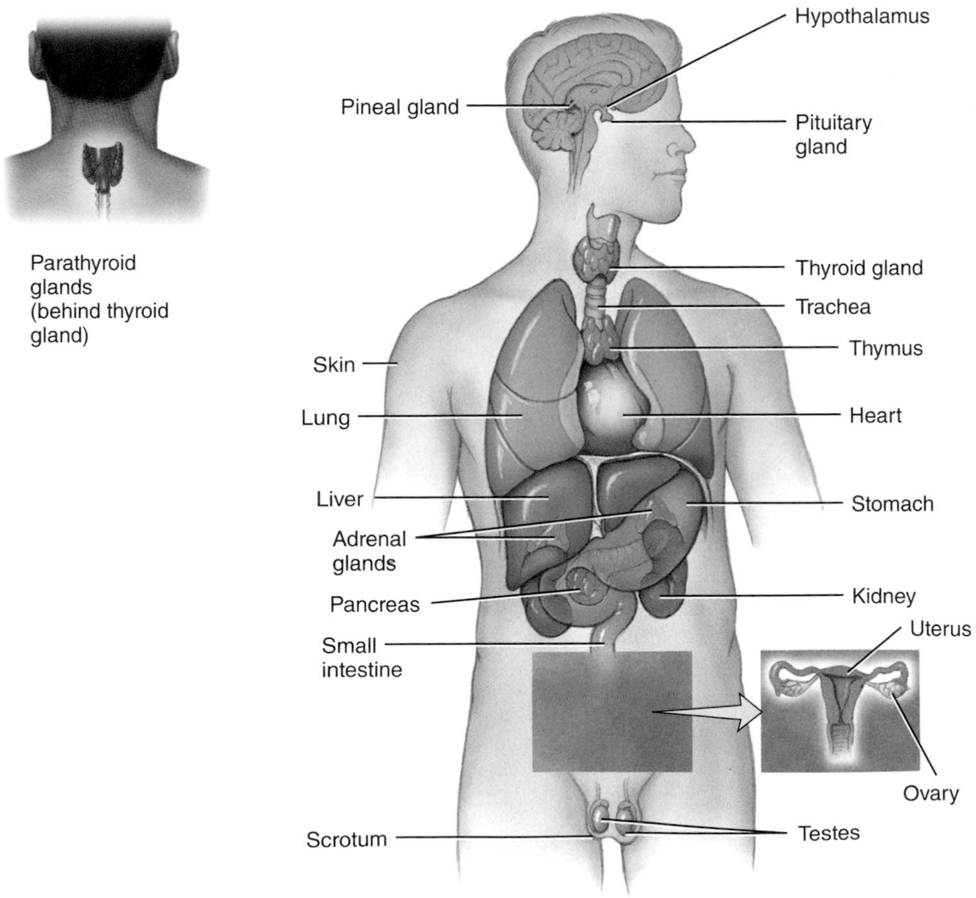
Parathyroid glands (behind thyroid gland)
Hypothalamus
Pineal gland
Pituitary gland
Thyroid gland
Trachea
Thymus
Skin
Lung
Heart
Liver
Stomach
Adrenal glands
Pancreas
Kidney
Small intestine
Uterus
Ovary
Scrotum
Testes

Figure 7.1 Location of the endocrine organs (Tortora and Derrickson 2009)

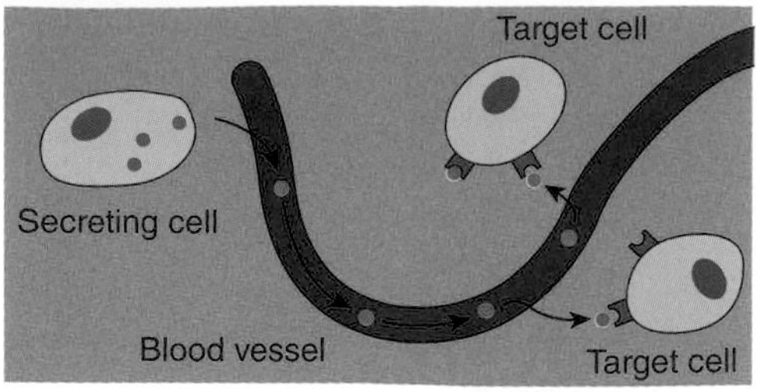
Target cell
Secreting cell
Blood vessel
Target cell

Figure 7.2 Transportation of hormones in the blood

Box 7.1 Endocrine, paracrine, exocrine and autocrine

Many words in anatomy and physiology have a similar ending to other words used about the same processes or areas of the body (Figure 7.3). It is important to be aware of these as confusion can quickly take over:

Endocrine is usually used to refer to hormones that are secreted into the blood and have an effect on cells distant from those that released the hormone. However, many endocrine hormones are known to act locally and even on the cells that secrete them.

Paracrine refers to hormones that act locally and diffuse to the cells in the immediate neighbourhood to produce their action.

Autocrine refers to hormones that act on the cells that produce it.

Exocrine refers to glands/organs that secrete substances into ducts that eventually lead to the outside of the body (for instance, the sweat glands, the part of the pancreas that secretes digestive juices, the gall bladder).

For the purposes of this chapter unless otherwise stated all discussions of hormone action will be with regards to endocrine activity.

supply. This arrangement of blood vessels and hormone-producing cells ensures that hormones enter into the blood stream rapidly and are then transported throughout the body to the target cells (see Figure 7.2).

Hormones

Hormones are chemical messengers that are secreted into the blood or the extracellular fluid by one cell and have an effect on the functioning of other cells. Unlike the nervous system which could be said to be based on wires (the neurones) like a telegraph the endocrine system is like a radio broadcast. As it is with a radio broadcast, it is necessary for there to be a receiver in order

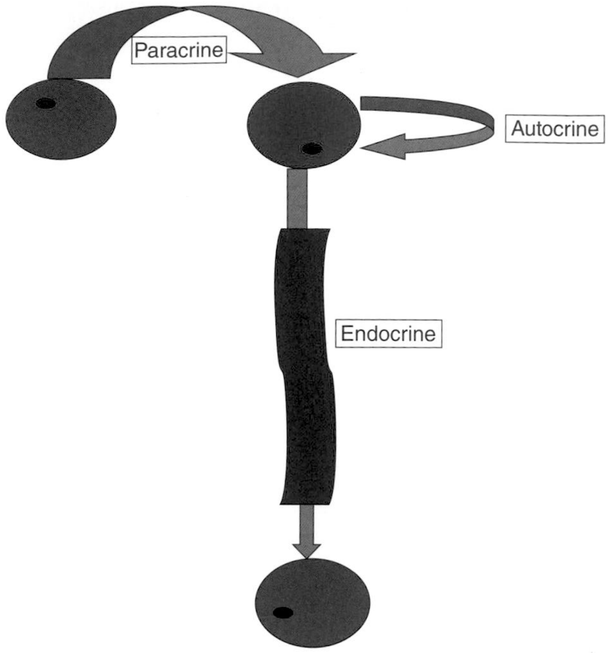
Paracrine
Autocrine
Endocrine

Figure 7.3 Endocrine, paracrine and autocrine

for the hormonal message to be received and acted upon. As hormones circulate in the blood they come into contact with virtually every cell in the body but they only exert their specific effect on those cells that have receptors for that hormone (the target cells). Like a lock and key mechanism, only the right key (hormone) can unlock a particular lock (receptor) (see Figure 7.4).

Hormone receptors are either found within the target cell or on its surface (as in Figure 7.4). The site of the receptor is dependent on the type of hormone the receptor is for. Most hormones are made from amino acids but some are made from cholesterol (the steroid hormones).

- Amino acid-based hormones cannot cross the cell membrane and thus their receptors are found on the cell wall. These hormones tend to exert their influence by activating enzymes and other molecules within the cell, which then affect the cell activity. This is often through a cascade of changes with the activation of the enzyme or molecule being the first step. The best understood example of this is cyclic AMP.
- The steroid hormones can cross the cell membrane because they are small and lipid-soluble and thus their receptors are found within the cell itself. These hormones usually exert their effect by stimulating the production of genes within the target cell. The genes then stimulate the synthesis of new proteins.
- One exception is thyroid hormone, which is very small and can diffuse easily across the cell membrane into the cell.

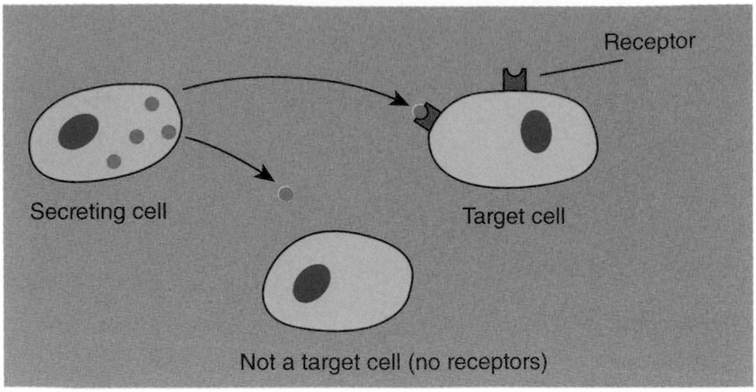
Receptor
Secreting cell
Target cell
Not a target cell (no receptors)

Figure 7.4 Target cell and non-target cell

The activation of a target cell depends on the concentration of the hormone in the blood; the number of receptors on the cell and the affinity of the receptor for the hormone. Changes in these factors can happen quickly in response to a change in stimuli.

The most important factor affecting the effect of a hormone on its target cell is its concentration in the blood and/or extracellular fluid. This concentration at the target cell is determined by three factors:

- Rate of production of the hormone – this is the most highly regulated aspect of the endocrine system
- Rate of delivery of the hormone – for instance, the blood flow to the organ or cell
- Rate of destruction and elimination of the hormone (half-life). Hormones with a short half-life will rapidly drop in concentration once production decreases. If the half-life of the hormone is long, then the hormone will still be present in significant concentrations for some time after its production stops.

Changes in the concentration of hormones can be a rapid mechanism of control, especially the rate of production, but longer-term adjustments to target cell sensitivity to a hormone will almost certainly include changes in the numbers of receptors as well. Changes in the number of receptors are known as up-regulation and down-regulation.

- Up-regulation is the creation of more receptors in response to low circulating levels of a hormone; the cell becomes more responsive to the presence of the hormone in the blood
- Down-regulation is the reduction in the number of receptors and is often the response of a cell to prolonged periods of high circulating levels of a hormone; the cell becomes less responsive (desensitised) to a hormone.

Effects of hormones

Hormones typically produce one of the following changes:

- Changes in cell membrane permeability and/or the cell's electrical state (membrane potential) by opening or closing ion channels in the cell membrane
- Synthesis of proteins or regulatory molecules (such as enzymes) within the cell
- Enzyme activation or deactivation
- Causing secretory activity
- Stimulation of mitosis.

Destruction and removal of hormones

Hormones are very powerful and can have a large effect at even low concentrations, therefore it is essential that active hormones are efficiently removed from the blood. Some hormones are rapidly broken down within the target cells. Most are inactivated by enzyme systems in the liver and kidneys and then excreted mostly in the urine, but some are excreted in the faeces.

Control of hormone release

The creation and release of most hormones are preceded by a stimulus which can be internal or external, for instance, a rise in blood glucose levels or a cold environment. The further synthesis and release of hormones is then usually controlled by a negative feedback system. As can be seen in Figure 7.5 the influence of a stimulus, from inside or outside the body (in this case a rise in blood glucose levels), leads to hormone release (insulin); following this some aspect of the target organ function then inhibits further reaction to the stimulus and thus further release of the hormone by the organ.

The initial stimulus for the release of a hormone is usually one of three types; though some organs respond to multiple stimuli (Marieb and Hoehn 2007).

- **Humoral.** A response to changing levels of certain ions and nutrients in the blood. For example, parathyroid hormone is stimulated by falling blood levels of calcium ions.

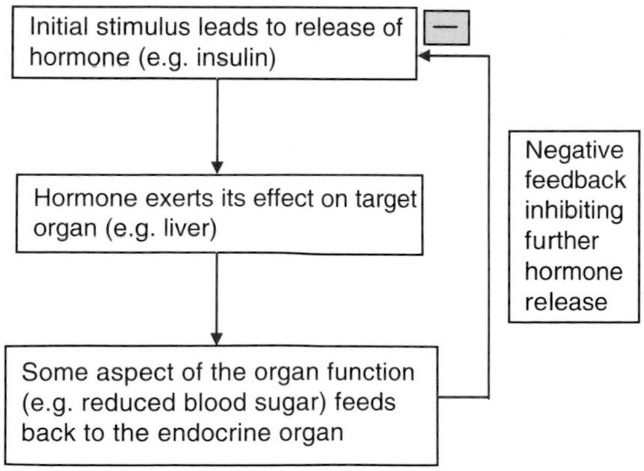
Initial stimulus leads to release of hormone (e.g. insulin)
—
Hormone exerts its effect on target organ (e.g. liver)
Some aspect of the organ function (e.g. reduced blood sugar) feeds back to the endocrine organ
Negative feedback inhibiting further hormone release

Figure 7.5 The negative feedback system (Nair and Peate 2009)

- **Neural.** A response to direct nervous stimulation. Very few endocrine organs are directly stimulated by the nervous system. An example is increased activity in the sympathetic nervous system which directly stimulates the release of catecholamines (adrenaline and noradrenaline) from the adrenal medulla.
- **Hormonal.** A response to hormones released by other organs. Hormones that are released in response to hormonal stimuli are usually rhythmical in their release (that is the levels rise and fall in a specific pattern). An example of hormonal control is the release of thyroid stimulating hormone (TSH) from the anterior pituitary gland directly stimulating the production and release of thyroxine from the thyroid gland.

The physiology of the endocrine organs

The hypothalamus and the pituitary gland

The hypothalamus is a portion of the brain with a variety of functions. It is a small (about 4 g), cone-like structure that is directly connected to the pituitary gland by the pituitary stalk (or infundibulum). One of the most important functions of the hypothalamus is to link the nervous system to the endocrine system via the pituitary gland. Almost all hormone secretion by the pituitary gland is controlled by either hormonal or electrical signals from the hypothalamus (Figure 7.6).

The hypothalamus receives signals from virtually all the potential sources within the nervous system but is also under negative feedback control by the hormones regulated by the pituitary gland. Thus when there is a low level of a hormone in the blood supplying the hypothalamus this leads to the release of the appropriate releasing hormone or factor which stimulates the release of the hormone by the pituitary, which in turn stimulates the release of the appropriate hormone. As the level of the target hormone rises in the blood this is detected by receptors in the hypothalamus and the stimulus for the release of the stimulating factor is removed and thus release of

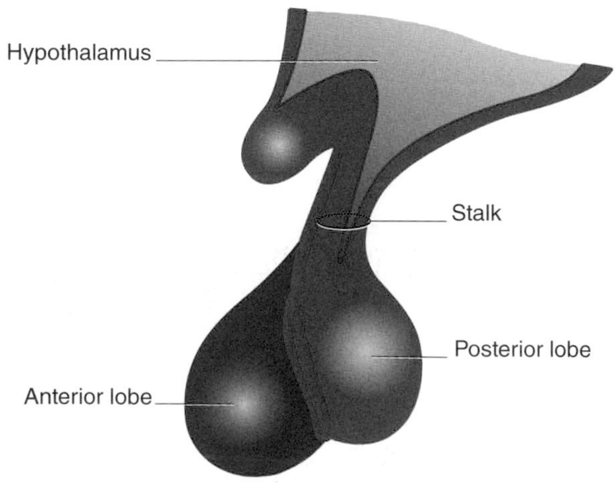
Hypothalamus
Stalk
Posterior lobe
Anterior lobe

Figure 7.6 The hypothalamus and pituitary gland

this factor is reduced. A classic example of this system is the release of thyrotrophin releasing hormone (TRH) and the subsequent release of thyroid stimulating hormone (TSH) by the anterior pituitary gland, which is described further on in this chapter.

The pituitary gland secretes at least nine major hormones and is the size and shape of a pea on a stalk. The pituitary gland is functionally and anatomically divided into two parts:

- The posterior lobe (neurohypophysis) is made up mostly of nerve fibres which originate in the hypothalamus and terminate on the surface of capillaries in the posterior lobe. The posterior lobe releases two hormones which it receives directly from the hypothalamus. In this sense it is in fact a storage area rather than a gland in the true sense of the term. The hypothalamus and the posterior pituitary are linked by a nerve bundle called the hypothalamic-hypophyseal tract
- The anterior lobe (adenohypophysis) is much larger than the posterior lobe and is made up of three parts which partly surround the posterior lobe and the infundibulum. It is made up of glandular tissue and produces and releases several hormones. The hypothalamus and the anterior pituitary have no direct nerve connections but do have a vascular (blood vessel) connection known as the hypothalamo-hypophyseal portal system whereby venous blood from the hypothalamus flows to the anterior lobe. Thus control of the anterior pituitary is by releasing and inhibiting factors (or hormones) released by the hypothalamus.

Hormones that are secreted by the posterior pituitary are:

- Oxytocin. Oxytocin has an effect on uterine contraction in childbirth and is responsible for the 'let down' response in breastfeeding mothers (the release of milk in response to suckling). In men and non-pregnant women it plays a role in sexual arousal and orgasm (Jenkins *et al.* 2007).
- Antidiuretic hormone (ADH). Under resting conditions large quantities of ADH accumulate in the posterior pituitary, excitation by nervous impulses leads to the release of the ADH from where it is stored into the adjacent blood vessels. The effects of ADH are that it increases water retention by the kidneys by increasing the permeability of the collecting ducts in the kidneys. The secretion of ADH is stimulated by:
  - Increased plasma osmolality – increased levels of certain substances in the plasma such as sodium
  - Decreased extracellular fluid volume
  - Pain and other stressed states
  - In response to certain drugs.

Hormones released by the anterior pituitary gland

Table 7.2 summarises the range of hormones released by the anterior pituitary gland and the releasing or inhibiting hormones (or factors) from the hypothalamus that influence this release.

There are five types of pituitary cell in the anterior lobe:

- Somatotropes, which secrete growth hormones
- Lactotropes, which secrete prolactin
- Thyrotropes, which secrete thyroid stimulating hormone (TSH)
- Gonadotropes, which secrete luteinising hormone and follicle stimulating hormone
- Corticotropes, which secrete adrenocorticotropic hormone (ACTH).

Table 7.2 Hormones released by the hypothalamus and the anterior pituitary gland (from Clare 2009)

Hypothalamus	Anterior pituitary gland	Target organ or tissues	Action
Growth hormone releasing factor	Growth hormone	Many (especially bones)	Stimulates growth of body cells
Growth hormone release inhibiting factor	Growth hormone (inhibits release)	Many	
Thyroid releasing hormone (TRH)	Thyroid stimulating hormone (TSH)	Thyroid gland	Stimulates thyroid hormone release
Corticotropin releasing hormone (CRH)	Adrenocorticotropic hormone (ACTH)	Adrenal cortex	Stimulates corticosteroid release
Prolactin releasing hormone	Prolactin	Breasts	Stimulates milk production
Prolactin inhibiting hormone	Prolactin (inhibits release)	Breasts	
Gonadotropin releasing hormone	Follicle stimulating hormone Luteinising hormone	Gonads	Various reproductive functions

Growth hormone

Effects

As its name suggests growth hormone promotes the growth of bone, cartilage and soft tissue by stimulating the production and release of insulin-like growth factor (IGF-1).

Regulation

Growth hormone release from the anterior pituitary is regulated by the release of growth hormone releasing hormone (GHRH) and growth hormone release inhibiting hormone (GHRIH or somata-ostatin) by the hypothalamus. Both growth hormone and IGF-1 produce a negative feedback effect on the hypothalamus.

Prolactin

Effects

Prolactin stimulates the secretion of milk in the breast.

Regulation

Secretion is inhibited by the release of dopamine from the hypothalamus. Secretion can be intermittently increased by the release of prolactin releasing hormone from the hypothalamus in response to the baby suckling at the breast.

Follicle stimulating hormone and luteinising hormone (gonadotrophins)

Effects

In males follicle stimulating hormone (FSH) stimulates sperm production. In females it leads to the early maturation of ovarian follicles and oestrogen secretion.

Luteinising hormone (LH) is responsible for the final maturation of the ovarian follicles and oestrogen secretion in females and in males it stimulates testosterone secretion.

Regulation

In males and females LH and FSH production is regulated by the release of gonadotrophin releasing hormone (GnRH). Testosterone and oestrogen exert a negative feedback effect on the release of GnRH from the hypothalamus.

Thyroid stimulating hormone (TSH)

Effects

TSH stimulates the activity of the cells of the thyroid gland leading to an increased production and secretion of thyroxine (T_4) and triiodothyronine (T_3).

Regulation

TSH is produced and released in response to the release of thyrotropin releasing hormone (TRH) from the hypothalamus. The hypothalamus can also inhibit the release of TSH through the action of somatostatin.

Free T3 and T4 in the blood have a direct negative feedback effect on the hypothalamus and the anterior pituitary gland.

Adrenocorticotrophic hormone (ACTH)

Effects

ACTH stimulates the production of cortisol and androgens from the cortex of the adrenal gland. It also leads to the production of aldosterone in response to increases concentrations of potassium ions, increased angtionesin levels or decreased total body sodium.

Regulation

ACTH is secreted from the anterior pituitary in response to the secretion of corticotrophin releasing hormone (CRH) from the hypothalamus. Excitation of the hypothalamus by any form of stress leads to the release of CRH and the subsequent release of ACTH and then cortisol. Cortisol exerts a direct negative feedback on the hypothalamus and the anterior pituitary gland.

The thyroid gland

The thyroid gland is a butterfly-shaped gland located in the front of the neck on the trachea just below the larynx (Figure 7.7). It is made up of two lobes joined by an isthmus (a narrow strip; isthmus = neck). The upper extremities of the lobes are known as the upper poles and the lower extremities the lower poles. Each lobe is made up of hollow, spherical, follicles surrounded by capillaries. This leads to an abundant blood supply, although the thyroid gland accounts for 0.4% of the total body weight it receives 2% of the circulating blood supply.

The follicles are comprised of a single layer of epithelial cells which form a cavity which contains thyroglobulin molecules with attached iodine molecules; the thyroid hormone is created from this. One unique factor of the thyroid gland is its ability to create and store large amounts hormone, this can be up to 100 days of hormone supply (Guyton and Hall 2006). The thyroid gland releases two forms of thyroid hormone; thyroxine (T_4) and triiodothyronine (T_3), both of which require iodine for their creation. Iodide taken in with the normal diet is concentrated by the

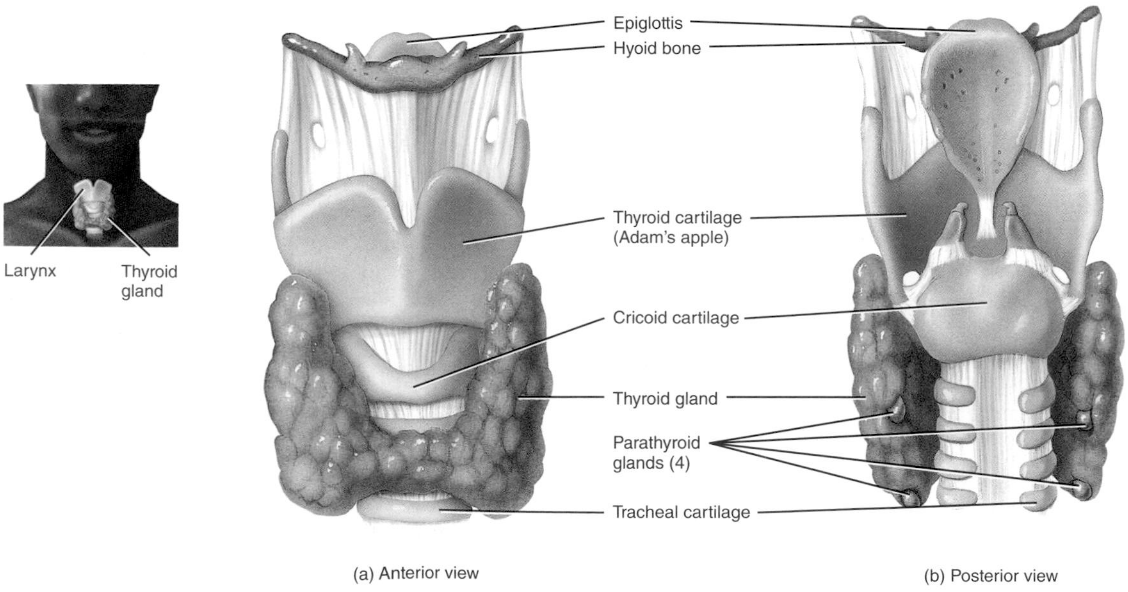
Larynx
Thyroid gland
Epiglottis
Hyoid bone
Thyroid cartilage (Adam's apple)
Cricoid cartilage
Thyroid gland
Parathyroid glands (4)
Tracheal cartilage
(a) Anterior view
(b) Posterior view

Figure 7.7 Position of the thyroid gland and parathyroid glands (Tortora and Derrickson 2009)

thyroid gland and is changed in the follicle cells into iodine. This iodine is then linked to tyrosine molecules and these iodinated tyrosine molecules are then linked together to create T_3 and T_4. All the steps in thyroid hormone production are stimulated by TSH. Thyroxine (T_4) is the primary hormone released by the thyroid gland; this is then converted into T_3 by the target cells. Most thyroid hormone is bound to transport proteins in the blood, very little is unbound (free) and T_3 is less firmly bound to transport proteins than T_4.

Thyroid hormone affects virtually every cell in the body, except:

- The adult brain
- Spleen
- Testes
- Uterus
- Thyroid gland.

Both T_4 and T_3 easily cross the cell membrane and interact with receptors inside the cell. In the target cells thyroid hormone stimulates enzymes that are involved with glucose oxidation. This is known as the calorigenic effect and its overall effects are:

- An increase in the basal metabolic rate
- An increase in oxygen consumption by the cell
- An increase in the production of body heat.

Basal metabolic rate is the amount of energy expended while at rest in a temperate environment (not hot or cold). The release of energy in this state is enough for the functioning of the vital organs. As basal metabolic rate is increased so oxygen consumption is increased as oxygen is required in the production of energy.

Thyroid hormone also has important role in the maintenance of blood pressure as it stimulates an increase in the number of receptors in the walls of the blood vessels.

The control of the release of thyroid hormone is mediated by a negative feedback system which involves the hypothalamus and cascades through the pituitary gland (Figure 7.8).

Plasma levels of thyroid hormone are monitored in the hypothalamus and by cells in the anterior lobe of the pituitary gland. Increased levels of T_4 in the blood inhibit the release of TRH from the hypothalamus thus reducing the stimulation for the release of TSH from the anterior pituitary gland. Thyroid hormones also have a direct negative feedback effect on the anterior pituitary gland. The effect of TSH on the thyroid gland is to promote the release of thyroid hormone into the blood; therefore a reduction in TSH reduces the release of T_3 and T_4. A reduced level of T_4 in the blood reduces the negative feedback and thus there is an increase in the release of TRH which leads to an increase in thyroid gland function. Conditions that increase the energy requirements of the body (such as pregnancy or prolonged cold) also stimulate the release of TRH from the hypothalamus and therefore lead to an increase in blood levels of thyroid hormone. In these situations the stimulating conditions override the normal negative feedback system (Marieb and Hoehn 2007). The negative feedback control of thyroid hormone can be likened to a central heating system. The hypothalamus and pituitary gland are the thermostat and the thyroid gland is the boiler. As the room temperature increases the thermostat turns off the central heating boiler, when the temperature decreases the thermostat turns the boiler on to increase the temperature.

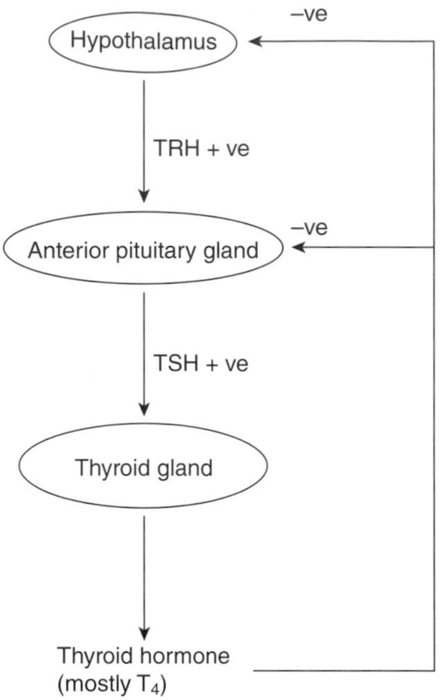
–ve
Hypothalamus
TRH + ve
–ve
Anterior pituitary gland
TSH + ve
Thyroid gland
Thyroid hormone
(mostly T4)

Figure 7.8 Negative feedback control of thyroid hormone production

Clinical considerations

Hypothyroidism and hyperthyroidism

A patient's blood level of thyroid hormone can be measured. Depending on whether the thyroid gland is overactive or underactive different levels of hormones will be shown by the test. Generally the patient would have their free T_4 and TSH levels assessed.

	TSH	Free T_4
Hyperthyroidism	Reduced	Elevated
Hypothyroidism	Elevated	Reduced

In the case of a patient with an overactive thyroid gland (hyperthyroidism) free T_4 will often be elevated but TSH levels will be reduced as the levels of thyroid hormone will be exerting a negative feedback effect on the hypothalamus and the pituitary gland. Despite the reduced TSH levels and the negative feedback effect on the pituitary gland as well hormone levels will remain elevated.

A patient with hypothyroidism (an underactive thyroid gland) will often present with a reduced free T_4 and an elevated TSH as the reduced hormone levels removes the negative feedback on the hypothalamus and the pituitary and thus TSH levels rise.

The half-life of T_4 is approximately seven days and the half-life of T_3 is one day. Thyroid hormones are broken down in the liver and the skeletal muscle and whilst much of the iodine is recycled some is lost in the urine and the faeces. Therefore, there is a need for daily replacement of iodide in the diet.

In addition to the thyroid epithelial cells are C cells which are found between the follicles and secrete calcitonin. Calcitonin is involved in the metabolism of calcium and phosphorous within the body. It decreases calcium levels in the blood by reducing the activity of osteoclasts (cells that 'digest' bone and thus release calcium and phosphorous into the blood). Calcitonin also inhibits the reabsorption of calcium from urine in the kidneys.

The parathyroid glands

The parathyroid glands (Figure 7.7) are small glands located on the back (posterior) of the thyroid gland. There are usually two pairs of glands, but the precise number varies and some patients have been reported to have up to four pairs (Marieb and Hoehn 2007). The cells that create and secrete parathyroid hormone (parathyroid chief cells) are arranged in cords or nests around a dense capillary network. Parathyroid hormone is the single most important hormone for the control of the calcium balance in the body. Its major target cells are in the bones and the kidneys:

- Increases intestinal calcium absorption
- Stimulates renal calcium absorption
- Stimulates osteoclast activity and therefore reabsorption of calcium from the bones.

Physiologically, calcium is important in the transmission of nerve impulses, is involved in muscle contraction and is also required in the creation of clotting factors in the blood. The regulation of parathyroid hormone synthesis and secretion is in response to the levels of calcium in the blood which is monitored by cells in the gland. A reduced blood calcium level leads to an increase in the synthesis and secretion of parathyroid hormone.

Calcitriol is a hormone released by the kidneys in response to a decrease in calcium ions in the blood; it is known to have some effect on parathyroid hormone secretion and also inhibits the release of calcitonin. Parathyroid hormone is a known stimulus for the release of calcitriol but when calcitriol levels achieve a high enough level its effect changes to that of inhibiting the release of parathyroid hormone. This prevents an uncontrollable increase in calcium in the blood.

The adrenal glands

The adrenal glands are complex, multifunctional organs whose secretions are essential for the maintenance of homeostasis. The two adrenal glands are found on the top of each of the two kidneys (Figure 7.9). The right gland is roughly triangular in shape and the left, which is commonly the larger of the two, is crescent-shaped. Both glands are encased in a connective tissue capsule and embedded in an area of fat. Adrenal glands are very vascular (have a rich blood supply from many blood vessels).

Functionally, each adrenal gland is actually two glands and is comprised of two major regions (Figure 7.10):

- Adrenal medulla
- Adrenal cortex.

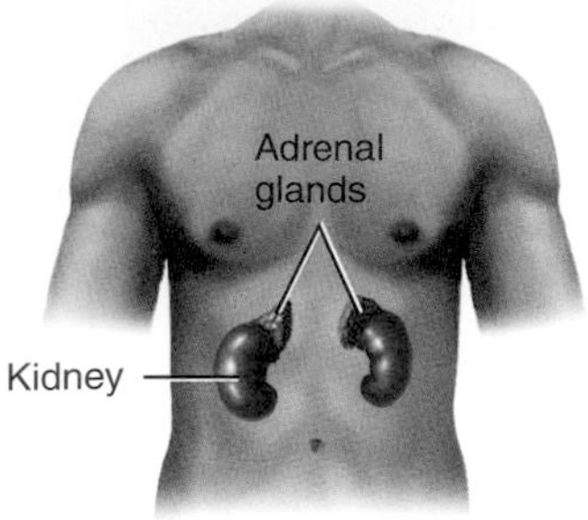
Adrenal glands
Kidney

Figure 7.9 Position of the adrenal glands (Tortora and Derrickson 2009)

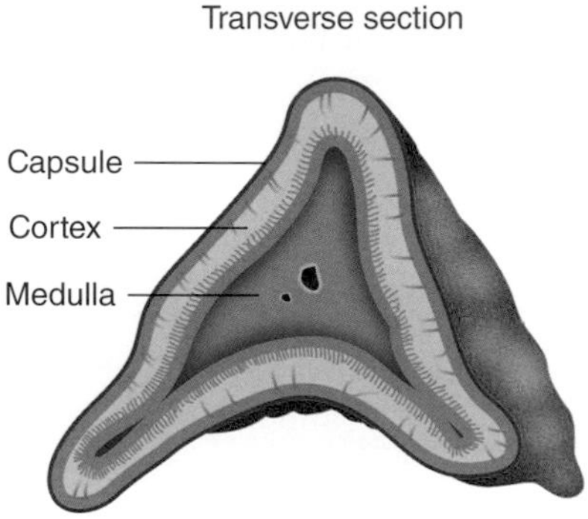
Transverse section
Capsule
Cortex
Medulla

Figure 7.10 Cross-section of an adrenal gland (Nair and Peate 2009)

Adrenal medulla

The adrenal medulla is the inner part of the adrenal gland; it makes up about 30% of the total mass of the adrenal gland. The function of the adrenal medulla is the secretion of catecholamines:

- Adrenaline
- Noradrenaline
- Dopamine.

The adrenal medulla is mostly a modified, densely innervated, sympathetic ganglion made up of granule-containing cells. Within the adrenal medulla approximately 90% of the cells secrete adrenaline and the remaining 10% secrete noradrenaline. It is unclear which cells secrete dopamine at this time.

The effects of the catecholamines are many and varied:

- Stimulate the nervous system
- Metabolic effects – for instance, glycogenolysis in the liver and skeletal muscle
- Increase metabolic rate
- Increase heart rate
- Increase alertness – though adrenaline frequently evokes anxiety and fear
- Noradrenaline causes significant, widespread, vasoconstriction
- Adrenaline causes vasoconstriction in the skin and viscera but vasodilation in skeletal muscles.

Although adrenaline and noradrenaline are essential for normal bodily functioning, adrenaline and the noradrenaline secreted by the adrenal medulla is not essential and serve only to intensify the effects of sympathetic nervous stimulation.

Secretion of catecholamines from the adrenal medulla is initiated by sympathetic nervous activity controlled by the hypothalamus and occurs in response to:

- Pain
- Anxiety
- Excitement
- Hypovolaemia
- Hypoglycaemia.

The medulla receives its blood supply from the adrenal cortex rich in corticosteroids. These regulate the production of the enzymes that convert noradrenaline to adrenaline. Thus an increase in corticosteroid production leads to an increase conversion of noradrenaline to adrenaline. With emergency stimulation of the hypothalamus there is a responding diffuse medullary activity preparing for fight or flight. Catecholamines have a very short half-life in the blood of less than two minutes as they are rapidly degraded by blood-borne enzymes.

Adrenal cortex

The outer part of each adrenal gland made up of three distinct functional layers (Figure 7.11).

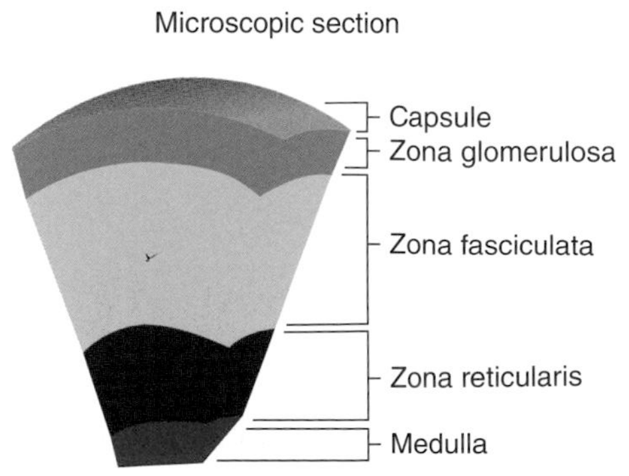
Microscopic section
Capsule
Zona glomerulosa
Zona fasciculata
Zona reticularis
Medulla

Figure 7.11 Cross-section of the adrenal cortex (Nair and Peate 2009)

Each layer is involved in the production of steroid-based hormones (known collectively as the corticosteroids).

- Zona glomerulosa – produces the mineralocorticoids
- Zona fasciculata – produces the glucocorticoids
- Zona reticularis – this zone is also involved in the production of glucocorticoids but also produces small amounts of adrenal sex hormones (the gonadocorticoids).

Mineralocorticoids

Mineralocorticoids are the group of hormones whose main function is the regulation of the concentration of the electrolytes in the blood. There are several known mineralocorticoids but the most common is aldosterone, which accounts for 95% of all the mineralocorticoids synthesised and is also the most potent.

The effect of aldosterone is to reduce the excretion of sodium in the urine by regulating the reabsorption of sodium from the urine in the distal portion of the renal tubules. Sodium is in effect exchanged for potassium and hydrogen, which results in the renal excretion of potassium and acidic urine. Aldosterone also has an effect on the levels of water in the body and several other ions (including potassium, bicarbonate and chloride) due to the fact that their regulation is coupled to the regulation of sodium in the body. The control of aldosterone secretion is primarily related to the blood concentrations of sodium (Na^+) and potassium (K^+), the mean arterial blood pressure (BP) and blood volume. Increased concentrations of potassium, reduced blood concentrations of sodium and a reduction in blood pressure and/or blood volume all stimulate the release of aldosterone, whilst the opposite inhibits release (Figure 7.12). High blood levels of potassium are also known to have a direct effect on the adrenal cortex in the stimulation of aldosterone production and secretion.

There are several mechanisms that regulate the release of aldosterone. The primary control mechanism is the production of angiotensin II by the renin angiotensin system in response to reduced blood pressure in the kidneys or reduced sodium delivery to the distal tubules of the kidneys. Raised levels of potassium and reduced levels of sodium in the blood are also known to have a direct effect on the adrenal cortex and stimulate the release of mineralocorticoids. However, in response to a severe, non-specific stressor hypothalamic release of CRH stimulates the increased release of ACTH. This increase in ACTH stimulates a slight increase in the release of aldosterone leading to a slight increase in blood volume and pressure which will help to maintain delivery of oxygen and nutrients to the tissues.

Glucocorticoids

There appears to be no cell within the body that does not have receptors for the glucocorticoid hormones. The glucocorticoid hormones have several effects:

- Influence the metabolism of most body cells
  - Promote glycogen storage in the liver
  - During fasting they stimulate the generation of glucose
  - Increase blood glucose levels
- Involved in providing resistance to stressors
- Potentiate the vasoconstrictor effect of catecholamines

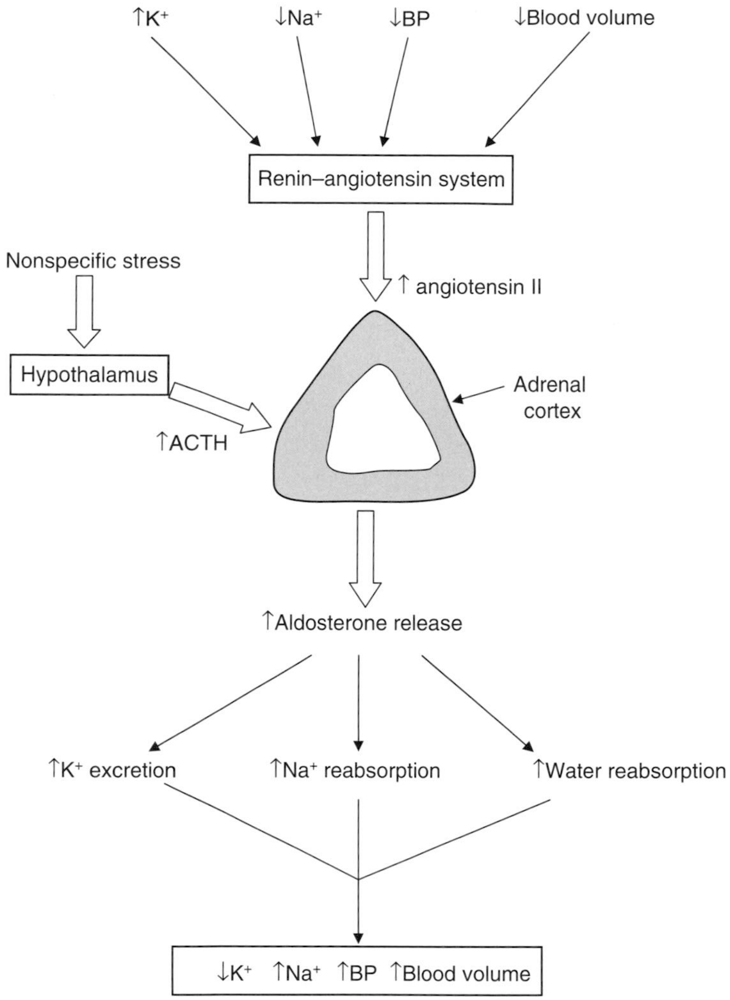
↑K⁺
↓Na⁺
↓BP
↓Blood volume
Renin–angiotensin system
Nonspecific stress
↑ angiotensin II
Hypothalamus
Adrenal cortex
↑ACTH
↑Aldosterone release
↑K⁺ excretion
↑Na⁺ reabsorption
↑Water reabsorption
↓K⁺ ↑Na⁺ ↑BP ↑Blood volume

Figure 7.12 Control of aldosterone secretion (Nair and Peate 2009)

- Decrease the permeability of vascular endothelium
- Promote the repair of damaged tissues by promoting the breakdown of stored protein to create amino acids
- Suppress the immune system
- Suppress inflammatory processes.

The glucocorticoid hormones include:

- Cortisol (hydrocortisone)
- Cortisone
- Corticosterone.

Only cortisol is secreted in any significant amounts. Cortisol is normally released in a rhythmical pattern, with most being released shortly after the person gets up from sleep and the lowest amount being released just before, and shortly after, sleep commences.

Cortisol release is stimulated by ACTH from the anterior pituitary gland. ACTH releases cholesterol from the cytoplasm in the cells which is then converted and modified to create the steroid hormones. ACTH secretion is regulated by the release of corticotropin releasing hormone (CRH) from the hypothalamus. Increasing levels of cortisol have a negative feedback effect on both the hypothalamus and the pituitary gland inhibiting further release of both CRH and ACTH. However, this negative feedback system can be overridden by acute physiological stress (for instance, trauma, infection or haemorrhage) and mental stress. The increase in sympathetic nervous system activity in response to an acute stress triggers greater CRH release and thus there is a significant increase in subsequent cortisol production (Figure 7.13).

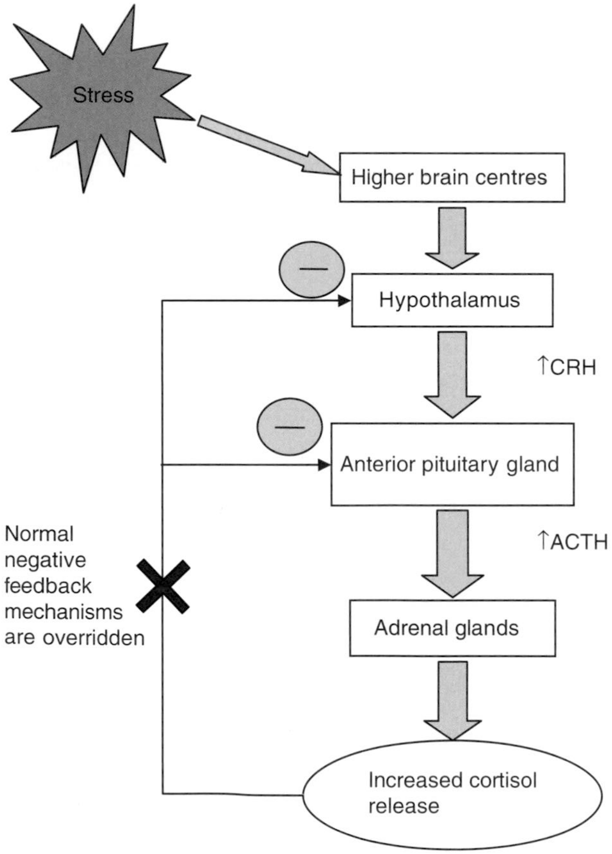
Stress
Higher brain centres
Hypothalamus
↑CRH
Anterior pituitary gland
↑ACTH
Adrenal glands
Increased cortisol release
Normal negative feedback mechanisms are overridden

Figure 7.13 Response of the endocrine system to stress (Nair and Peate 2009)

Clinical considerations

Glucocorticoid steroids and inflammatory diseases

Synthetic glucocorticoid steroid hormones are used widely in health care for the suppression of inflammation in diseases such as arthritis, ulcerative colitis and acute severe asthma. However, after taking glucocorticoid steroids such as prednisolone for more than a few days (except in asthma inhalers) the patient should carry a 'steroid card' and treatment should be gradually reduced not stopped suddenly.

The constant intake of synthetic steroids leads to a reduction in the production of steroids by the adrenal cortex (probably due to reduced CRH and ACTH secretion because of negative feedback to the hypothalamus and pituitary gland) and suddenly stopping the medication may leave the patient with reduced levels of glucocorticoid steroids in their blood and may lead to a life-threatening hypoadrenal crisis.

Pancreas

The pancreas is an elongated organ and is found next to the first part of the small intestine. The pancreas is composed of two different types of tissues. The majority of the pancreas is made up of exocrine tissue and the associated ducts. This tissue produces and secretes a fluid rich with digestive enzymes into the small intestine. Scattered throughout the exocrine tissue are many small clusters of cells called islets of Langerhans (islets). These islets are the site of the endocrine cells of the pancreas. Each islet has three major cell types, each of which produces a different hormone:

- Alpha cells, which secrete glucagon
- Beta cells, the most abundant of the three cell types and which secrete insulin
- Delta cells, which secrete somatostatin.

The different cell types within each islet are distributed in a set pattern with the beta cells being the central portion of the islet, surrounded by alpha and delta cells. The islets are highly vascularised ensuring rapid transit of the hormones into the bloodstream. Although the islets only account for 1–2% of the mass of the pancreas they receive about 10–15% of the pancreatic blood flow. The pancreas is innervated by the parasympathetic and sympathetic nervous systems and it is clear that nervous stimulation influences the secretion of insulin and glucagon.

Insulin

Insulin is well known for its effect in reducing the blood glucose levels and it does this by:

- Facilitating the entry of glucose into muscle, adipose tissue and several other tissues. Note that the brain and the liver do not require insulin to facilitate the uptake of glucose
- Stimulating the liver to store glucose in the form of glycogen.

However, as well as its effects on glucose, insulin is known to have an effect on protein and mineral metabolism. Finally, insulin has an effect on lipid metabolism. As has been noted, insulin promotes the synthesis of glycogen in the liver. As glycogen accumulation in the liver rises to higher levels (5% of the total liver mass) further glycogen synthesis is suppressed. Further uptake of glucose is then diverted by insulin into the production of fatty acids and insulin inhibits the breakdown of fat in adipose tissue and facilitates the production of triglycerides from glucose for further storage in these tissues. From a whole body perspective insulin has a fat-sparing effect in that it promotes the use of glucose instead of fatty acids and stimulates the storage of fat in the adipose tissue.

The stimulation of insulin synthesis and secretion is primarily a response to a rise in blood glucose levels, but rises in blood levels of amino acids and fatty acids also have a stimulating effect. Some neural stimuli, for instance the sight and smell of food, also increase insulin secretion. The pancreas is innervated by the sympathetic and parasympathetic nervous systems and nervous stimulation clearly influences the secretion of insulin (and glucagon).

As blood glucose levels fall there is a corresponding fall in the production and secretion of insulin. When insulin levels in the blood fall glycogen synthesis in the liver reduces and enzymes that break down glycogen become active. The half-life of insulin is approximately five minutes and it is destroyed in the liver.

Glucagon

Glucagon has an important role in maintaining normal blood glucose levels, especially as the brain and neurones can only use glucose as a fuel. Glucagon has the opposite effect on blood glucose levels to insulin (Figure 7.14):

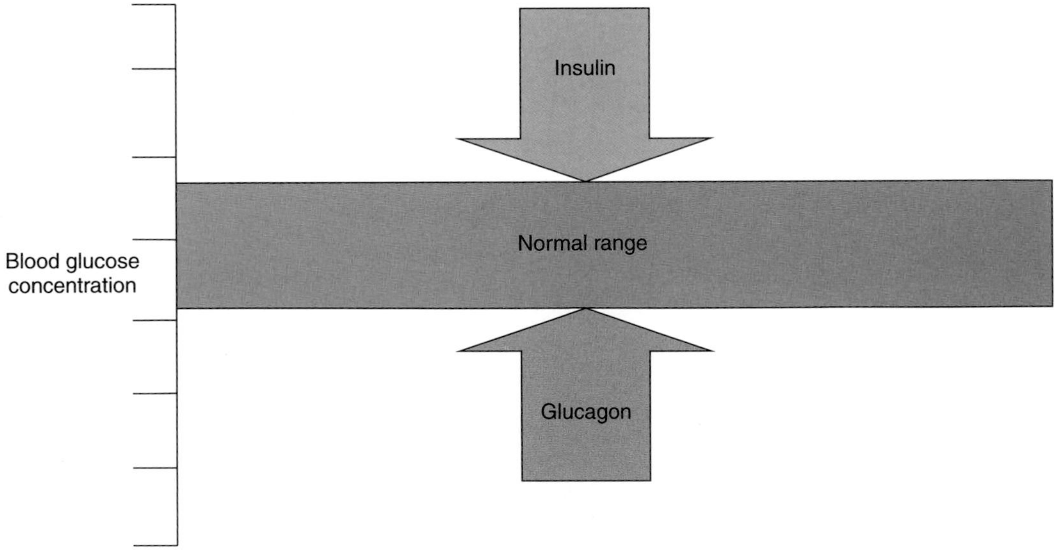
Insulin
Normal range
Blood glucose concentration
Glucagon

Figure 7.14 Effects of insulin and glucagon on blood glucose concentrations

- Stimulates the breakdown of glycogen stored in the liver
- Activates hepatic gluconeogenesis (the creation of glucose from substrates such as amino acids)
- Has a minor effect enhancing triglyceride breakdown in adipose tissue – providing fatty acid fuel for most cells and thus conserving glucose for the brain and neurones.

The production and secretion of glucagon are stimulated in response to a reduction in blood glucose concentrations and elevated blood levels of amino acids (for instance, after a protein-rich meal). It has also been found that glucagon levels in the blood rise in response to exercise but it is unclear whether this is a response to the exercise itself or a response to the reduced blood glucose levels that exercise creates.

Glucagon production and secretion are inhibited when there is increased glucose levels in the blood, however it is unknown whether this is a direct effect of the glucose levels or a response to rising levels of insulin, as insulin is known to inhibit the release of glucagon.

Clinical considerations

Hypoglycaemia

When a patient becomes hypoglycaemic (has a low blood sugar level), one of the treatments that can be used is the injection of a synthetic version of glucagon. The action is the same as that of natural glucagon – it stimulates the production of glucose in the liver both by gluconeogenesis and glycogenolysis.

Once glucagon has been administered, however, it is important to check the patient's blood sugar regularly as the glucagon injection can use up the patient's glycogen stores and a 'rebound' hypoglycaemia may occur. It is often advisable to get the patient to eat some carbohydrates to help to maintain a stable blood sugar level.

Somatostatin

Somatostatin is actually released by a broad range of tissues. Its physiological effect in the pancreas is to inhibit the release of insulin and glucagon; it does this in a paracrine fashion, that is the hormone is released and has its effect locally. The exact mechanism of control of this hormone is unknown.

Conclusion

This chapter has introduced the reader to the endocrine system, a diverse system that is one of the two necessary for the maintenance of haemostasis. Whilst often working in close conjunction with the nervous system the endocrine system is often responsible for the control of longer-term processes. The major functions of the endocrine system are based on four main areas:

- The maintenance of homeostasis (especially electrolyte levels and fluid balance)
- Metabolism

- Growth and development
- Responses to stress.

The secretion of hormones can be stimulated by nervous impulses, hormones or changes in the body levels of ions and nutrients and further regulation of hormone release is then often controlled by negative feedback loops. Hormones can only have an effect on a cell if that cell has a receptor for the hormone; however there appears to be virtually no cell within the body that is not affected by the endocrine system.

Glossary

Amino acid: Chemical compound that is the basic building block of proteins and enzymes.

Carbohydrate: A group of compounds (including starches and sugars) that are a major food source.

Catecholamines: A collective term for adrenaline, noradrenaline and dopamine.

Cortex: The outermost layer of an organ.

Corticosteroids: Steroid hormones released by the adrenal cortex, further divided into glucocorticoids and mineralocorticoids.

Cortisol: The major glucocorticoid steroid released by the adrenal gland.

Cytoplasm: The part of the cell enclosed within the cell membrane.

Down regulation: The reduction in the number of hormone receptors of a cell, often the response of a cell to prolonged periods of high circulating levels of a hormone.

Electrolytes: A group of chemical elements or compounds that includes sodium, potassium, calcium, chloride and bicarbonate.

Fatty acids: Dietary fats that have broken down into elements that can be absorbed into the blood.

Free T_4: Thyroxine in the blood that is not bound to proteins.

Ganglion: A mass, or group, of nerve cells.

Gland: Any organ in the body that secretes substances not related to its own, internal, functioning.

Glucocorticoids: A group of hormones that exert their major effect on the metabolism of carbohydrates.

Gluconeogenesis: Creation of new glucose from non-carbohydrate substrates.

Glycogen:	A carbohydrate (complex sugar) made from glucose.
Glycogenolysis:	Breakdown of glycogen to create glucose.
Hormonal stimulation:	Stimulation of a gland that produces a change in the activity of that gland in response to hormones released by other organs.
Hormone:	Chemical substance that is released into the blood by the endocrine system, and has a physiological control over the function of cells or organs other than those that created it.
Humoral stimulation:	Stimulation of a gland that produces a change in the activity of that gland in response to changing levels of certain ions and nutrients in the blood.
Hyperglycaemia:	High blood levels of glucose.
Hypoglycaemia:	Low blood levels of glucose.
Hypovolaemia:	Low levels of fluid in the circulation.
Ion:	An atom or group of atoms that carry an electrical charge.
Lipids:	A group of organic compounds, including the fats, oils, waxes, sterols and triglycerides.
Medulla:	The most internal part of an organ.
Mineralocorticoids:	A group of hormones released by the adrenal glands that exert their effect on the electrolytes and water balance in the body.
Neural stimulation:	Stimulation of a gland which produces a change in the activity of that gland in response to direct nervous activity.
Up regulation:	The increase of hormone receptors of a cell, usually in response to low circulating levels of a hormone.
Osmotic:	The movement of water through a semi-permeable barrier from an area of low concentration of a chemical to an area of high concentration of a chemical.
Osteoclasts:	A type of cell that breaks down bone tissue and thus releases the calcium used to create bones.
Substrate:	A molecule on which an enzyme acts.
Triglycerides:	A form of fatty acid having three fatty acid components.

References

Clare, C. (2009) The endocrine system and associated disorders. In: Nair, M. and Peate, I. (eds) *Fundamentals of Applied Pathophysiology: An Essential Guide for Nursing Students*. Chichester: John Wiley & Sons, pp. 318–348.

Guyton, A.C. and Hall, J. (2006) *Textbook of Medical Physiology*, 11th edn. Philadelphia: Elsevier Saunders.

Jenkins, G.W., Kemnitz, C.P. and Tortora, G.J. (2007) *Anatomy and Physiology: From Science to Life*. Hoboken, NJ: John Wiley & Sons.

Marieb, E.N. and Hoehn, K. (2007) *Human Anatomy and Physiology. International Edition*, 7th edn. San Francisco: Pearson Benjamin Cummings.

Tortora, G.J. and Derrickson, B.H. (2009) *Principles of Anatomy and Physiology*, 12th edn. Hoboken, NJ: John Wiley & Sons.

Activities

www.wiley.com/go/peate

Multiple choice questions

1. The receptors for amino acid-based hormones are found:
   - (a) on the cell wall
   - (b) inside the cell
   - (c) inside the cell nucleus
   - (d) none of the above

2. What stimulates the release of glucagon from the pancreas?
   - (a) high levels of blood glucose
   - (b) high levels of amino acids in the blood
   - (c) high levels of calcium in the blood
   - (d) high levels of sodium in the blood.

3. Where in the body are the adrenal glands?
   - (a) in the chest
   - (b) behind the thyroid gland
   - (c) next to the stomach
   - (d) on top of the kidneys

4. The concentration of a hormone at the target cell is determined by:
   - (a) the rate of hormone production
   - (b) the rate of delivery of the hormone
   - (c) the half-life of the hormone
   - (d) all of the above

5. Adrenaline and noradrenaline are released in response to stimulation from:
   (a) the parasympathetic nervous system
   (b) the sympathetic nervous system
   (c) the enteric nervous system
   (d) somatic nervous system

6. The connection between the hypothalamus and the anterior pituitary gland is:
   (a) lymphatic
   (b) neural
   (c) vascular
   (d) humoral

7. The average person has how many parathyroid glands?
   (a) 2
   (b) 4
   (c) 6
   (d) 8

8. Thyroid hormone requires what to be produced?
   (a) amino acids
   (b) iodine
   (c) lipids
   (d) proteins

9. Which cells in the pancreas produce insulin?
   (a) alpha
   (b) beta
   (c) delta
   (d) gamma

10. ACTH is secreted by:
   (a) the posterior pituitary gland
   (b) the anterior pituitary gland
   (c) the hypothalamus
   (d) the adrenal glands

Test your learning

1. What effect does insulin have on lipid metabolism?
2. What is the most common form of thyroid hormone?
3. Name the three cell types in the pancreas.

Label the diagram

From the lists of words, label the diagrams below:

Parathyroid glands (behind thyroid gland), Pineal gland, Skin, Lung, Liver, Adrenal glands, Pancreas, Small intestine, Scrotum, Hypothalamus, Pituitary gland, Thyroid gland, Trachea, Thymus, Heart, Stomach, Kidney, Uterus, Ovary, Testes

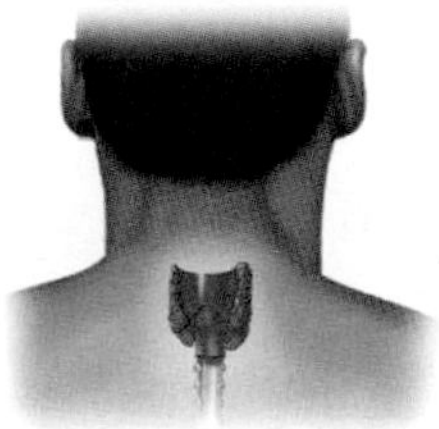

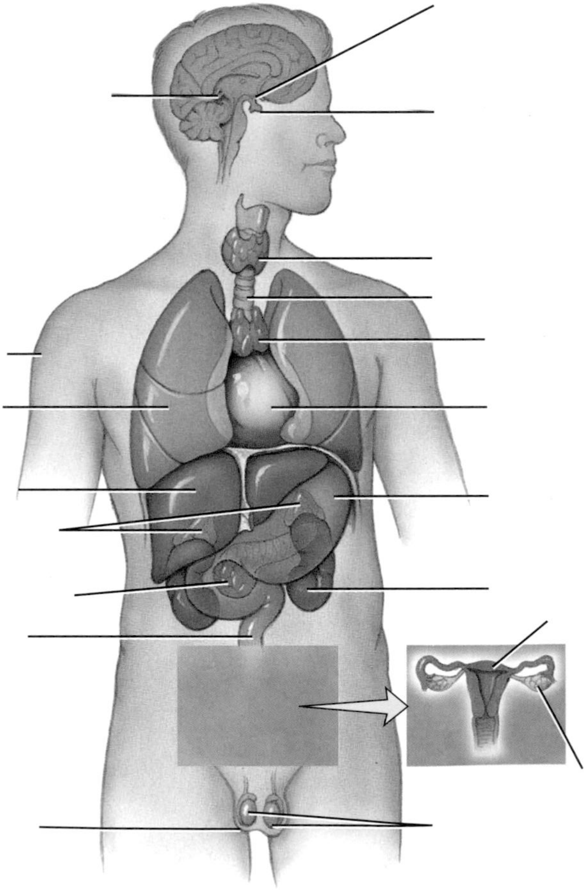

Larynx, Thyroid gland, Epiglottis, Hyoid bone, Thyroid cartilage (Adam's apple), Cricoid cartilage, Thyroid gland, Parathyroid glands (4), Tracheal cartilage

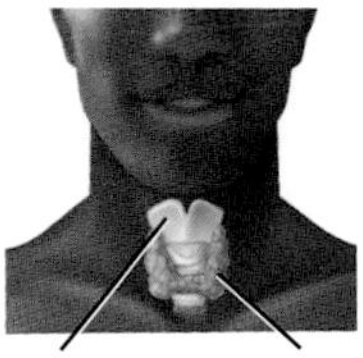

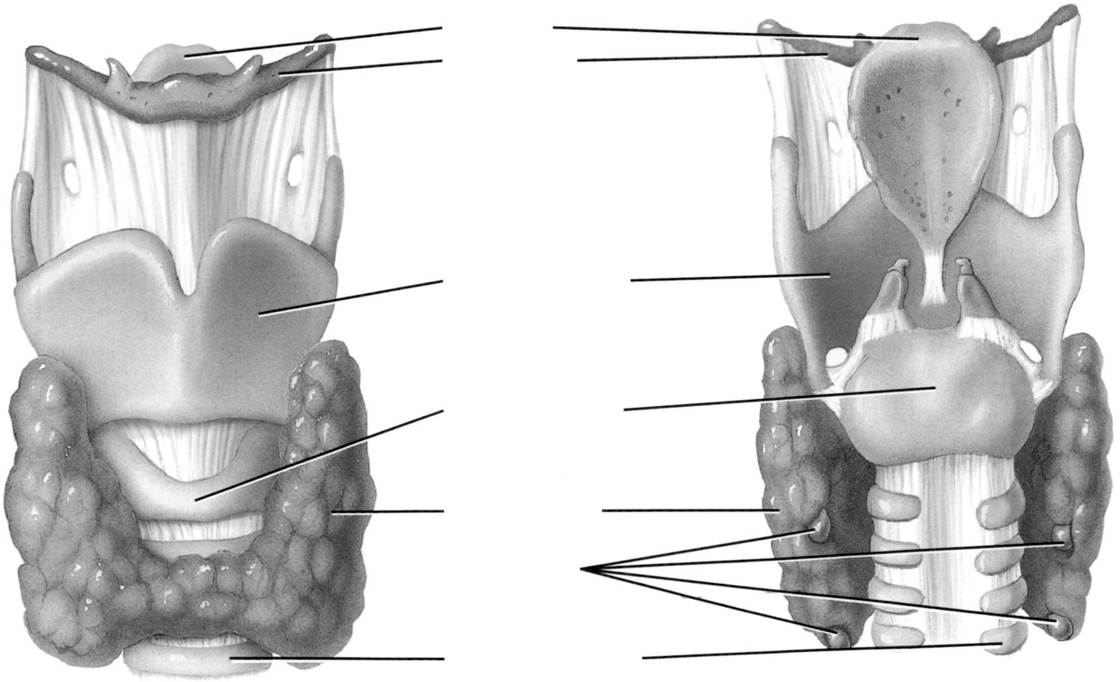

↑K^+, ↓Na^+, ↓BP, ↓Blood volume, Renin angiotensin system, Nonspecific stress, ↑angiotensin II, Hypothalamus, ↑ACTH, Adrenal cortex, ↑Aldosterone release, ↑K^+ excretion, ↑Na^+ reabsorption, ↑Water reabsorption, ↓K^+, ↑Na^+, ↑BP, ↑ Blood volume

Insert the gland/organ names and the hormones into the following diagram showing the bodily response to stress: gland/organ; hormone; anterior pituitary gland; ACTH; higher brain centres; CRH; hypothalamus; cortisol; adrenal glands.

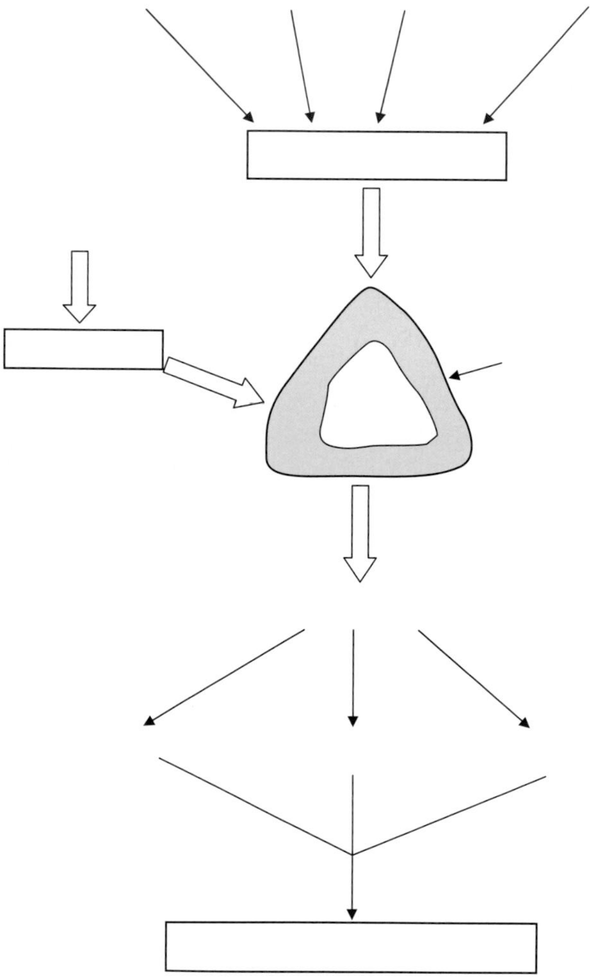

Crossword

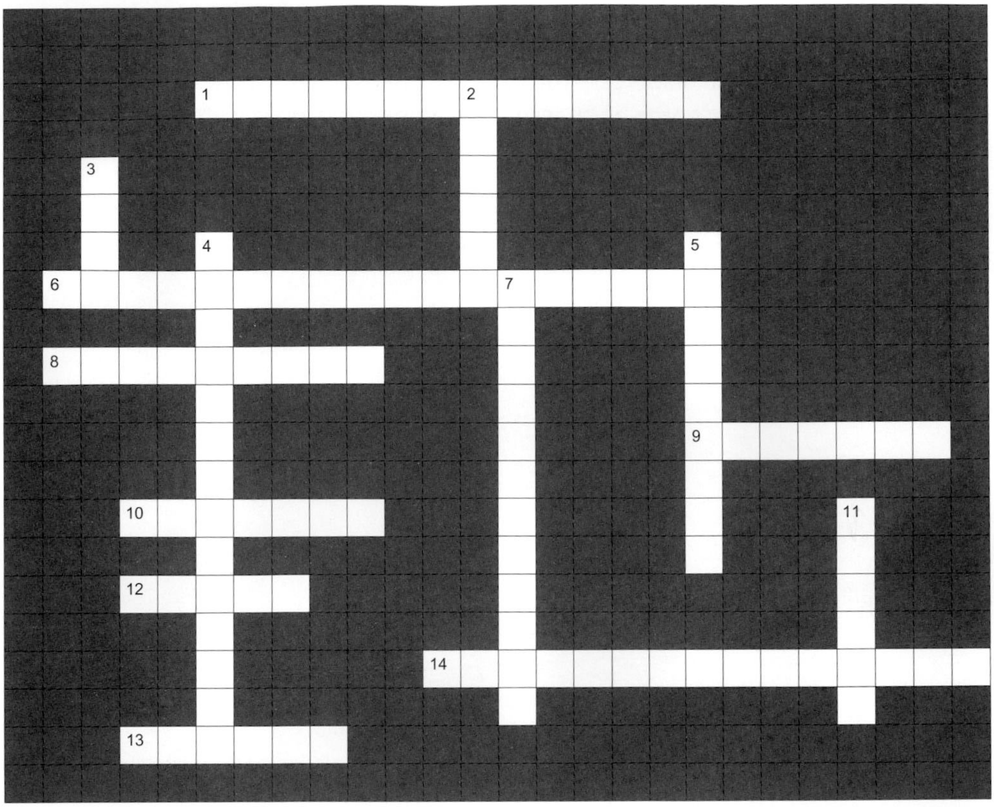
1
2
3
4
5
6
7
8
9
10
11
12
13
14

Across:

1. The breakdown of glycogen to create glucose (14).
6. The amount of energy expended while at rest in a temperate environment (5, 9, 4).
8. Hormone having an effect on the cell that produced it (9).
9. Endocrine gland found in the neck (7).
10. Endocrine gland that produces mineralocorticoids (7).
12. _____ acid. Chemical compound that is the basic building block of proteins and enzymes (5).
13. Required for the creation of thyroid hormone (6).
14. Creation of new glucose from non-carbohydrate substrates (15).

Down:

2. Stimulation for initial hormone release by direct nervous stimulation (6).
3. ____ glomerulosa (for instance) (4).
4. Adrenal hormone group (for instance cortisol) (14).
5. A cell must have these for a hormone to have an effect on it (9).
7. Pituitary stalk (12).
11. A cell that has 5 down for a hormone is a ________ cell for that hormone (6).

Conditions

Below is a list of conditions that are associated with the endocrine system. Take some time and write notes about each of the conditions. You may make the notes taken from text books or other resources, for example, people you work with in a clinical area, or you may make the notes as a result of people you have cared for. If you are making notes about people you have cared for you must ensure that you adhere to the rules of confidentiality.

Addison's disease	
Cushing's disease	
Diabetes insipidus	
Diabetes mellitus	
Graves' disease	
Hashimoto's thyroiditis	
Hyperparathyroidism	
Hypoparathyroidism	
Hypopituitarism	
Thyroid storm	
Viral thyroiditis	

Answers

MCQs

1a; 2b; 3d; 4d; 5b; 6c; 7b; 8b; 9b; 10b

Crossword

Across:

1. Glycogenolysis

6. Basal metabolic rate

8. Autocrine

9. Thyroid

10. Adrenal

12. Amino

13. Iodine

14. Gluconeogenesis

Down:

2. Neural

3. Zona

4. Glucocorticoid

5. Receptors

7. Infundibulum

11. Target

8

The skeletal system

Ian Peate

Contents

Introduction	*226*
The axial and appendicular skeleton	**226**
The axial skeleton	226
The appendicular skeleton	226
Bone and its functions	**226**
Support	229
Movement	229
Storage	229
Protection	229
Production	229
Bone formation and growth (ossification)	**230**
Embryonic formation	**231**
Intramembranous ossification	231
Endochondral ossification	231
Bone length and thickness	234
Bone remodelling	234
Bone fractures	**235**
Bone structure and blood supply (histology)	**236**
Blood supply	237
Organisation of bone based on shape	**237**
Long bones	237
Short bones	238
Flat bones	238
Irregular bones	241
Sesamoid bones	241
Joints	**241**
Fibrous joints	242
Cartilaginous joints	242
Synovial joints	243
Conclusion	*243*
Glossary of terms	*247*
References	*249*
Activities	*250*

Test your knowledge

- Why is calcium an important mineral in respect to bone?
- What do you understand by the skeletal system?
- What are the functions of the skeletal system?

Fundamentals of Anatomy and Physiology for Student Nurses, First Edition. Edited by Ian Peate, Muralitharan Nair.

- Why do babies have more bones than adults?
- What makes bones so strong?
- How does spongy bone differ from compact bone?
- Compare the appendicular and axial skeletons.
- What are the regions of the vertebral column?
- How many bones make up the cranium?
- What is synovial fluid and where is it found?

Learning outcomes

After reading the chapter you will be able to:

- Discuss the function of the skeletal system
- Describe the divisions of the skeleton
- List the four general bone categories
- Discuss bone composition
- Describe the various joints
- Understand the organisation of bone based on shape

Body map

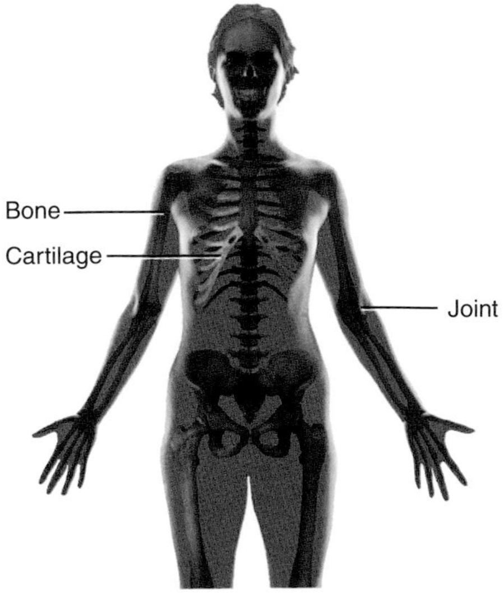
Bone
Cartilage
Joint

Introduction

Despite what seems to be a solid, dry, inert material, bone is in fact a complex living organism that is being recreated constantly; bone is metabolically active. As old bone dies new bone is being rebuilt. There are a number of complex activities occurring as bone is destroyed and re-formed. Bones are therefore living organs that are made up of a number of different tissues and this includes bone tissue.

The human skeleton, in contrast to other skeletons, is built to move erect as opposed to walking on all fours. The skeleton provides us with shape and the power to move, but it cannot do this in isolation, it needs many other systems of the body for it to function properly, for example, the nervous system and the muscles and for the body to move in its various and complex ways (the spine, for example, allows us to twist and bend); this is attributed to the joints and their ability to articulate.

Like a house, the human body needs a framework but the framework for the body is not made of wood and steel as is the case with the house. The skeletal system is made up of bones, ligaments and tendons. The human skeleton is built to take the hard knocks of life; it is an engineering wonder: for its weight, bone is nearly as strong as steel.

The skeleton produces blood cells. The bones also act as storage areas for minerals, vital for blood clotting, nerve function and contraction of muscles. The bones begin to form *in utero* and continue to grow into adulthood. Bones develop from cartilage, so infants are born with large amounts of cartilage as well as has having more bones than adults. As the child ages the bones usually fuse together and the child ends up with the normal adult number of bones. The bones of babies are soft, but as more minerals are deposited they become harder – this is known as ossification.

The axial and appendicular skeleton

There are 206 named bones in the adult human skeleton. For classification purposes the skeleton is divided into two parts – the axial skeleton and the appendicular skeleton; both have their own purposes.

The axial skeleton

The axial skeleton forms the central axis of the body and consists of 80 bones. This part of the skeleton supports the head (including the bones in the ear), neck and the torso (this is also referred to as the trunk). It consists of the skull, the vertebral column, the ribs and the sternum. There are 80 bones in the axial skeleton and these bones are noted in Table 8.1.

The appendicular skeleton

The bones of the appendicular skeleton are those bones of the upper and lower extremities – the arms and the legs as well as the bones that attach them to the axial skeleton. There are 126 bones in the appendicular skeleton and these bones are shown in Table 8.2.

Bone and its functions

The skeletal system – and this includes the bones of the skeleton, the ligaments, cartilage and connective tissues that provide stability or attach the bones – has a number of key functions:

Table 8.1 The bones of the axial skeleton

Structure	Number of bones
Skull	
Cranium	8
Face	14
Total	**22**
Hyoid	1
Auditory ossicles (bones)	6
Vertebral column	26
Thorax	
Sternum	1
Ribs	24
Total	**25**
Total number of bones in the axial skeleton	**80**

Table 8.2. The bone of the appendicular skeleton

Structure	Number of bones
Pectoral girdle	
Clavicle	2
Scapula	2
Total	**4**
Upper limbs	
Humerus	2
Ulna	2
Radius	2
Carpals	16
Metacarpals	10
Phalanges	28
Total	**60**
Pelvic girdle	
Pelvic bone	2
Lower limbs	
Femur	2
Patella	2
Fibula	2
Tibia	2
Tarsals	14
Metatarsals	10
Phalanges	28
Total	**62**
Total number of bones in the appendicular skeleton	**126**
Total number of bones in the adult human skeleton	**206**

See Figure 8.1, the human skeleton.

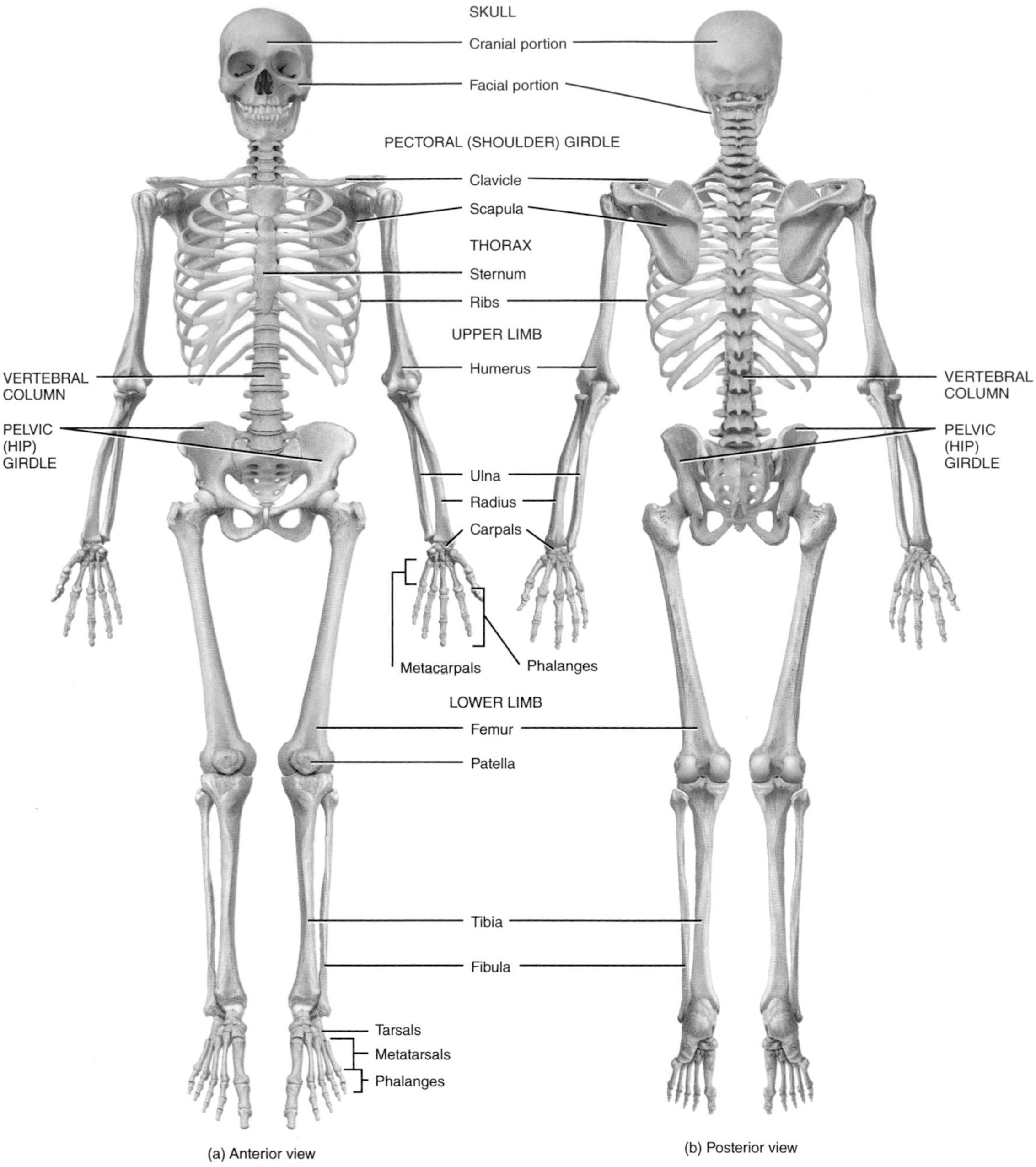
SKULL
Cranial portion
Facial portion
PECTORAL (SHOULDER) GIRDLE
Clavicle
Scapula
THORAX
Sternum
Ribs
UPPER LIMB
Humerus
VERTEBRAL COLUMN
PELVIC (HIP) GIRDLE
Ulna
Radius
Carpals
Metacarpals
Phalanges
LOWER LIMB
Femur
Patella
Tibia
Fibula
Tarsals
Metatarsals
Phalanges
(a) Anterior view
(b) Posterior view

Figure 8.1 The human skeleton. Axial skeleton blue and appendicular skeleton white (Tortora and Derrickson 2009)

(1) Provides support
(2) Enables movement
(3) Stores minerals and lipids
(4) Protects the body
(5) Produces blood cells.

Support

Apart from bone and cartilage, all body tissue is soft and without the skeleton the body would be jelly-like and would not be able to stand up. The way the bones are arranged provides the body with its shape/form. The skeletal system provides structural support for the body providing a bony framework for the attachment of soft tissues and organs.

Movement

The skeleton allows and enables movement. The bones act as levers providing the transmission of muscular forces. A number of bones can (through leverage, contracting and pulling) change the extent and direction of the forces generated by skeletal muscles, through the work of the tendons and the ligaments. These movements can be very intricate, such as the ability to write, the ability to thread a needle (the coordination of fine movement), to gross movement, such as the ability to change body posture. The skeleton with the interaction of muscles permits breathing to occur. Movement becomes possible through articulation.

Storage

The bones are capable of storing essential minerals such as calcium, magnesium and phosphorous; calcium is the most abundant mineral in the human body. The bone also has the ability to release stored minerals in response to the body's demands, for example, when the amount of calcium in the blood is high (a high concentration) the calcium can be deposited in the bones. When calcium in the blood is low or it decreases the bones give up calcium into the bloodstream. This ability to provide an internal homeostasis is regulated by hormones. Lipids are also stored in the yellow marrow of some bones; lipids are stored or released depending on the body's needs when providing energy.

Protection

Bone, a rigid structure, protects most of the soft tissues of the body and the internal organs, for example, the skull protects the brain, the sternum and ribs protect the lungs and heart, the spinal cord is protected by the vertebrae, the orbit protects the eyes and the periosteum protects the red bone marrow. The pelvis shields and protects the delicate internal abdominal digestive and reproductive organs.

Production

There are some bones in the body that produce red and white blood cells; this is known as haematopoiesis. Haematopoiesis mainly occurs in red bone marrow. The red bone marrow fills the internal cavity of most bones, yellow bone marrow can also be found in some bones, but this is made up mainly of fat.

Clinical considerations

Red bone marrow

Understanding the role and function of bone marrow can assist the nurse to help people being cared for who may experience any condition affecting the bone marrow or its production.

Bone marrow is a spongy material that fills the bones. There are two types: yellow and red. Red bone marrow contains cells called stem cells; these are early blood cells. In the healthy person these blood cells grow and divide, providing the basis for the formation of new blood cells. Red bone marrow is only found in certain bones, for example, the pelvis, the sternum, the end of the thigh and arm bones.

Some cancer drugs act on the bone marrow by slowing down the production of blood cells by killing them off as they grow and divide. Hence, some cancer-treating drugs – chemotherapy (and some biological therapies) – have the potential to help and to harm.

When white blood cells (the cells primarily responsible for fighting infection), for example, are killed off this means the person may be at risk of developing an infection. When the red cells are killed off (these are the cells that have a key role to play in transporting oxygen around the body) a person may experience anaemia. The platelets, the cells responsible for helping the blood to clot, are also formed within the red bone marrow. A disruption in the production of platelets can also have health and wellbeing implications for the person being cared. The person may bruise easily, bleed more than they usually do, even from small cuts or grazes (when shaving, for example) and experience nose bleeds.

When caring for a person who has problems with the bone marrow (for example, those with cancer), the nurse must be aware of the issues discussed above in order to provide safe and effective care.

Bone formation and growth (ossification)

The strength of bone comes from the protein matrix which provides it with resilience and elasticity. This allows bone to give a little as it is comes under pressure. Within the bone are a number of minerals that have been deposited there, these add to the strength of bone protecting it and supporting it as pressure and force are applied. It is important to understand how bone develops as this can help understand its strengths and boundaries.

By the end of the third month of pregnancy the skeleton of a foetus is completely formed (Rizzo 2006). Most of the skeleton at this stage is primarily cartilage; ossification occurs as the pregnancy develops and the formation of bone takes place. The process of bone formation is known as ossification. Bone formation takes place during various phases of a person's life. Tortora and Derrickson (2010) discuss four principal situations in a person's life when bone formation occurs (see Table 8.3).

Table 8.3 Bone formation throughout a person's life (Adapted from Tortora and Derrickson 2010)

Stage	Activity
One	The initial formation of bone *in utero* in the foetus
Two	The growth of bones during infancy, childhood and adolescents
Three	The replacement of old bone with new bone (bone remodelling) – this occurs throughout an individual's life
Four	The repair of fractures that can occur throughout a person's life

Embryonic formation

As the foetus develops an embryonic skeleton is forming; at first this appears as mesenchyme which is shaped similar to bones and in the sites where ossification will take place. Bone formation at this stage goes through a number of stages and changes. Hyaline cartilage develops from the mesenchyme. Osteoblasts converge on the cartilage and then the process of ossification begins.

Intramembranous ossification

The mesenchymal cells at the site of ossification – the ossification centre – cluster together and differentiate at first into osteogenic cells and then into osteoblasts. The extracellular matrix of bones is secreted by the osteoblasts. Secretion of extracellular matrix ceases and the cells, now known as osteocytes, sit within the lacunae. These cells have narrow cytoplasmic processes that extend into the canaliculi radiating in many different directions. After a few days the extracellular matrix calcifies (hardens) as a result of calcium and other minerals being deposited.

When the bone and the extracellular matrix form these develop into trabeculae; the trabeculae fuse with one another and spongy bone is formed. Angiogenesis (blood vessel formation) occurs between the trabeculae spaces. Red bone marrow is formed as the connective tissue within the trabeculae differentiates and periosteum is formed as mesenchyme condenses along with the formation of trabeculae. Spongy bone remains in the centre despite a thin layer of compact bone forming on the surface of the spongy bones. The process outlined above is known as intramembranous ossification. The process described next is called endochondral ossification.

Figure 8.2 provides an illustration of intramembranous ossification.

Endochondral ossification

Cartilage that is replaced by bone is called endochondral ossification, the majority of bones in the body are formed in this way. Mesenchymal cells crowd together at the site where bone is going to form and they take on the shape of the future bone and develop into chondroblasts. These chondroblasts secrete the extracellular matrix and produce a cartilage model that is made up of hyaline cartilage. The perichondrium – a membrane – develops around the cartilage model.

As the chondroblasts become buried deep into the cartilage matrix they change their name and become chondrocytes. As growth continues through cell division the chondrocytes also grow

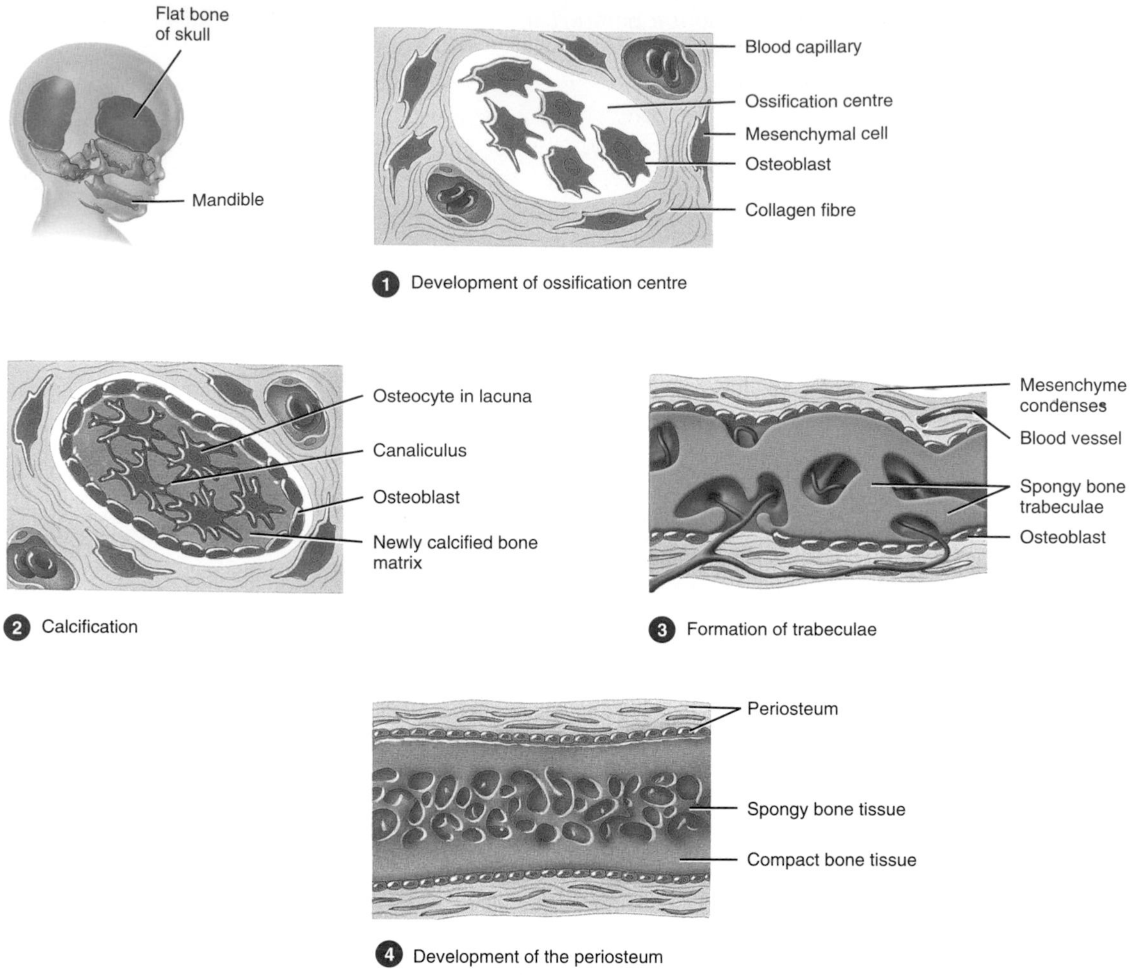
Flat bone of skull
Mandible
Blood capillary
Ossification centre
Mesenchymal cell
Osteoblast
Collagen fibre
1 Development of ossification centre
Osteocyte in lacuna
Canaliculus
Osteoblast
Newly calcified bone matrix
2 Calcification
Mesenchyme condenses
Blood vessel
Spongy bone trabeculae
Osteoblast
3 Formation of trabeculae
Periosteum
Spongy bone tissue
Compact bone tissue
4 Development of the periosteum

Figure 8.2 Intramembranous ossification (Tortora and Derrickson 2009)

and the extracellular matrix starts to calcify. The chondrocytes also start to die as they are unable to receive nutrients through the extracellular matrix; as death occurs lacunae form and merge into small cavities.

A nutrient artery enters the perichondrium and the matrix that is calcifying; ossification occurs inwardly from the external surface of the bone. This activity encourages osteogenic bone cell production within the perichondrium to become (through differentiation) osteoblasts. The formation of bone is called perositeum, towards the centre the blood vessels grow and eventually bone replaces most of the cartilage.

The bone marrow is developed as the primary ossification centre grows towards the ends of the bone, here osteoblasts break down some of the newly formed spongy bone. As this action continues it produces a cavity, the medullary cavity (bone marrow), in the shaft of the bone (called the diaphysis).

Secondary ossification centres frequently develop prior to or just after birth when the blood vessels enter the epiphyses. Bone formation in secondary ossification is similar to that in primary ossification; however, there are no medullary cavities left. In secondary ossification the process occurs outwardly from the centre of the epiphysis towards the surface of the bone.

The articular cartilage and the epiphyseal plates are formed from the hyaline cartilage that covers the epiphyses. Before a person reaches adulthood hyaline cartilage remains between the diaphysis and epiphysis.

Figure 8.3 provides an illustration depicting endochondral ossification.

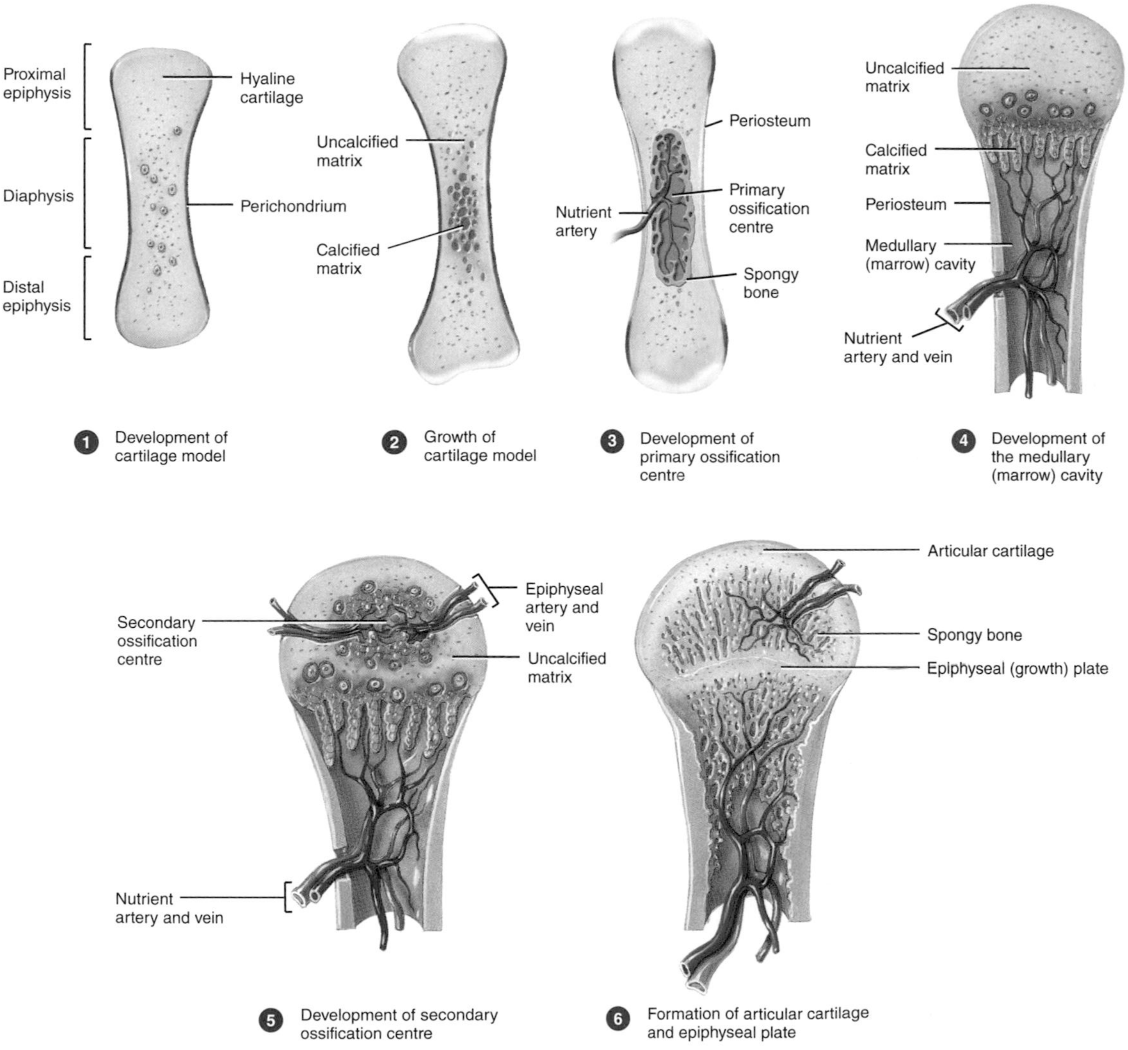
Proximal epiphysis
Diaphysis
Distal epiphysis
Hyaline cartilage
Perichondrium
Uncalcified matrix
Calcified matrix
Periosteum
Nutrient artery
Primary ossification centre
Spongy bone
Uncalcified matrix
Calcified matrix
Periosteum
Medullary (marrow) cavity
Nutrient artery and vein
1 Development of cartilage model
2 Growth of cartilage model
3 Development of primary ossification centre
4 Development of the medullary (marrow) cavity
Secondary ossification centre
Epiphyseal artery and vein
Uncalcified matrix
Nutrient artery and vein
Articular cartilage
Spongy bone
Epiphyseal (growth) plate
5 Development of secondary ossification centre
6 Formation of articular cartilage and epiphyseal plate

Figure 8.3 Endochondral ossification of the tibia (Tortora and Derrickson 2009)

Bone length and thickness

As the person grows, for example, during infancy, childhood and adolescence, long bone grows in length and thickness. This longtitudinal growth and expansion of thickness continues until the person is usually 15 and 16 years of age in girls and boys respectively.

The chondrocytes present in the epiphyseal plate are constantly dividing and this activity is related to the length of bone growth. As adolescence ends the formation of new cells decreases and between the ages of 18 and 25 years this activity ceases altogether.

Growth of bone (thickness) occurs as the cells in the perichondrium differentiate into osteoblasts; the osteoblasts then develop into osteocytes. Lamella are added to the bone surface and osteons (the basic units of structure of the adult compact bone) are formed. Osteoblastic and osteoclastic activity occurs and the result is an enlarged medullary cavity and thicker bone is formed.

Bone remodelling

As adolescence ends between the ages of 18 and 25 years formation of new cells occurs and bone continually renews itself through bone remodelling. This happens when ongoing replacement of old bone is renewed by new bone. Remodelling takes place at different rates in different parts of the body. When bones reach their adult shapes old bones are being repeatedly demolished and new bone is formed in its place, this clearly demonstrates that bone is a living, metabolising organ.

A fine balance must exist between the breakdown and buildup of bone: if bone is built up too quickly, then an abnormally thick and heavy bone will be formed. Weak bone, as a result of too much calcium or bone tissue loss can result in bone that breaks easily.

Clinical consideration

Osteoarthritis

As a person ages the action of bone breakdown and buildup continues. As well as breakdown and rebuilding, the bone also thickens and bone mass increases. Damage to joints, tissues surrounding the joints and the bones themselves can also occur as the ageing process occurs.

The condition osteoarthritis is a degenerative non-inflammatory condition. It is more common in people aged over 50 years, but younger people can also be affected and women suffer with osteoarthritis more than men.

The joints are characteristically affected, damage appears to the cartilage, bony growths occur at the ends of the bones and around the joints and synovitis (inflammation of the tissues around the joints) may occur.

The impact of osteoarthritis will differ from person to person and so the care of those with osteoarthritis will depend on the assessment of individual needs. There is no cure for osteoarthritis, but there are many interventions that can be implemented to help improve the health and wellbeing of the person being cared for.

A multidisciplinary approach to care is required whether in a hospital setting or in the person's own home. Adjustments to lifestyle, for example, an increase in exercise and the modification of footwear, can help. The administration of medicines to control pain and inflammation can also help the person carry out their activities of living in a more effective way, promoting independence.

Bone fractures

Tucker (2008) defines a fracture as the breakage of bone due either to an injury or disease. There are a number of types of fracture including:

(1) Simple
(2) Compound
(3) Comminuted
(4) Greenstick (incomplete).

The repair of a bone that has been broken (fractured) goes through a number of stages (see Figure 8.4). Although bone has a rich blood supply, healing can sometimes take many months. The break in the bone will interfere with the blood supply to the bone temporarily and this will result in a delay in healing.

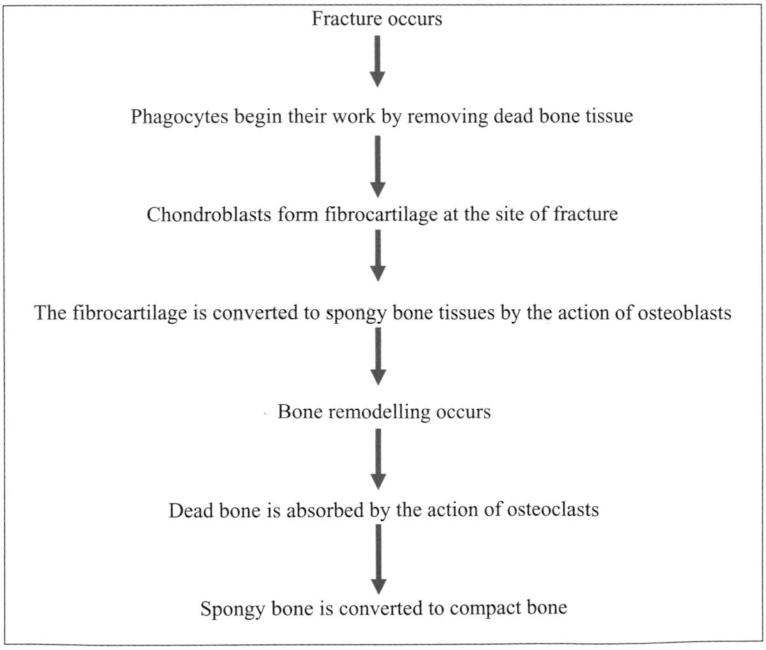
Fracture occurs
Phagocytes begin their work by removing dead bone tissue
Chondroblasts form fibrocartilage at the site of fracture
The fibrocartilage is converted to spongy bone tissues by the action of osteoblasts
Bone remodelling occurs
Dead bone is absorbed by the action of osteoclasts
Spongy bone is converted to compact bone

Figure 8.4 The stages a broken bone goes through for repair to occur

As a fracture occurs phagocytes remove any dead bone tissues. Osteocytes will proliferate when a break in bone occurs as the fracture stimulates production. The bone will heal gradually as calcium and phosphorus (needed to strengthen and harden new bone) is deposited and bone cells slowly grow and duplicate. McRae (2006) suggests that full bone healing can take months to take place.

Bone has the capacity to regenerate and heal itself; the action of osteoblasts and osetoclasts produce new cells and remove those cells that have died. Tortora and Grabowski (2009) suggest that the balance of calcium is an essential requirement in bone growth and repair; this is affected by the level of vitamin D in the body as well as renal and intestinal functioning, parathyroid gland functioning and the ability of the adrenal glands to work effectively.

Bone structure and blood supply (histology)

There are a number of factors that will impinge upon bone growth (and therefore its structure) (see Table 8.4).

All of the factors cited in Table 8.4 are required for bone growth and an alteration in any of them will impact on bone structure as well as a number of other bodily functions.

Table 8.4 Some factors that impact on bone structure (Adapted from Rizzo 2006; Tortora and Derrickson 2009)

Factor	Comment
Vitamins	A, C, D, K and B_{12}. There are a number of sources of these vitamins and their roles and functions vary. Too high amounts can be toxic and too low amounts can, for example, stunt growth.
Hormones	Human growth hormone (hGH), insulin-like growth factors (IGFs), oestrogens, androgens and thyroid hormones (for example, parathyroid hormone). Some of these hormones are produced in the pituitary gland, hence any condition affecting this gland could result in problems related to bone formation and structure. Insulin-like growth factors are produced by the liver in response to hGH. If oestrogen (the sex hormone produced in the ovaries) and androgens (the sex hormone produce in the testes) are not released, there are potential complications associated with a number of body functions, including bone.
Minerals	Calcium, phosphorus, magnesium and fluoride. Calcium is a mineral that becomes available to the rest of the body when remodelling occurs. The amount of calcium in the blood stream must be within precise limits otherwise serious problems can occur (the heart may stop if there is too much circulating calcium).
Exercise	All exercise is beneficial to the body, but weight-bearing exercise is particularly important for the stimulation of bone growth, particularly those exercises that places stress on the bones. When placed under stress bone tissue becomes stronger as remodelling occurs; without this stress the bone will weaken and demineralisation occurs.

Blood supply

Blood supply to the bone comes via three routes:

- The haversian canals
- The Volkmann's canals
- The vessels.

The haversian canals are minute channels that are laid down parallel to the axis of the bone and are the passages for arterioles; they allow for the efficient metabolism of bone cells. These are central canals that contain blood vessels, nerves and lymphatic vessels. The canals are surrounded by lamellae which are made up of rings of hard, calcified extracellular matrix. Lying between the lamellae are the lacunae which contain the osteocytes and radiating in all directions are the canaliculi filled with extracellular fluid. These various interconnecting structures provide nutrients and oxygen to the bones as well as providing a route for waste to be removed.

The periosteum provides the route for the blood vessels, nerves and lymphatic vessels to penetrate the compact bones through the Volkmann's canals. These blood vessels, lymph vessels and nerves connect with those of the bone marrow, periosteum and haversian canals. The fluid present in the Volkmann's canals bathes the osteocytes bringing in oxygen and removing waste (including carbon dioxide), helping to keep the osteocytes alive and healthy (Rizzo 2006). Figure 8.5 provides an illustration of the haversian system in compact bone and trabeculae in spongy bone.

Organisation of bone based on shape

There are, according to Rizzo (2006), five categories that individual bones of the body can be divided into:

- Long
- Short
- Flat
- Irregular
- Sesamoid.

Long bones

Some examples of long bones are the humerus, clavicle, radius, ulna, femur, tibia and fibula. The metacarpals, metatarsals and phalanges are also classed as long bones (despite their shortness) as the length of these bones exceeds their width. They allow movement, particularly in the limbs (for example, the femur and the humerus).

Long bones consist of a diaphysis composed primarily of compact bone and a metaphysis which is composed mainly of cancellous or spongy bone. There are two extremities that are separated from the metaphysis called the epiphysis; the separating line is called the epiphyseal line. The diaphysis is thickest towards the middle of the bone. There is a reason for this: it is where most strain on the bone occurs. The long bone has a slight curve to it – this also aids strength – distributing weight. The interior of the shaft contains the bone marrow (the medullary cavity). Figure 8.6 shows a long bone.

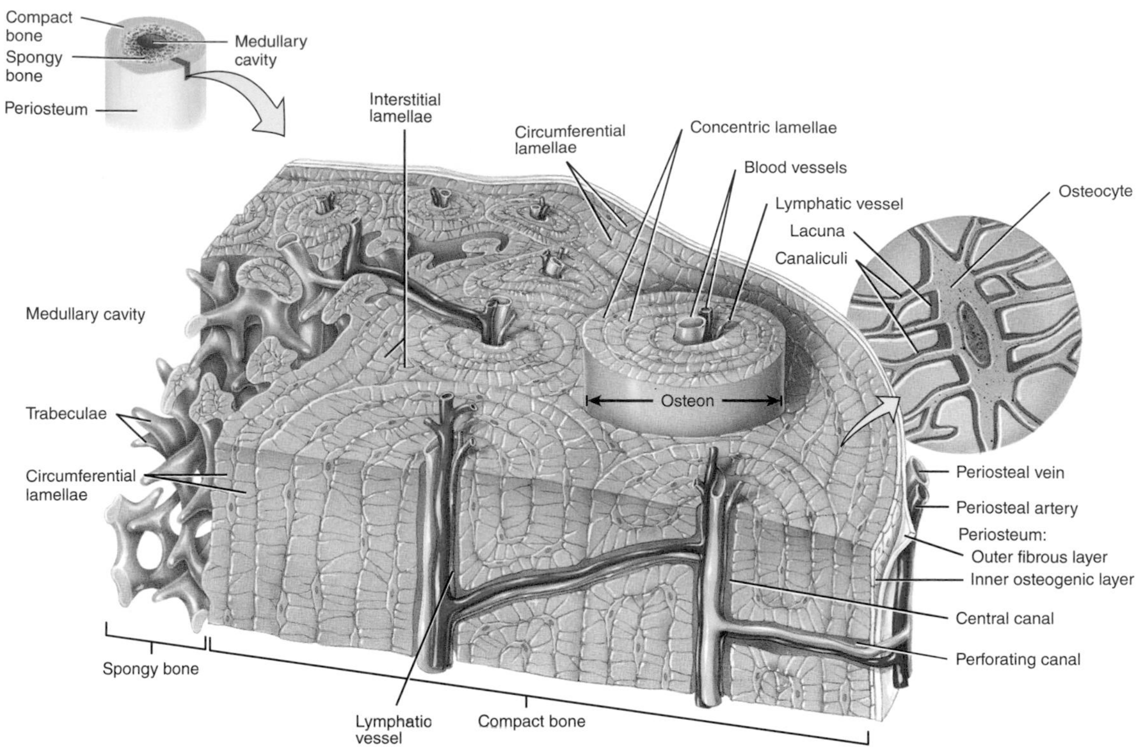

Compact bone
Spongy bone
Medullary cavity
Periosteum
Interstitial lamellae
Circumferential lamellae
Concentric lamellae
Blood vessels
Lymphatic vessel
Lacuna
Canaliculi
Osteocyte
Medullary cavity
Trabeculae
Circumferential lamellae
Osteon
Periosteal vein
Periosteal artery
Periosteum:
Outer fibrous layer
Inner osteogenic layer
Central canal
Perforating canal
Spongy bone
Lymphatic vessel
Compact bone

Figure 8.5 The haversian system in compact bones and trabeculae in spongy bone (Tortora and Derrickson 2009)

Short bones

These bones are usually grouped in pairs; they are strong and compact. Often they are found in parts of the body where little movement is needed. Examples of short bones include the carpal bones of the wrist and the tarsal bones of the foot (see Figure 8.7). Short bones are not just shorter versions of long bones, they do not have a long axis and are irregular in shape. They have thin a layer of compact tissue over a predominantly spongy or cancellous bone.

Flat bones

These are thin bones that are found where there is a need for muscle attachment or for protection of soft or important aspects of the body. Their broad flat surface allows for extensive muscle attachment. Examples of flat bones are the sternum, ribs, scapula, some bones of the skull and some bones of the pelvis (see Figure 8.8). These bones are often curved and are made up of compact tissues enclosing a layer of cancellous bone.

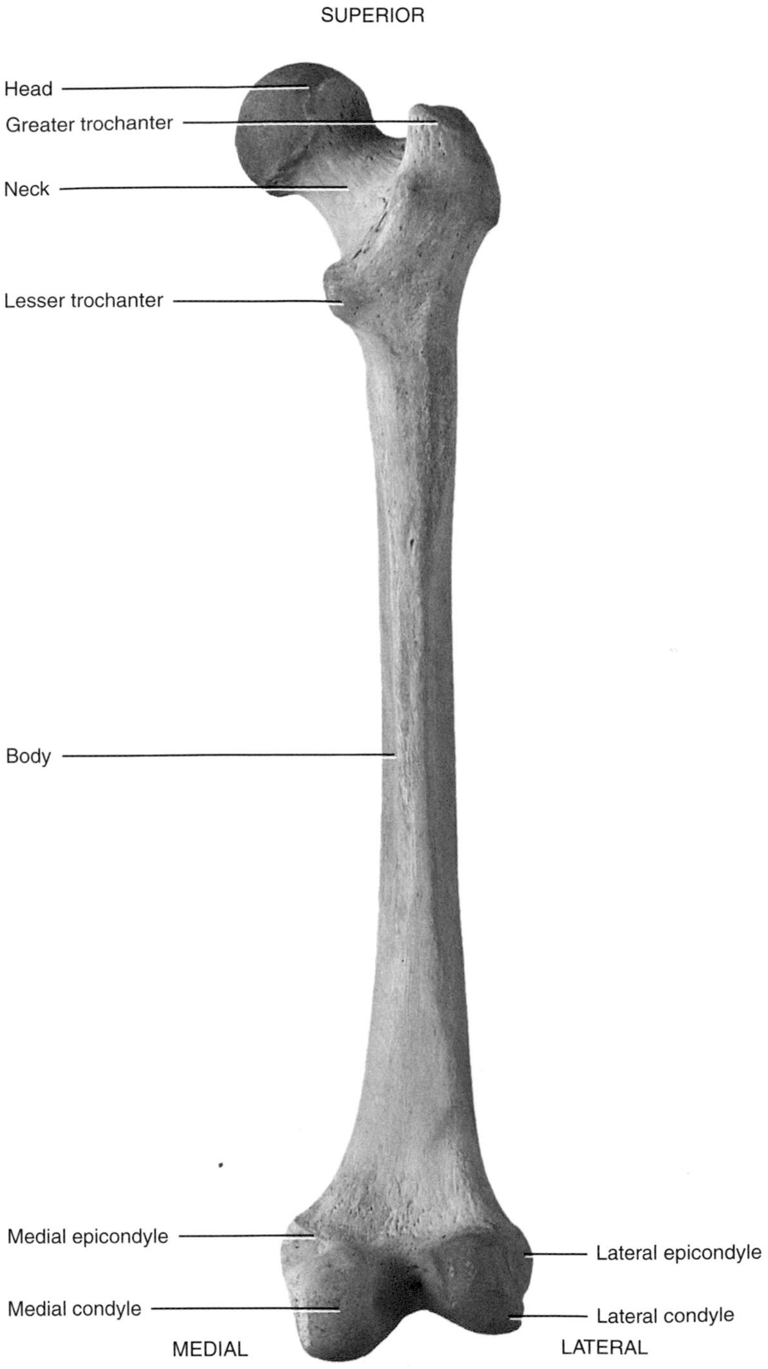
SUPERIOR
Head
Greater trochanter
Neck
Lesser trochanter
Body
Medial epicondyle
Medial condyle
MEDIAL
Lateral epicondyle
Lateral condyle
LATERAL

Figure 8.6 A long bone – the femur (Tortora 2008)

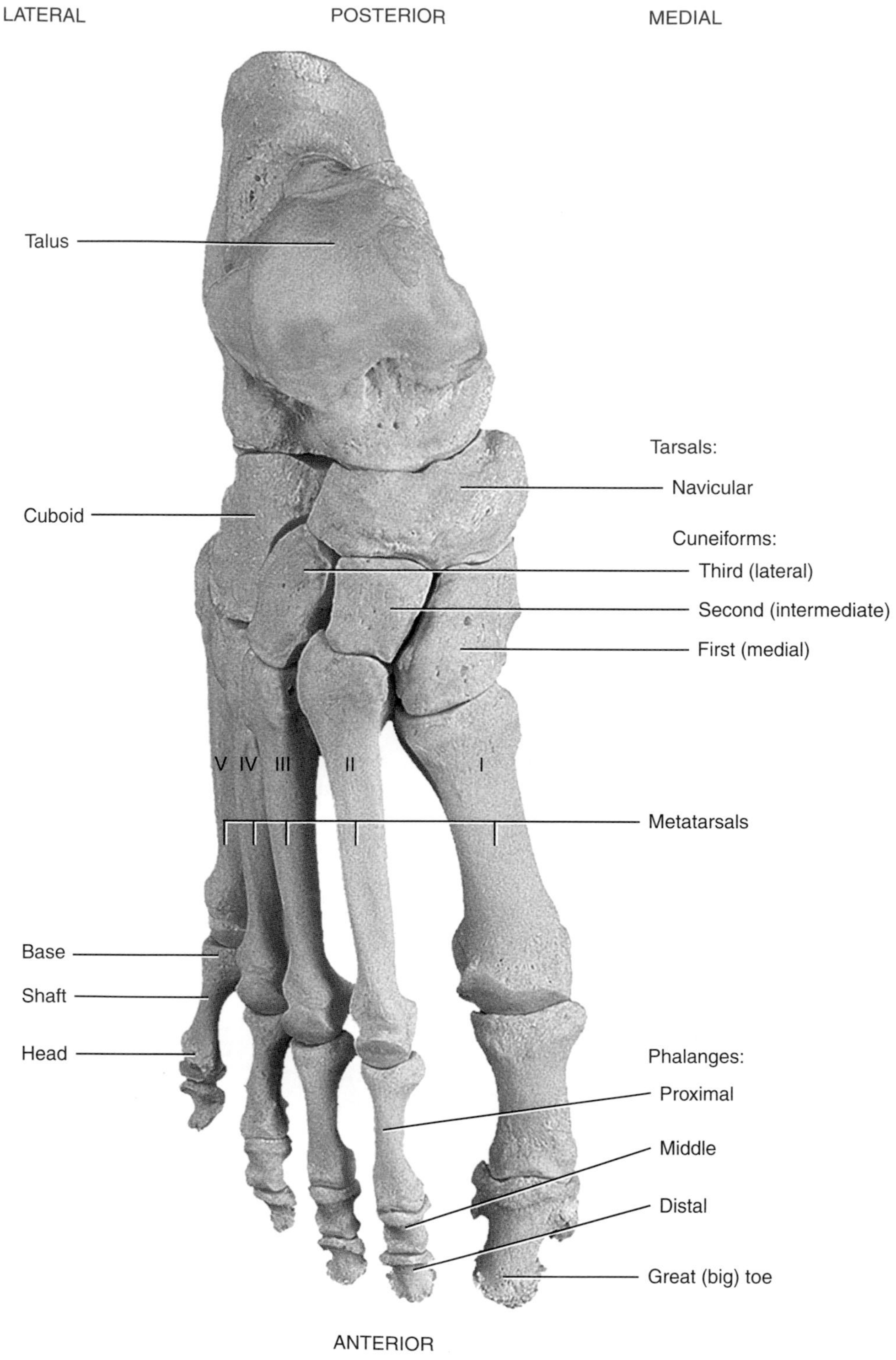
LATERAL
POSTERIOR
MEDIAL
Talus
Tarsals:
Navicular
Cuboid
Cuneiforms:
Third (lateral)
Second (intermediate)
First (medial)
V IV III II I
Metatarsals
Base
Shaft
Head
Phalanges:
Proximal
Middle
Distal
Great (big) toe
ANTERIOR

Figure 8.7 The tarsal bones – short bones (Tortora 2008)

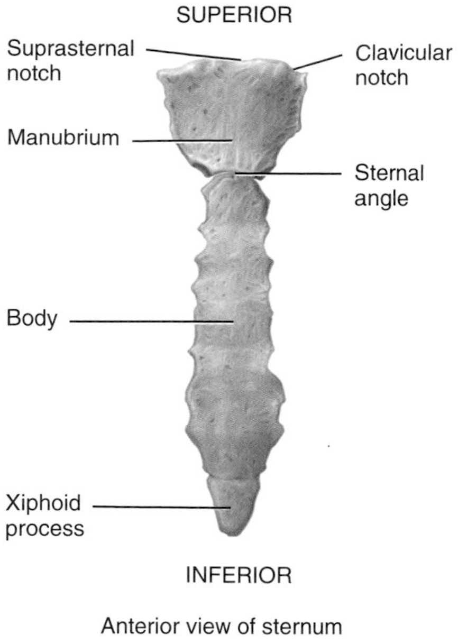
SUPERIOR
Suprasternal notch
Clavicular notch
Manubrium
Sternal angle
Body
Xiphoid process
INFERIOR
Anterior view of sternum

Figure 8.8 A flat bone – the sternum (Tortora and Derrickson 2009)

Irregular bones

These bones do not fit into the categories described above as they have a number of different characteristics. As the name suggests, they are irregular, different and peculiar. These bones consist of spongy bone which is enclosed by thin layers of compact bones. These bones include the vertebrae, coccyx, sphenoid, zygomatic, the ossicles of the ear and the vertebrae (see Figure 8.9).

Sesamoid bones

The human body has only two sesamoid bones: the patella and the hyoid bone (this is located at the base of the tongue), although some of the bones of the wrist or ankle could be classed as sesamoid. Sesamoid bones are bones within tendons; they are small and round, and assist in the functioning of muscles. Figure 8.10 shows the patella.

Joints

A joint is the point at which two or more bones meet. Joints are sometimes also called articulations. There are a number of ways of classifying joints, for example:

- Fibrous
- Cartilaginous
- Synovial.

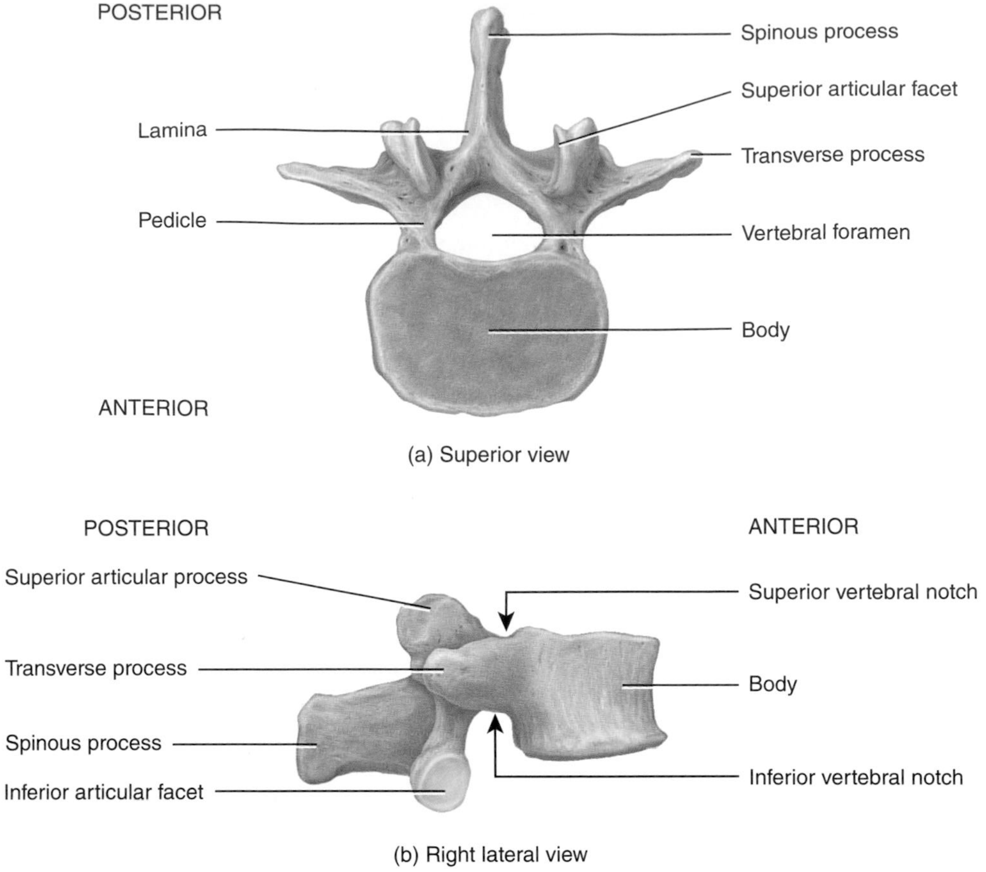
POSTERIOR
Spinous process
Superior articular facet
Lamina
Transverse process
Pedicle
Vertebral foramen
Body
ANTERIOR
(a) Superior view
POSTERIOR
ANTERIOR
Superior articular process
Superior vertebral notch
Transverse process
Body
Spinous process
Inferior articular facet
Inferior vertebral notch
(b) Right lateral view

Figure 8.9 The vertebrae – an irregular bone (Tortora and Derrickson 2009)

Fibrous joints

These joints are also called synarthrodial joints and are held together by only a ligament, a dense irregular tissue that is made up of collagen-rich fibres. There is no synovial cavity in this type of joint. Examples of synarthrodial joints are where the teeth are held to their bony sockets; other examples include both the radioulnar and tibiofibular joints.

Cartilaginous joints

These joints are also called synchondroses and symphyses (singular symphysis). They occur where the connection between the articulating bones are made up of cartilage with no synovial cavity, for example, the joints occurring between vertebrae in the spine.

The synchondroses are temporary joints and are only present in children until the end of puberty, by which stage the hyaline cartilage converts to bone, for example the epiphyseal plates of long bones. Symphysis joints are permanent cartilagenous joints which have an intervening pad of fibrocartilage, for example, the symphysis pubis.

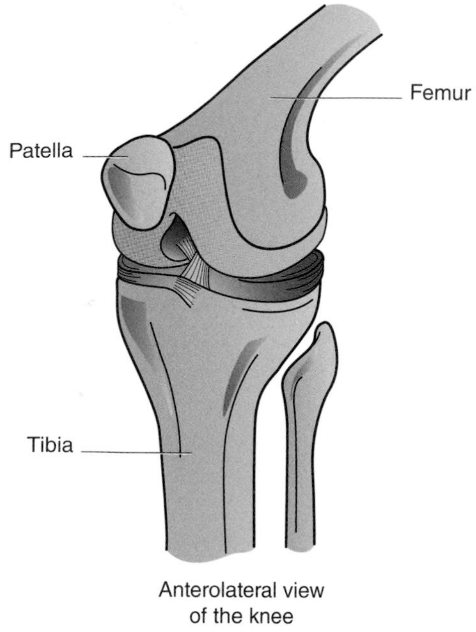
Femur
Patella
Tibia
Anterolateral view
of the knee

Figure 8.10 The patella – a sesamoid bone

Synovial joints

Synovial joints, also called diarthrosis joints, are by far the most common classification of joint within the human body. They are extremely moveable joints with a synovial cavity and all have an articular capsule enclosing the whole joint, a synovial membrane (the inner layer of the capsule) which produces synovial fluid (a lubricating solution) and cartilage known as hyaline cartilage, which pads the ends of the articulating bones.

Synovial fluid is a thin film that is usually viscous, clear or yellowish. This fluid helps to prevent friction by providing the joint with lubrication, supplying nutrients and removing waste products. If the joint becomes immobile for a period of time the fluid becomes gel-like and returns to its normal viscous consistency when the joint begins to move again.

There are six types of synovial joints and these are classified by the shape of the joint and the movement available (see Table 8.5).

Conclusion

All activities that people perform are related to movement, for example, verbal communication, moving the mouth (jaw) to speak, requires the skeleton. In order to perform in the best possible way the skeleton and the bones of the body are required. When gases are exchanged during breathing mobility is required for this life-sustaining activity to occur. The intact skeletal system permits these activities to occur. Mobility is an essential activity of living.

Table 8.5 Six types of joint

Type of joint	Movement at joint	Examples	Structure
Hinge	A convex portion of one bone fits into a concave portion of another bone. The movement reflects the hinge and bracket movement of a household hinge and bracket, movement is limited to flexion and extension. The joint produces an open and closing motion. These joints are uniaxial.	Elbow Knee 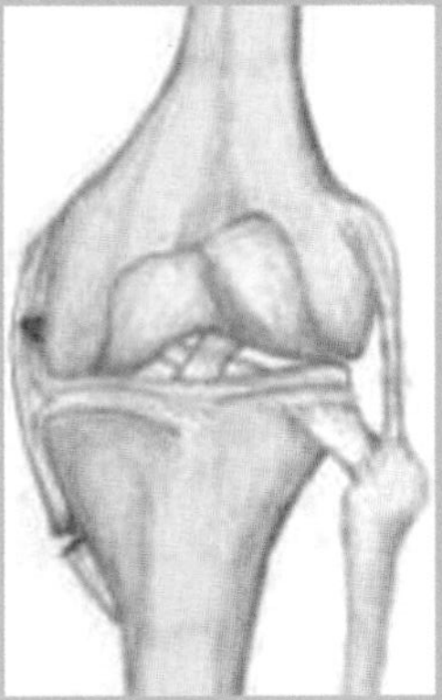	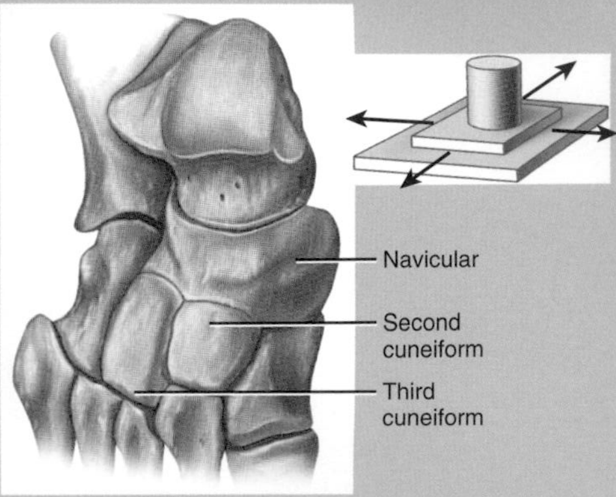Navicular Second cuneiform Third cuneiform
Pivot	A rounded part of one bone fits into grove of another bone. These joints will only permit movement of one bone around another – uniaxial movement.	Radius and ulna The atlas and the axis 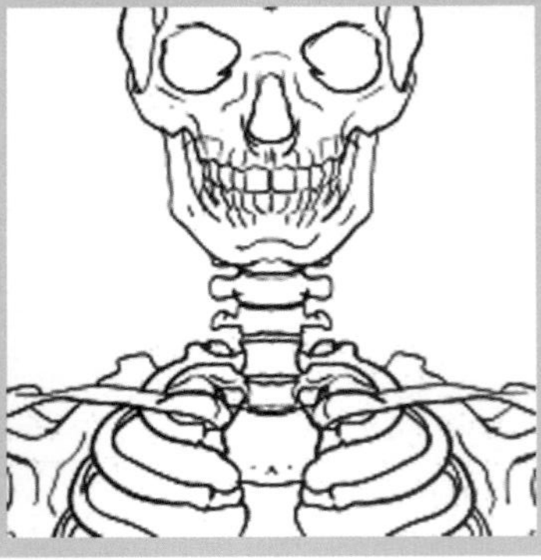	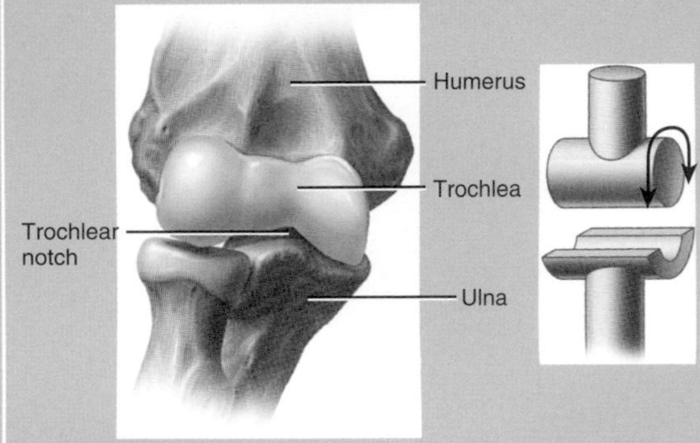Humerus Trochlea Trochlear notch Ulna

<table>
<tr>
<td>Ball and socket</td>
<td>The spherical end of one bone fits into a concave socket of another bone, hence, ball and socket. Movement occurs through flexion, extension and adduction. This is triaxial joint.</td>
<td>Hip
Shoulder
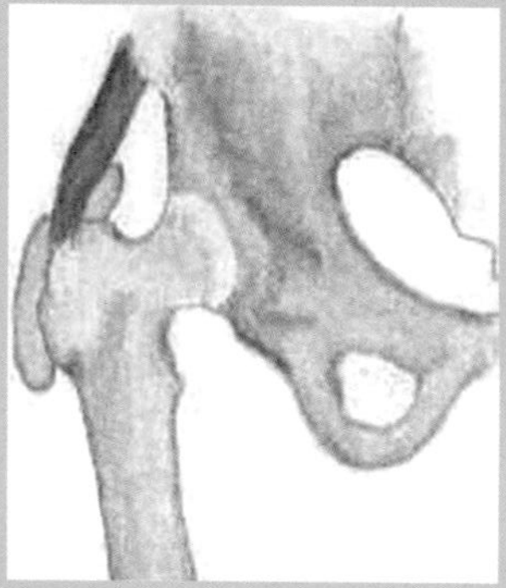</td>
<td>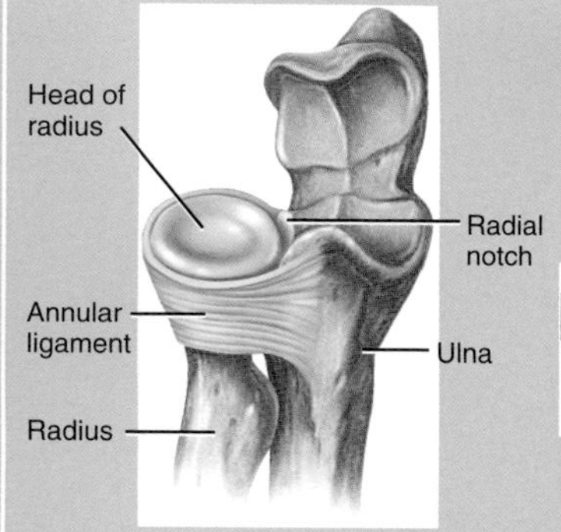
Head of radius
Radial notch
Annular ligament
Ulna
Radius
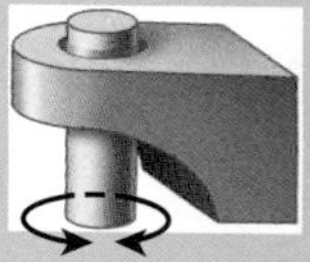</td>
</tr>
<tr>
<td>Saddle</td>
<td>Similar to condyloid joints, but these joints permit greater movement. Allow flexion, extension and adduction. The joint is classed as triaxial.</td>
<td>The carpometacarpal joints of the thumb
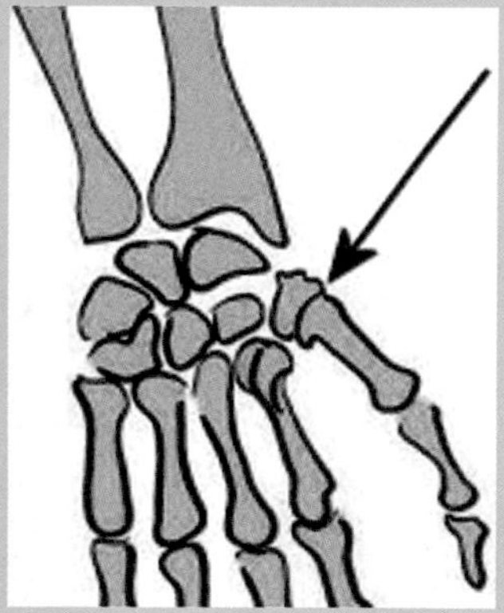</td>
<td>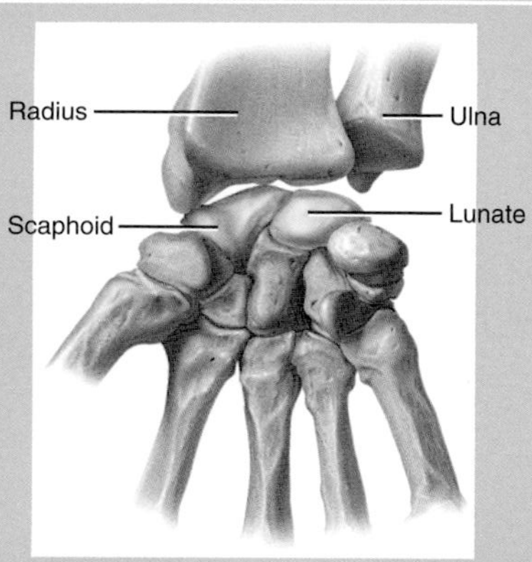
Radius
Ulna
Scaphoid
Lunate
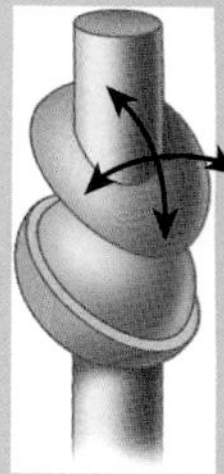</td>
</tr>
</table>

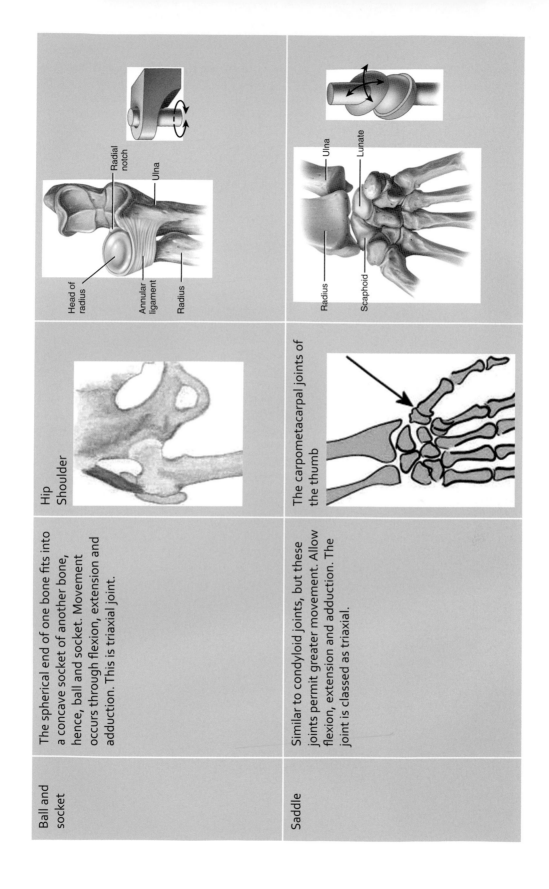

Table 8.5 *Continued*

Type of joint	Movement at joint	Examples	Structure
Condyloid	Where an oval surface of one bone fits into a concavity of another bone and where condyloid joints are found. Allows flexion, extension and adduction. This is a biaxial joint.	The radiocarpal and metacarpophalangeal joints of the hand 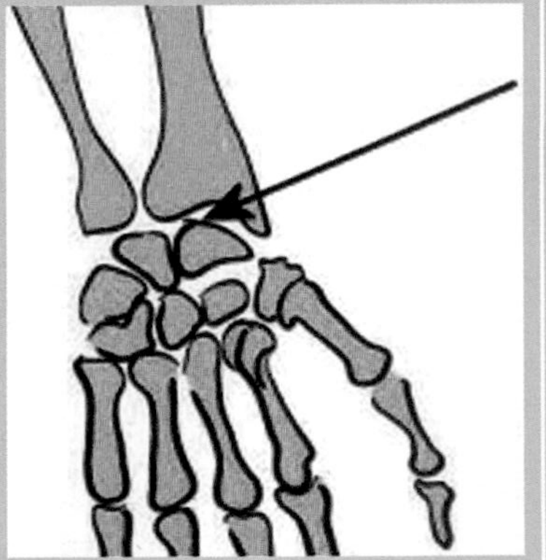	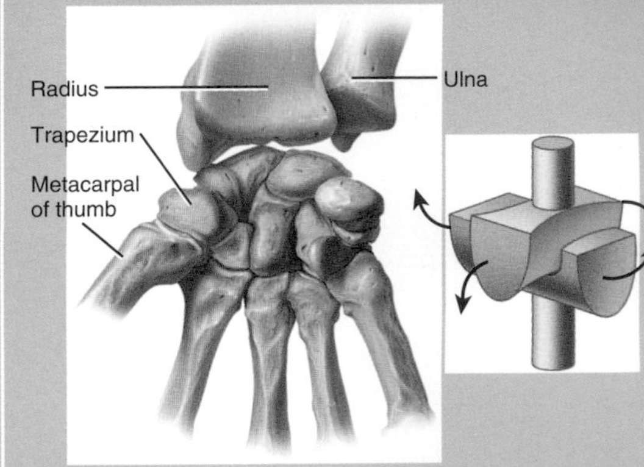 Radius Ulna Trapezium Metacarpal of thumb
Gliding	These joints have a flat or slightly curved surface permitting gliding movements. The joints are bound by ligaments and movement in all directions is restricted. The joint moves back and forth and side to side.	Intertarsal and intercarpal joints of the hands and feet 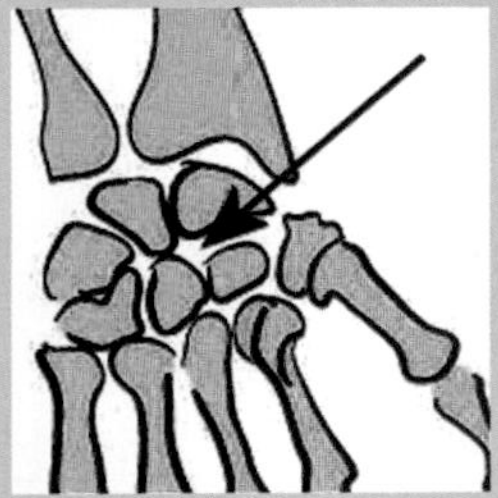	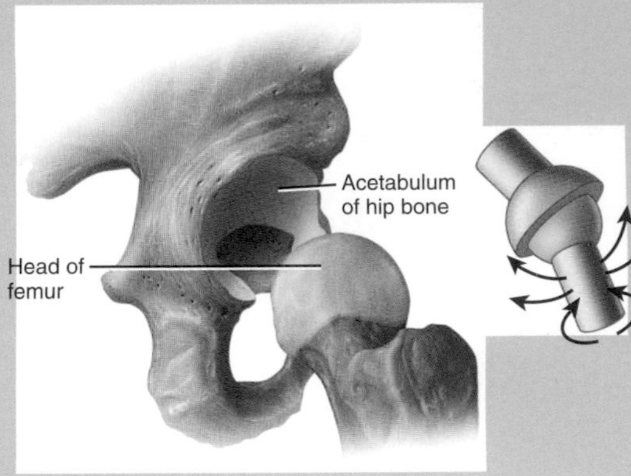 Acetabulum of hip bone Head of femur

The human skeleton is a living organism that is constantly metabolising. The skeletal system links very closely to muscles; muscles provide leverage and movements and the skeleton provides the framework. The long bones are responsible for the production of erythrocytes (haemopoiesis); production (or failure to produce erythrocytes) can have an impact on the person's health and wellbeing. The nervous system is closely related to the skeletal system as muscles require a nerve impulse to contract, this then results in skeletal movement. The digestive system enables food to be broken down to such a level that the nutrients can be used for bone production. Hormones produced by the kidneys help to stimulate the production of bone marrow in the long bones.

The skeletal system is essential for life, providing support and protection of the internal organs. The bones store, and when needed release, calcium, a mineral that is essential to ensure safe bodily functioning.

Glossary of terms

Abduction:	Movement away from the body's midline.
Adduction:	Movement towards the body's midline.
Anatomy:	The study of body structures and their relation to other structures in the body.
Artery:	A blood vessel that carries blood away from the heart.
Articulation:	Sometimes called a joint, where bones meet.
Ball and socket joint:	A synovial joint in which the rounded surface of one bone fits within the cup-shaped depression of the socket of the other bone.
Calcification:	Deposition of mineral salts in a framework formed by collagen fibres in which tissue hardens.
Cancellous:	A type of structure as seen in spongy bone tissue, resembles a latticework structure.
Cartilage:	Strong, tough material on the bone ends that helps to distribute the load within the joint, the slippery surface allows smooth movement between the bones, a type of connective tissue.
Cartilaginous joint:	A joint where the bones are held together tightly by cartilage, little movement occurs in this joint. This joint does not have a synovial cavity.
Collagen:	A protein that makes up most of the connective tissue.
Condyloid joint:	A synovial joint that allows one oval-shaped bone to fit into an elliptical cavity of another.
Diaphysis:	The shaft of a long bone.
Epiphysis:	The ends of long bone.
Fibrous joint:	A type of joint that allows little or no movement.

Flexion:	Movement where there is a decrease in the angle between two bones.
Fracture:	A break in a bone.
Gliding joint:	A synovial joint whose articulating surfaces are usually flat, allowing only side to side or back and forth movement.
Haemopoiesis:	The formation and development of blood cells in the bone marrow after birth.
Histology:	The microscopic study of tissue.
Homeostasis:	A state whereby the body's internal environment remains relatively constant within physiological limits.
Hormone:	The secretion of endocrine cells that have the ability to alter the physiological activity of target cells in the body.
Insulinlike growth factor (IGF):	Produced by the liver and other tissues this is a small protein that is produced in response to hGH.
In utero:	Within the uterus.
Kinesiology:	The study of movement of the body.
Lacuna:	A small, hollow space found in the bones where osteocytes lie.
Lamellae:	Rings of hard, calcified martrix found in compact bones.
Ligaments:	Tough fibrous bands of connective tissue that hold two bones together in a joint.
Macrophage:	Cells that engulf and the digest cellular debris and pathogens.
Marrow:	A sponge-like material found in the cavities of some bones.
Mesenchyme:	Embryonic connective tissue from which nearly all other connective tissue arises.
Metaphysis:	The aspect of long bone that lies between the diaphysis and the epiphysis.
Ossification:	The formation of bone, sometimes called osteogenesis.
Osseous:	Bony.
Ossicle:	Small bones of the middle ear – the malleus, the incus, the stapes.
Osteoblasts:	Cells that arise from osteogenic cells; these cells participate in bone formation.
Osteoclasts:	Large cells that are associated with absorption and removal of bone.
Osteocytes:	Mature bone cells.
Osteon:	The basic unit of structure in adult compact bone.

Osteophytes:	Overgrowth of new bone around the side of osteoarthritic joints; also known as spur growth.
Periosteum:	Membrane covering bone consisting of osteogenic cells, connective tissue and osteoblasts. This is vital for bone growth, repair and nutrition.
Pivot joint:	A joint where a rounded or conical-shaped surface of a bone articulates with a ring formed partly by another bone or ligament.
Remodelling:	Replacement of old bone by new.
Resorption:	Absorption of what has been excreted.
Saddle joint:	A synovial joint articulates the surface of a bone that is saddle-shaped on the other bone that is said to be shaped like the legs of the rider.
Spongy (cancellous) bone tissue:	Bone tissue comprised of an irregular latticework of thin plates of bone known as trabeculae. Some bones are filled with red bone marrow and these are found in short, flat and irregular bones as well as the epiphyses of long bones.
Synovial cavity:	The space between the articulating bones of a synovial cavity, filled with synovial fluid.
Synovial fluid:	The sections of the synovial membranes that lubricate the joints and nourishes the articular cartilage.
Trabeculae:	A network of irregular latticework of thin plates of spongy bones.

References

McRae, R. (2006) *Pocket Book of Orthopaedics and Fractures*, 2nd edn. Edinburgh: Churchill Livingstone.

Rizzo, D.C. (2006) *Fundamentals of Anatomy and Physiology*. New York: Thompson.

Tortora, G.J. and Derrickson, B. (2009) *Principles of Anatomy and Physiology*, 12th edn. Hoboken, NJ: John Wiley & Sons.

Tortora, G.J. and Derrickson, B. (2010) *Essentials of Anatomy and Physiology*, 8th edn. New York: John Wiley & Sons.

Tortora, G.J. and Grabowski, S.R. (2009) *Principles of Anatomy and Physiology*, 11th edn. New York: John Wiley & Sons.

Tortora, G.J. (2008) *A Brief Atlas of the Human Skeleton, Surface Anatomy and Selected Medical Images*. New York: John Wiley & Sons.

Tucker, L. (2008) *An Introductory Guide to Anatomy and Physiology*, 3rd edn. London: EMS Publishing.

Activities

www.wiley.com/go/peate

Multiple choice questions

1. What is an osteophyte?
   (a) a bone cell
   (b) a small bony outgrowth
   (c) a bone cancer cell
   (d) a lymph cell

2. Where would you find the medial melleolus?
   (a) the hip
   (b) in the thoracic cavity
   (c) the fibula
   (d) the cranium

3. What is another name for the clavicle?
   (a) the rib
   (b) the breast bone
   (c) the collar bone
   (d) the pelvis

4. What does the term kinesiology mean?
   (a) the study of light
   (b) the study of brain
   (c) the study of art
   (d) the study of movement of the body

5. A joint that allows free movement is known as:
   (a) diarthrosis
   (b) haemathrosis
   (c) synarthrosis
   (d) amphiarthroses

6. The jaw bone is the:
   (a) calcaneus
   (b) maxilla
   (c) ischium
   (d) mandible

7. A joint such as the elbow joint that only moves in one plane is known as a:
   (a) hinge joint
   (b) socket joint
   (c) arthritic joint
   (d) saddle joint

8. Bone is covered by a protective tissue membrane called the:
   (a) lacunae
   (b) diaphysis
   (c) peritoneum
   (d) periosteum

9. The skull and ribs are part of the:
   (a) appendicular skeleton
   (b) external skeleton
   (c) axial skeleton
   (d) internal skeleton

10. The ribs are attached to:
   (a) the cervical vertebrae
   (b) the thoracic verebrae
   (c) the lumbar verebrae
   (d) the skull

True or false

1. The skeleton is a living organism.
2. There are more bones in adults than in babies.
3. Bone stores and releases calcium.
4. The ribs protect the pancreas.
5. Yellow bone marrow produces red blood cells.
6. There is no difference in the weight and size of male and female bones.
7. The patella is located in the humerus.
8. Osteoblasts build up bone.
9. Replacement of old bone by new is called remodelling.
10. The axial skeleton has more bones that the appendicular skeleton.

Label the diagram

From the lists of words, label the diagrams below:

Head, Greater trochanter, Neck, Lesser trochanter, Body, Medial epicondyle, Medial condyle, Lateral epicondyle, Lateral condyle

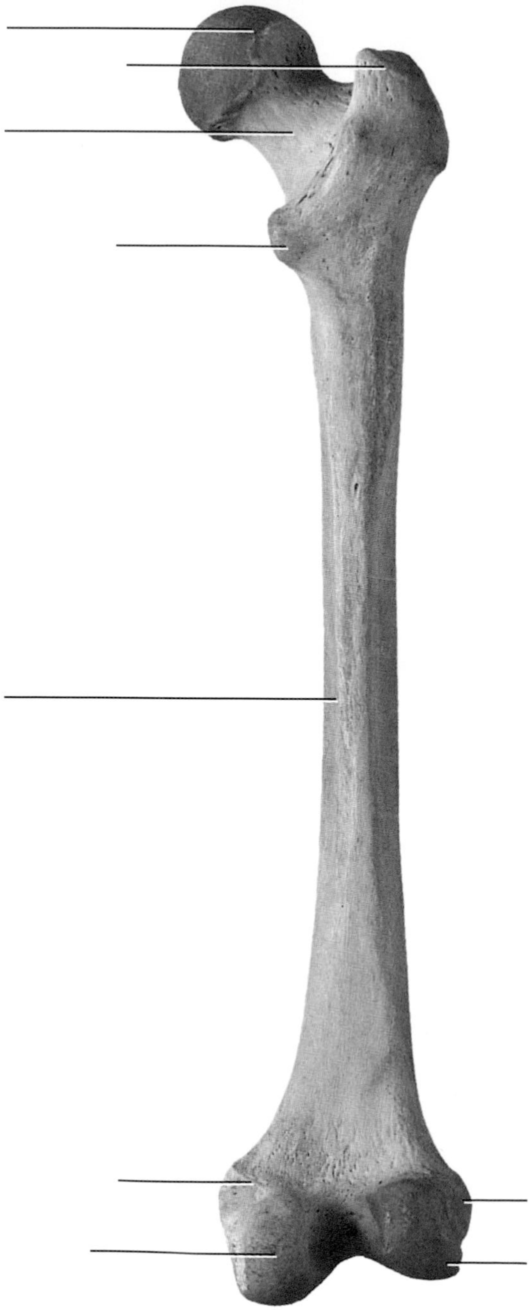

Femur, Tibia, Patella

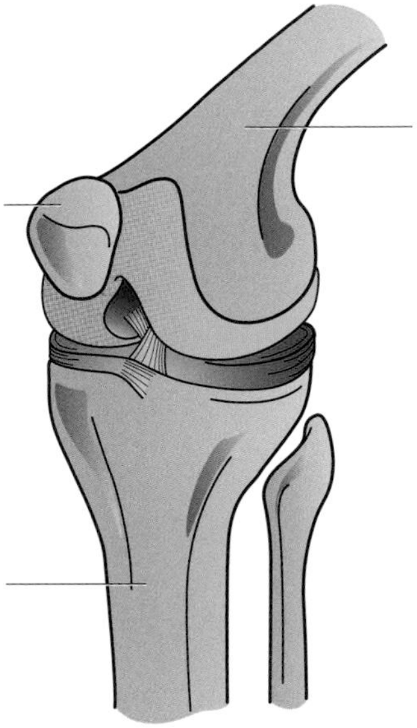

Word search

In the grid below there are 15 words that you will have seen in this chapter. Can you find them all?

O	P	C	H	T	S	A	L	B	O	E	T	S	O	W	J
N	E	A	R	B	E	T	R	E	V	R	F	I	T	O	I
O	L	T	D	I	O	M	H	T	E	O	P	P	I	P	E
T	A	A	K	L	U	C	O	B	O	N	E	N	O	A	R
E	S	L	I	N	S	Y	S	R	S	C	T	Y	D	T	U
L	R	F	R	C	R	O	O	S	S	E	O	U	S	E	T
E	A	E	P	I	P	H	Y	S	E	A	L	A	N	L	U
K	T	I	B	I	A	B	M	L	O	M	A	X	E	L	S
S	O	S	T	E	O	C	L	A	S	T	N	D	I	A	O

Fill in the blanks

The ____________ is the ____________ and ____________ bone of the ____________ arm. The head of the humerus is _________ and _________ to the rest of the bone by the anatomic ____________. The upper aspect of the bone has two prominences the _________ and ___________ tubercles. The ulna is ____________________ than the radius. The bones of the wrists are called the ______________ and arranged in ____________ rows of four each. The palms of the hand are made up of the ___________ ___________ bones. Metatarsals are small _____________ bones they each have a ___________ and a ___________. The thumb has only a ___________ and ___________ phalanx.

Match the bone to the shape:

1. **Irregular bone**
2. **Long bone**
3. **Flat bone**
4. **Short bone**

A. Sternum
B. Zygomatic
C. Metacarpal
D. Hyoid
E. Tarsal
F. Femur
G. Ethmoid
H. Scapula

Find out more

1. Why do healthy bones require exercise?
2. Describe the composition of bone.
3. How does the skeletal system help to maintain homeostasis?
4. In bone remodelling how do osteoblasts and osteoclasts work together?
5. What happens to bone as we age?
6. What is synovial fluid?
7. Describe the healing that occurs after a fracture has been sustained.
8. Discuss intramembranous ossification.
9. What factors are essential for bone remodelling?
10. Where in the body are the two sesamoid bones and what are they called?

Conditions

Below is a list of conditions that are associated with the skeletal system. Take some time and write notes about each of the conditions. You may make the notes taken from text books or other resources, for example, people you work with in a clinical area, or you may make the notes as a result of people you have cared for. If you are making notes about people you have cared for you must ensure that you adhere to the rules of confidentiality.

Fractured neck of femur	
Osteoarthritis	
Osteoporosis	

Gout	
Osteomyelitis	
Osteosarcoma	

Answers

MCQs

1b; 2c; 3c; 4d; 5a; 6b; 7a; 8d; 9c; 10b

True or false

1T; 2F; 3T; 4F; 5F; 6F; 7F; 8F; 9T; 10F

Word search

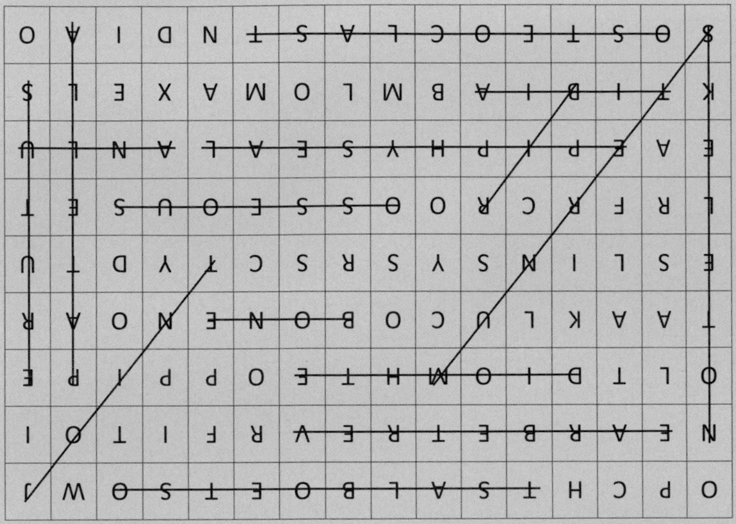

Fill in the blanks

The humerus is the largest and longest bone of the upper arm. The head of the humerus is rounded and joined to the rest of the bone by the anatomic neck. The upper aspect of the bone has two prominences, the greater and lesser tubercles. The ulna is longer than the radius. The bones of the wrists are called the carpals and arranged in two rows of four each. The palms of the hand are made up of the five metatarsal bones. Metatarsals are small long bones they each have a shaft and a head. The thumb has only a proximal and distal phalanx.

Match the bones to the shape

1. B, D, G
2. F
3. A, H, C, E

9

The muscular system

Janet G Migliozzi

Contents

Introduction	*260*
Types of muscle tissue	**260**
Smooth	260
Cardiac	260
Skeletal	260
Functions of the muscular system	**260**
Maintenance of body posture	261
Production of movement	261
Stabilisation of joints	261
Protection and control of internal tissue structures/organs	261
Generation of heat	261
Composition of skeletal muscle tissue	**261**
Gross anatomy of skeletal muscles	**262**
Microanatomy of skeletal muscle fibre	**263**
The sarcolemma and transverse tubules	264
The sarcoplasm	264
The myofibrils	264
The sarcomeres	264
Types of muscle fibres	**264**
Blood supply	**265**
Skeletal muscle contraction and relaxation	**266**
Energy sources for muscle contraction	**267**
Aerobic respiration	**269**
Oxygen debt	**269**
Muscle fatigue	**269**
Organisation of the skeletal muscular system	**270**
Skeletal muscle movement	**271**
The effects of ageing	**285**
Conclusion	*285*
Glossary	*286*
References	*286*
Activities	*287*

Fundamentals of Anatomy and Physiology for Student Nurses, First Edition. Edited by Ian Peate, Muralitharan Nair.

Test your knowledge

- List the functions of the muscular system.
- Name the different types of muscles found in the human body.
- Describe the energy sources that enable muscles to contract.
- List the stages involved in muscle contraction.
- List the different types of body movement.

Learning outcomes

After reading this chapter you will be able to:

- Describe the structure and functions of the muscular system
- Describe the different types of muscles in the human body
- Name the major muscles of the body and their functions
- Describe how a muscle contracts
- Describe the energy sources that muscles use

Body map

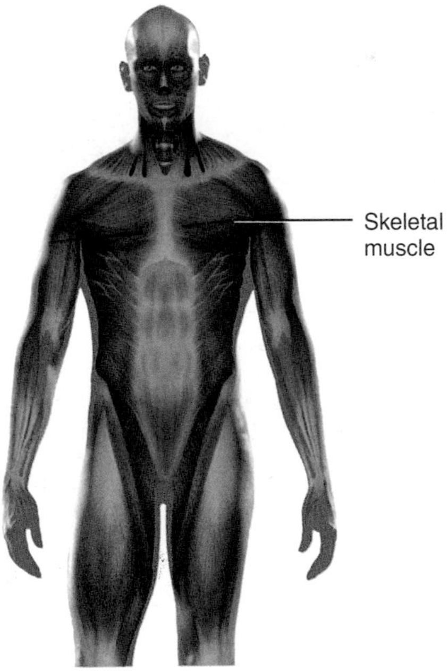
Skeletal
muscle

Introduction

All physical function of the body involves muscular activity and as muscles are responsible for all body movement, they can be considered the 'machines' of the body (Marieb 2006). This chapter will discuss the structure and function of the muscular system.

Types of muscle tissue

The body contains three types of muscle tissue: smooth, cardiac and skeletal.

Smooth

Smooth or visceral muscle is located in the walls of hollow internal organs and blood vessels of the body, e.g. the small intestine, throat, blood vessels (arteries, arterioles, venules and veins), bronchioles of the respiratory tract, urinary bladder and ureters, uterus and fallopian tubes but not the heart. Smooth muscle fibres have a single nucleus, are usually arranged in parallel lines and are not striated. Smooth muscles are involuntary, do not fatigue easily and are controlled by the medulla oblongata in the brain which is responsible for controlling involuntary action throughout the body. Smooth muscle is discussed in more detail in Chapter 13.

Cardiac

Cardiac muscle, found only in the heart, is also a form of involuntary muscle and forms the walls of the heart. Its main function is to propel blood into the circulation by making the right atrium contract. Cardiac muscles also have a single nucleus, are striated, branched and tubular. Cardiac muscle is discussed in more detail in Chapter 10.

Skeletal

The skeletal muscles make up the muscular system of the body (composed of over 600 muscles) and account for 40–50% of the body weight in an adult. The skeletal muscles are the only voluntary muscles of the body (i.e. are consciously controlled) and are the muscles involved in moving bones and generating external movement. Skeletal muscle is also referred to as striped or striated muscle because of the banded patterns of the cells seen under the microscope.

Table 9.1 provides a summary of the different types of muscle tissue.

As both smooth and cardiac muscle are discussed in more detail elsewhere, the rest of this chapter will focus on skeletal muscle only.

Functions of the muscular system

The muscular system plays four important roles in the body:

- Maintains posture
- Produces movement
- Stabilises joints
- Generates heat.

Table 9.1 Different types of muscle tissue

Skeletal muscle	Smooth muscle	Cardiac muscle
Attached to bones or the skin (facial muscles only)	Found in the walls of hollow visceral organs and blood vessels	Located in the walls of the heart
Single, long cylindrical cells	Single, narrow, rod-shaped cells	Branching chains of cells
Striated, multinucleated cells	Non-striated, uninucleated cells	Non-striated, uninucleated cells
Under voluntary control	Involuntary control	Involuntary control

Maintenance of body posture

Despite the continuous downward pull of gravity, the body is able to maintain an erect or seated posture because of the continuous tiny adjustments that the skeletal muscles make.

Production of movement

The body's ability to mobilise is a result of skeletal muscle activity and muscle contraction as when muscles contract they pull on the tendons and bones of the skeleton to produce movement.

Stabilisation of joints

Muscle tendons play a vital role in stabilising and reinforcing the joints of the body. During movement the skeletal muscles pull on bones which stabilise the joints of the skeleton.

Protection and control of internal tissue structures/organs

Skeletal muscle plays an important role in protecting the internal organs as the visceral organs and internal tissues contained within the abdominal cavity are protected by layers of skeletal tissue within the abdominal wall and floor of the pelvic cavity. Similarly the orifices contained within the digestive and urinary tract are encircled by skeletal muscle and this allows for voluntary control over swallowing, urination and defaecation (Martini and Bartholomew 2003).

Generation of heat

Heat generation is vital in maintaining normal body temperature and skeletal muscles which account for 40% of the body's mass are the muscle type mostly responsible for the body's heat generation. During muscle contraction, adenisotriphosphate (ATP) is used to release the needed energy with nearly three-quarters of its energy escaping as heat.

Composition of skeletal muscle tissue

As muscles contain other types of tissues such as blood vessels, connective and nervous tissue, they are considered to be organs (Logenbaker 2008). Each cell in skeletal muscle tissue is known as a single muscle fibre which, due to their large size, contain hundreds of nuclei (i.e. are multinucleate). A skeletal muscle consists of individual muscle fibres which are markedly different from a 'typical' cell (not least by their size) bundled into fascicles and surrounded by three layers of connective tissue.

Gross anatomy of skeletal muscles

Muscle is separated from skin by the hypodermis which consists of adipose tissue (which provides insulation and protects the muscle from physical damage) and a dense, broad band of connective tissue known as fascia, which supports and surrounds muscle tissue and provides a pathway for nerves, lymphatic and blood vessels to enter and exit a muscle. Extending from the fascia are three layers of connective tissue which also play a role in supporting and protecting the muscle and are necessary to ensure that the force of contraction from each muscle cell is transmitted to its points of attachment to the skeleton (see Figure 9.1). These include the:

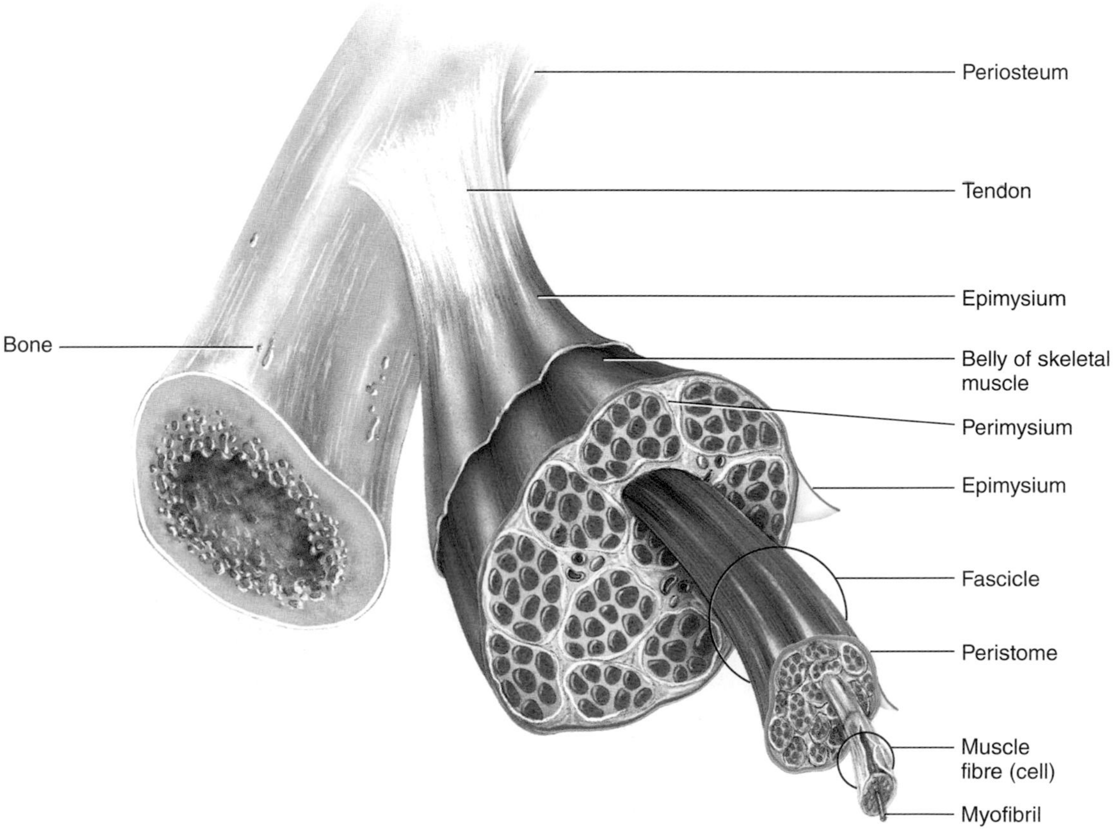
Periosteum
Tendon
Epimysium
Bone
Belly of skeletal muscle
Perimysium
Epimysium
Fascicle
Peristome
Muscle fibre (cell)
Myofibril

Figure 9.1 Gross anatomy of a skeletal muscle (Tortora and Derrickson 2009)

- **Epimysium** which is wrapped around the entire muscle
- **Perimysium** which surrounds bundles of muscle fibres known as fascicles
- **Endomysium** which is wrapped around each individual muscle cell.

The epimysium, perimysium and endomysium blend into either strong, cord-like tendons or into sheet-like aponeuroses which attach muscles indirectly to bones, cartilages or connective tissue coverings of each other (Marieb 2006).

Microanatomy of skeletal muscle fibre

When examined microscopically, skeletal muscle cells appear cylindrical in shape, have a distinctive banded appearance of alternate light and dark stripes and lie parallel to each other (see Figure 9.2).

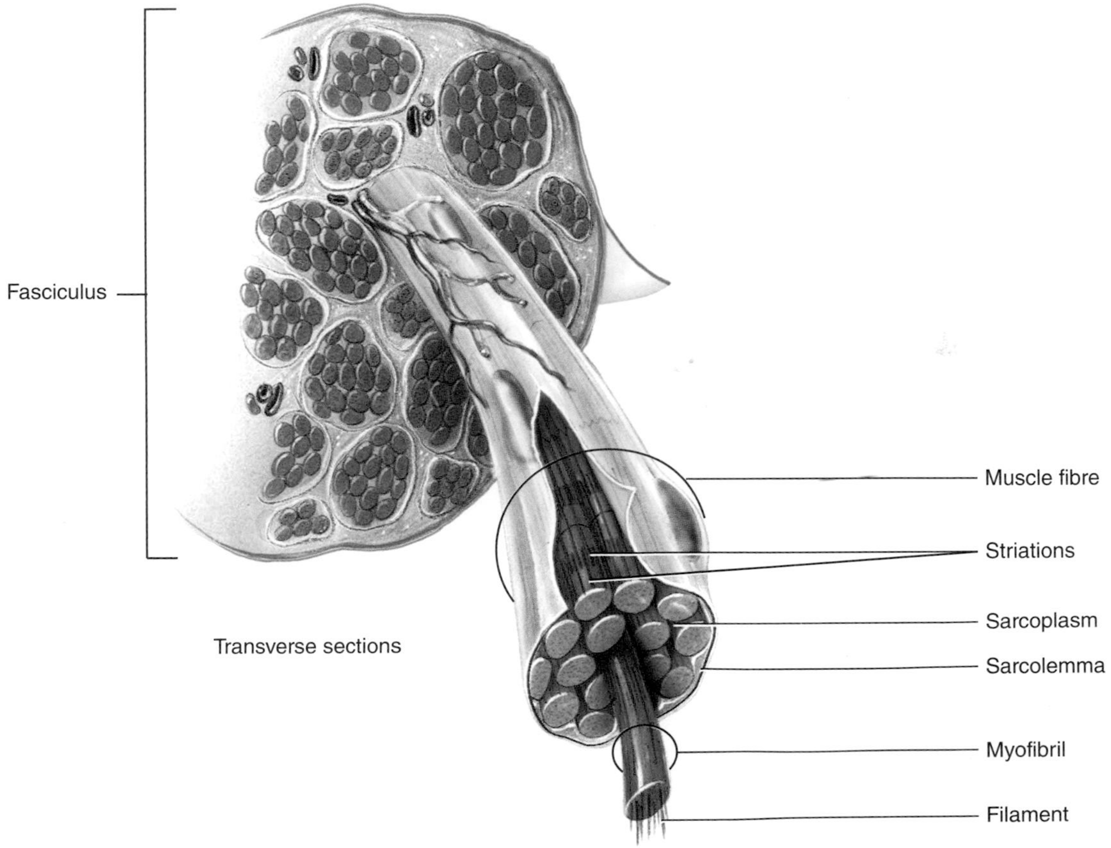
Fasciculus
Transverse sections
Muscle fibre
Striations
Sarcoplasm
Sarcolemma
Myofibril
Filament

Figure 9.2 Diagram showing a skeletal muscle fibre

The sarcolemma and transverse tubules

Each muscle fibre is covered by a plasma membrane called the sarcolemma and cylindrical structures called myofibrils which are suspended inside the muscle fibre in a matrix called the sarcoplasm (cytoplasm), which extends along the entire length of the muscle fibre. The surface of the sarcolemma is scattered with openings that lead into a network of narrow tubules called transverse or 'T' tubules which are filled with extracellular fluid and form passageways though the muscle fibre (Martin and Bartholomew 2003).

The sarcoplasm

The sarcoplasm contains multiple mitochondria which produce large amounts of ATP during muscle contraction (Tortora and Derrickson 2010) and it is here that the T tubules makes contact with a membranes known as the sarcoplasmic reticulum (SR). The SR stores calcium ions (essential for muscle contraction) in structures called cisternae and myoglobin (a reddish-brown pigment which is similar to haemoglobin) which stores oxygen until needed to generate ATP.

The myofibrils

Myofibrils (which are bundles of myofilaments) are thread-like structures which are found in abundance in the sarcoplasm. The myofibrils plays a key role in the muscle contraction mechanism and contain two types of protein filaments – thick filaments composed of myosin and thin filaments composed of actin and two other proteins, tropomyosin and troponin. These filaments form compartments know as sarcomeres, which are the basic functional units of striated muscle fibres (Tortora and Derrickson 2010) and each myofibril contains approximately 10,000 sarcomeres arranged end to end. The sarcomeres are separated from each other by dense zig-zagging protein-based structures called Z discs.

The sarcomeres

Extending across each of the thick filaments found within the sarcomere is a dark area known as the A band in the centre of which is a narrow H zone. On either side of the A band there is a lighter coloured area consisting of thin filaments called the I band. The alternating A and I bands give skeletal muscles their striated (striped) appearance. Table 9.2 provides a summary of the cellular components of a muscle fibre.

Types of muscle fibres

Three types of muscle fibres are found in skeletal muscles and are found in varying proportions throughout the body:

- **Slow oxidative (SO) fibres** which are small, dark-red fibres (due to containing large amounts of myoglobin) that generate ATP by aerobic respiration make up approximately 50% of skeletal muscle and are capable of slow, prolonged contractions and not easily fatigued
- **Fast oxidative-glycolytic (FOG) fibres** which are medium, dark-red fibres that also generate ATP by aerobic respiration but due to their high glycogen content are also able to generate ATP by anaerobic glycolysis. FOG fibres are able to contact and relax more quickly than SO fibres

Table 9.2 Cellular components of a muscle fibre

Name	Function
Sarcolemma	Plasma membrane of a muscle fibre that forms T tubules
Sarcoplasm	Cytoplasm of the muscle fibre which contains myofibrils
Myofibril	Consists of bundles of myofilament and plays a key role in muscle contraction
Myofilament	Consists of thick and thin filaments that gives muscle tissue its striated appearance and plays a role in muscle contraction
Myoglobin	A reddish-brown pigment (gives muscle tissue its dark-red colour) which stores oxygen for muscle contraction
T tubule	Fluid-filled tubular structure that releases calcium from the sarcoplasmic reticulum
Sarcoplasmic reticulum	Storage site for calcium ions

- **Fast glycolytic (FG) fibres** which are large white fibres (low myoglobin content) that generate ATP mainly by anaerobic glycolysis and provide the most rapid and powerful muscle contractions but fatigue easily.

Blood supply

Skeletal muscles have a very extensive blood supply and receive a total of 1 litre of blood each minute which equates to 20% of the resting cardiac output. This increases to 15–20 litres per minute when exercising intensively. As a general rule, each skeletal muscle is supplied by an artery and one or two veins and each muscle fibre is in close contact with a network of microscopic capillaries within the endomysium.

Clinical considerations

Intramuscular injection

An intramuscular (IM) injection is given directly into a selected muscle and whilst there are several sites on the body that are suitable for IM injections, the most common areas used are:

- The deltoid muscle of the upper arm
- The vastus lateralis muscle which forms part of the quadriceps muscle group of the upper leg
- The gluteus medius (ventrogluteal site) muscle which runs beneath the gluteus maximus from the ilium to the femur.

IM injections are used for the delivery of certain drugs that (for various reasons) cannot be given via an oral, intravenous or subcutaneous route. The IM route enables a large amount (up to 5 ml) of drug to be introduced at one time, minimises tissue irritation and provides a faster route than subcutaneous/intradermal injections.

Skeletal muscle contraction and relaxation

The ability of skeletal muscle to contract is controlled by the body's nervous system and each muscle fibre is controlled by a motor neurone (nerve cell) which may stimulate a few muscle cells or several hundred depending on the particular muscle and the work it does (Marieb 2006). Skeletal muscle contracts in response to stimulation by an electrical signal (muscle action potential) delivered by the motor neurone which is found halfway along the muscle cell where it terminates at the neuromuscular junction. Here the muscle fibre membrane is specialised to form a motor end plate.

Although a muscle fibre normally has a single motor end plate, the densely branched motor neurone axons (see Figure 9.3) mean that one motor neurone axon can connect and control many muscle fibres. The motor neurone and the muscle fibres it controls are known as a motor unit.

When a nerve impulse reaches the axon terminals, the neurotransmitter that stimulates skeletal muscle acetylcholine (ACh) is released into the synaptic cleft, which is a small gap that separates the membrane of the nerve cell from the membrane of the muscle fibre (Shier *et al.* 2004). The synaptic cleft and motor end plate contain acetylcholinesterase (AChE) which breaks down molecules of ACh. The release of ACh results in changes to the sarcolemma that trigger the contraction of the muscle fibre.

Skeletal muscle fibres are stimulated by neurones that control the production of an action potential (electrical impulse) in the sarcolemma by:

- **The release of acetylcholine** – an action potential travels along a motor neurone until it reaches the synaptic terminal where vesicles contained within the synaptic terminal release acetycholine (ACh) into the synaptic cleft between the motor neurone and the motor end plate.
- **The binding of ACh at the motor end plate** – the ACh molecules diffuse across the synaptic cleft and bind to ACh receptors on the sarcolemma. This changes the permeability of the

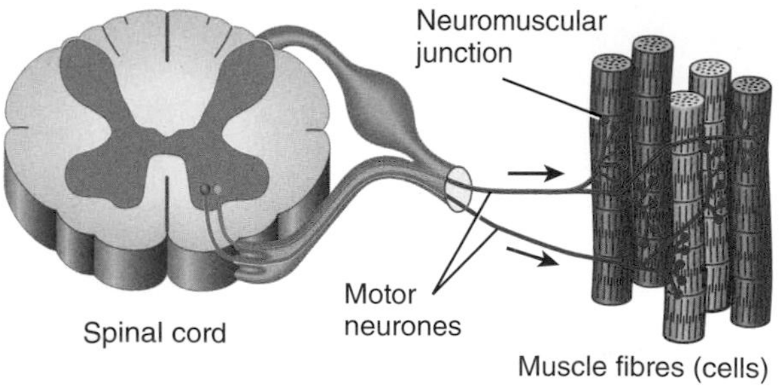
Neuromuscular
junction
Spinal cord
Motor
neurones
Muscle fibres (cells)

Figure 9.3 Motor unit (Tortora and Derrickson 2009)

membrane and allows sodium ions (Na^+) into the sarcoplasm which triggers the production of a muscle action potential in the sarcolemma.

- **The conduction of action potentials by the sarcolemma** – the action potential spreads across the entire surface of the sarcolemma and then travels down the transverse tubules to the cisternae which encircle the sarcomeres of the muscle fibre. As a result of the action potential travelling across it, the cisternae releases significant amounts of calcium ions (Ca^{2+}) which leads to the initiation of a muscle contraction. Each nerve impulse normally results in one muscle action potential and stages 2 and 3 are repeated if more ACh is released by another nerve impulse.
- **Muscle relaxation** – action potential generation ceases as ACh is broken down by **acetylcholinesterase (AchE)** and the concentration of calcium ions in the sarcoplasm declines. Once calcium ions return to normal resting levels, muscle contraction will end and muscle relaxation occurs.

Figure 9.4 provides a summary of the steps involved in skeletal muscle contraction and relaxation.

Clinical considerations

Pharmacology

Pyridostigmine is an anticholinesterase agent or AChE inhibitor and is used mainly to enhance neuromuscular transmission and improve muscle strength in voluntary and in voluntary muscles of patients with myasthenia gravis. AChE inhibitors inhibit AChE raising the concentration of ACh at the neuromuscular junction. In so doing they prolong the action of acetycholine by inhibiting the action of the enzyme acetylcholinesterase (British National Formulary 2010).

Cautions and contraindications

The drug should be used with caution in patients who have asthma, heart disease, epilepsy, parkinsonism, thyroid disease or stomach ulcer. AChE inhibitors should not be given to patients with intestinal or urinary obstruction.

Adverse effects

Adverse effects of pyridostigmine include nausea, vomiting, abdominal cramps, diarrhoea, excessive salivation, sweating, bradycardia and bronchospasm. Adverse effects of the drug may be minimised by precise dosage adjustment.

Energy sources for muscle contraction

Muscle fibres require an energy source to enable them to contract as and when needed. This is provided initially in the form of adenisotriphosphate (ATP) which is stored in the muscle fibre.

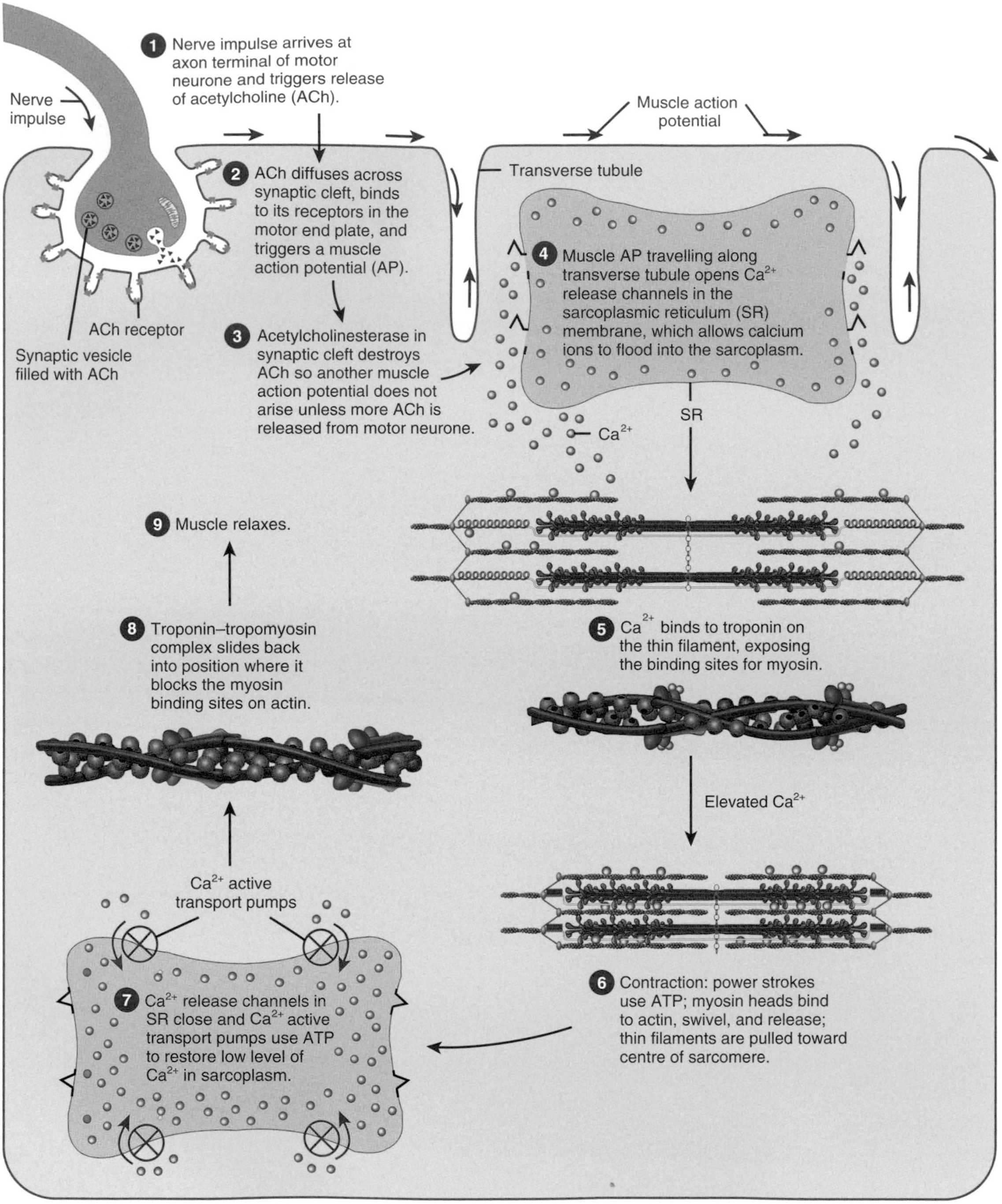

Nerve impulse
1 Nerve impulse arrives at axon terminal of motor neurone and triggers release of acetylcholine (ACh).
2 ACh diffuses across synaptic cleft, binds to its receptors in the motor end plate, and triggers a muscle action potential (AP).
3 Acetylcholinesterase in synaptic cleft destroys ACh so another muscle action potential does not arise unless more ACh is released from motor neurone.
ACh receptor
Synaptic vesicle filled with ACh
Muscle action potential
Transverse tubule
4 Muscle AP travelling along transverse tubule opens Ca^{2+} release channels in the sarcoplasmic reticulum (SR) membrane, which allows calcium ions to flood into the sarcoplasm.
SR
Ca^{2+}
5 Ca^{2+} binds to troponin on the thin filament, exposing the binding sites for myosin.
Elevated Ca^{2+}
6 Contraction: power strokes use ATP; myosin heads bind to actin, swivel, and release; thin filaments are pulled toward centre of sarcomere.
7 Ca^{2+} release channels in SR close and Ca^{2+} active transport pumps use ATP to restore low level of Ca^{2+} in sarcoplasm.
Ca^{2+} active transport pumps
8 Troponin–tropomyosin complex slides back into position where it blocks the myosin binding sites on actin.
9 Muscle relaxes.

Figure 9.4 Summary of muscle contraction and relaxation (Tortora and Derrickson 2009)

However, as only small amounts of ATP are stored in the muscle fibre, it is quickly depleted when the muscle is used and needs to be continuously available to power muscles. Therefore, working muscles require additional pathways to produce ATP and these include:

- **Creatine phosphate** (CP) broken down into creatine, phosphate and energy is the energy that is used to synthesise more ATP. Most of the creatine formed is used to resynthesise creatine phosphate and the creatine not used is converted to the waste product creatinine which is excreted by the kidneys.
- **Anaerobic respiration** Glycogen is the most abundant energy source found in muscle fibres and is broken down into glucose when it is needed to provide energy for muscle contraction. Glucose is initially broken down into pyruvic acid without the need for oxygen – a process known as glycolysis – and the small amounts of energy that are created by this process are captured by the bonds of ATP molecules.

During intensive muscle activity or when glucose and oxygen delivery is (temporarily) insufficient to meet the muscle requirements, the pyruvic acid generated during glycolysis converts to lactic acid. This pathway is much faster than that provided by aerobic respiration and can provide sufficient ATP for short spells of intensive exercise.

Aerobic respiration

Approximately 95% of the ATP used at rest and during moderate exercise comes from aerobic respiration involving a series of metabolic pathways that use oxygen – collectively known as oxidative phosphorylation (Marieb 2006). In order to release energy from glucose, oxygen is necessary and muscles receive this either from the haemoglobin in red blood cells or from myoglobin, a protein which stores some oxygen within the muscle cells. During aerobic respiration, glucose is broken down into carbon dioxide and water. The energy produced by the breakdown of these compounds is captured by the bonds of ATP molecules. Whilst a rich source of ATP is obtained this way, it is a slow process which requires a continuous oxygen and fuel supply to the muscles.

Figure 9.5 provides an overview of the different ATP sources available for muscles.

Oxygen debt

When the body is moderately active or at rest, the cardiovascular and respiratory systems of the body can usually supply sufficient oxygen to skeletal muscles to support the aerobic reactions of cellular respiration (Shier *et al.* 2004). However, when more strenuous activity is undertaken and a muscle relies on anaerobic respiration to supply its energy needs, it incurs an oxygen debt (Longenbaker 2008) which requires the body to dispose of lactic acid and replenish creatinine phosphate in order to repay the debt.

Muscle fatigue

Muscle fatigue occurs when a muscle fibre can no longer contract despite continued neural stimulation and occurs as a result of the oxygen debt which occurs during prolonged muscle activity.

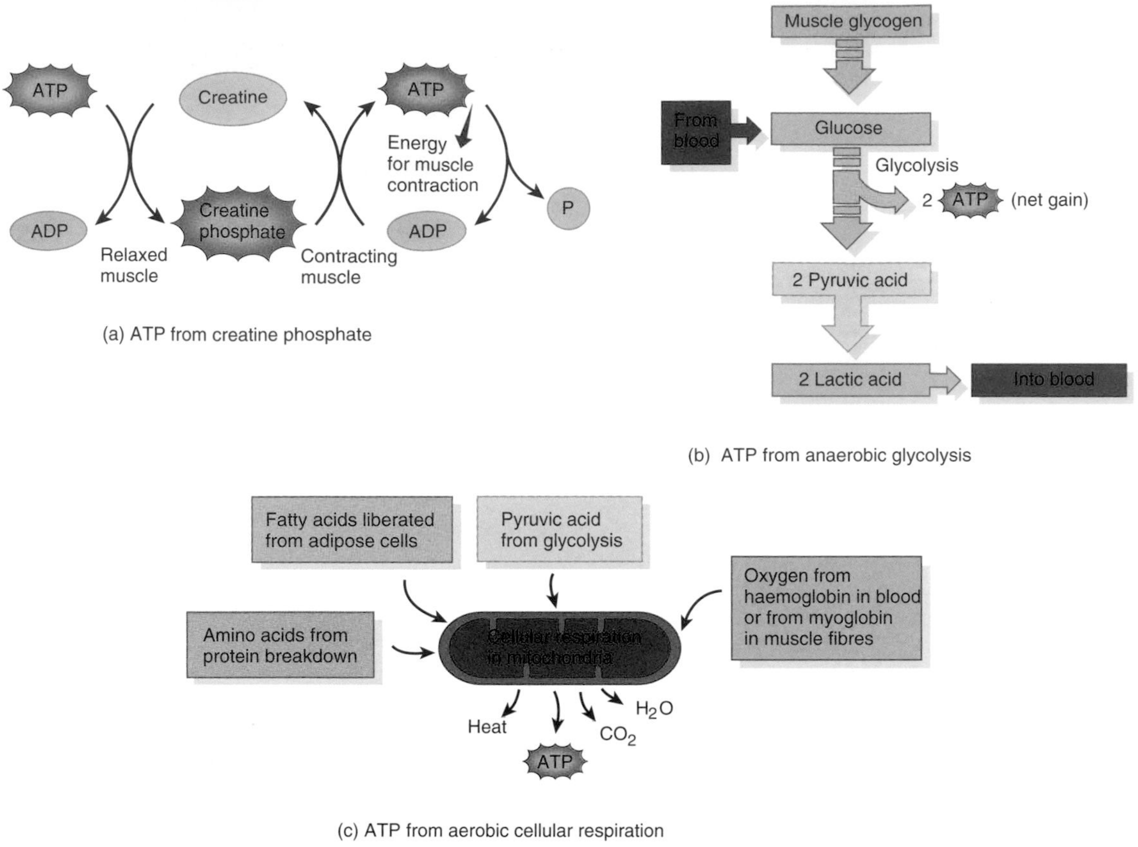
ATP
Creatine
ATP
Energy for muscle contraction
ADP
Creatine phosphate
ADP
P
Relaxed muscle
Contracting muscle
(a) ATP from creatine phosphate
Muscle glycogen
From blood
Glucose
Glycolysis
2 ATP (net gain)
2 Pyruvic acid
2 Lactic acid
Into blood
(b) ATP from anaerobic glycolysis
Fatty acids liberated from adipose cells
Pyruvic acid from glycolysis
Oxygen from haemoglobin in blood or from myoglobin in muscle fibres
Amino acids from protein breakdown
Cellular respiration in mitochondria
Heat
H_2O
CO_2
ATP
(c) ATP from aerobic cellular respiration

Figure 9.5 Sources of ATP for muscle energy (Tortora and Derrickson 2009)

Organisation of the skeletal muscular system

Every one of the body's skeletal muscles is attached at a minimum of two points to bone or other connective tissue. When one part of the skeleton is moved by muscle contraction, related parts have to be steadied by other muscles for the movement to be effective. The origin of a muscle is on the stationary bone where it begins, and the muscle ends at an insertion on the bone that moves (Longenbaker 2008).

Muscles can be named according to size, shape, location and number of origins, associated bones and the action of the muscle. Table 9.3 provides examples of the criteria used to name muscles.

The body's skeletal muscles can be divided into four areas:

- Head and neck muscles
- Muscles of the upper limbs (shoulder, arm, forearm)

Table 9.3 Muscle names

Character/Term	Definition	Example
DIRECTION		
Transverse	Across	Transversus abdominis
Oblique	Diagonal	External oblique
Rectus	Straight	Rectus abdominis
SHAPE		
Trapezius	Trapezoid	Trapezius
Deltoid	Triangular	Deltoid
Obicularis	Circular	Obicularis oculi
Rhomboid	Diamond-shaped	Rhomboideus
Platys	Flat	Platysma
SIZE		
Major	Larger	Pectoralis major
Minor	Smaller	Pectoralis minor
Maximus	Largest	Gluteus maximus
Minimus	Smallest	Gluteus minimus
Longus	Longest	Adductor longus
Latissimus	Widest	Latissimus dorsi
NUMBER OF ORIGINS		
Biceps	Two origins	Biceps brachii
Triceps	Three origins	Triceps brachii
Quadriceps	Four origins	Quadriceps femoris

- Trunk (thorax and abdomen)
- Muscles of the lower limbs (hip, pelvis/thigh, leg).

The major muscles of the body are listed according to body area in Tables 9.4–9.7 and illustrated in Figures 9.6–9.9.

Figures 9.10 and 9.11 provide an overview of the major muscles of the body.

Skeletal muscle movement

Skeletal muscle movement occurs as a result of more than one muscle moving and muscles invariable move in groups. As a general rule, when a muscle contracts at a joint, one bone remains fairly stationary and the other one moves. The origin of a muscle is on the stationary bone and the insertion of a muscle is on the bone that moves. The action of each muscle is dependent upon how the muscle is attached to either side of a joint and also the kind of joint it is associated with. When a muscle contracts it produces a specific action, however, muscles can only pull, they cannot push as when a muscle contracts, it becomes shorter. Usually there are at

Table 9.4 Muscles of the head and neck

Muscle	Origin	Insertion	Function
Frontalis	Skin and muscles around eye	Skin of eyebrow and bridge of nose	Wrinkles forehead Raises eyebrows
Occipitalis	Occipital bone	Galea aponeurotica (tendinous sheet)	Tenses and retracts scalp
Obicularis oculi	Maxillary and frontal bones	Skin around eye	Closes eye
Buccinator	Maxillary bone and mandible	Fibres of orbicularis oris	Compresses cheeks
Zygomaticus	Zygomatic bone	Obicularis oculi	Raises corner of mouth
Obicularis oris	Muscles near the mouth	Skin of central lip	Closes and protrudes lips
Masseter	Zygomatic arch/ mandible	Lateral surface of mandible	Closes jaw
Temporalis	Temporal bone		Closes jaw
Pterygoids (medial and lateral)	Sphenoid and maxillary bones	Medial and anterior surface of mandible	Elevates and depresses mandible Moves mandible from side to side
Platysma	Fascia in upper chest	Lower mandible	Draws mouth downward
Stylohyoid	Temporal bone	Hyoid bone	Depresses hyoid bone and larynx
Mylohyoid	Mandible	Hyoid bone	Depresses mandible Elevates floor of mouth
Sternocleidomastoid	Margins of sternum of clavicle	Mastoid region of skull	Flexes the neck Rotates head

Table 9.5 Muscles of the upper limbs (shoulder, arm and hand)

Muscle	Origin	Insertion	Function
Levator scapulae	Transverse processes of cervical vertebrae	Scapula	Elevates scapula
Trapezius	Occipital bone and cervical and thoracic vertebrae	Clavicle, spine and scapula	Help to extend the head Adduct the scapulae when shoulders are shrugged or pulled back
Rotator cuff muscles: Supraspinatus Infraspinatus Subscapularis Teres minor Teres major	Posterior surface above and below Scapula	Humerus	A group of muscles that are responsible for angular and rotational movements of the arm
Pectoralis major	Clavicle, sternum and upper ribs	Humerus	Flexes and adducts the arm
Muscles that move the forearm			
Biceps brachii	Between the scapula and forearm	Radius	Flexes and supinates the forearm
Triceps brachii	Between the scapula and forearm	Ulna	Extends the elbow/ forearm
Brachialis	Between humerus and ulna	Ulna	Flexes forearm
Muscles that move the hand and fingers			
Flexor and extensor carpi	Base of 2nd and 3rd metacarpal bones	Base of second and third metacarpals	Flexion, extension abduction and adduction at wrist
Flexor and extensor digitorum	Posterior and distal phalanges	Base and surface of phalanges in fingers 2–5	Flexion and extension at finger joints and wrist
Palmaris longus	Distal end of Humerus	Fascia of palm	Flexes the wrist

Table 9.6 Muscles of the trunk (thorax and abdomen)

Muscle	Origin	Insertion	Function
Internal intercostals	Superior border of each rib	Inferior border of preceding rib	Depress the rib cage and contract during forced expiration
External intercostals	Inferior border of each rib	Superior border of next rib	Elevate the ribs during inspiration
Diaphragm	Ribs 4–10, lumbar vertebrae	Tendon near to centre of diaphragm	Contracts to allow inhalation Relaxes to allow exhalation
Internal and external obliques	Between the lower ribs and pelvic girdle	Lower ribs, iliac crest and crest of pubis	Compress the abdominal cavity and protect and support the abdominal organs Rotation of the trunk
Transversus abdominis	Lower ribs, iliac crest and inguinal ligament	Extend horizontally across the abdomen from sternum to crest of pubis	Compress the abdominal cavity, protect and support the abdominal organs Rotation of the trunk
Rectus abdominis	Crest of pubic bone and symphysis pubis	Sternum and ribs	Compress the abdominal cavity, protect and support the abdominal organs Assists with flexing and rotating the lumbar spine

Table 9.7 Muscles of the lower limbs (hip, pelvis/thigh and leg)

Muscle	Origin	Insertion	Function
Psoas major	Lumbar vertebrae	Femur	Flexes thigh
Gluteus maximus	Sacrum, coccyx and surface of Ilium	Femur and fascia of thigh	Extends thigh at hip
Gluteus medius and minimus	Surface of Ilium	Femur	Abducts and rotates thigh
Adductor group	Pubic bone and Ischial tuberosity	Posterior surface of femur	Adducts, flexes, extends and rotates thigh
Quadriceps femoris group • Rectus femoris • Vastus lateralis • Vastus medialis • Vastus intermedius • Sartorius	Ilium, acetabulum and femur Ilium	Patella Tibia	Extends leg at knee Flexes, abducts and rotates thing to allow crossing of legs
Hamstring group • Biceps femoris • Semitendinosus • Semimembranosus	Femur, Ischial tuberosity, iliac spine	Tibia and head of fibula	Flexes and rotates leg, abducts, rotates and extends thigh
Posterior compartment • Gastocnnemius • Soleus • Tibialis posterior	Femur Fibula and tibia Tibia and fibula	Calcaneus (by means of the Achilles tendon) Calcaneus (by means of the Achilles tendon) 2nd, 3rd and 4th metatarsals	Flexes foot and leg at knee joint Flexes foot Flexes and inverts foot
Anterior compartment • Tibialis anterior • Extensor digitorum longus	Tibia Tibia and fibula	1st metatarsal Middle and distal phalanges of each toe	Dorsiflexes and inverts foot Dorsiflexes and everts foot, extends toes
Lateral compartment • Fibularis longus	Fibula and tibia	1st metatarsal	Flexes and everts foot

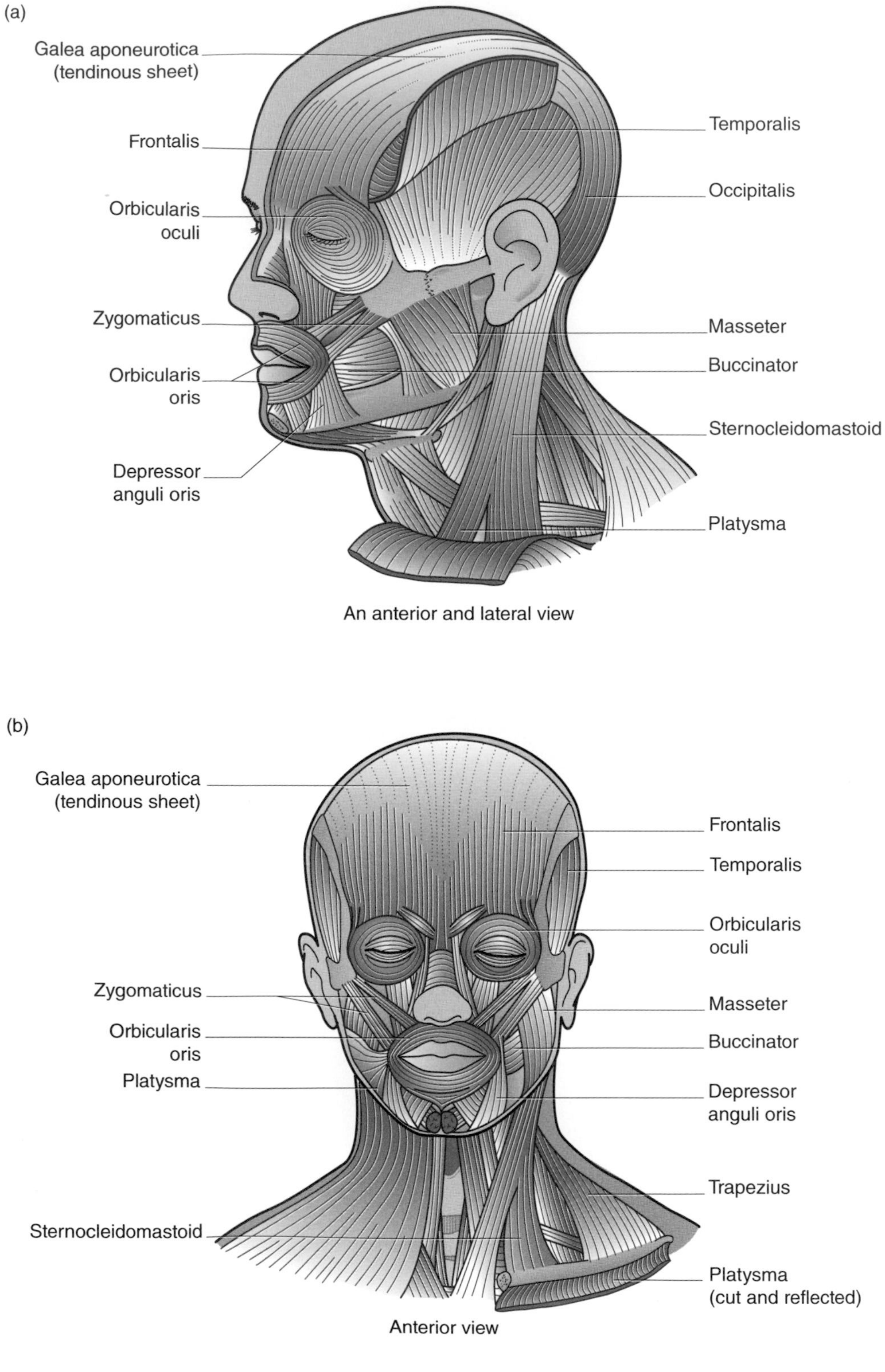
(a)
Galea aponeurotica
(tendinous sheet)
Frontalis
Orbicularis
oculi
Zygomaticus
Orbicularis
oris
Depressor
anguli oris
Temporalis
Occipitalis
Masseter
Buccinator
Sternocleidomastoid
Platysma
An anterior and lateral view
(b)
Galea aponeurotica
(tendinous sheet)
Zygomaticus
Orbicularis
oris
Platysma
Sternocleidomastoid
Frontalis
Temporalis
Orbicularis
oculi
Masseter
Buccinator
Depressor
anguli oris
Trapezius
Platysma
(cut and reflected)
Anterior view

Figure 9.6 Head and neck muscles

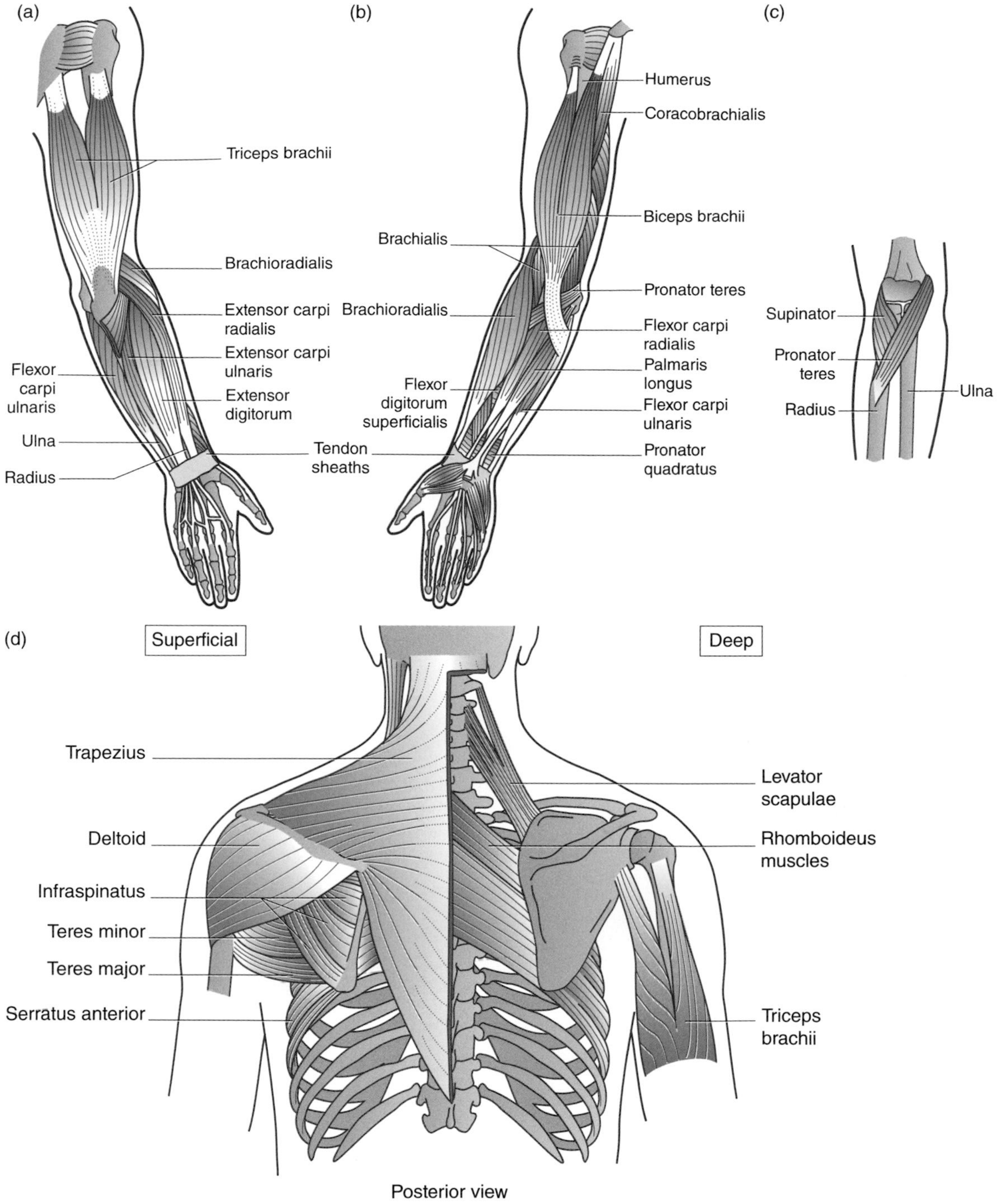
(a)
Triceps brachii
Brachioradialis
Extensor carpi radialis
Extensor carpi ulnaris
Flexor carpi ulnaris
Extensor digitorum
Ulna
Radius
Tendon sheaths
(b)
Humerus
Coracobrachialis
Biceps brachii
Brachialis
Pronator teres
Brachioradialis
Flexor carpi radialis
Palmaris longus
Flexor digitorum superficialis
Flexor carpi ulnaris
Pronator quadratus
(c)
Supinator
Pronator teres
Radius
Ulna
(d)
Superficial
Deep
Trapezius
Levator scapulae
Deltoid
Rhomboideus muscles
Infraspinatus
Teres minor
Teres major
Serratus anterior
Triceps brachii
Posterior view

Figure 9.7 Muscles of the upper limbs (shoulder, arm and hand)

(e)

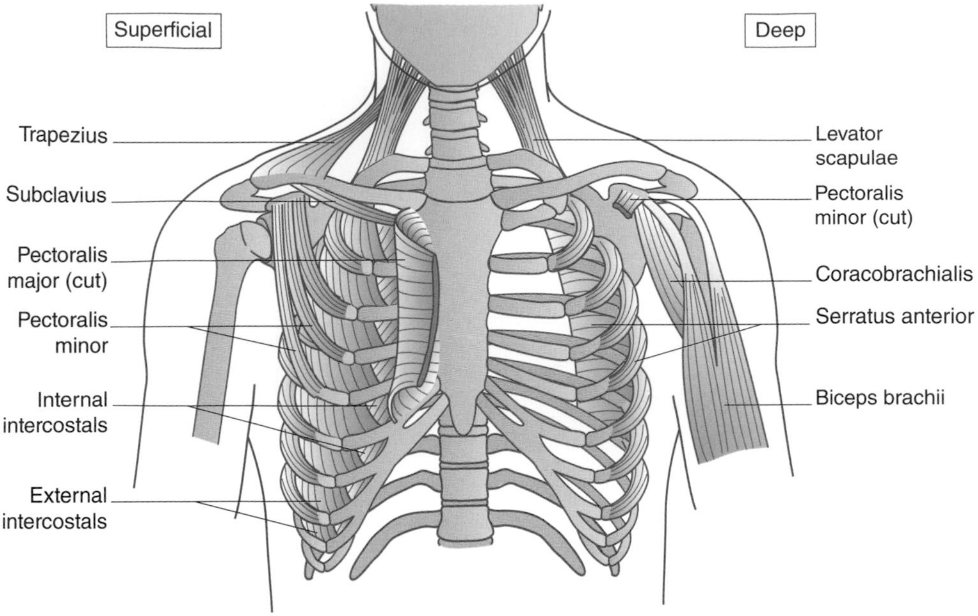
Superficial
Deep
Trapezius
Subclavius
Pectoralis major (cut)
Pectoralis minor
Internal intercostals
External intercostals
Levator scapulae
Pectoralis minor (cut)
Coracobrachialis
Serratus anterior
Biceps brachii

Anterior view

(f)

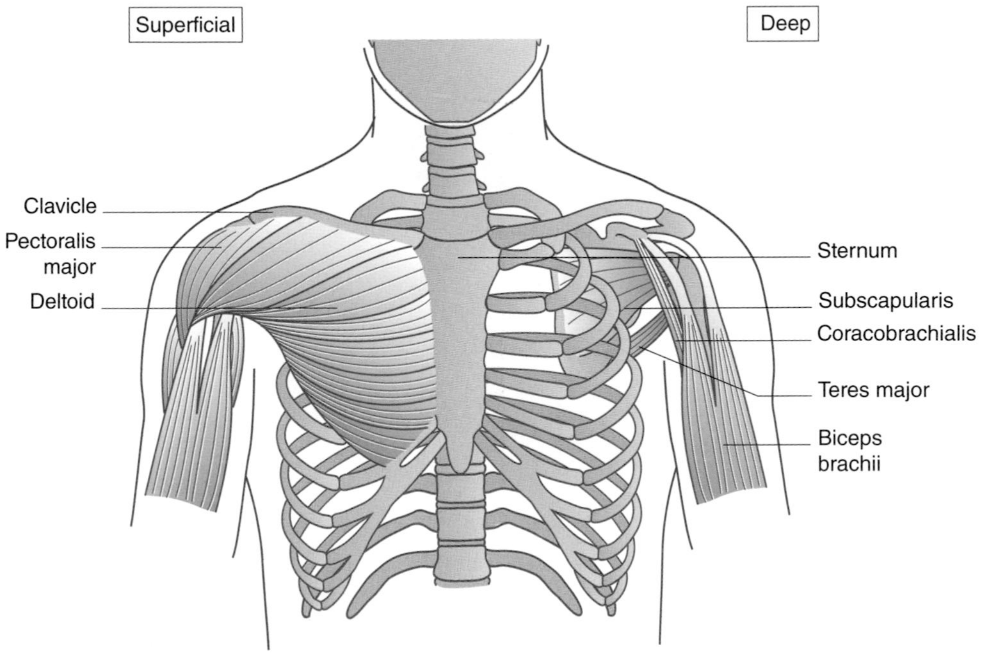
Superficial
Deep
Clavicle
Pectoralis major
Deltoid
Sternum
Subscapularis
Coracobrachialis
Teres major
Biceps brachii

Anterior view

Figure 9.7 *Continued*

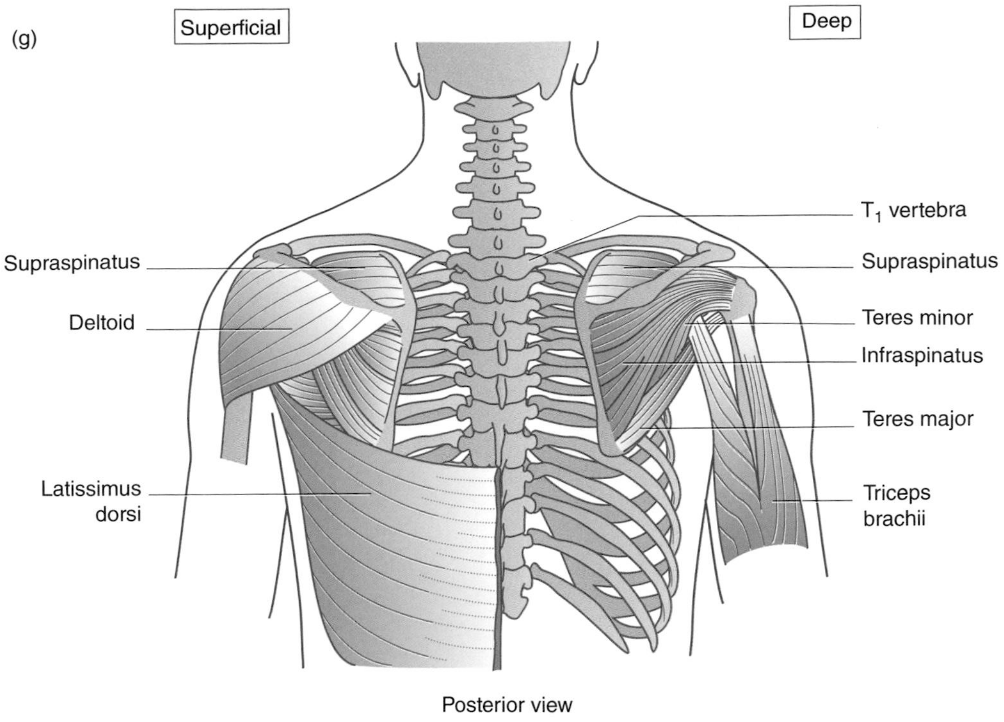
(g)
Superficial
Deep
T$_1$ vertebra
Supraspinatus
Supraspinatus
Deltoid
Teres minor
Infraspinatus
Teres major
Latissimus dorsi
Triceps brachii
Posterior view

Figure 9.7 *Continued*

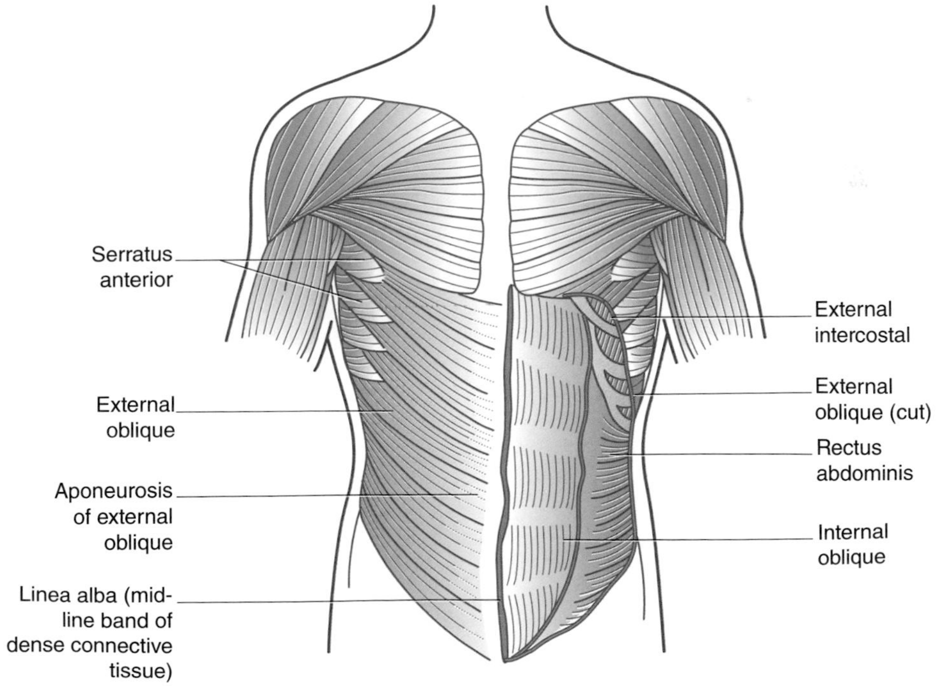
Serratus anterior
External oblique
Aponeurosis of external oblique
Linea alba (mid-line band of dense connective tissue)
External intercostal
External oblique (cut)
Rectus abdominis
Internal oblique

Figure 9.8 Trunk (thorax and abdomen)

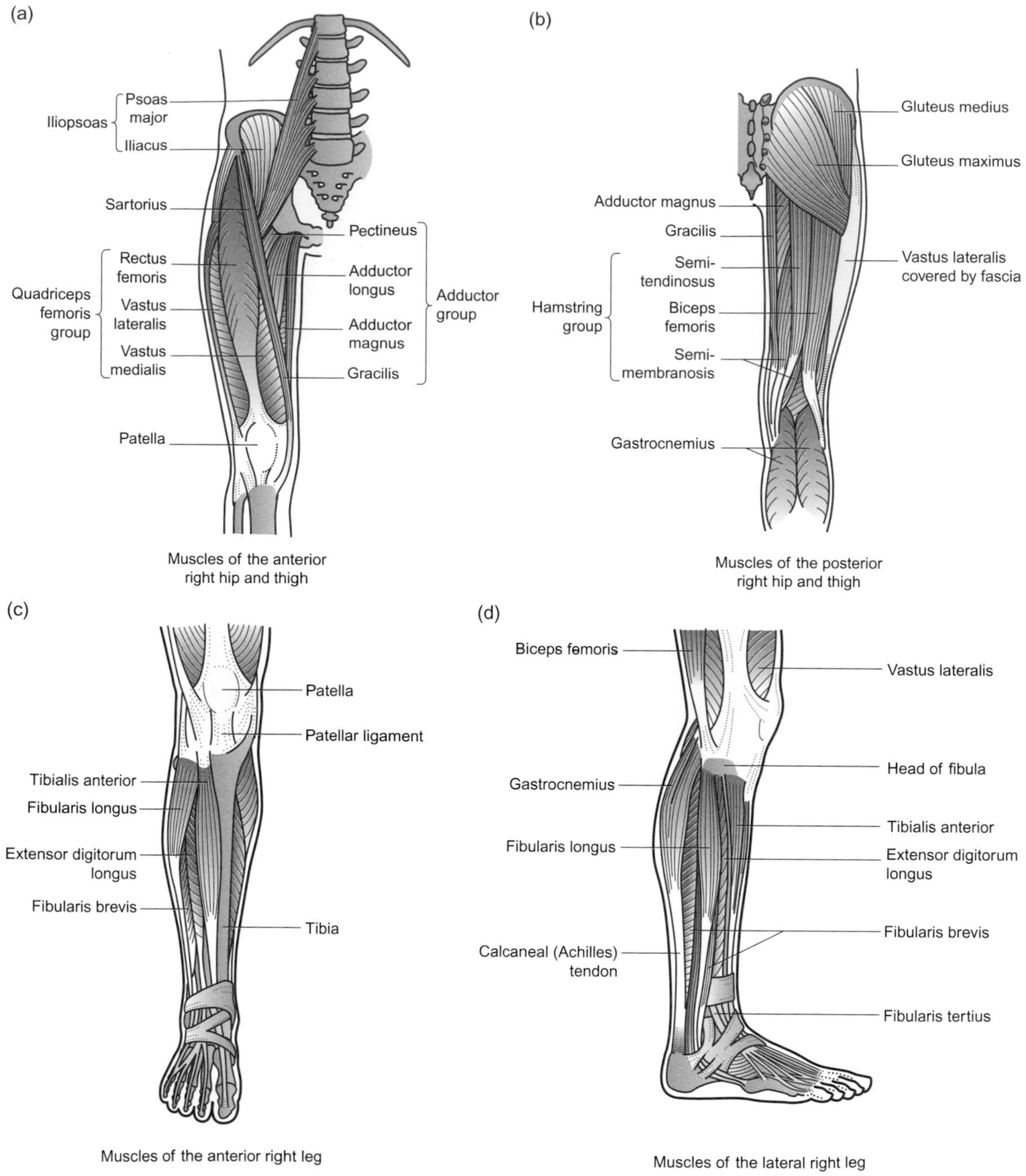
(a)
Iliopsoas
Psoas major
Iliacus
Sartorius
Quadriceps femoris group
Rectus femoris
Vastus lateralis
Vastus medialis
Patella
Pectineus
Adductor longus
Adductor magnus
Gracilis
Adductor group
Muscles of the anterior right hip and thigh
(b)
Gluteus medius
Gluteus maximus
Adductor magnus
Gracilis
Hamstring group
Semi-tendinosus
Biceps femoris
Semi-membranosis
Vastus lateralis covered by fascia
Gastrocnemius
Muscles of the posterior right hip and thigh
(c)
Patella
Patellar ligament
Tibialis anterior
Fibularis longus
Extensor digitorum longus
Fibularis brevis
Tibia
Muscles of the anterior right leg
(d)
Biceps femoris
Vastus lateralis
Head of fibula
Gastrocnemius
Tibialis anterior
Fibularis longus
Extensor digitorum longus
Fibularis brevis
Calcaneal (Achilles) tendon
Fibularis tertius
Muscles of the lateral right leg

Figure 9.9 Muscles of the lower limbs (hip, pelvis/thigh and leg)

(e)

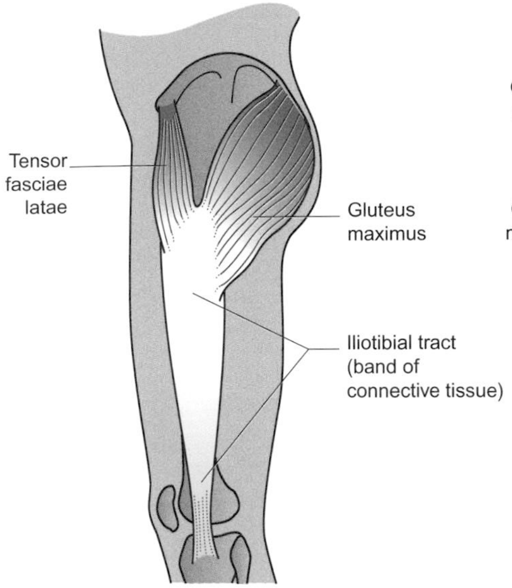
Tensor
fasciae
latae
Gluteus
maximus
Iliotibial tract
(band of
connective tissue)

Muscles that move the thigh

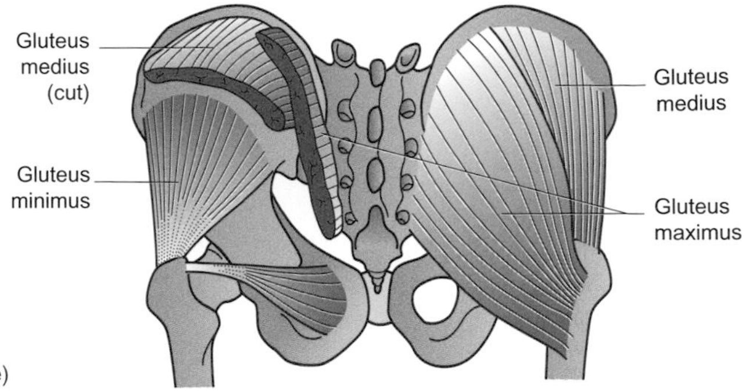
Gluteus
medius
(cut)
Gluteus
minimus
Gluteus
medius
Gluteus
maximus

The gluteal muscle group

(f)

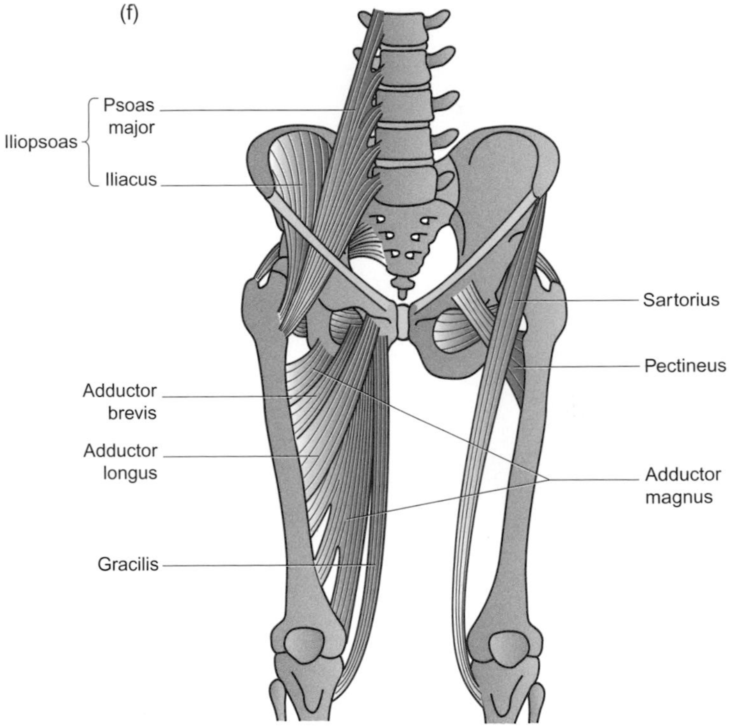
Iliopsoas
Psoas
major
Iliacus
Sartorius
Pectineus
Adductor
brevis
Adductor
longus
Adductor
magnus
Gracilis

The iliopsoas muscle and the adductor group

Figure 9.9 *Continued*

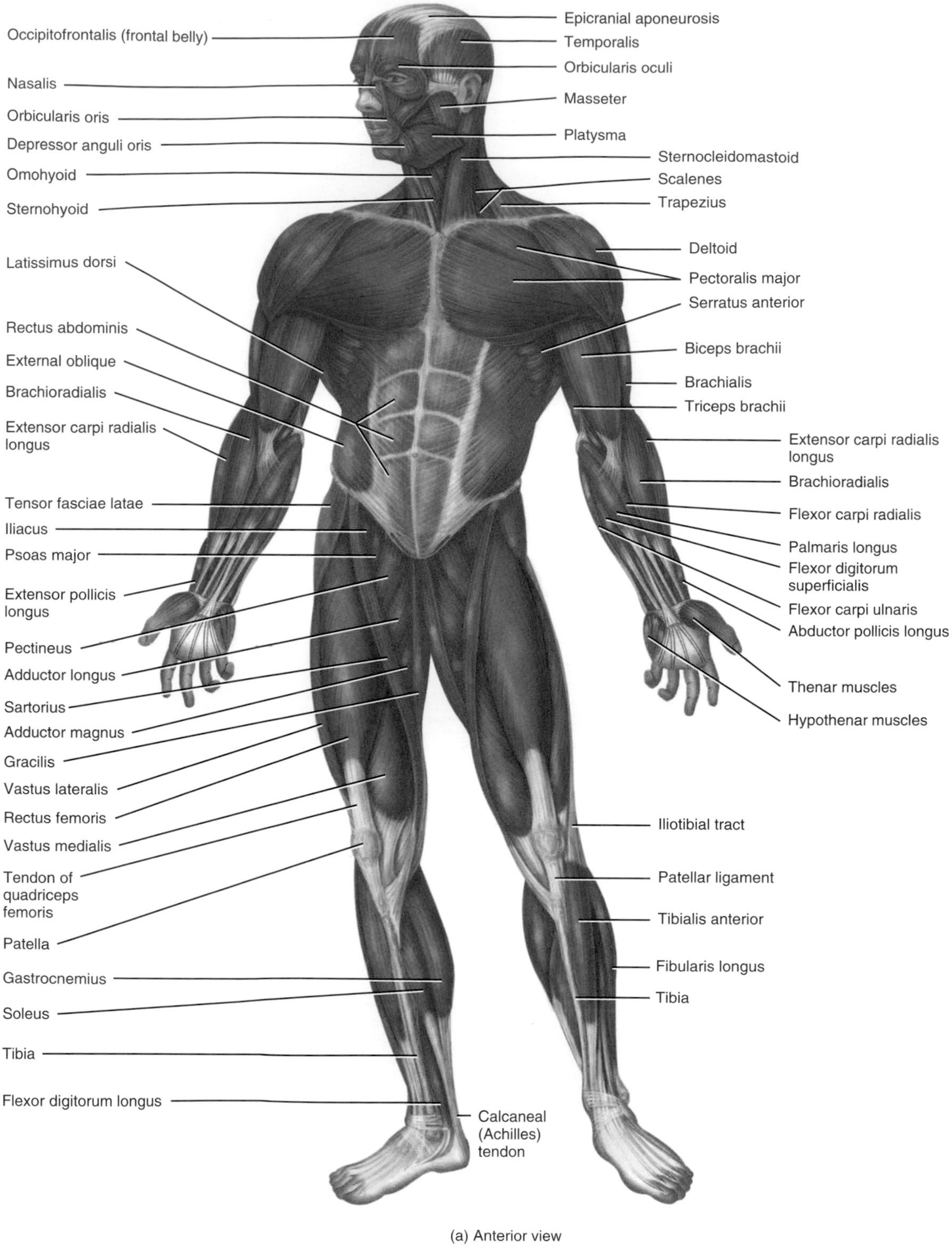
Epicranial aponeurosis
Occipitofrontalis (frontal belly)
Temporalis
Orbicularis oculi
Nasalis
Masseter
Orbicularis oris
Platysma
Depressor anguli oris
Sternocleidomastoid
Omohyoid
Scalenes
Sternohyoid
Trapezius
Deltoid
Latissimus dorsi
Pectoralis major
Serratus anterior
Rectus abdominis
Biceps brachii
External oblique
Brachialis
Brachioradialis
Triceps brachii
Extensor carpi radialis longus
Extensor carpi radialis longus
Brachioradialis
Tensor fasciae latae
Flexor carpi radialis
Iliacus
Palmaris longus
Psoas major
Flexor digitorum superficialis
Extensor pollicis longus
Flexor carpi ulnaris
Abductor pollicis longus
Pectineus
Adductor longus
Thenar muscles
Sartorius
Hypothenar muscles
Adductor magnus
Gracilis
Vastus lateralis
Rectus femoris
Iliotibial tract
Vastus medialis
Tendon of quadriceps femoris
Patellar ligament
Tibialis anterior
Patella
Fibularis longus
Gastrocnemius
Tibia
Soleus
Tibia
Flexor digitorum longus
Calcaneal (Achilles) tendon
(a) Anterior view

Figure 9.10 Anterior view of the major muscles of the body (Tortora and Derrickson 2009)

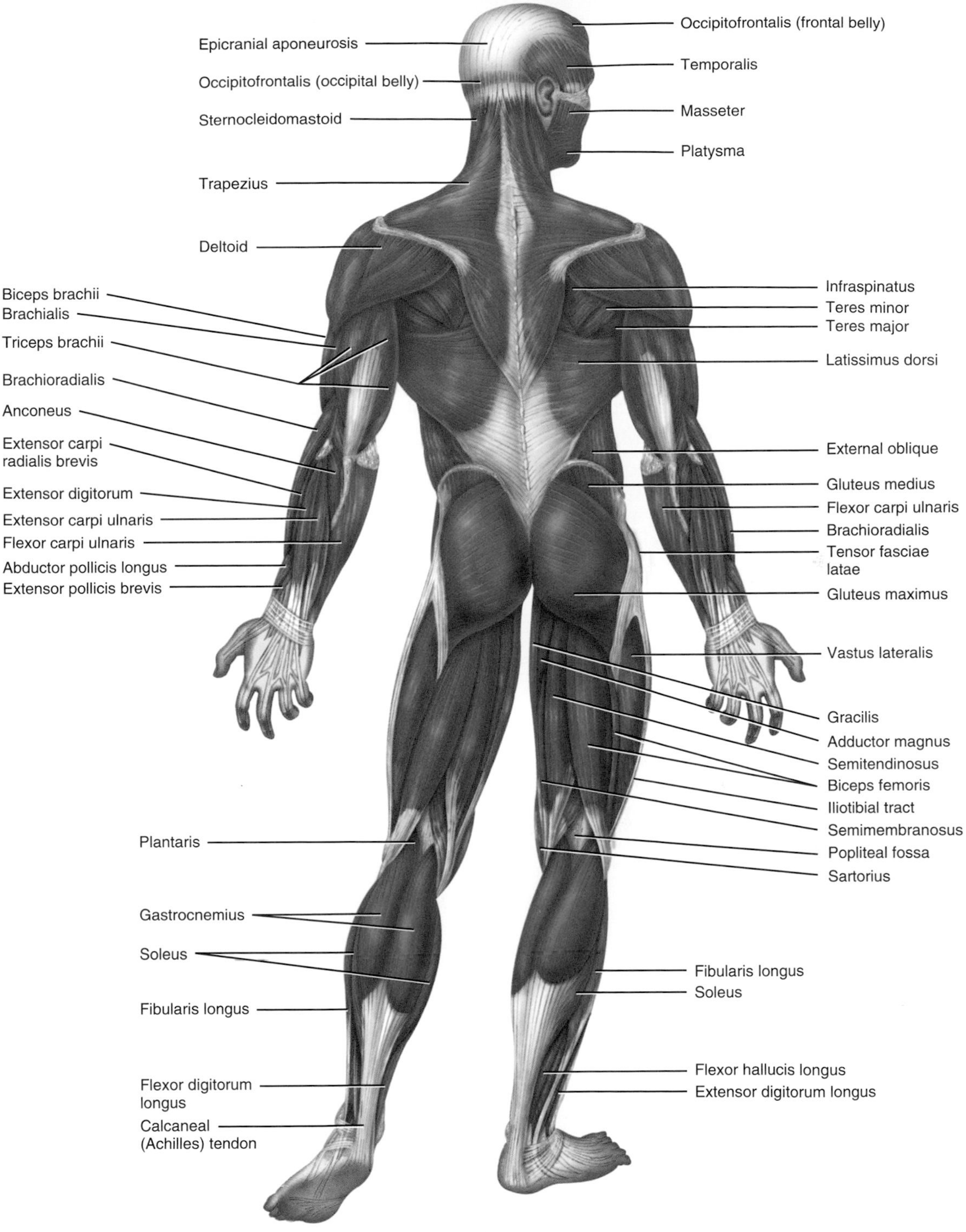
Epicranial aponeurosis
Occipitofrontalis (occipital belly)
Sternocleidomastoid
Trapezius
Deltoid
Biceps brachii
Brachialis
Triceps brachii
Brachioradialis
Anconeus
Extensor carpi radialis brevis
Extensor digitorum
Extensor carpi ulnaris
Flexor carpi ulnaris
Abductor pollicis longus
Extensor pollicis brevis
Plantaris
Gastrocnemius
Soleus
Fibularis longus
Flexor digitorum longus
Calcaneal (Achilles) tendon
Occipitofrontalis (frontal belly)
Temporalis
Masseter
Platysma
Infraspinatus
Teres minor
Teres major
Latissimus dorsi
External oblique
Gluteus medius
Flexor carpi ulnaris
Brachioradialis
Tensor fasciae latae
Gluteus maximus
Vastus lateralis
Gracilis
Adductor magnus
Semitendinosus
Biceps femoris
Iliotibial tract
Semimembranosus
Popliteal fossa
Sartorius
Fibularis longus
Soleus
Flexor hallucis longus
Extensor digitorum longus

(b) Posterior view

Figure 9.11 Posterior view of the major muscles of the body (Tortora and Derrickson 2009)

least two opposing muscles (agonist and antagonist) acting on a joint which bring about movement in opposite directions. An agonist or prime mover is a muscle primarily responsible for producing an action, whilst an antagonist of a prime mover causes muscle movement in the opposite direction, for example an agonist may cause an arm to bend whilst the antagonist will cause it to straighten.

Common types of body movements include:

- Extension – a movement that *increases* the angle or distance between two bones or parts of the body
- Hyperextension – an extension angle greater than 180°
- Flexion – the opposite of extension in that it is a movement that *decreases* the angle or distance between two bones and brings the bones closer together and is a common movement of hinge joints – for example bending the elbow or knee
- Abduction – moving a limb *away* from the midline of the body
- Adduction – (the opposite of abduction) the movement of a limb *towards* the midline of the body
- Rotation – a movement common to ball and socket joints and is the movement of a bone around its longitudinal axis.
- Circumduction – a combination of abduction adduction, extension and flexion.

Table 9.8 provides a summary of the different actions of muscle movement.

Table 9.8 Types of muscle movement

Action	Definition
Extension	Increases the angle or distance between two bones or parts of the body
Flexion	Decreases the angle of a joint
Abduction	Moves away from the midline
Adduction	Moves closer to the midline
Circumduction	A combination of flexion, extension, abduction and adduction
Supination	Turns the palm up
Pronation	Turns the palm down
Plantar flexion	Lowers the foot (point the toes)
Dorsiflexion	Elevates the foot
Rotation	Moves a bone around its longitudinal axis

The effects of ageing

Generally, the size and power of all muscle tissues within the body decrease as the body ages. This can be attributed to:

- Loss of elasticity to skeletal muscle – as muscles age they lose their elasticity due to a process called fibrosis (Martini and Bartholomew 2003). Fibrosis causes ageing muscles to develop increasing amounts of fibrous connective tissue which results in a loss of flexibility, movement and circulation
- Decrease in size of muscle fibres – as the muscle ages, the number of myofibrils decreases and results in a loss of muscle strength and an increased tendency for the muscle to fatigue more quickly. This tendency for rapid fatigue also means that with age, there is a lower tolerance for exercise
- Age-related reduction in cardiovascular performance – means that blood flow to muscles does not increase with exercise and the ability to recover from muscular injuries decreases and is likely to result in scar tissue formation.

Clinical considerations

Muscular dystrophy

Muscular dystrophy is a broad term applied to an inherited group of disorders that destroy the muscles by causing muscle fibres to degenerate, shrink in size and eventually die. The muscle fibres that die are replaced with fat and connective tissue.

The most common form of the disease is Duchenne's muscular dystrophy which is inherited via a flawed gene carried by the mother and results in a lack of protein called dystrophin which plays a part in the structure and function of muscle fibres. The lack of dystrophin causes calcium to leak into muscle fibres and activate an enzyme that causes the muscle fibre to dissolve.

The condition occurs predominately in males and manifests itself between the ages of 2 and 6 years. The disease is progressive and most sufferers are wheelchair bound by the age of 12 years and do not live beyond young adulthood (Marieb 2006). Whilst treatment in the form of injections of immature muscle cells that produce dystophin provides some relief (Longenbaker 2008), there is no known cure.

Conclusion

Muscular tissue is either smooth, cardiac or skeletal and is a specialised tissue that is structured to contract. In so doing, it causes movement of bones at a joint or in soft tissues. Through its ability to sustain partial contraction of muscle, the muscular system also play an important role in maintaining body posture for a long period of time. Skeletal muscle also plays an important role in heat production and is able to adjust heat production in extremes of environmental temperatures.

Glossary

Acetylcholine (ACh):	Neurotransmitter responsible for the transmission of a nerve impulse across a synaptic cleft.
Acetylcholinesterase (AChE):	Enzyme that breaks down acetylcholine.
Actin:	One of the two major proteins of muscle that makes up the myofibrils of muscle cells.
Adenosinetriphosphate (ATP):	Molecule used by cells when energy is needed.
Aerobic:	With oxygen.
Anaerobic:	Without oxygen.
Antagonist:	Muscle that acts in opposition to a prime mover.
Anterior:	Pertaining to the front.
Aponeurosis:	Membranous sheet connecting a muscle and the part it moves.
Glycogen:	A polysaccharide that stores energy for muscle contraction.
Ligament:	Strong connective tissue that connects bone.
Myofibril:	A bundle of myofilaments that contracts
Myasthenia gravis:	Muscle weakness due to an inability to respond to the neurotransmitter acetycholine.
Myofibril:	Portion of a muscle fibre that contracts.
Myoglobin:	A red pigment that stores oxygen for muscle contraction.
Posterior:	Pertaining to the back.
Sarcolemma:	Plasma membrane of a muscle fibre that forms T tubules.
Sarcoplasm:	Cytoplasm of a muscle fibre that contains organelles, including myofibrils.
Tendon:	Tissue that connects muscle to bone.
T tubule:	Extension of the sarcolemma that extends into the muscle fibre.

References

British National Formulary (2010) http://www.medicinescomplete.com/mc/bnf

Longenbaker, S.N. (2008) *Mader's Understanding Human Anatomy and Physiology*, 6th edn. Maidenhead: McGraw-Hill.

Marieb, E.N. (2006) *Essentials of Human Anatomy and Physiology*, 8th edn. London: Pearson Benjamin Cummings.
Martini, F.H. and Bartholomew, E.F. (2003) *Essentials of Anatomy and Physiology*, 3rd edn. Upper Saddle River, NJ: Pearson Education.
Shier, D., Butler, J. and Lewis, R. (2004) *Hole's Human Anatomy and Physiology*, 10th edn. Maidenhead: McGraw-Hill.
Tortora, G.J. and Derrickson, B.H. (2009) *Principles of Anatomy and Physiology*, 11th edn. Hoboken, NJ: John Wiley & Sons.
Tortora, G.J. and Derrickson, B.H. (2010) *Essentials of Anatomy and Physiology*, 8th edn. Chichester: John Wiley & Sons.

Activities

www.wiley.com/go/peate

Multiple choice questions

1. How much of the average adult human body is made up of skeletal muscle?
   (a) 40–50%
   (b) 10%
   (c) 30%
   (d) 70%

2. In an isotonic muscle contraction:
   (a) Movement of bones does not occur
   (b) Both muscle tension and length are changed
   (c) The length of the muscle remains constant
   (d) The muscle tension remains constant

3. The innermost layer of connective tissue surrounding a skeletal muscle is:
   (a) hypodermis
   (b) perimysium
   (c) endomysium
   (d) epimysium

4. Which of the following statement is **NOT** true of skeletal muscle?
   (a) is under voluntary control
   (b) is not striated
   (c) can have long muscle fibres
   (d) is usually attached to the skeleton

5. The energy for muscle contraction is most *directly* obtained from:

   (a) aerobic respiration
   (b) phosphocreatinine
   (c) anaerobic respiration
   (d) ATP

6. Extension of a muscle:

   (a) decreases the angle
   (b) increases the angle
   (c) renal column
   (d) renal corpuscle

7. The movable attachment of muscle to bone is referred to as the:

   (a) joint
   (b) origin
   (c) rotator
   (d) insertion

8. Skeletal muscles move the body by:

   (a) means of neural stimulation
   (b) pulling on the bones of the skeleton
   (c) using the energy of ATP to form ADP
   (d) activation of enzyme pathways

9. If additional ATP is required, which of the following can be used as an alternative energy source?

   (a) myosin
   (b) troponin
   (c) creatine phosphate
   (d) myoglobin

10. Relaxing and contracting the masseter muscle would mean that you were:

   (a) blinking
   (b) running
   (c) chewing
   (d) bending downwards

True or false

1. The skeletal muscles are under involuntary control.
2. Each muscle begins at an origin and ends at an insertion.
3. Anaerobic respiration provides 95% of the ATP required by a muscle cell.
4. Skeletal muscle appears non-striated when looked at under the microscope.
5. The number of myofibrils in a muscle cell decreases with age.

Label the diagram

From the list of words, label the diagrams below:

Muscle glycogen, From blood, Glucose, Glycolysis, 2 ATP (net gain), 2 Pyruvic acid, 2 Lactic acid, Into blood

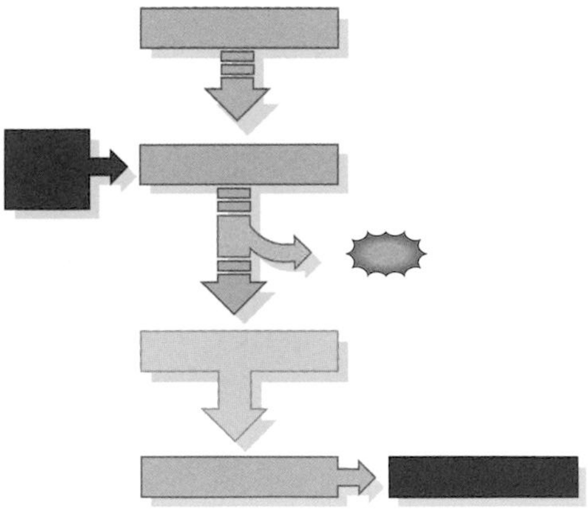

Serratus anterior, External oblique, Aponeurosis of external oblique, Linea alba (midline band of dense connective tissue), External intercostal, External oblique (cut), Rectus abdominis, Internal obique

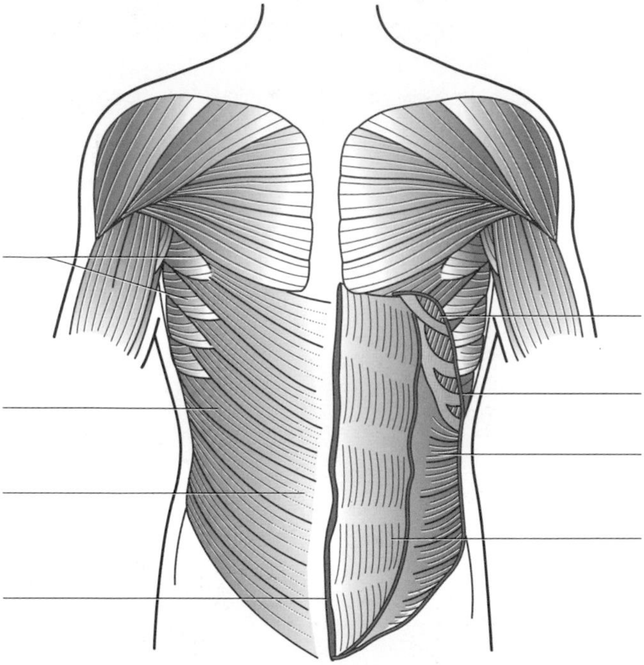

Crossword

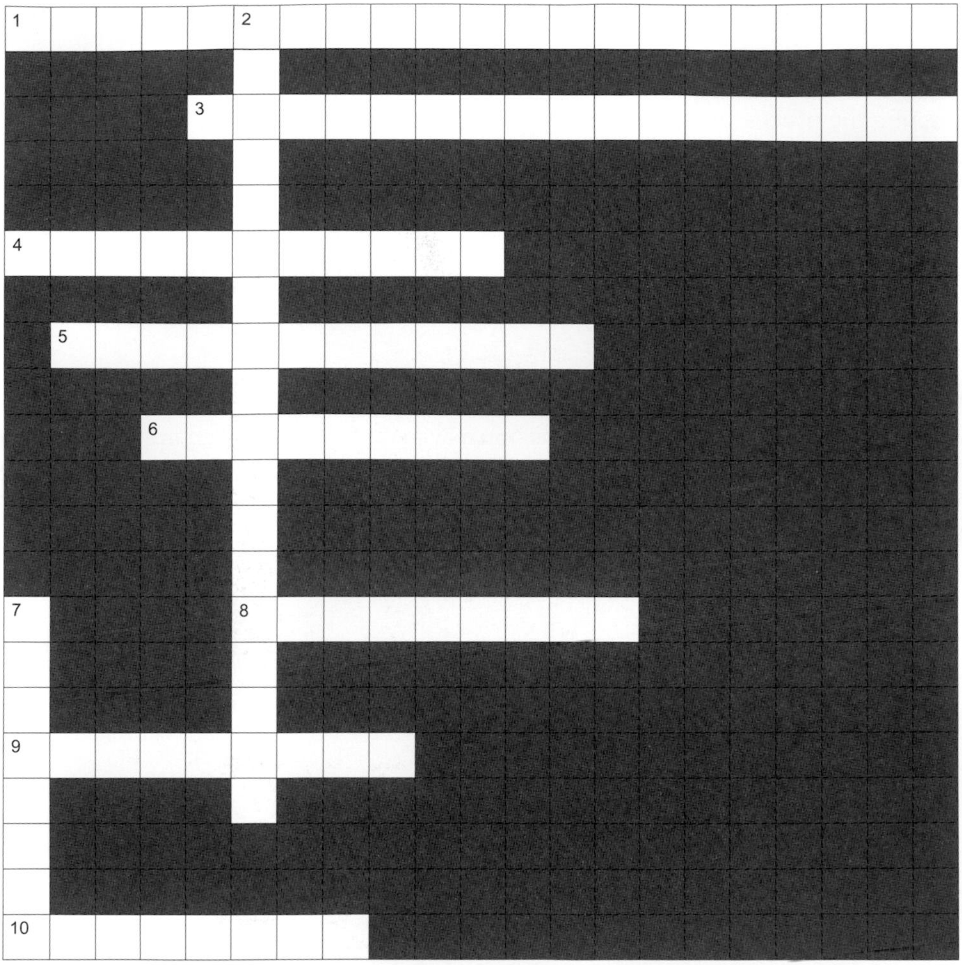
1
2
3
4
5
6
7
8
9
10

Across:

1. Produce the striations in skeletal muscle (5, 3, 4, 9).
3. Network of tubes that stores calcium (10, 7).
4. Glucose is converted to this during anaerobic respiration (7, 4).
5. One of the functions of the muscular system (8, 4).
6. The ________ of a muscle is on the bone that moves (9).
8. Movement away from the midline (9).
9. Reddish-brown pigment that stores oxygen (9).
10. Ageing results in this in muscle strength (8).

Down:

2. Provides 95% of the ATP required for moderate exercise (7, 11).
7. Diamond-shaped muscle (8).

Find out more

1. Name and describe the three forms of human muscle tissue and list where they are found in the body.
2. Outline how ATP is supplied to muscles.
3. Describe the processes that enable a muscle to contract.
4. Explain how ageing affects skeletal muscle.
5. Describe a neuromuscular junction.
6. Why does skeletal muscle appear striated when looked at under the microscope?

Conditions

Below is a list of conditions that are associated with the muscular system. Take some time and write notes about each of the conditions. You may make the notes taken from text books or other resources, for example, people you work with in a clinical area, or you may make the notes as a result of people you have cared for. If you are making notes about people you have cared for you must ensure that you adhere to the rules of confidentiality.

Muscular dystrophy	
Myasthesia gravis	
Fibromyalgia	
Tetanus	
Rigor mortis	
Muscle cramps	
Poliomyelitis	
Rhabdomyosis	
Sarcoma	
Fibrosis	
Botulism	

Answers

MCQs

1a; 2d; 3c; 4b; 5a; 6b; 7d; 8b; 9; d; 10c

True/false

1F; 2T; 3F; 4F; 5T

Crossword

Across:

1. Thick and thin filaments

3. Transverse tubules

4. Pyruvic acid

5. Generate heat

6. Insertion

8. Abduction

9. Myoglobin

10. Decrease

Down:

2. Aerobic respiration

7. Rhomboid

10

The cardiac system

Carl Clare

Contents

Introduction *296*

Size and location of the heart **296**

The structures of the heart **297**
Heart wall 297
The heart chambers 299

The blood supply to the heart **302**

Blood flow through the heart **304**

The electrical pathways of the heart **306**

The cardiac cycle **309**

Factors affecting cardiac output **312**

Regulation of stroke volume **313**
Preload 313
Force of contraction 313
Afterload 314

Regulation of heart rate **314**
Autonomic nervous system activity 314
Baroreceptors and the cardiovascular centre 315
Hormone activity 315

Conclusion *315*
Glossary *317*
References *321*
Activities *321*

Test your knowledge

- Name the chambers of the heart.
- Describe blood flow through the heart.
- Name one of the valves in the heart.
- Describe the position of the heart in the body.

Fundamentals of Anatomy and Physiology for Student Nurses, First Edition. Edited by Ian Peate, Muralitharan Nair.

Learning outcomes

On completion of this chapter the reader will be able to:

- Describe the structure of the heart
- List the arteries that supply blood to the heart muscle
- Describe the electrical excitation of the heart
- Describe the cardiac action potential
- Discuss the cardiac cycle

Body map

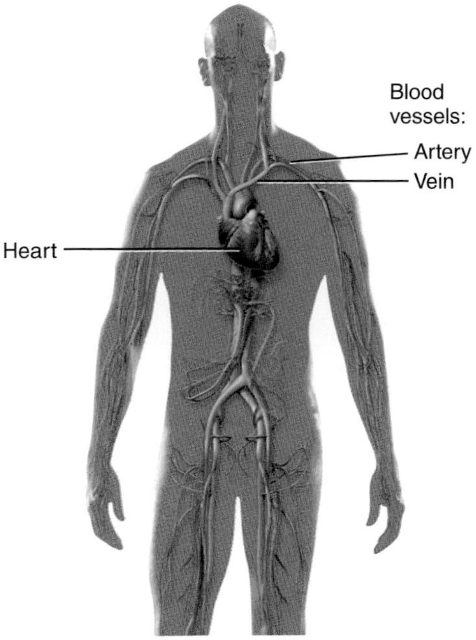
Blood vessels:
Artery
Vein
Heart

Introduction

The heart is a muscular organ containing four chambers. Its main function is to pump blood around the circulatory system of the lungs and the systemic circulation of the rest of the body. In the average day the heart beats about 100,000 times and never rests. It must continue its cycle of contraction and relaxation in order to provide a continuous blood supply to the tissues and ensure the delivery of nutrients and oxygen and the removal of waste products. The purpose of this chapter is to review the structure and function of the heart including:

- The size and location of the heart
- The overall structure of the heart
- The heart muscle and the cells of the heart
- The blood supply to the heart muscle
- The flow of blood through the heart
- The electrical pathways of the heart
- The cardiac cycle
- Factors affecting cardiac output.

Size and location of the heart

The heart weighs 250–390 g in men and 200–275 g in women (Marieb and Hoehn 2007) and is a little larger than the owner's closed fist, being approximately 12 cm long and 9 cm wide. It is located in the thoracic cavity (chest) in the mediastinum (between the lungs), behind and to the left of the sternum (breast bone) (see Figure 10.1).

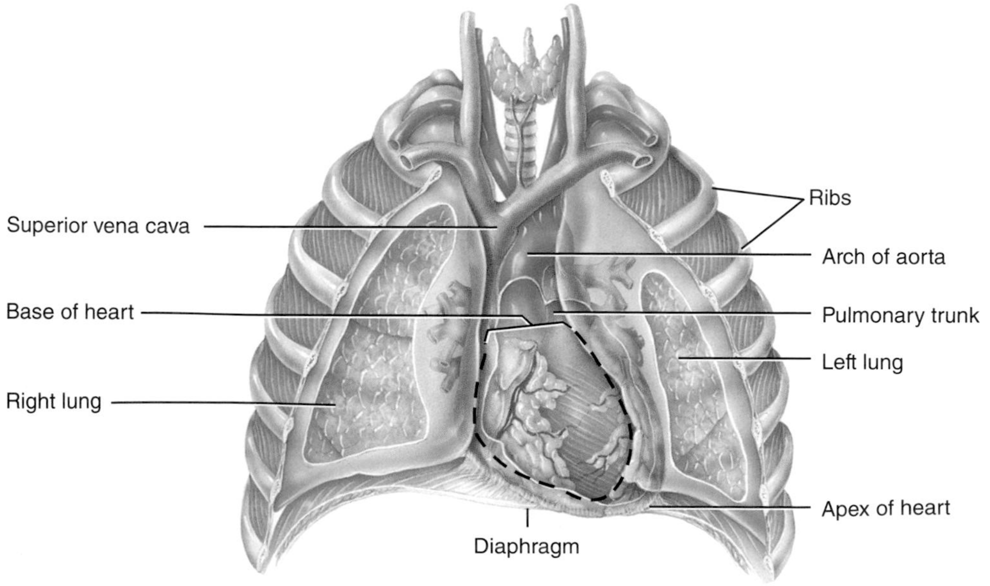
Superior vena cava
Base of heart
Right lung
Ribs
Arch of aorta
Pulmonary trunk
Left lung
Apex of heart
Diaphragm

Figure 10.1 Location of the heart (Tortora and Derrickson 2009)

As can be seen the apex of the heart (the pointed end) is below the base of the heart and lies on the diaphragm. The base of the heart is itself made up of two of the chambers of the heart known as the atria.

The structures of the heart

Heart wall

Pericardium

The heart is surrounded by a membrane called the pericardium (peri = around). This is often referred to as a single sac surrounding the heart but is in fact made up of two sacs (the fibrous pericardium and the serous pericardium) which are closely connected to each other (see Figure 10.2). These two sacs have very different structures (Jenkins *et al.* 2007):

- The fibrous pericardium, a tough, inelastic layer made up of dense, irregular, connective tissue. The role of this layer is to prevent the overstretching of the heart. It also provides protection to the heart and anchors it in place.
- The serous pericardium, a thinner, more delicate, layer that forms a double layer around the heart.
  - The parietal pericardium, the outer layer fused to the fibrous pericardium.
  - The visceral pericardium (otherwise known as the epicardium) adheres tightly to the surface of the heart.

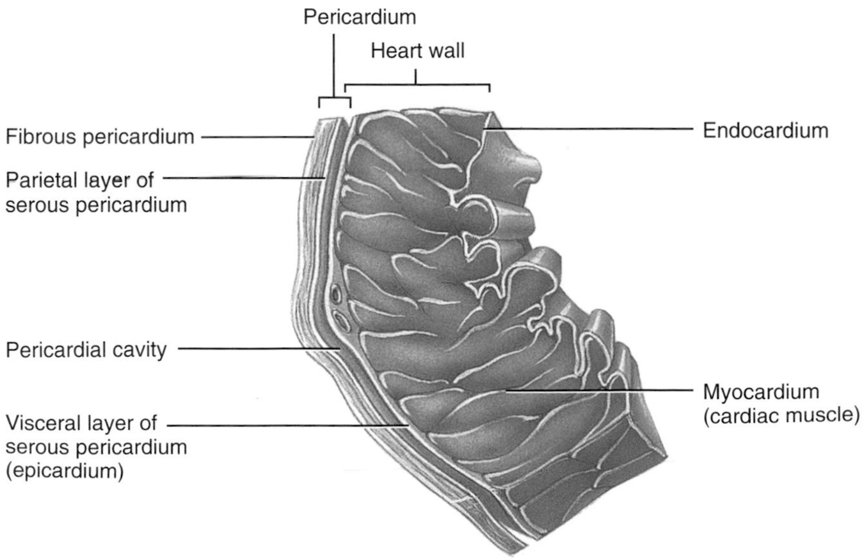
Pericardium
Heart wall
Fibrous pericardium
Parietal layer of serous pericardium
Pericardial cavity
Visceral layer of serous pericardium (epicardium)
Endocardium
Myocardium (cardiac muscle)

Figure 10.2 Heart wall (Tortora and Derrickson 2009)

Between the parietal and visceral pericardium is a thin film of fluid (pericardial fluid) which reduces the friction between the membranes as the heart moves during its cycle of contraction and relaxation. The space containing the pericardial fluid is known as the pericardial cavity, however it must be noted that this 'space' is so small it is normally considered to be a 'virtual' space.

Myocardium

Underlying the pericardium is the heart muscle known as the myocardium (myo = muscle). The myocardium makes up the majority of the bulk of the heart. It is a type of muscle only found within the heart and is specialised in its structure and function. The myocardium can be divided into two categories, the majority are specialised to perform mechanical work (contraction); the remainder are specialised to the task of initiating and conducting electrical impulses (this second type of cardiac muscle cell will be reviewed later in the chapter). The cardiac muscle cells (myocytes) are held together in interlacing bundles of fibres that are arranged in a spiral or circular bundles. Compared with skeletal muscle fibres, cardiac muscle fibres are shorter in length and have branches (see Figure 10.3). The ends of the cardiac myocytes are attached to the adjacent cells in an end-to-end fashion. At this point there is a thickening of the sarcolemma (plasma membrane) known as intercalated discs. These discs contain two types of junction:

- Desmosomes hold the cells together so that the fibres do not pull apart
- Gap junctions allow the rapid passage of action potentials (electrical current) between cells.

Compared to skeletal muscle cells the cardiac myocyte contains one (occasionally two) nuclei and the mitochondria are larger, and more numerous, making cardiac muscle cells less prone to fatigue. However, cardiac muscle requires a large supply of oxygen and is less able to cope with reductions in the amount of available oxygen.

The cardiac muscle cells are divided into two, discrete networks separated by a fibrous layer, the atria and the ventricles, and these two networks contract as separate units. Thus the atria

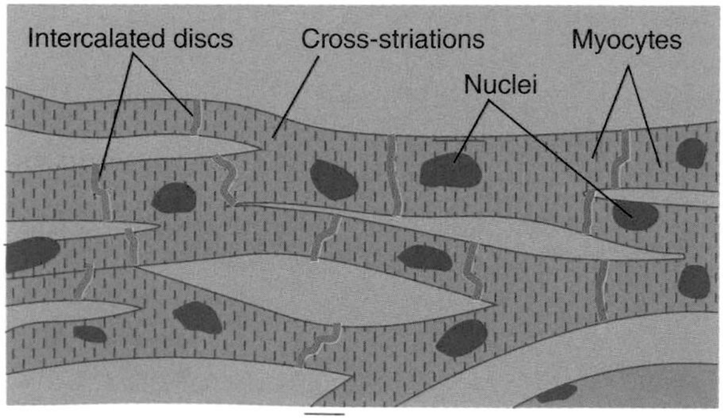
Intercalated discs
Cross-striations
Myocytes
Nuclei

Figure 10.3 Cardiac muscle cells (cardiac myocytes)

contract separately from the ventricles (see later). Within each myocyte are long contractile bundles of myofibrils. Myofibrils are in turn made up of smaller units known as sarcomeres. Contraction of the cardiac muscle is by the shortening of its sarcomeres.

The cardiac action potential

Unlike the normal skeletal muscle, in response to a single action potential a cardiac muscle fibre develops a prolonged contraction which is approximately 10–15 times longer in duration than a skeletal muscle contraction due to a plateau phase. Cardiac muscle fibres also have a longer refractory period and thus a new contraction cannot be initiated until muscle relaxation is well advanced. Thus a maintained contraction (tetany) cannot occur in cardiac muscle (Figure 10.4).

Endocardium

The endocardium (endo = within) is a layer of smooth simple epithelium lining the inside of the heart muscle (see Figure 10.2) and the heart valves. It is connected seamlessly with the lining of the large blood vessels that are connected to the heart.

The heart chambers

The heart is divided into four chambers (see Figure 10.5): the atria (entry halls or chambers) and the ventricles (little bellies). Even though the heart is referred to as a pump it is better to think of it as two pumps:

- The right heart pump receives deoxygenated blood (blood that has given up some of its oxygen to the cells) from the tissues and pumps it out into the pulmonary circulation (the lungs).
- The left heart pump receives oxygenated blood from the pulmonary circulation and pumps it out to the rest of the body (the systemic circulation).

Atria

The atria are the smaller chambers of the heart and lie superior to (above) the ventricles. There are two atria (atrium is the singular of atria):

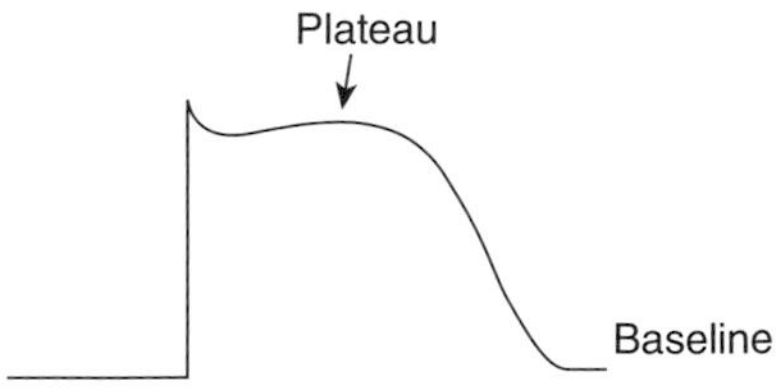
Plateau
Baseline

Figure 10.4 Cardiac action potential

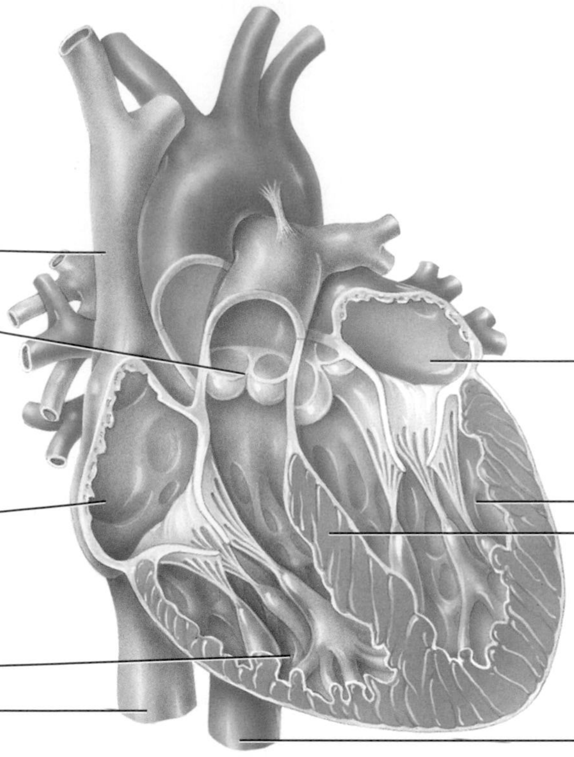
Superior vena cava
Pulmonary valve
Left atrium
Left ventricle
Interventricular septum
Right atrium
Right ventricle
Inferior vena cava
Descending aorta

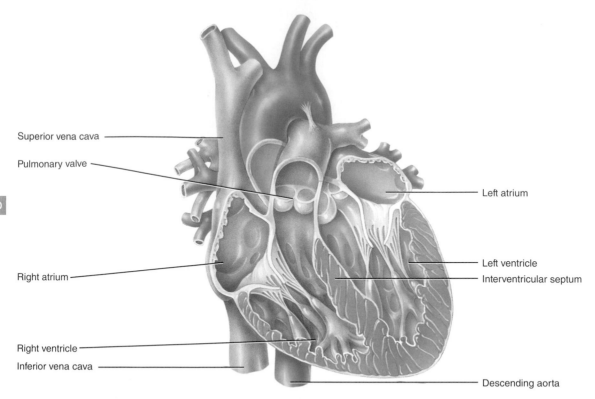

Figure 10.5 The chambers of the heart (Tortora and Derrickson 2009)

- The right atrium receives blood from three veins – the superior vena cava, the inferior vena cava and the coronary sinus. The superior vena cava drains blood from the upper parts of the body, the inferior vena cava drains blood from the lower parts of the body and the coronary sinus drains blood from the circulation of the heart itself
- The left atrium forms most of the base of the heart and receives blood from the lungs through four pulmonary veins.

Between the atria is a thin dividing wall, the interatrial septum (inter = between, septum = dividing wall).

The thickness of a chamber's wall varies according to the work the chamber has to perform. As the atria are only pumping blood into the ventricles they have much thinner walls than the ventricles which have to pump blood around the pulmonary and systemic circulation.

Between the atria and the ventricles are two valves (the atrioventricular valves):

- The tricuspid valve is made up of three cusps (leaflets) and lies between the right atrium and the right ventricle
- The bicuspid (mitral) valve is made up of two cusps and lies between the left atrium and the left ventricle.

The purpose of the atrioventricular valves is to prevent the backward flow of blood from the ventricles into the atria.

Ventricles

There are two ventricles, the right ventricle and the left ventricle. Each ventricle pumps the same amount of blood per beat but they have very different pressures.

- The right ventricle receives blood from the right atrium and pumps this blood out into the pulmonary circulation (the lungs). As the pressure in the pulmonary circulation is quite low the right ventricle has a thinner wall than the left ventricle
- The left ventricle receives blood from the left atrium and pumps this blood out into the systemic circulation (the rest of the body) via the aorta. As the left ventricle has to pump against a higher pressure and over a greater distance it has a much thicker (more muscular) wall.

Between the ventricles is a dividing wall, the interventicular septum. Thus with the septum between the atria and the septum between the ventricles there is no mixing of blood between the two sides.

At the outlet of each ventricle is a valve. Both of these valves are made up of three semilunar (half-moon shaped) cusps (leaflets):

- The pulmonary valve lies between the right ventricle and the pulmonary arteries and prevents the backward flow of blood into the right ventricle from the pulmonary arteries
- The aortic valve lies between the left ventricle and the aorta (the main artery leading to the systemic circulation) and prevents the backward flow of blood into the left ventricle from the systemic circulation.

Clinical considerations

Valve disease

Any of the four valves of the heart can become disordered in their functioning. There are two main processes that can affect the valves (Clare 2007):

- Valvular incompetence (regurgitation). The valve becomes unable to close properly and thus there is backward flow of blood into the heart chamber behind the valve. Incompetence is most common in the mitral and aortic valves; it is very rare in both the tricuspid and pulmonary valves. Common causes of incompetence include age-related degeneration of the valve, infection of the valve and coronary heart disease.
- Valve stenosis. The valve becomes stiff and the leaflets of the valve may fuse together, thus narrowing the opening that blood can pass through. Stenosis is rare in the pulmonary valve and is usually only found in the tricuspid valve in conjunction with aortic and/or mitral valve stenosis. Common causes of stenosis are rheumatic fever, and in the case of aortic valve stenosis age-related changes.

The blood supply to the heart

Although small the heart receives about 5% of the body's blood supply. Ensuring that the heart receives a plentiful supply of blood is essential to ensure the constant supply of oxygen and nutrients and the efficient removal of waste products required by the myocardium.

Only the inner part of the endocardium (about 2 mm in thickness) is supplied with blood directly from the inside of the heart chambers. The rest of the heart is supplied by the coronary arteries. The coronary arteries come directly off the aorta just after the aortic valve. They continuously divide into smaller branches, forming a web of blood vessels to supply the heart muscle. Figure 10.6 shows the main coronary arteries.

Each artery (and its branches) supplies different areas of the heart muscle, Table 10.1 gives a summary of the main arteries, their branches and the areas of the heart they supply. It is important to note that the table gives the anatomy as it pertains to most people but there are normal variations in this pattern of blood supply in as much as 30% of the population. These variations have no significance in the normal, healthy person but can be important in the treatment of cardiac patients.

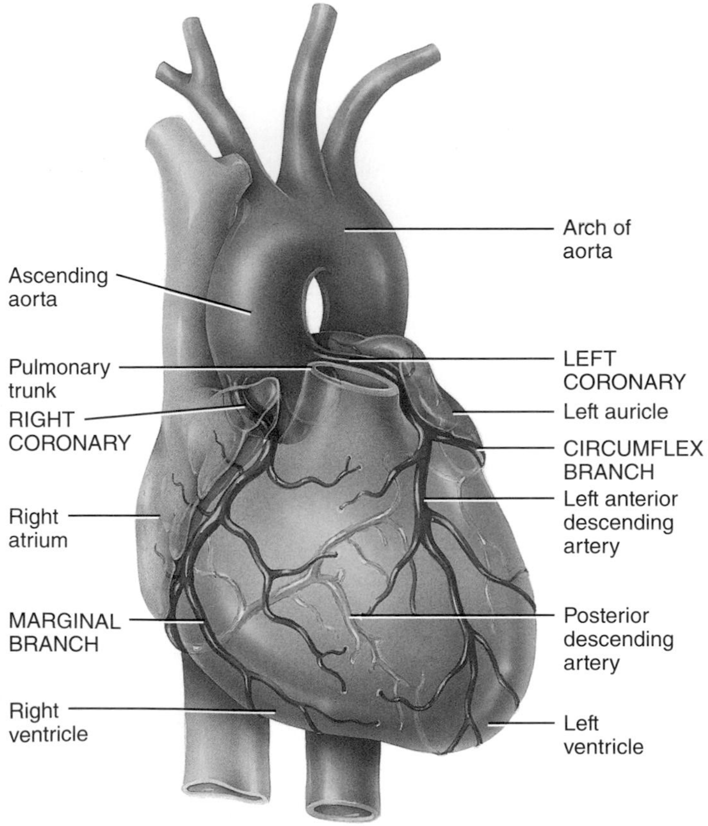
Arch of aorta
Ascending aorta
Pulmonary trunk
LEFT CORONARY
Left auricle
RIGHT CORONARY
CIRCUMFLEX BRANCH
Left anterior descending artery
Right atrium
MARGINAL BRANCH
Posterior descending artery
Right ventricle
Left ventricle

Figure 10.6 Coronary arteries (Tortora and Derrickson 2009)

Each of the main coronary arteries has branches coming off it and supplies different areas of the heart. Table 10.1 gives a summary of the major arteries, their branches and the areas of the heart they supply in the majority of people. Other (normal) variations can occur with each artery supplying a greater or lesser area of the heart.

As the coronary arteries are compressed during each heart beat blood does not flow through the coronary arteries at this time. Thus blood flow to the myocardium occurs during the relaxation phase; this is the opposite of every other part of the body.

Table 10.1 Names of the coronary arteries, their major branches and the areas of the heart they supply.

Artery	Area of the heart supplied	Major branches
Left anterior descending (LAD)	Front and side of the left ventricle, apex of the heart	Diagonals Septals
Circumflex artery	Back and side of the left ventricle	Oblique marginal
Right coronary artery (RCA)	Right ventricle, base of the heart and interventricular septum	Posterior descending artery

Clinical considerations

Myocardial infarction

When one of the arteries supplying the heart muscle with blood becomes blocked by a thrombus (blood clot) the patient needs rapid treatment in order to try to limit the damage to the heart muscle. There are two main treatment options available:

- Thrombolysis – The administration of a thrombolytic drug in order to try to break up the clot and return blood flow through the artery. This form of treatment is very common and requires no specialist equipment to administer. However, patients are closely monitored for side effects, including bleeding, hypotension and disturbances in the heart rhythm.
- Percutaneous coronary intervention (PCI). This is a specialist procedure requiring a dedicated cardiac catheterisation suite (a form of operating theatre with special imaging equipment), trained staff and various cardiac catheters, balloons and stents. The patient has a

catheter inserted through a hole made in the femoral artery and the catheter is manoeuvred to the artery where the blockage is situated. A balloon is then passed through and inflated to push the thrombus into the walls of the artery and if necessary a metal cage (a stent) is inserted into the artery to keep the artery open. Though a specialist procedure PCI is becoming more common in the UK.

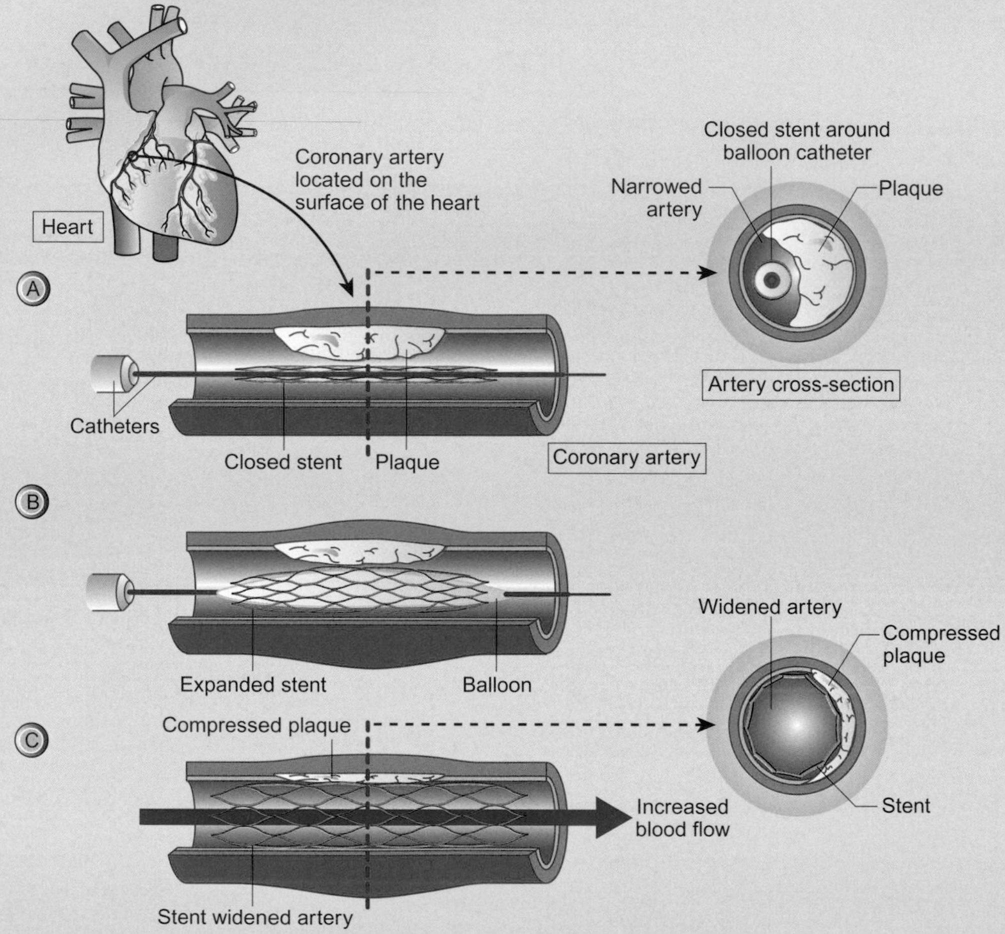
Heart
Coronary artery located on the surface of the heart
A
Catheters
Closed stent
Plaque
Coronary artery
Closed stent around balloon catheter
Narrowed artery
Plaque
Artery cross-section
B
Expanded stent
Balloon
Widened artery
Compressed plaque
C
Compressed plaque
Increased blood flow
Stent
Stent widened artery

National Heart Lung and Blood Institute 2010

Blood flow through the heart

As noted earlier in the chapter, though the heart is a single organ it is best to think of it as two pumps, the right and the left heart pumps. Each pump is made up of two chambers (atrium and ventricle) and their associated valves.

- The right heart pump receives blood from the systemic circulation (the body) and pumps it through the pulmonary circulation (the lungs)
- The left heart pump receives blood from the pulmonary circulation and pumps it out around the systemic circulation.

Figure 10.7 gives a simplified explanation of the flow of blood through the heart. In this diagram deoxygenated blood is in blue and oxygenated blood is in red. It is important to note that 'deoxygenated blood' does not refer to blood that has no oxygen in it but blood that has given up some of its oxygen to the tissues. Typically deoxygenated blood contains 75% of the oxygen that oxygenated blood carries.

So as can be seen, deoxygenated blood returns from the body to the right atrium and then into the right ventricle from where it is pumped out to the lungs. In the lungs the waste gases are exchanged for oxygen and the oxygenated blood flows into the left atrium and into the left ventricle. From the left ventricle the blood is then pumped into the circulation of the body.

A more detailed and anatomical view can be seen in Figure 10.8. Blood enters the right atrium via the superior vena cava and inferior vena cava and leaves the right ventricle via the pulmonary arteries. Note that even though it is deoxygenated blood leaving the right ventricle it is the vessels that the blood is carried in that makes it arterial or venous. Thus:

- Blood entering the atria is carried in veins and is therefore venous blood
- Blood leaving the ventricles is carried in arteries and is arterial blood.

Blood is transported through the pulmonary circulation and returned to the left atrium through the pulmonary veins, it is then pumped out by the left ventricle into the aorta.

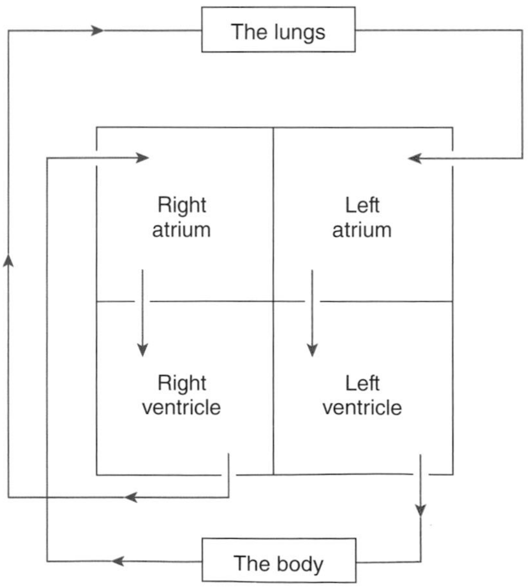
The lungs
Right atrium
Left atrium
Right ventricle
Left ventricle
The body

Figure 10.7 A simplified diagram of the flow of blood though the heart

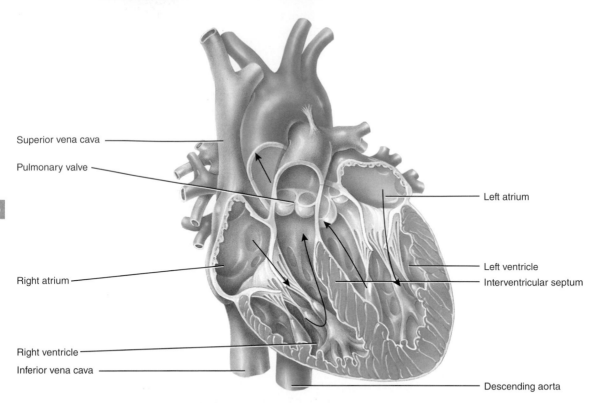

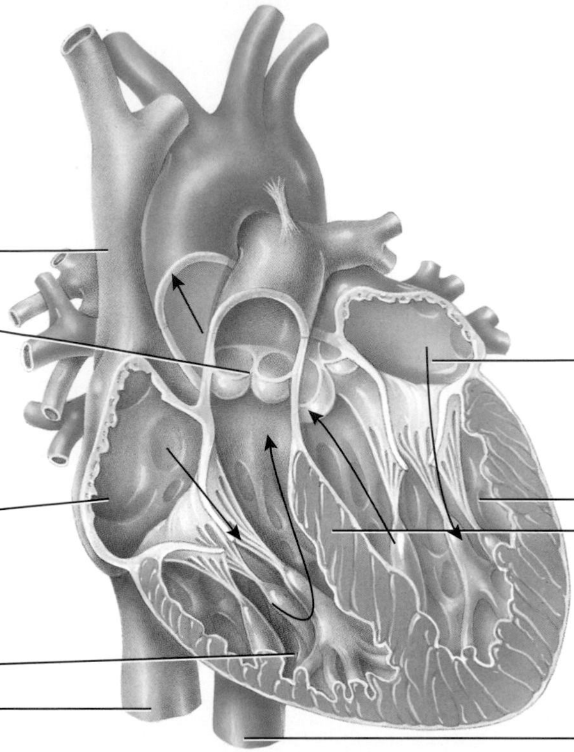
Superior vena cava
Pulmonary valve
Right atrium
Right ventricle
Inferior vena cava
Left atrium
Left ventricle
Interventricular septum
Descending aorta

Figure 10.8 Anatomical view of the blood flow through the heart (Tortora and Derrickson 2009)

The electrical pathways of the heart

Within the heart there is a specialised network of electrical pathways dedicated to ensuring the rapid transmission of electrical impulses. This ensures that the myocardium is excited rapidly in response to an initiating impulse so that the chambers contract and relax in the right order and the different pairs of chambers (atria and ventricles) contract at the same time. So, for instance, the left and right ventricles will contract simultaneously in response to an impulse (but after the atria). Also, the way in which the conduction system is organised means that the ventricles contract in a certain way to ensure they eject blood effectively. For example, if you wanted to empty out a tube of toothpaste you would squeeze from the base to ensure maximum effect. Likewise the ventricles contract in such a way to push blood towards and through the semilunar valves.

The cardiac muscles have a specialised property not seen in any other part of the body. All cells within the myocardium have the ability to create their own action potential without external excitation from another cell or a hormone (Colbert *et al.* 2009). This is known as automaticity (or auto-rhythmicity). The problem with this ability is that, uncontrolled, the cells would all act inde-

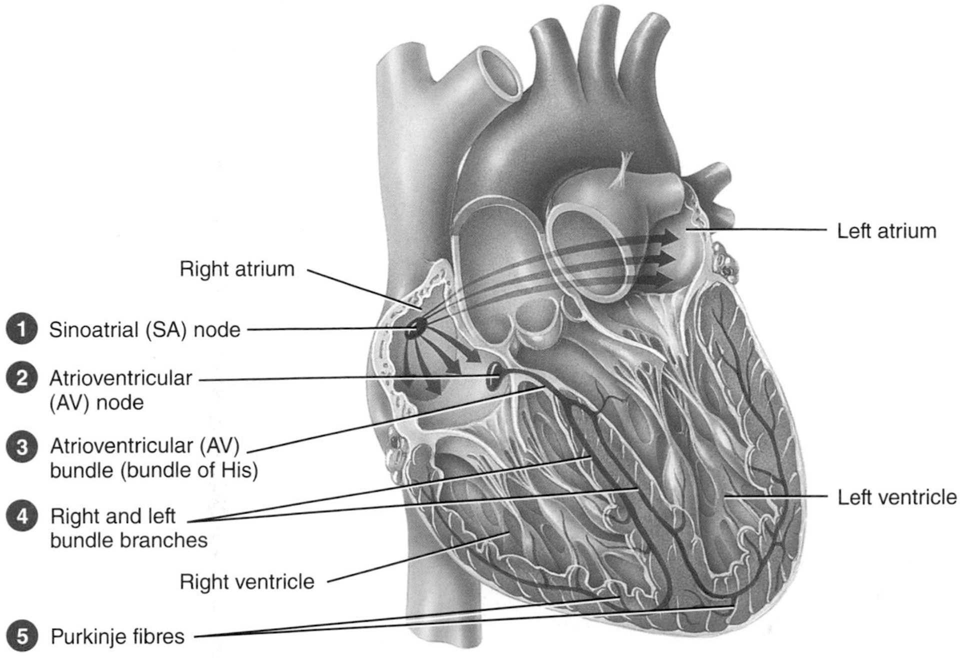
Left atrium
Right atrium
1 Sinoatrial (SA) node
2 Atrioventricular (AV) node
3 Atrioventricular (AV) bundle (bundle of His)
4 Right and left bundle branches
Left ventricle
Right ventricle
5 Purkinje fibres

Figure 10.9 Conduction system of the heart (Tortora and Derrickson 2009)

pendently and the heart would not beat effectively as there would be no coordination of the electrical activity and the subsequent muscle contractions. This is overcome by the use of the specialised cells in the conduction system. These cells create and distribute an electrical current that leads to a controlled and effective heart contraction. An overview of the anatomy of the conduction system can be seen in Figure 10.9.

Normal electrical excitation/distribution begins in the sinoatrial (SA) node, which is located in the right atrium, and is rapidly transmitted across the atria by fast pathways. This ensures that the right and left atria are excited together and beat as one unit. The impulse is transmitted to the atrioventricular (AV) node where further transmission is delayed for approximately 0.1 seconds (Martini and Nath 2009). This ensures that the atria have completely contracted before ventricular contraction is initiated. It should be noted that the atria and the ventricles are electrically isolated from each other by a band of non-conducting fibrous tissue and thus the only electrical connection between the two is the bundle of His (Figure 10.10).

Once the impulse has been 'held' in the AV node it is then transmitted down the bundle of His to the fast pathways of the two bundle branches (one bundle branch per ventricle). The bundles then divide into the smaller and smaller branches of the purkinje system which transmits the impulses to the muscles of the ventricles.

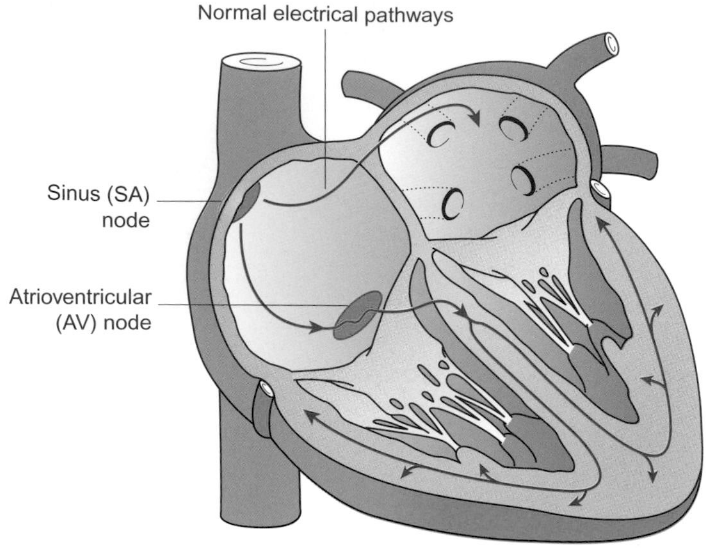
Normal electrical pathways
Sinus (SA) node
Atrioventricular (AV) node

Figure 10.10 Normal electrical conduction

Box 10.1 Nodal cells

Otherwise known as pacemaker cells, these are specialised cells that not only create electrical impulses but create them at regular intervals.

Nodal cells are divided into two groups:

- The sinoatrial node located in the right atrium, which generates electrical impulses at approximately 70–80 impulses per minute
- The atrioventricular node located just above the point where the atria and ventricles meet. This node generates impulses at 40–60 impulses per minute.

The difference in the rate of impulse creation is important in the normal functioning of the heart as every time an impulse is transmitted down the electrical system it 'resets' the cells 'lower down'. Hence the SA node is the normal pacemaker of the heart as it creates impulses faster than the AV node.

Thus like a military command structure the SA node could be seen to be a general who commands a captain (AV node) but if the general no longer issues commands, then the captain will take over.

Clinical considerations

Pacemakers

Sometimes the conduction system of the heart stops working properly and the patient can become very unwell. For instance, if the AV node no longer transmits impulses into the bundle of His, the cells in the lower parts of the conduction system can produce action potentials of their own, but this will be at a slow rate. In order to deal with this problem the patient would need to have a permanent pacemaker fitted.

The 'generator' (battery and circuitry) is contained in a small box that is buried beneath the skin of the chest wall. Wires lead from the generator through a vein into the patient's heart. Depending on the type of pacemaker fitted there may be one or two wires. So, for instance, in the case of a failed AV node the pacemaker would have two wires, one in the right atrium and one in the right ventricle. The pacemaker would sense the atrial action potential and then (after a short delay to mimic the action of the AV node) the ventricle would receive an electrical impulse causing it to contract. Thus the pacemaker acts as a replacement AV node.

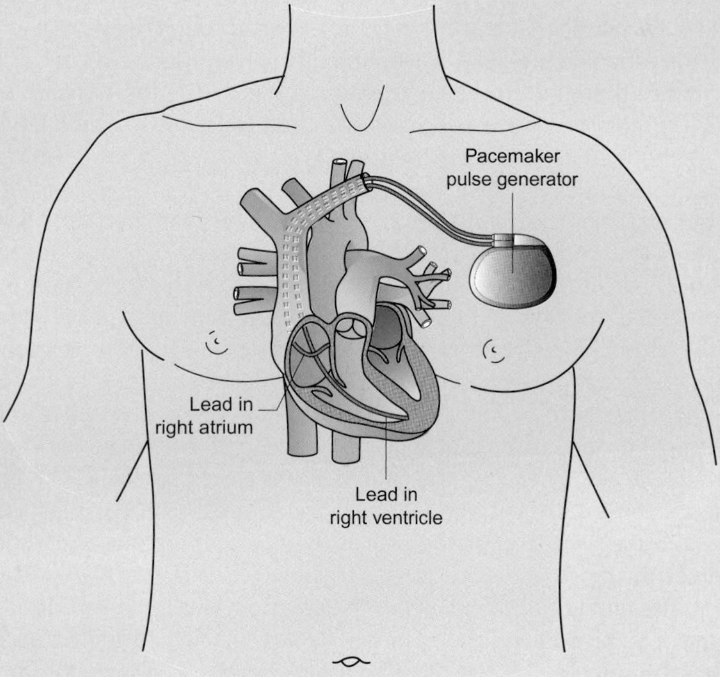
Pacemaker
pulse generator
Lead in
right atrium
Lead in
right ventricle

The cardiac cycle

The cardiac cycle is the name given to the mechanical activity of the heart and is best understood by looking at the pressure changes in the heart chambers and the aorta and relating these to the mechanical activity of the heart and its chambers.

Box 10.2 Systole and diastole

These are two terms that require definition as they are unique in anatomy and physiology to the functioning of the heart.

Systole: The contraction of a heart chamber (atrium or ventricle)
Diastole: The relaxation of a heart chamber (atrium or ventricle).

The cardiac cycle can be seen in Figure 10.11. Note the diagram refers to the pressures in the left side of the heart (atrium and ventricle); the cardiac cycle is the same on the right side but the pressures are lower. The cardiac cycle can be broken down into a series of steps that are detailed below. The flow of blood in the heart and the circulatory system is always from a point of higher pressure to a point of lower pressure. The cardiac cycle is usually divided into three phases.

(1) A period of ventricular filling in mid-to-late relaxation (ventricular diastole). Pressure in the ventricle is low. Blood that is returning to the heart through the vena cava is flowing passively through the atria and the open atrioventricular valves into the ventricle. The pressure in the atria is higher than that in the ventricles and this forces the bicuspid and tricuspid valves open. As the pressure in the ventricles rises due to the increased amount of blood ion the ventricles the leaflets of the atrioventricular valves begin to drift upwards to their closed positions. The semilunar valves (the aortic and the pulmonary valves) are closed; the pressure in the aorta and the pulmonary arteries is greater than that in the ventricles thus forcing these valves shut. About 70% of ventricular filling happens during this phase.

(2) Late in this phase the atria begin to contract (atrial systole) in response to excitation by an action potential from the SA node; this compresses the blood in the atria leading to a slight rise in the pressure in the atria. This rise in pressure leads to a greater flow of blood into the ventricles from the atria. The ventricles remain in diastole as the electrical excitation that led to atrial contraction is delayed in the AV node. By the end of this point in time the ventricles are in the last part of their relaxation phase and contain the largest amount of blood they will contain during the cardiac cycle. This is known as the end diastolic volume (EDV) and is about 130 ml of blood (Tortora and Derrickson 2009), that is the volume of blood contained in the ventricles at the end of their relaxation phase (diastole). The EDV is the main factor in the creation of the end diastolic pressure (EDP) as the pressure is directly related to the amount of blood within the ventricle when the ventricle is relaxed.

(3) Ventricular contraction (systole). The atria relax, leading to a drop in atrial pressure. The ventricles begin to contract as the electrical excitation is transmitted from the AV node to the ventricles through the bundle of His, then the bundle branches and finally the purkinje fibres; this leads to a sharp rise in ventricular pressure without any change in ventricular volume (i.e. the amount of blood in the ventricles does not change). Once this pressure rises above the pressure in the atria the atrioventricular valves are forced closed. As the semilunar valves remain closed at this point (the ventricular pressure is still lower than the pressure in the aorta and the pulmonary arteries) the ventricles are completely closed off and blood volume in the ventricles remains the same whilst pressure rises. This is known as the

isovolumetric contraction phase ('iso' means remaining the same). Eventually, the pressure in the ventricles becomes greater than the pressure in the aorta and the pulmonary arteries. At this point the semilunar valves are forced open and blood is ejected form the ventricles.

(4) Early ventricular diastole (relaxation). The ventricles begin to relax. The blood in the ventricles is no longer compressed by the action of the heart muscle and the pressure within the ventricles drops rapidly. As the blood volume in the ventricles remains constant (the atrioventricular valves are closed) the pressure in the aorta and the pulmonary arteries becomes greater than the pressure in the ventricles and the semilunar valves are forced closed. This is the ventricular isovolumetric relaxation phase. Closure of the semilunar valves causes a brief rise in the pressure in the aorta as backflowing blood rebounds off the closed aortic valve, this can be seen as a slight 'bump' in the pressure tracing known as the 'dicrotic notch'.

(5) During the period of ventricular systole the atria have been in diastole and filling with blood from the veins. When the pressure in the atria is greater than the pressure in the ventricles the atrioventricular valves are forced open and blood begins to flow into the ventricles again.

Despite this appearing to be a long process if we assume a heart rate of 75 beats per minute, then the average cardiac cycle would take approximately 0.8 seconds (Marieb 2001). The atria are in systole for 0.1 seconds and then in diastole for 0.7 seconds, while the ventricles are in systole for 0.3 seconds and diastole for 0.5 seconds. As heart rate increases the cardiac cycle becomes shorter, all of this change in the time taken by the cardiac cycle is due to the shortening of the diastolic phase. As noted above, the heart muscle is supplied with blood during the diastolic

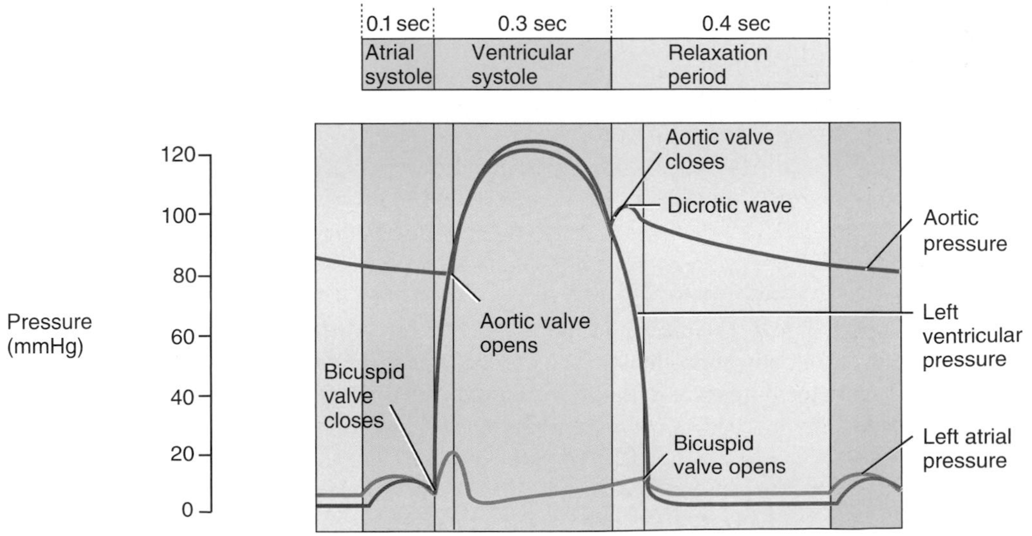
0.1 sec
0.3 sec
0.4 sec
Atrial systole
Ventricular systole
Relaxation period
Pressure (mmHg)
120
100
80
60
40
20
0
Aortic valve closes
Dicrotic wave
Aortic pressure
Aortic valve opens
Left ventricular pressure
Bicuspid valve closes
Bicuspid valve opens
Left atrial pressure

Figure 10.11 The cardiac cycle (Tortora and Derrickson 2009)

Box 10.3 Electrocardiogram and the cardiac cycle

Though the cardiac cycle refers to the mechanical action of the heart the electrical activity that stimulates this mechanical action can be seen by the use of an electrocardiogram (ECG), an electrical tracing produced by attaching electrodes to the patient's skin and generated by an ECG machine, though it is possible for the electrical tracing to be present without mechanical activity in certain types of cardiac arrest.

The normal ECG of one cycle of the heart is shown below with relation to the cardiac cycle (pressure changes) of the left side of the heart.

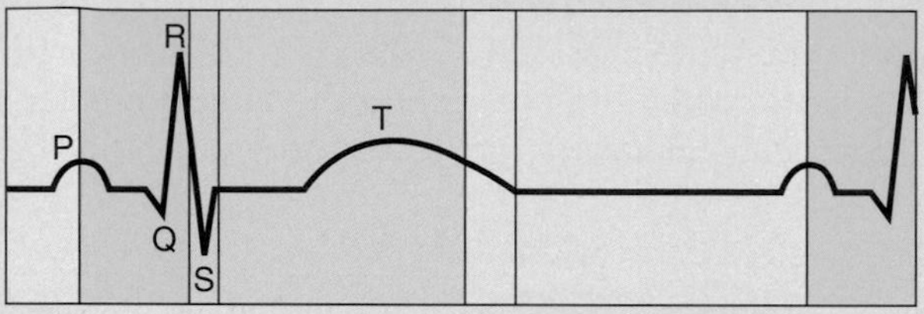
R
T
P
Q
S

Tortora and Derrickson 2009

The changes from the baseline on the ECG are labelled by letters of the alphabet:

P – atrial depolarisation. Corresponds to atrial contraction

QRS – ventricular depolarisation. Corresponds approximately to ventricular contraction (though this happens just after the peak of the R wave).

T – ventricular repolarisation. Corresponds to the relaxation phase of the ventricle, atrial repolarisation cannot be seen as it is hidden by the greater electrical activity of ventricular depolarisation.

(relaxation) phase, as blood cannot flow in the coronary arteries when the heart is contracting, and thus as heart rate increases blood flow in the coronary arteries (and blood supply to the heart muscle) is reduced.

Factors affecting cardiac output

This section gives an overview of the factors affecting the cardiac output. 'Cardiac output' is a term relating to the amount of blood the heart pumps out in one minute and is defined by the following equation.

Cardiac output (CO) = stroke volume (SV) × heart rate (HR)

Thus the amount of blood the heart pumps out in a minute is made up of the amount of blood ejected from the ventricle in one beat (SV) times the heart rate (HR) in beats per minute. This gives a total volume. Thus if we said that SV is 70 ml and the heart rate is 75, then cardiac output is 70 × 75 = 5250 ml (or 5.25 litres) per minute.

To review the factors affecting cardiac output this section will look at the factors regulating stroke volume and the factors regulating heart rate separately.

Regulation of stroke volume

Stroke volume is effectively the difference between the end diastolic volume (EDV), that is the amount of blood in the ventricle at the end of relaxation, and the end systolic volume (ESV), the amount of blood in the ventricle at the end of systole. The factors that affect stroke volume are preload, force of contraction and afterload (Marieb and Hoehn 2007).

Preload

The amount of stretch that the cardiac muscle fibres are subjected to relates to the force with which they contract during systole (the Frank–Starling law). This stretch is related to the amount of blood in the ventricle at the end of diastole (EDV) which is, in turn, dependent on the amount of blood returned to the ventricles by the veins (venous return). Anything that affects the speed or volume of venous return affects EDV. So for instance:

- A slower heart rate allows for more time for blood to fill the ventricle, increasing the volume of blood in the ventricle at the end of diastole
- Exercise increases venous return as the increase in heart rate increases the pressure in the veins and the speed of venous return and the effect of skeletal muscle activity squeezes the veins 'pushing' blood back to the heart. Conversely, standing still means that venous return is reduced. Thus the guardsmen who have to stand still outside Buckingham Palace are taught to contract and relax their feet to aid venous return and prevent fainting
- Hormonal and nervous influences. The release of adrenaline or the exc1tation of the sympathetic nervous system leads to the contraction of the veins and the 'squeezing' of blood back to the heart
- Very fast heart rates reduce the diastolic filling time and thus there is less time for the ventricle to receive blood before systole starts
- Certain heart arrhythmias stop the atria contracting effectively and thus atrial systole is no longer effective at 'pushing' the last bit of blood into the ventricles
- A reduced blood volume (for instance, due to a haemorrhage) reduces venous return.

Force of contraction

Though end diastolic volume is a major component of the force of contraction (because of the Frank–Starling law), force of contraction can also be affected by other factors. The contractility of the heart can be affected by several factors:

- Hormones such as adrenaline, glucagon and thyroxine all increase the force of contraction
- Sympathetic nervous system activity increases the force of contraction through the action of noradrenaline
- Contractility can be reduced by acidaemia (excess hydrogen ions in the blood) and high potassium levels in the blood.

Afterload

Afterload refers to the pressure in the arteries leading from the ventricles (aorta or pulmonary arteries) that the ventricle must overcome in order to eject blood. In the normal adult the pressure is 80 mm Hg in the aorta and 8 mm Hg in the pulmonary arteries (Marieb and Hoehn 2007). This difference in the pressure to be overcome is reflected in the relative thickness of the ventricular walls with the left ventricular wall being thicker (more muscular) than the right (see previous discussion on the structure of the heart).

In the average adult aortic and pulmonary pressure is not an important factor in determining afterload as it is constant, but changes in anatomy and/or physiology such as hypertension or aortic valve disease can increase afterload. Increased afterload increases the amount of blood left in the ventricle after each systole and thus also has an effect in increasing the preload (by increasing ventricular end diastolic volume and therefore pressure).

Regulation of heart rate

Heart rate is controlled by two main mechanisms:

- Autononomic nervous system activity
- Hormone activity.

Resting heart rate is also affected by factors such as age, gender, temperature and physical fitness (Tortora and Derrickson 2009).

Autonomic nervous system activity

When activated by a stimulus, such as exercise or stress, the sympathetic nerve fibres release noradrenaline at their cardiac endings as a neurotransmitter. This leads to the excitation of the sinoatrial node and an increase in its production of action potentials and thus an increase in heart rate.

Alternatively, when the parasympathetic nervous system is stimulated this results in the release of acetylcholine at the parasymapathetic cardiac nerve endings which has the effect of reducing the rate of action potential generation in the sinoatrial node and thus reducing heart rate.

Both the sympathetic and parasympathetic nervous systems are active at all times, but the parasympathetic nervous system normally has the dominant influence. This can be seen if the vagus nerve (cranial nerve X) is cut, for instance in heart transplant patients. In these situations the sinoatrial node will normally produce action potentials at a rate of 100 a minute and therefore the heart rate increases to 100 beats per minute. The removal of the influence of the parasympathetic nervous system (by the disconnection of the vagus nerve) removes the heart rate, reducing effect of this system.

Baroreceptors and the cardiovascular centre

Baroreceptors are specialised mechanical receptors located in the carotid sinus and the aortic arch. They are sensitive to the amount of stretch in these blood vessels (Jenkins *et al.* 2007) and have direct outflow via the autonomic nervous system to the cardiovascular centre in the medulla oblongata.

The cardiovascular centre of the medulla oblongata is the main centre for the control of autonomic nervous activity that affects the heart. As can be seen in Figure 10.12 the cardiovascular centre is made up of two sub-centres:

- The cardioinhibitory centre directly controls parasymapathetic outflow to the heart (especially the sinoatrial node), thus increased outflow from this centre has the effect of reducing heart rate
- The vasomotor centre is further divided into the pressor area and the depressor area. The pressor area has a relatively constant outflow of action potentials to the heart via the symapathetic nervous system. This has a direct effect on both heart rate and the force of ventricular contraction (and therefore stroke volume) as well as effects on the vasculature which subsequently will affect heart function by changing preload and afterload. Outflow from the pressor area is moderated by nerves transmitting impulses from the depressor area which have a directly inhibiting effect on the transmission of impulses from the pressor area. Thus it can be thought that the nerve impulses of the depressor area act like a 'collar' or tap; the greater the number of impulses from the depressor area the tighter the collar or tap is made, reducing the number of impulses from the pressor area to the heart and thus the effect on heart rate and force of contraction.

Hormone activity

Two hormones are normally associated with the control of heart rate:

- Adrenaline – from the adrenal medulla. Adrenaline has the same effect as noradrenaline released by the sympathetic nervous system
- Thyroxine – from the thyroid gland. Released in large quantities thyroxine has the effect of increasing the heart rate.

Conclusion

The heart is a single organ situated in the thoracic cavity between the lungs. Though a single organ, the heart is effectively two separate pumps made up of four chambers:

- The right heart pump, comprised of the right atrium and right ventricle, pumps blood through the pulmonary circulation
- The left heart pump, comprised of the left atrium and the left ventricle, this pumps blood through the systemic circulation.

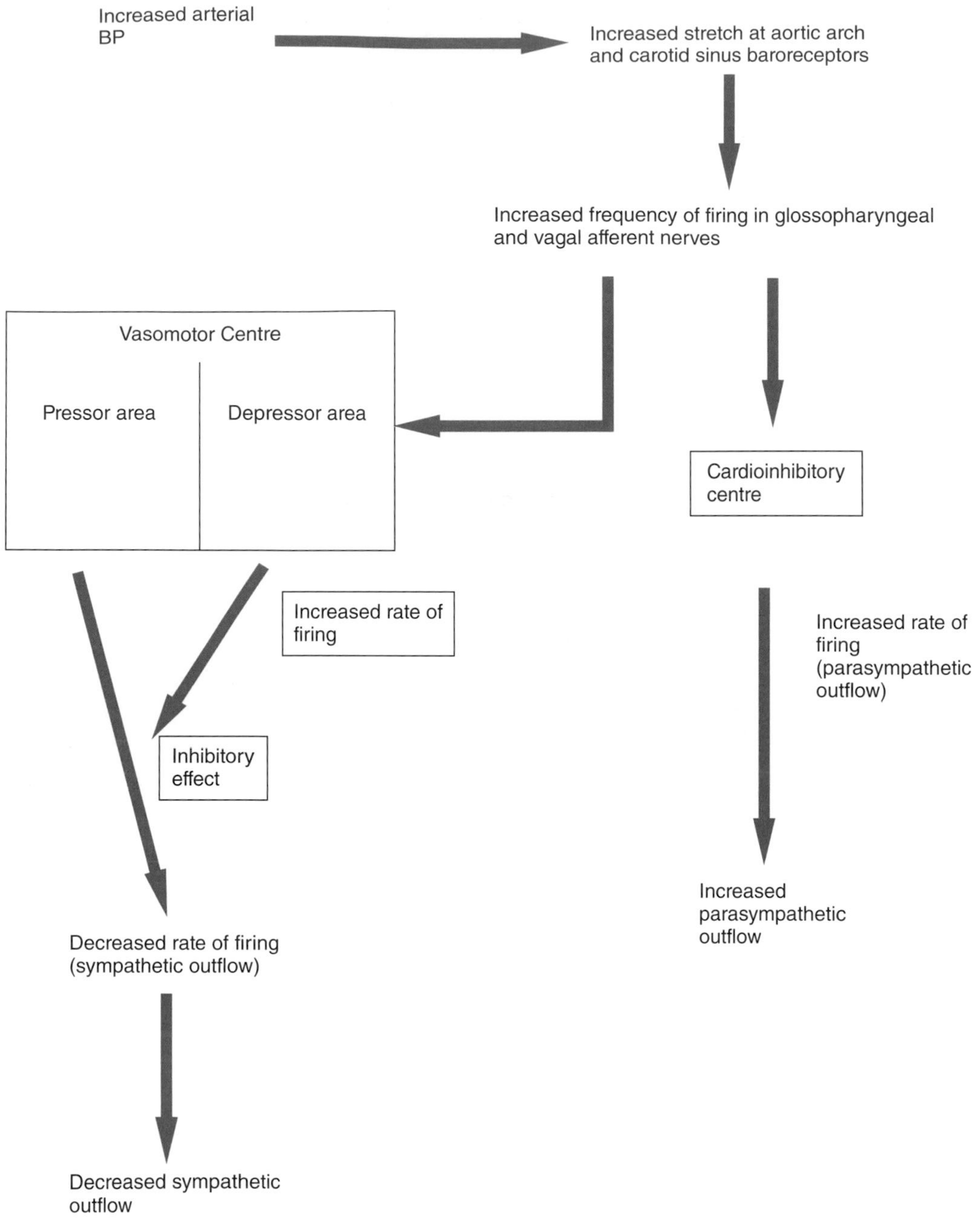

Increased arterial BP
Increased stretch at aortic arch and carotid sinus baroreceptors
Increased frequency of firing in glossopharyngeal and vagal afferent nerves
Vasomotor Centre
Pressor area
Depressor area
Cardioinhibitory centre
Increased rate of firing
Inhibitory effect
Increased rate of firing (parasympathetic outflow)
Decreased rate of firing (sympathetic outflow)
Increased parasympathetic outflow
Decreased sympathetic outflow

Figure 10.12 Baroreceptor reflex

Surrounding the heart is a double protective sac called the pericardium. Underlying the pericardium is the heart muscle (myocardium), which is a specialised type of muscle that is branched in its structure and is laid down in spiral bundles to make up the walls of the various heart chambers.

Control of the heart muscle is achieved by the use of a specialised series of nerve cells that make up the conduction system of the heart including:

- The sinoatrial (SA) node, the pacemaker of the heart
- The atrioventricular (AV) node, an area of the heart's conduction system that controls the delivery of the action potential to the ventricles
- Purkinje fibres, conductive fibres that aid rapid distribution of the action potential throughout the ventricles.

Blood flow through the heart is based on changes of pressure in the cardiac cycle. These pressure changes also lead to the opening and closing of the cardiac valves, thus further controlling blood flow.

Regulation of the heart's activity is based on the actions of:

- Hormones, especially adrenaline
- Autonomic nervous system activity, for instance via the cardiovascular centres.

Glossary

Action potential: Momentary change in the electrical status of a cell wall.

Afterload: The 'load' which the heart has to pump against, mostly created by the blood pressure in the arteries.

Aorta: Main artery leading from the left ventricle.

Aortic valve: Semilunar valve that lies between the left ventricle and the aorta.

Arterial: Pertaining to the arteries.

Arterial blood: Blood carried in the arteries.

Atria: Upper chambers of the heart (singular = atrium)

Atrioventricular bundle: Bundle of conductive nerve fibres that transmit action potentials from the AV node to the ventricular conduction system. Otherwise known as the bundle of His.

Atrioventricular node: Otherwise known as the AV node. Specialised area of cardiac cells located just above the point where the right atrium and right ventricle meets.

Atrioventricular valve:	Collective name for the two valves that lie between the atria and the ventricles (bicuspid and tricuspid).
Automaticity:	The ability of certain cells to generate their own action potential without an external stimulus.
Baroreceptors:	Specialised mechanical receptors located in the aortic arch and the carotid sinus.
Bicuspid valve:	The atrioventricular valve that lies between the left atrium and the left ventricle. Also known as the mitral valve.
Bundle of His:	See atrioventricular bundle.
Cardiac action potential:	Specialised action potential of the heart muscle cells, it is of longer duration than normal cellular action potentials.
Cardiac cycle:	The sequence of events that occur when the heart beats.
Cardiac output:	The amount of blood pumped out by a ventricle in ml per minute.
Cardioinhibitory centre:	Part of the cardiovascular centre, when stimulated the major effect is to slow down the heart rate.
Cardiovascular centre:	Located in the medulla oblongata this centre controls most of the nervous activity that affects the heart.
Coronary arteries:	Arteries that supply the myocardium with oxygenated blood.
Coronary sinus:	Collection of veins that come together to form a single large vessel that returns blood from the myocardium to the right atrium.
Depolarisation:	Change in the electrical potential of a cell membrane to a more positive charge.
Desmosomes:	A specialised cell structure whose function is to hold cells together.
Diastole:	The relaxation of a heart chamber (atrium or ventricle).
Dicrotic notch:	A small bump in the pressure tracing of the arteries created by a backflow of blood after the closure of the aortic valve.
End diastolic pressure:	The pressure created by the blood in a named chamber (usually the left ventricle) at the end of diastole.
End diastolic volume:	The volume of blood in a named chamber (usually the left ventricle) at the end of diastole.
Endocardium:	Innermost layer that lines the chambers of the heart and also lines the cardiac valves.
Epithelium:	Layer of body tissue that lines the inside of cavities and the surface of many structures.

Fibrous pericardium: The outer, tough layer of the pericardium that provides protection to the heart, prevents overstretching of the heart and helps to anchor the heart in place.

Gap junction: A specialised connection between cell membranes that allow the passage of ions and molecules.

Hormone: Chemical substance that is released into the blood by the endocrine system, and has a physiological control over the function of cells or organs other than those that created it.

Inferior vena cava: Large vein that returns blood to the right atrium from the lower parts of the body.

Interatrial septum: Dividing wall between the atria.

Interventricular septum: Dividing wall between the ventricles.

Ion: An electrically charged atom or molecule.

Isovolumetric: No change in volume (amount).

Medulla oblongata: The lower half of the brainstem.

Mitral valve: See bicuspid valve.

Myocardium: Muscle layer of the heart.

Myocyte: Cardiac muscle cell.

Nodal cells: Otherwise known as pacemaker cells, these are specialised cells that not only create electrical impulses but create them at regular intervals. The two main groupings of these cells are located in the sinoatrial node and the atrioventricular node.

Parietal pericardium: The outer layer of the serous pericardium, it is fused to the fibrous pericardium.

Pericardial fluid: A thin film of fluid which reduces the friction between the pericardial membranes as the heart moves during its cycle of contraction and relaxation.

Pericardium: Double layered sac that surrounds the heart.

Pulmonary circulation: Circulatory system of the lungs.

Pulmonary valve: Semilunar valve that lies between the right ventricle and the pulmonary circulation.

Pulmonary veins: Veins of the pulmonary circulation that return blood from the lungs to the left atrium.

Purkinje fibres (system): Specialised conductive fibres that rapidly transport action potentials through the ventricle walls.

Repolarisation: Return of the electrical potential of a cell membrane to a negative resting state.

Sarcolemma: Cell membrane of a muscle cell.

Semilunar valves: The valves that lie between the ventricles and the pulmonary or systemic circulation (aortic valve and pulmonary valve).

Septum: A dividing wall.

Serous pericardium: Inner (double) layer of the pericardium comprised of the parietal and visceral pericardial layers.

Sinoatrial node: Otherwise known as the SA node. Specialised area of cardiac cells located in the upper part of the right atrium. Usually referred to as the pacemaker of the heart.

Stroke volume: The amount of blood ejected by a ventricle in one beat.

Superior vena cava: The large vein that returns blood to the right atrium from the upper part of the body.

Systemic circulation: The circulatory system of the body (excluding the lungs).

Systole: The contraction of a heart chamber (atrium or ventricle).

Tetany: Sustained involuntary contraction of a muscle.

Tricuspid valve: The atrioventricular valve that lies between the right atrium and ventricle.

Vasomotor centre: Part of the cardiovascular centre, has effects on heart rate and the force of contraction of the heart.

Venous: Pertaining to the veins.

Venous blood: Blood carried in the veins.

Ventricles: The large lower chambers of the heart.

Visceral pericardium: The inner layer of the serous pericardium (otherwise known as the epicardium) adheres tightly to the surface of the heart.

References

Clare, C. (2007) Valve disorders. In: Hatchett, R. and Thompson, D.R. (eds) *Cardiac Nursing: A Comprehensive Guide*. London: Churchill Livingstone Elsevier, pp. 357–382.

Colbert, B., Ankey, J., Lee, K., Steggall, M. and Dingle, M. (2009) *Anatomy and Physiology for Nursing and Health Professionals*. Harlow: Pearson Education.

Jenkins, G.W., Kemnitz, C.P. and Tortora, G.J. (2007) *Anatomy and Physiology: From Science to Life*. Hoboken, NJ: John Wiley & Sons.

Marieb, E.N. (2001) *Human Anatomy and Physiology*, 5th edn. San Francisco: Pearson Benjamin Cummings.

Marieb, E.N. and Hoehn, K. (2007) *Human Anatomy and Physiology. International Edition*, 7th edn. San Francisco: Pearson Benjamin Cummings.

Martini, F.H. and Nath, J.L. (2009) *Fundamentals of Anatomy and Physiology. Pearson International Edition*, 8th edn. San Francisco: Pearson Benjamin Cummings.

National Heart, Lung and Blood Institute (2010) Coronary Balloon Angioplasty. [Online] Retrieved 19.04.2010 from www.nhlbi.nih.gov/health/dci/Diseases/Angioplasty/Angioplasty_howdone.htm

Tortora, G.J. and Derrickson, B.H. (2009) *Principles of Anatomy and Physiology. Vol 2. Maintenance and Continuity of the Human Body. International Student Version*, 12th edn. Hoboken, NJ: John Wiley & Sons.

Activities

www.wiley.com/go/peate

Multiple choice questions

1. The double sac surrounding the heart is the:
   (a) myocardium
   (b) pericardium
   (c) endocardium
   (d) epicardium

2. Which heart chamber has the thickest muscle wall?
   (a) right ventricle
   (b) right atrium
   (c) left ventricle
   (d) left atrium

3. Blood flowing into the right atrium comes from:
   (a) the lungs
   (b) the body (systemic circulation)
   (c) the left heart
   (d) the right heart

4. Blood pumped out from the left heart is carried by the:

(a) vena cava
(b) pulmonary arteries
(c) aorta
(d) coronary arteries

5. The contraction of a heart chamber is known as:

(a) automaticity
(b) diastole
(c) isovulmetric
(d) systole

6. The blood flow through the heart is caused by changes in:

(a) pressure
(b) electricity
(c) transport molecules
(d) oxygen

7. The artery supplying blood to the front of the left ventricle is the:

(a) posterior descending artery
(b) circumflex artery
(c) right coronary artery
(d) left anterior descending artery

8. Normal electrical excitation of the heart begins in:

(a) the bundle of His
(b) the purkinje fibres
(c) the atrioventricular node
(d) the sinoatrial node

9. The effect of increased parasympathetic nervous system activity is to:

(a) increase heart rate
(b) decrease heart rate
(c) increase force of contraction
(d) decrease force of contraction

10. Preload is mostly a factor of:

(a) end systolic volume
(b) end diastolic volume
(c) the Frank-Starling law
(d) adrenaline release

Test your learning

1. Describe the path that an action potential takes through the conduction system of the heart.
2. Describe the effect of increased sympathetic nervous system activity on the heart.
3. Complete the following equation: Cardiac output = SV × HR

Label the diagram

From the list of words, label the diagram below:

Superior vena cava, Pulmonary valve, Right atrium, Right ventricle, Inferior vena cava, Left atrium, Left ventricle, Interventricular septum, Descending aorta

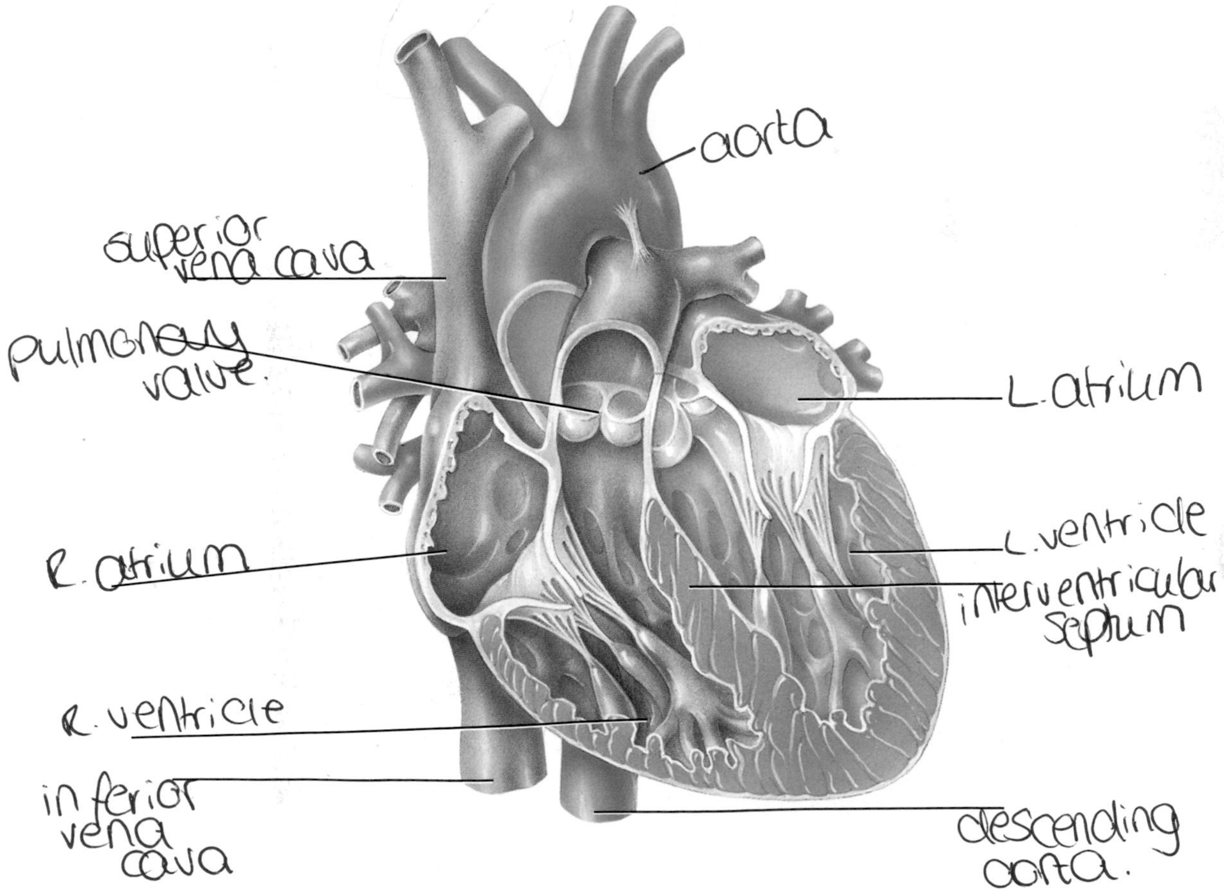
aorta
superior vena cava
pulmonary valve.
L.atrium
R.atrium
L.ventricle
interventricular septum
R.ventricle
inferior vena cava
descending aorta.

Draw arrows on the diagram below to show blood flow through the heart.

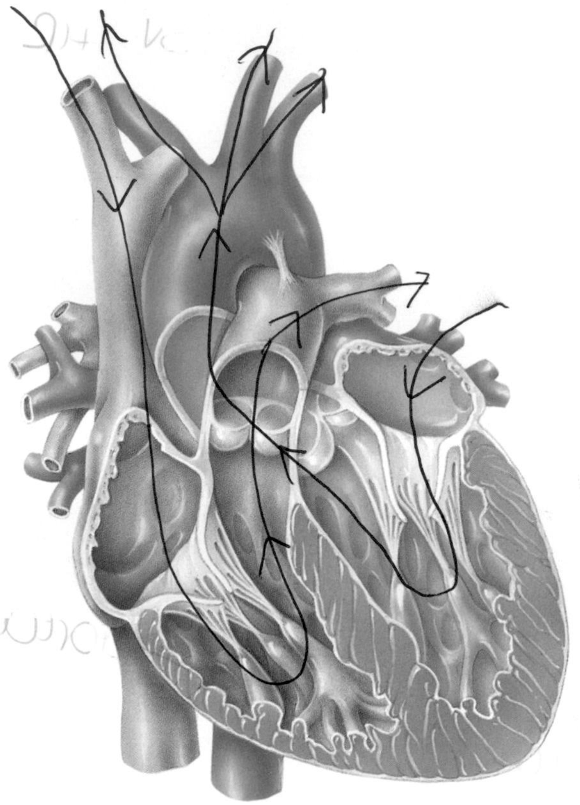

Crossword

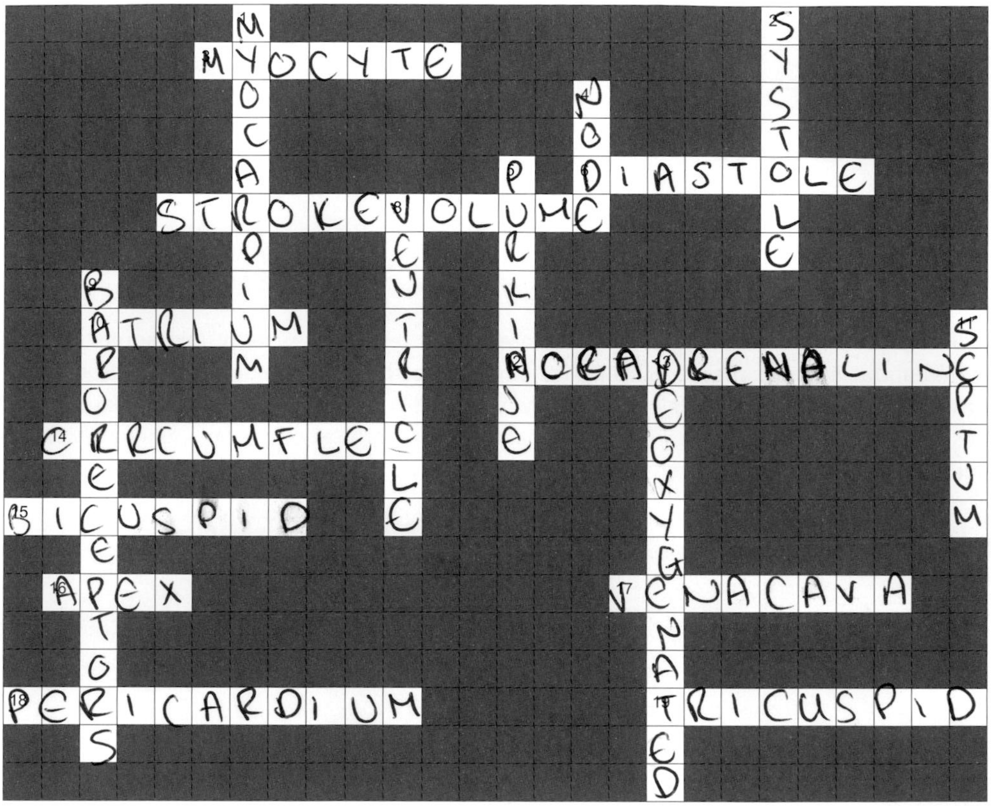

Across:

3. Cardiac muscle cell (7).
6. Relaxation of a heart chamber (8).
7. Amount of blood pumped out by a ventricle in one beat (6,6).
10. Upper chamber of the heart – singular (6).
12. Neurotransmitter of the sympathetic nervous system (13).
14. Coronary artery supplying the back and side of the left ventricle (10).
15. Valve situated between the left atrium and left ventricle (otherwise known as the mitral valve) (8).
16. The pointed end of the heart resting on the diaphragm (4).

Down:

1. Name given to all the cardiac muscle together, i.e. the heart walls (10).
2. Contraction of a heart chamber (7).
4. Sinoatrial _______, pacemaker of the heart (4).
5. Fibres that transport the action potential around the ventricles (8).
8. 'Little belly', main pumping chamber of the heart (9).
9. Specialised mechanical receptors in the carotid sinus and aortic arch (13).
11. Dividing wall between two heart chambers (i.e. the ventricles) (6).

Across:

17. Large vein returning blood to the heart from the systemic circulation (inferior or superior) (4,4).

18. Double thickness sac that surrounds the heart (11).

19. Valve located between the right atrium and the right ventricle (9).

Down:

13. Type of blood returned to the right atrium (12).

Conditions

Below is a list of conditions that are associated with the cardiac system. Take some time and write notes about each of the conditions. You may make the notes taken from text books or other resources, for example, people you work with in a clinical area, or you may make the notes as a result of people you have cared for. If you are making notes about people you have cared for you must ensure that you adhere to the rules of confidentiality.

Angina	
Myocardial infarction	
Aortic stenosis	
Mitral regurgitation	
Pericarditis	
Infective endocarditis	
Complete heart block	
Atrial fibrillation	
Heart failure	
Hypertensive heart disease	

Answers

MCQs

1b; 2c; 3b; 4c; 5d; 6a; 7d; 8d; 9b; 10b

Crossword

Across:		**Down:**	
3.	Myocyte	**1.**	Myocardium
6.	Diastole	**2.**	Systole
7.	Stroke volume	**4.**	Node
10.	Atrium	**5.**	Purkinje
12.	Noradrenaline	**8.**	Ventricle
14.	Circumflex	**9.**	Baroreceptors
15.	Bicuspid	**11.**	Septum
16.	Apex	**13.**	Deoxygenated
17.	Vena cava		
18.	Pericardium		
19.	Tricuspid		

11

The respiratory system

Anthony Wheeldon

Contents

Introduction	*330*
Organisation of the respiratory system	**330**
The upper respiratory tract	**330**
The lower respiratory tract	**331**
Larynx	332
Trachea	333
Bronchial tree	334
Blood supply	**336**
Respiration	**336**
Pulmonary ventilation	**337**
Mechanics of breathing	337
Work of breathing	**339**
Volumes and capacities	**340**
Control of breathing	**342**
External respiration	**343**
Gaseous exchange	343
Factors affecting diffusion	344
Ventilation and perfusion	**345**
Transport of gases	**345**
Transport of oxygen (O_2)	345
Transport of carbon dioxide (CO_2)	347
Acid base balance	**348**
Internal respiration	**350**
Conclusion	*350*
Glossary	*352*
References	*357*
Activities	*357*

Fundamentals of Anatomy and Physiology for Student Nurses, First Edition. Edited by Ian Peate, Muralitharan Nair.

Test your knowledge

- List five major structures of the upper and lower respiratory tract.
- What is the main function of the respiratory system?
- Describe the physiological process of breathing – which muscles are utilised?
- What factors may increase or decrease a person's rate and depth of breathing?

Learning outcomes

On completion of this section the reader will be able to:

- List the main anatomical structures of both the upper and lower respiratory tract
- Describe the events of pulmonary ventilation
- Explain how the body is able to control the rate and depth of breathing
- Discuss the principles of external respiration
- Describe how oxygen and carbon dioxide are transported around the body

Body map

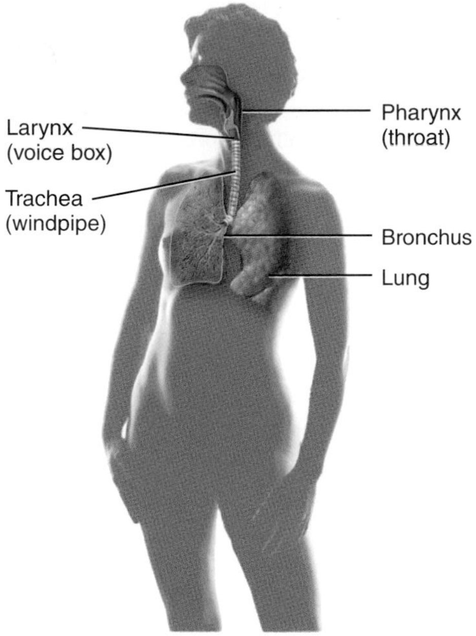
Larynx
(voice box)
Trachea
(windpipe)
Pharynx
(throat)
Bronchus
Lung

Introduction

Human cells can only survive if they receive a continuous supply of oxygen. As cells use oxygen a waste gas, carbon dioxide, is produced. If allowed to build up, carbon dioxide can affect cellular activity and disrupt homeostasis. The principal function of the respiratory system therefore is to ensure that the body extracts enough oxygen from the atmosphere and disposes of the excess carbon dioxide. The collection of oxygen and removal of carbon dioxide is referred to as respiration. Respiration involves the following four distinct processes: pulmonary ventilation, external respiration, transport of gases and internal respiration. Although all four are examined in this chapter only pulmonary ventilation and external respiration are the sole responsibility of the respiratory system. As oxygen and carbon dioxide are transported around the body in blood, effective respiration is also reliant upon a fully functioning cardiovascular system.

Organisation of the respiratory system

The respiratory system is divided into the upper and lower respiratory tract (see Figure 11.1). All structures found below the larynx form part of the lower respiratory tract. The respiratory system can also be said to be divided into conduction and respiratory regions. The upper respiratory tract and the uppermost section of lower respiratory tract form the conduction region, in which air is conducted through a series of tubes and vessels. The respiratory region is the functional part of the lungs, in which oxygen diffuses into blood. The structures within the respiratory region are microscopic, very fragile and easily damaged by infection. For this reason both the upper and lower respiratory tracts are equipped to fight off any invading airborne bacterial or viral pathogens.

The upper respiratory tract

Air enters the body via the nasal and oral cavities. The nasal cavity is divided into two equal sections by the nasal septum, a structure formed out of the ethmoid bones and the vomer of the skull. The space where air enters the nasal cavity just inside the nostrils is referred to as the vestibule. Beyond each vestibule the nasal cavities are subdivided into three air passageways, the meatuses, which are formed by three shelf-like projections called the superior, middle and inferior nasal conchae (see Figure 11.2). The region around the superior conchae and upper septum contains olfactory receptors, which are responsible for our sense of smell. The pharynx connects the nasal and oral cavity with the larynx. The pharynx is divided into three regions called the nasopharynx, the oropharynx and the laryngopharynx. The nasopharynx sits behind the nasal cavity and contains two openings that lead to the auditory (Eustachian) tubes. The oropharynx and laryngopharynx sit underneath the nasopharynx and behind the oral cavity. The oropharynx and oral cavity are divided by the fauces (see Figure 11.2). Both the oropharynx and the laryngopharynx are passageways for food and drink as well as air. To protect them from abrasion by food particles they are lined with non-keratinised stratified squamous epithelium.

As well as providing the sense of smell the upper respiratory tract also ensures that the air entering the lower respiratory tract is warm, damp and clean. The vestibule is lined with coarse hairs that filter incoming air, ensuring that large dust particles do not enter the airways. The conchae are lined with a mucous membrane made from pseudostratified ciliated columnar epithelium, which contains a network of capillaries and a plentiful supply of mucus-secreting goblet cells. The blood flowing through the capillaries warms the passing air while the mucus moistens

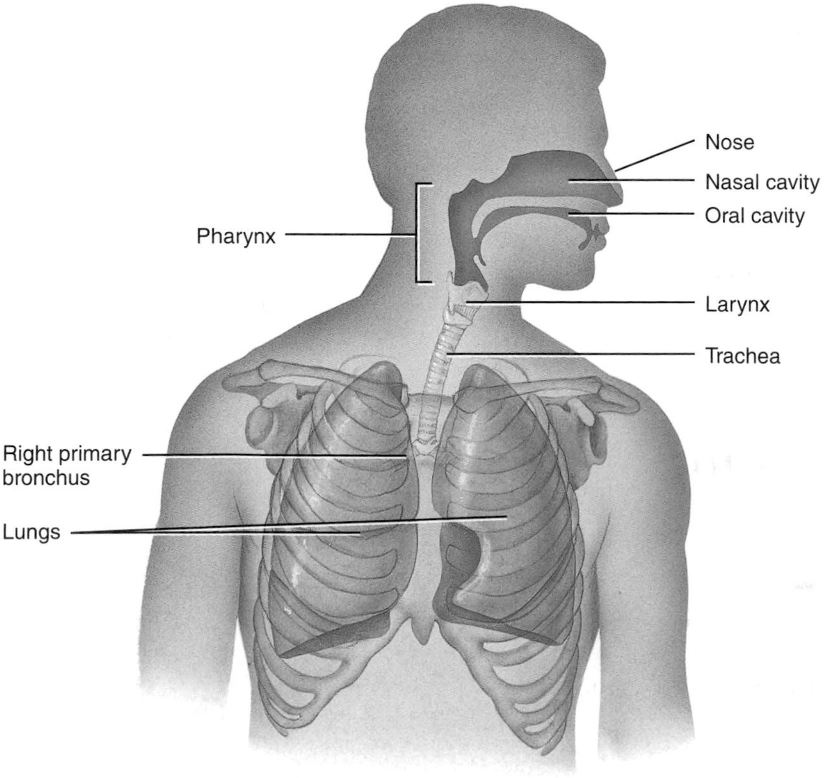
Nose
Nasal cavity
Oral cavity
Pharynx
Larynx
Trachea
Right primary bronchus
Lungs

Anterior view showing organs of respiration

Figure 11.1 Major structures of the upper and lower respiratory tract (Tortora and Derrickson 2009)

it and traps any passing dust particles. The mucus-covered dust particles are then propelled by the cilia towards the pharynx where they can be swallowed or expectorated.

To add further protection the upper respiratory tract is lined with irritant receptors, which when stimulated by invading particles (dust or pollen for example) force a sneeze, ensuring the offending material is ejected through the nose or mouth. The pharynx also contains five tonsils. The two tonsils visible when the mouth is open are the palatine tonsils, behind the tongue lie the lingual tonsils and the pharyngeal tonsil or adenoid sits on the upper back wall of the pharynx. Tonsils are lymph nodules and part of the body's defence system. The epithelial lining of their surface has deep folds, called crypts. Inhaled bacteria or particles become entangled within the crypts and are then engulfed and destroyed.

The lower respiratory tract

The lower respiratory tract includes the larynx, the trachea, the right and left primary bronchi and all the constituents of both lungs (see Figure 11.3). The lungs are two coned-shaped organs that

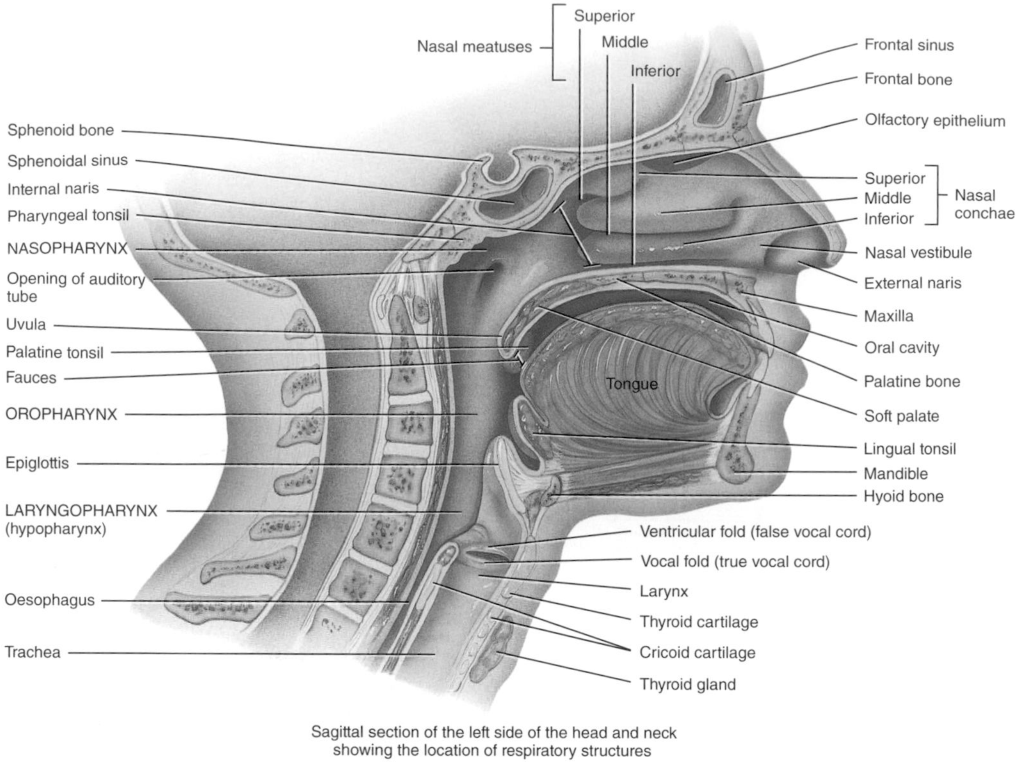
Nasal meatuses
Superior
Middle
Inferior
Frontal sinus
Frontal bone
Olfactory epithelium
Sphenoid bone
Sphenoidal sinus
Internal naris
Pharyngeal tonsil
NASOPHARYNX
Opening of auditory tube
Uvula
Palatine tonsil
Fauces
OROPHARYNX
Epiglottis
LARYNGOPHARYNX (hypopharynx)
Oesophagus
Trachea
Superior
Middle
Inferior
Nasal conchae
Nasal vestibule
External naris
Maxilla
Oral cavity
Palatine bone
Soft palate
Tongue
Lingual tonsil
Mandible
Hyoid bone
Ventricular fold (false vocal cord)
Vocal fold (true vocal cord)
Larynx
Thyroid cartilage
Cricoid cartilage
Thyroid gland
Sagittal section of the left side of the head and neck showing the location of respiratory structures

Figure 11.2 Structures of the upper respiratory tract (Tortora and Derrickson 2009)

almost fill the thorax. They are protected by a framework of bones, the thoracic cage, which consists of the ribs, sternum (breast bone) and vertebrae (spine). The tip of each lung, the apex, extends just above the clavicle (collar bone) and their wider bases sit just above a concave muscle called the diaphragm. The larynx (voice box) connects the trachea and the laryngopharynx. The remainder of the lower respiratory tract divides into branches of airways. For this reason the structure of the lower respiratory tract is often referred to as the bronchial tree.

Larynx

The larynx consists of nine pieces of cartilage tissue, three single pieces and three pairs (see Figure 11.4). The single pieces of cartilage are the thyroid cartilage, the epiglottis and the cricoid cartilage. The thyroid cartilage is more commonly known as the Adam's apple and, together with the cricoid cartilage, protects the vocal cords. The cricothyroid ligament, which connects the thyroid and cricoid cartilage, is the landmark of an emergency airway or tracheostomy (Russell and Matta 2004). The epiglottis is a leaf-shaped piece of elastic cartilage attached to the top of the larynx. Its function is to protect the airway from food and water. On swallowing, the epiglottis blocks entry to the larynx and food and liquids are diverted towards the oesophagus, which sits nearby. Inhalation of solid or liquid substances can block the lower respiratory tract and cut off the body's

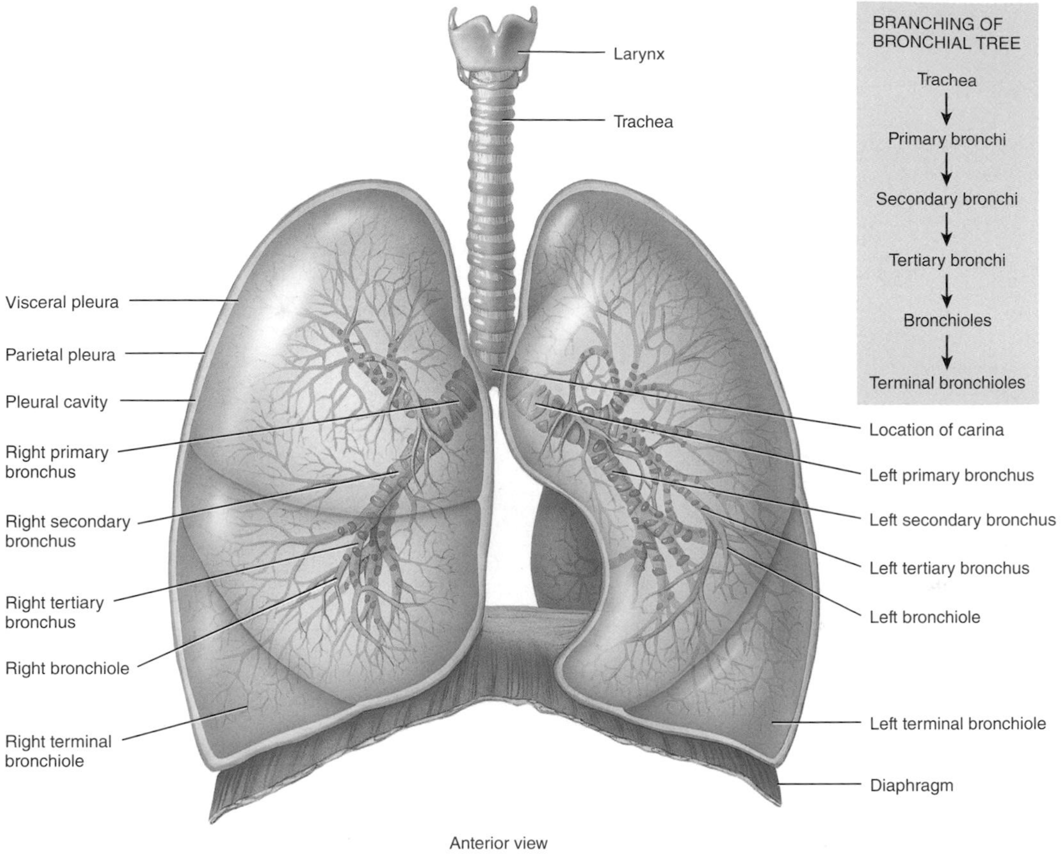
Larynx
Trachea
BRANCHING OF BRONCHIAL TREE
Trachea
Primary bronchi
Secondary bronchi
Tertiary bronchi
Bronchioles
Terminal bronchioles
Visceral pleura
Parietal pleura
Pleural cavity
Right primary bronchus
Right secondary bronchus
Right tertiary bronchus
Right bronchiole
Right terminal bronchiole
Location of carina
Left primary bronchus
Left secondary bronchus
Left tertiary bronchus
Left bronchiole
Left terminal bronchiole
Diaphragm
Anterior view

Figure 11.3 Gross anatomy of the lower respiratory tract (Tortora and Derrickson 2009)

supply of oxygen – this medical emergency is referred to as aspiration and necessitates the swift removal of the offending substance.

The three pairs of cartilage are the arytenoid, cuneiform and corniculate cartilages (see Figure 11.4). The arytenoid cartilages are the most significant as they influence the movement of the mucous membranes (true vocal folds) that generate the voice. Speaking therefore is reliant upon a fully functioning respiratory system. Many obstructive lung disorders, such as asthma, reduce a person's ability to speak a full sentence without drawing a new breath (Corbridge and Corbridge 2004).

Trachea

The trachea (or windpipe) is a tubular vessel that carries air from the larynx down towards the lungs. The trachea is also lined with pseudostratified ciliated columnar epithelium so that any inhaled debris is trapped and propelled upwards towards the oesophagus and pharynx to be swallowed or expectorated. The trachea and the bronchi also contain irritant receptors, which stimulate a cough, forcing larger invading particles upwards. The outermost layer of the trachea

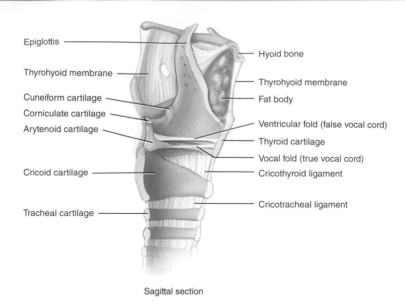

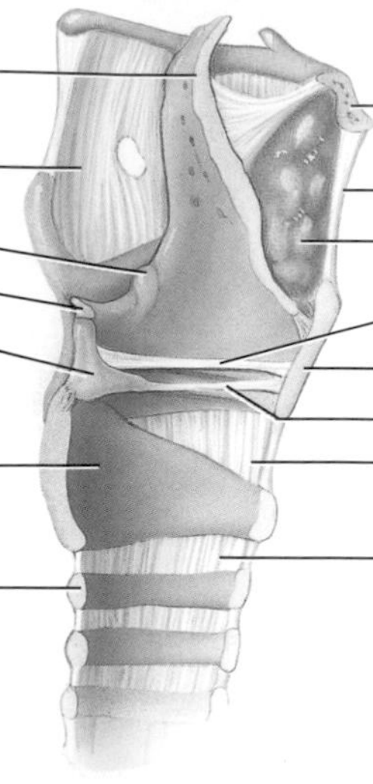
Epiglottis
Thyrohyoid membrane
Cuneiform cartilage
Corniculate cartilage
Arytenoid cartilage
Cricoid cartilage
Tracheal cartilage
Hyoid bone
Thyrohyoid membrane
Fat body
Ventricular fold (false vocal cord)
Thyroid cartilage
Vocal fold (true vocal cord)
Cricothyroid ligament
Cricotracheal ligament
Sagittal section

Figure 11.4 Anatomy of the larynx (Tortora and Derrickson 2009)

contains connective tissue that is reinforced by a series of 16–20 C-shaped cartilage rings. The rings prevent the trachea from collapsing during an active breathing cycle.

Bronchial tree

The lungs are divided into distinct regions called lobes. There are three lobes in the right lung and two in the left. The heart, along with its major blood vessels, sits in a space between the two lungs called the cardiac notch. Each lung is surrounded by two thin protective membranes called the parietal and visceral pleura (see Figure 11.3). The parietal pleura lines the wall of the thorax whereas the visceral pleura lines the lungs themselves. The space between the two pleura, the pleural space, is minute and contains a thin film of lubricating fluid. This reduces friction between the two pleura, allowing the two layers to slide over one another during breathing. The fluid also helps the visceral and parietal pleura to adhere to each other, in the same way two pieces of glass stick together when wet.

Within the lungs the primary bronchi divide into the secondary bronchi, each serving a lobe (three secondary bronchi on the right and two on the left). The secondary bronchi split into tertiary bronchi (see Figure 11.3 and Figure 11.5) of which there are 10 in each lung. Tertiary bronchi continue to divide into a network of bronchioles, which eventually lead to a terminal bronchiole. The section of the lung supplied by a terminal bronchiole is referred to as a lobule and each lobule has its own arterial blood supply and lymph vessels. The bronchial tree continues to subdivide, with the terminal bronchiole leading to a series of respiratory bronchioles, which in turn generate several alveolar ducts. The airways terminate with numerous sphere-like structures called alveoli, which are clustered together to form alveolar sacs (see Figure 11.6). There is an average of 480

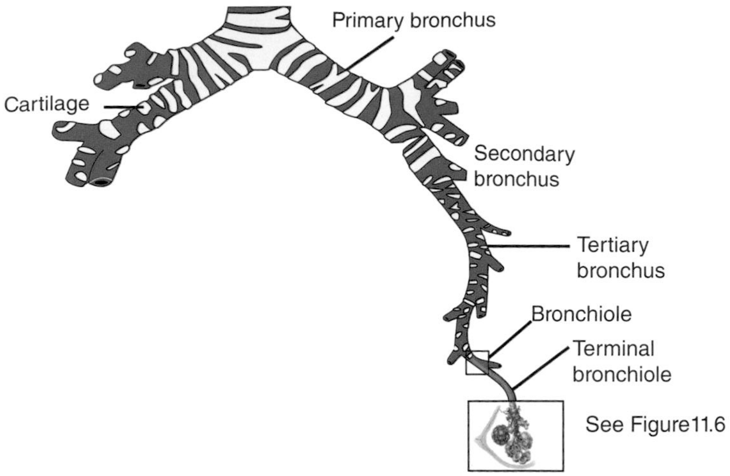
Primary bronchus
Cartilage
Secondary bronchus
Tertiary bronchus
Bronchiole
Terminal bronchiole
See Figure11.6

Figure 11.5 The bronchial tree (Nair and Peate 2009)

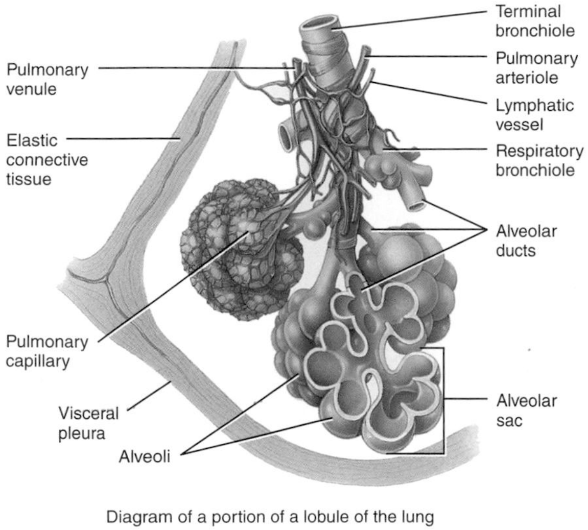
Terminal bronchiole
Pulmonary venule
Pulmonary arteriole
Lymphatic vessel
Elastic connective tissue
Respiratory bronchiole
Alveolar ducts
Pulmonary capillary
Visceral pleura
Alveolar sac
Alveoli
Diagram of a portion of a lobule of the lung

Figure 11.6 Microscopic anatomy of a lobule (Tortora and Derrickson 2009)

million alveoli in human lungs (Ochs *et al.* 2004). The transfer of oxygen from air to blood only occurs from the respiratory bronchiole onwards. All of the airways from the trachea to the respiratory bronchioles form the conduction region of the lungs. The lobules from the respiratory bronchioles onwards constitute the functional respiratory region of the lungs. The respiratory region accounts for two-thirds of the lungs' surface area (Tortora and Grabowski 2003).

Blood supply

The conduction and respiratory regions of the lungs receive blood from different arteries. Deoxygenated blood is delivered to the lobules via capillaries that originate from the right and left pulmonary arteries. Once re-oxygenated, blood is sent back to the left-hand side of the heart via one of four pulmonary veins, ready to be ejected into systemic circulation (see Figure 11.7). The conduction region of the lungs receives oxygenated blood from capillaries that stem from the bronchial arteries, which originate from the aorta. Some of the bronchial arteries are connected to the pulmonary arteries but the majority of blood returns to the heart via the pulmonary or bronchial veins.

Respiration

The process by which oxygen and carbon dioxide are exchanged between the atmosphere and body cells is called respiration. Respiration follows the following four distinct phases:

- Pulmonary ventilation – how air gets in and out of the lungs
- External respiration – how oxygen diffuses from the lungs to the bloodstream and how carbon dioxide diffuses from blood and to the lungs

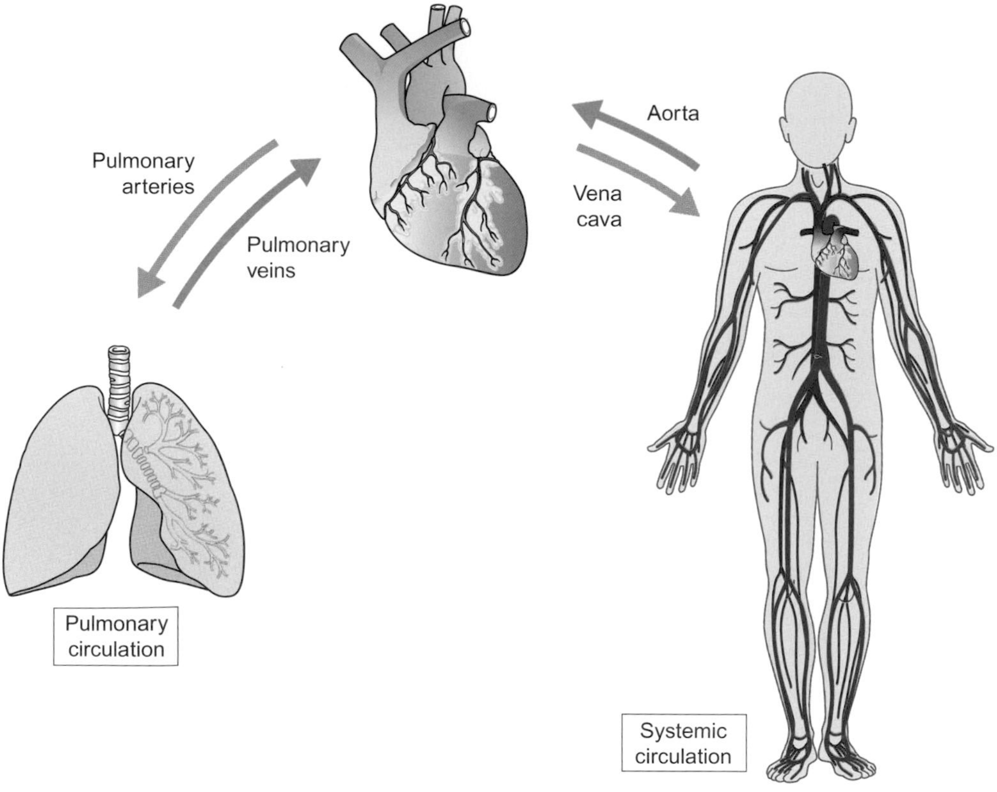
Pulmonary arteries
Pulmonary veins
Aorta
Vena cava
Pulmonary circulation
Systemic circulation

Figure 11.7 The flow of blood between the lungs, the heart and the body

Table 11.1 Summary of important gas laws (Davies and Moores 2003)

Gas law	Summary	Clinical application
Boyle's law	The pressure exerted by gas is inversely proportional to its volume	As the thorax expands intrapulmonary pressure falls below atmospheric pressure
Dalton's law	In a mixture of gases each gas will exert its own individual pressure, as if no other gases are present	Differences in partial pressure govern the movement of oxygen and carbon dioxide between the atmosphere, the lungs and blood
Henry's law	The quantity of gas that will dissolve in a liquid is proportional to its pressure and its solubility	Oxygen and carbon dioxide are soluble in water and are transported in blood. Nitrogen is highly insoluble and despite accounting for 79% of the atmosphere very little is dissolved in blood
Fick's law	The rate a gas will diffuse across a permeable membrane will depend upon pressure difference, surface area, diffusion distance and molecular weight and solubility	Helps explain how altitude, exercise and respiratory disease can influence the amount of oxygen that is diffused into blood

- Transport of gases – how oxygen and carbon dioxide are transported between the lungs and body tissues
- Internal respiration – how oxygen is delivered to and carbon dioxide collected from body cells.

The understanding of all four processes is reliant upon the appreciation of a series of gas laws, which are summarised in Table 11.1.

Pulmonary ventilation

Mechanics of breathing

Pulmonary ventilation describes the process more commonly known as breathing. In order for air to pass in and out of our lungs a change in pressure needs to occur. Before inspiration intrapulmonary pressure, the pressure within the lungs, is the same as atmospheric pressure. During inspiration the thorax expands and intrapulmonary pressure falls below atmospheric pressure. Because intrapulmonary pressure is now less than atmospheric pressure air will naturally enter our lungs until the pressure difference no longer exists. This phenomenon is explained by Boyle's law and Dalton's law. Gases exert pressure and Boyle's law states that the amount of pressure exerted is inversely proportional to the size of its container. Larger volumes provide greater space for the circulation of gas molecules and therefore less pressure is exerted. In smaller volumes gas molecules are more likely to collide with the walls of the container and exert a greater pressure as a result (see Figure 11.8). Dalton's law explains that in a mixture of gases each gas exerts its own individual pressure proportional to its size. For example, atmospheric air contains a mixture of gases. Each individual gas will exert its own pressure dependent upon its quantity. Nitrogen, for example, will exert the greatest pressure as it is the most abundant gas. Collectively, all the gases in the atmosphere exert a pressure, atmospheric pressure, which is 101.3 Kilopascals (kPa) at sea level (see Table 11.2). On inhalation the thorax expands, intrapulmonary pressure falls below 101.3 kPa and air enters the lungs because air flows from areas of high pressure to low pressure (McGowan *et al.* 2003).

A range of respiratory muscles are used to achieve thoracic expansion during inspiration (see Figure 11.9). The major muscles of inspiration are the diaphragm and external intercostal muscles.

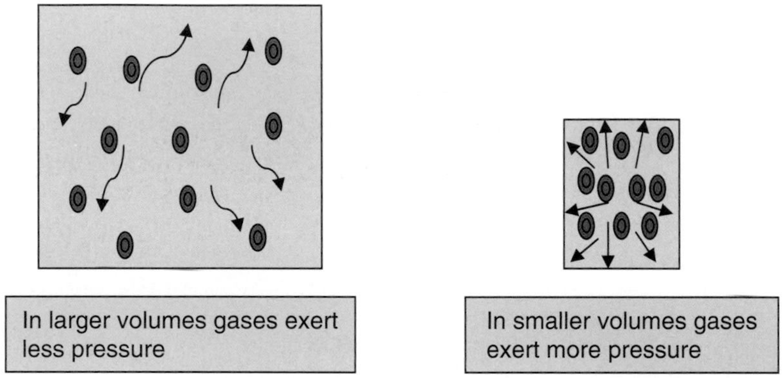
In larger volumes gases exert less pressure
In smaller volumes gases exert more pressure

Figure 11.8 Boyle's law – The volume of a gas varies inversely with its pressure

Table 11.2 The proportion of gases that constitute the atmosphere (partial pressures are expressed as P_{gas} (Brimblecombe 1986; Lutgens and Tarbuck 2001; Lumb 2005)

Gas	Volume	Pressure
Nitrogen (P_{N_2})	78.084%	79.055 kPa
Oxygen (P_{O_2})	20.946%	21.218 kPa
Carbon dioxide (P_{CO_2})	0.035%	0.0355 kPa
Argon (P_{AR})	0.934%	0.946 kPa
Other gases (neon, helium, methane, krypton, nitrous oxide, hydrogen, ozone, xenon)	0.001%	0.001 kPa
Total		
atmospheric pressure (P_B)	100%	101.3 kPa

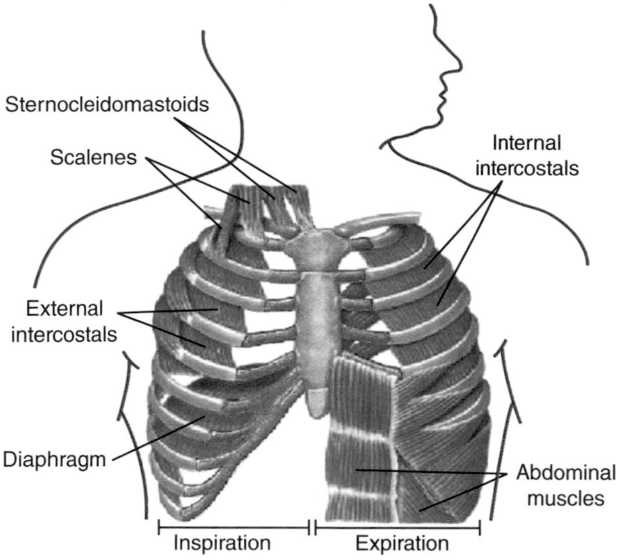
Sternocleidomastoids
Scalenes
Internal intercostals
External intercostals
Diaphragm
Abdominal muscles
Inspiration
Expiration

Figure 11.9 The muscles involved in pulmonary ventilation (Nair and Peate 2009)

The diaphragm is a dome-shaped skeletal muscle found beneath the lungs at the base of the thorax. There are 11 external intercostal muscles, which sit in the intercostal spaces – the spaces between the ribs. During inspiration the diaphragm contracts downwards, pulling the lungs with it. Simultaneously, the external intercostal muscles pull the rib cage outwards and upwards. The thorax is now bigger than before and intrapulmonary pressure is reduced below atmospheric pressure as a result. The most important muscle of inspiration is the diaphragm, 75% of the air that enters the lungs is as a result of diaphragmatic contraction. Expiration is a more passive process. The external intercostal muscles and the diaphragm relax allowing the natural elastic recoil of the lung tissue to spring back into shape, forcing air back into the atmosphere (see Figure 11.10).

Other respiratory muscles can be also be utilised. The abdominal wall muscles and internal intercostal muscles, for instance, are utilised to force air out beyond a normal breath, when playing a musical instrument or blowing out candles on a birthday cake, for example. The sternocleidomastoids, the scalenes and the pectoralis can also be used to produce a deep forceful inspiration. These muscles are referred to as accessory muscles, so called because they are rarely used in normal, quiet breathing (Simpson 2006).

Work of breathing

During inspiration respiratory muscles must overcome various factors that hinder thoracic expansion. The natural elastic recoil of lung tissue, the resistance to airflow through narrow airways and the surface tension forces at the liquid/air interface in the lobule all oppose thoracic expansion. The energy required by the respiratory muscles to overcome these hindering forces is referred to as work of breathing. The amount of energy expended is kept to a minimum by the ease with which lungs can be stretched. This ease of stretch is called lung compliance. Because of lung

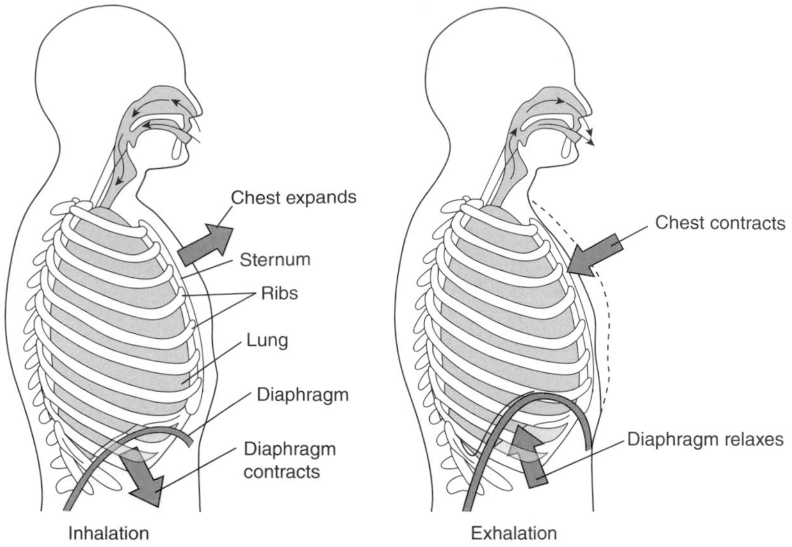
Chest expands
Sternum
Ribs
Lung
Diaphragm
Diaphragm contracts
Inhalation
Chest contracts
Diaphragm relaxes
Exhalation

Figure 11.10 Movements of inspiration and expiration (Nair and Peate 2009)

compliance an inhalation of around 500 ml of air is achievable without any noticeable effort. Blowing a similar amount of air into a balloon would take a much greater effort. Lung compliance is aided by the production of a detergent-like substance called surfactant. Whenever a liquid and gas come into close contact with one another surface tension is generated. Surfactant reduces the surface tension that occurs where the alveoli meet pulmonary capillary blood flow in the lobule, thereby reducing the amount of energy required to inflate the alveoli. Surfactant is manufactured by type II alveolar cells, found in the alveoli.

Work of breathing is also required to overcome airway resistance. As air flows through the bronchial tree resistance to airflow occurs as the gas molecules begin to collide with one another in the increasingly narrow airways. Despite these opposing forces work of breathing accounts for less than 5% of total body energy expenditure. However, many lung diseases can affect lung compliance and airway resistance and therefore increase work of breathing. In asthma, for example, airway inflammation reduces the diameter of the airways and increases airway resistance. If the diameter of an airway is halved, resistance increases 16-fold. Lung diseases that damage lung tissue can also affect lung compliance. Any increase in airway resistance and lung compliance will inevitably increase work of breathing. In acute respiratory disease work of breathing could account of up to 30% of total body energy expenditure (Levitzky *et al.* 1990).

Volumes and capacities

Lung volumes and capacities measure or estimate the amount of air passing in and out of the lungs. Each individual has a total lung capacity (TLC), which is the total amount of air their lungs are capable of housing. Each individual's TLC will be dependent upon their age, sex and height. Total lung capacity can be subdivided into a range of potential or actual volumes of air. For example, the amount of air that passes in and out of the lungs during one breath is called the tidal volume (V_T). After a normal, quiet breath the lungs will still have room for a deeper inspiration that could fill the lungs. This potential capacity for inspiration is referred to as inspiratory reserve volume (IRV). Likewise, after a normal, quiet breath, there remains the potential for a larger exhalation. This potential capacity of exhalation is referred to as expiratory reserve volume (ERV). If tidal volume increases, due to exercise for example, IRV and ERV would be reduced. Tidal volume, inspiratory reserve volume and expiratory reserve volume can all be measured. However, because a small volume of air always remains in the lungs, total lung capacity can only be estimated, even after a maximal exhalation. This small volume of remaining air is called residual volume (RV). Because RV cannot be exhaled the total amount of air that could possibly pass in and out of an individual's lungs is a combination of tidal volume, inspiratory reserve volume and expiratory reserve volume, collectively referred to as vital capacity (see Figure 11.11).

Other important measures of lung volume include minute volume (V_E), alveolar minute ventilation (V_A) and anatomical dead space (V_D) (see Table 11.3). Minute volume (V_E) is the amount of air breathed in each minute and is calculated by multiplying tidal volume (V_T) by respiration rate. In health minute volume is around 6–8 litres per minute. However, only the air that travels beyond the terminal bronchioles will actually take part in gaseous exchange. For this reason the air present in the rest of the lungs is referred to as anatomical dead space (V_D). In order to ascertain exactly how much air is available for gaseous exchange each minute anatomical dead space must be accounted for. Alveolar minute ventilation (V_A) is calculated by subtracting anatomical dead space from minute volume, which in health would be approximately 4–6 litres per minute (McGowan *et al.* 2003).

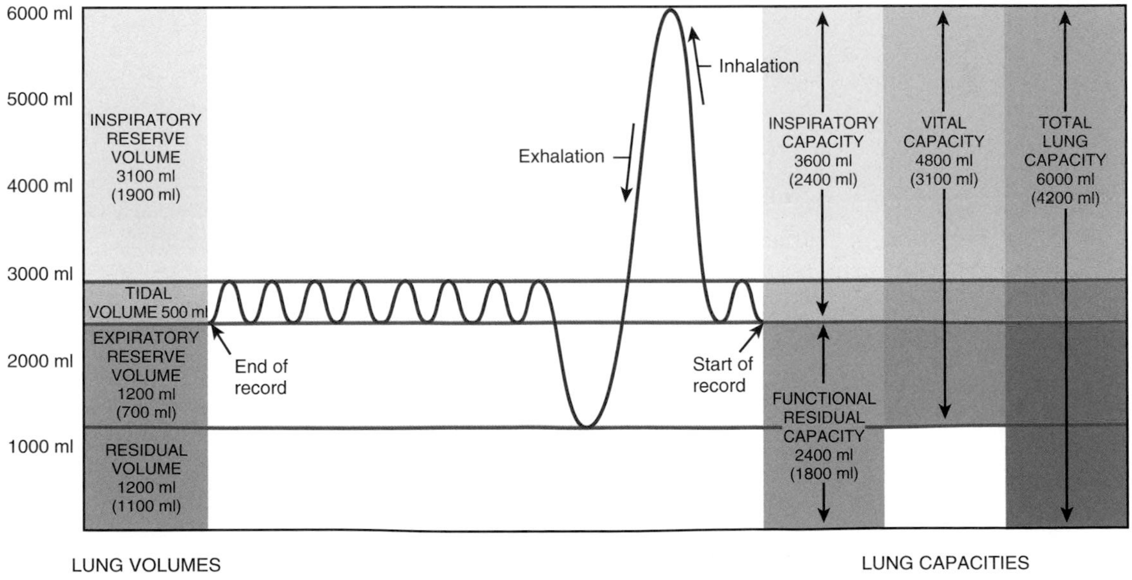
6000 ml
5000 ml
4000 ml
3000 ml
2000 ml
1000 ml
INSPIRATORY RESERVE VOLUME 3100 ml (1900 ml)
TIDAL VOLUME 500 ml
EXPIRATORY RESERVE VOLUME 1200 ml (700 ml)
RESIDUAL VOLUME 1200 ml (1100 ml)
End of record
Exhalation
Inhalation
Start of record
INSPIRATORY CAPACITY 3600 ml (2400 ml)
VITAL CAPACITY 4800 ml (3100 ml)
TOTAL LUNG CAPACITY 6000 ml (4200 ml)
FUNCTIONAL RESIDUAL CAPACITY 2400 ml (1800 ml)
LUNG VOLUMES
LUNG CAPACITIES

Figure 11.11 Diagrammatic description of the major lung volumes and capacities (Tortora and Derrickson 2009)

Table 11.3 Important lung volumes (Martini and Nath 2009)

Volume	Calculation
Minute volume (V_E)	Tidal volume (T_V) × Respiration rate e.g. 500 (T_V) × 12 = 6000 ml (V_E)
Alveolar minute ventilation (V_A)	(Tidal volume (T_V) – Anatomical dead space (V_D)) × Respiration rate e.g. (500 (T_V) – 150 (V_D) × 12 = 4000 ml (V_A)

Clinical considerations

Spirometry and peak flow

Spirometry measures the force and volume of a maximum expiration after a full inspiration. The air the patient forces out is referred to forced vital capacity (FVC). The volume the patient expired after 1 second is called forced expiratory volume in the first second (FEV_1). By comparing FEV_1 with FVC, the FEV_1:FVC ratio, the severity of airway obstruction can be ascertained. An FEV_1:FVC ratio of less than 80% is indicative of obstructive airways disease (Sheldon 2005).

Peak expiratory flow rate (PEFR) or 'peak flow' measures the extent of airway resistance. PEFR is the force of expiration in litres per minute. It measures the patient's maximum expiratory flow rate via their mouth. An inability to meet a predicted value based on age, sex and height could indicate increased airway resistance as occurs during an asthma attack. Peak expiratory flow rates provide a quick and simple assessment of the airways; however regular peak flow measurements are more revealing than single arbitrary readings and nurses should be mindful that peak expiratory flow rates are effort dependent (Talley and O'Connor 2001).

Control of breathing

The rate and depth of breathing are controlled by the respiratory centres, which are found in the brain stem, within the areas called the medulla oblongata and pons (see Figure 11.12). The rate of breathing is set by the inspiratory centre of the medulla oblongata. The expiratory centre is thought to play a role in forced expiration. Also within the medulla oblongata there are specialised chemoreceptors, which continually analyse carbon dioxide levels within cerebrospinal fluid (CSF). As levels of carbon dioxide rise messages are sent via the phrenic and intercostal nerves to the diaphragm and intercostal muscles instructing them to contract. Another set of chemoreceptors found in the aorta and carotid arteries analyse levels of oxygen as well as carbon dioxide. If oxygen falls or carbon dioxide rises, messages are sent to the respiratory centres via the glossopharyngeal and vagus nerves, stimulating further contraction. Breathing is refined by the actions of the pneumotaxic and apneustic centres of the pons (see Figure 11.12). The pneumotaxic centre sends inhibitory signals to the medulla to slow breathing down, while the apneustic centre stimulates the inspiratory centres, lengthening inspiration. Both these actions fine-tune breathing and prevent the lungs from becoming overinflated. Throughout the day, whether at work, rest or play, respiration rate will change in order to meet the body's oxygen needs.

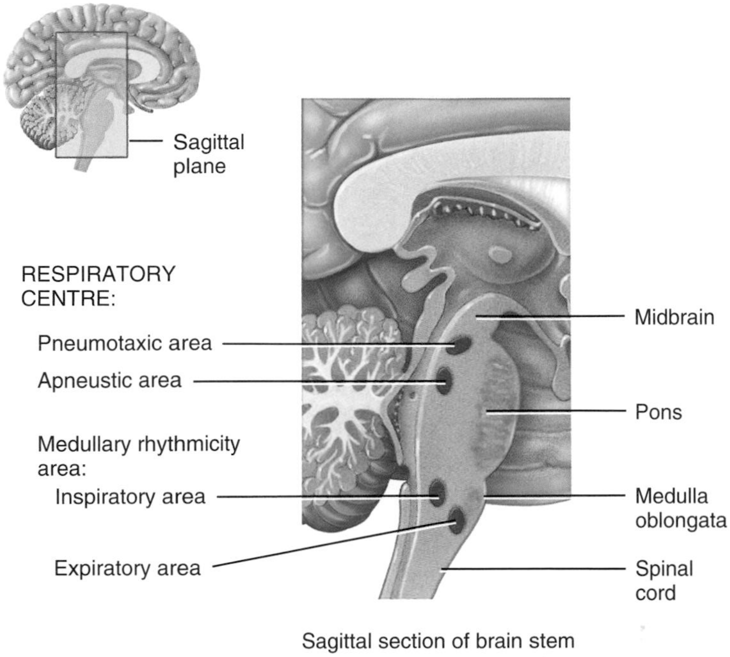
Sagittal plane
RESPIRATORY CENTRE:
Pneumotaxic area
Apneustic area
Medullary rhythmicity area:
Inspiratory area
Expiratory area
Midbrain
Pons
Medulla oblongata
Spinal cord
Sagittal section of brain stem

Figure 11.12 The respiratory centres of the brain stem (Tortora and Derrickson 2009)

Clinical considerations

Respiratory rate

In health, an adult's respiratory rate is normally between 12 and 16 respirations per minute. Although breathing is essentially a subconscious activity the rate and depth of breathing can be controlled voluntarily or even stopped altogether, when swimming underwater for example. However, this voluntary control is limited as the respiratory centres have a strong urge to keep breathing. Breathing can also be influenced by state of mind. The inspiratory area of the respiratory centres can be stimulated by both the limbic system and hypothalamus, two areas of the brain responsible for processing emotion. Fear, anxiety or even the anticipation of stressful activities can cause an involuntary increase in the rate and depth of breathing. Other factors that can affect breathing include pyrexia and pain. Because breathing is largely beyond an individual's control any changes in respiration rate are clinically significant (Hogan 2006).

External respiration

Gaseous exchange

External respiration only occurs beyond the respiratory bronchioles. External respiration is the diffusion of oxygen from the alveoli into pulmonary circulation (blood flow through the lungs) and the diffusion of carbon dioxide in the opposite direction. Diffusion occurs because gas molecules always move from areas of high concentration to low concentration. Each lobule of the lung has its own arterial blood supply; this blood supply originates from the pulmonary artery, which stems from the right ventricle of the heart. The blood present in the pulmonary artery has been collected from systemic circulation and is therefore low in oxygen and relatively high in carbon dioxide. The amount (and therefore pressure) of oxygen in the alveoli is far greater than in the passing arterial blood supply. Oxygen therefore moves passively out of the alveoli and into pulmonary circulation and on towards the left-hand side of the heart. Because there is less carbon dioxide in the alveoli than in pulmonary circulation carbon dioxide transfers into the alveoli ready to be exhaled (see Figure 11.13).

Factors affecting diffusion

It takes approximately 0.25 seconds for an oxygen molecule to diffuse from the alveoli into pulmonary circulation. However, there are various influencing factors that determine the rate by which oxygen and carbon dioxide diffuse between alveoli and pulmonary circulation. This is best explained by the use of Fick's law of diffusion, which uses an equation to determine the rate of diffusion (see box 11.1). According to Fick's law the rate of diffusion is determined by gas solubility/molecular weight, surface area, concentration difference and membrane thickness. The more soluble a gas is in water the easier it is for diffusion to occur. Oxygen (O_2) and carbon dioxide (CO_2) are both soluble in water and therefore easily diffused; indeed, CO_2 is 20 times more soluble than O_2. The most abundant gas in the atmosphere is nitrogen (N_2), however nitrogen is highly insoluble in water and therefore very little diffuses into the bloodstream. The larger the surface area available for diffusion the greater the rate of diffusion will be. Large inhalations will recruit more alveoli and a greater rate of diffusion occurs as a result. The greater the gas concentration difference between the alveoli and pulmonary circulation the faster that gas will diffuse. Because blood travelling towards the alveoli is deoxygenated there always remains a large difference in concentration of oxygen between the alveoli and pulmonary circulation. However, the rate of diffusion can be enhanced if this concentration difference is increased, by administering prescribed oxygen therapy for example. The final factor for consideration is membrane thickness. The further the distance gases have to travel the slower diffusion will be. Conditions such as pulmonary oedema, in which fluid collects in the alveoli, result in an increased distance between alveoli and pulmonary circulation and diffusion is slowed down as a result (Bassett and Makin 2000).

Box 11.1 Fick's law of diffusion (McGowan *et al.* 2003)

$J = (S/wt_{mol}) \times A \times \Delta C/t$

$J =$ rate of diffusion

$S/Wt_{mol} =$ solubility/molecular weight

$A =$ surface area

$\Delta C =$ concentration difference

$t =$ membrane thickness

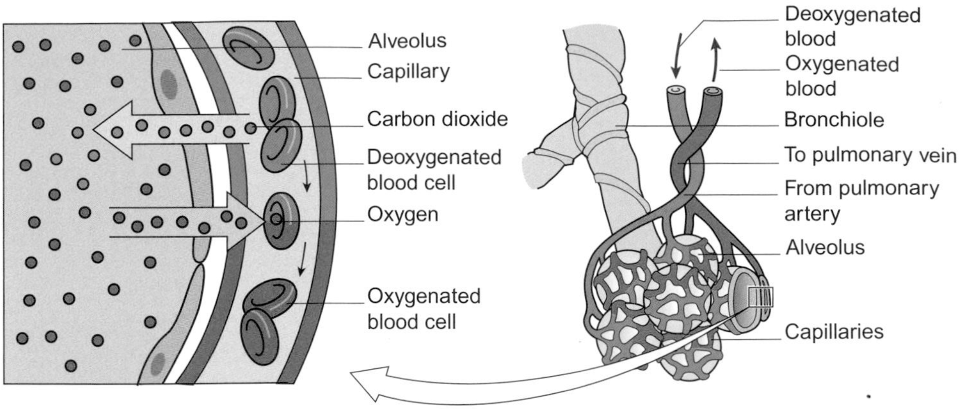
Alveolus
Capillary
Carbon dioxide
Deoxygenated blood cell
Oxygen
Oxygenated blood cell
Deoxygenated blood
Oxygenated blood
Bronchiole
To pulmonary vein
From pulmonary artery
Alveolus
Capillaries

Figure 11.13 External respiration – exchange of oxygen and carbon dioxide within the lungs

Ventilation and perfusion

External respiration is most effective where there is an adequate supply of both oxygen and blood. In order to ensure a good enough supply of oxygen the alveoli have to be adequately ventilated. In health an alveolar minute ventilation (V_A) of around 4 litres is required. In order to ensure that an adequate supply of blood is re-oxygenated a plentiful supply of blood must be delivered to the lungs from the right ventricle of the heart, in other words a pulmonary blood flow of around 5 litres per minute. This ideal delivery of adequate amounts of both air and blood is referred to as the ventilation V_A:perfusion Q ratio. A normal V_A:Q ratio would be 4:5 or 0.8. Any disruption to either ventilation or pulmonary blood flow would lead to a V_A:Q mismatch and less oxygen diffusing into blood. For example, if someone hypoventilates and V_A falls below 4 litres, then less blood would be re-oxygenated. This would be described as a low V_A:Q ratio – i.e. 3:5 or 0.3. Another potential problem would be an inadequate pulmonary blood flow due to an embolism for example. In such an instance less blood is available to be re-oxygenated and the V_A:Q ratio would become high – i.e. 4:3 or 1.34. In reality, however, the V_A:Q ratio differs throughout the lungs and depends upon a person's position (Margereson 2001).

Transport of gases

Both oxygen and carbon dioxide are transported from the lungs to body tissues in blood. Both gases travel in blood plasma and haemoglobin, which is found within erythrocytes (red blood cells). Key gas transport terminology is summarised in Table 11.4.

Transport of oxygen (O_2)

The vast majority of oxygen, around 98.5%, is transported attached to haemoglobin in the erythrocyte (red blood cell). Each erythrocyte contains around 280 million haemoglobin and each haemoglobin has the potential to carry for oxygen (O_2) molecules. The percentage of haemoglobin carrying oxygen is measured as an oxygen saturation (SaO_2). The remaining 1.5% of oxygen is dissolved in blood plasma, and is often measured in kilopascals (PaO_2), which in health is around

Table 11.4 Definitions of important gas transport terminology

Gas transport term	Definition
Oxygen saturation	SaO_2 The percentage of arterial haemoglobin carrying oxygen molecules SpO_2– SaO_2 measured by a pulse-oximeter
Partial pressure of arterial oxygen (PaO_2)	The amount of oxygen dissolved in arterial blood plasma measured in kilopascals (kPa)
Partial pressure of carbon dioxide ($PaCO_2$)	The amount of carbon dioxide dissolved in arterial blood plasma measured in kilopascals (kPa)
Oxygen capacity	The potential space for oxygen transport by haemoglobin (Hb) per 100 ml of blood Hb × 1.39 = oxygen capacity per 100 ml of blood
Arterial oxygen content (CaO_2)	The actual amount of oxygen in arterial blood carried by haemoglobin (Hb) per 100 ml of arterial blood Arterial oxygen saturation (SaO_2) × oxygen capacity = oxygen content per 100 ml of arterial blood
Oxygen delivery (DO_2)	The actual amount of oxygen being delivered to body tissues based on cardiac output. Arterial oxygen content (CaO_2) × cardiac output = oxygen delivery (DO_2)
Oxygen consumption (VO_2)/ oxygen extraction ratio	The amount of oxygen utilised by body tissues each minute

11–13.5 kPa (82–101 mmHg). The delivery of oxygen, therefore, is also reliant upon the presence of an adequate supply of erythrocytes and haemoglobin (Hb). In health the average male would possess between 15 and 18 g of haemoglobin (Hb) for every 100 ml of blood. Each gram of haemoglobin can carry approximately 1.39 ml of oxygen. Therefore a male with an Hb of 16 g/dl would have the capacity to carry 22.24 ml of oxygen for every 100 ml of blood ($16 \times 1.39 = 22.24$). This volume of oxygen is referred to as oxygen capacity. However, it is rare for an individual's haemoglobin to be fully saturated with oxygen. The actual amount of oxygen being transported by haemoglobin is called oxygen content (CaO_2). Oxygen content is determined by oxygen saturation levels. In health an individual's oxygen saturation level (SaO_2) would normally be between 97% and 99%. Therefore a male with an Hb of 16 g/dl and an SaO_2 of 98% would have an oxygen content of 21.8 ml (0.98×22.24). CaO_2 only provides the amount of available oxygen per 100 ml of blood. Multiplying CaO_2 by cardiac output will provide the amount of oxygen being delivered to all body tissues each minute. This volume of oxygen is called oxygen delivery (DO_2). In other words, if cardiac output is 5000 ml per minute, the aforementioned individual would have an oxygen delivery (DO_2) of 1090 ml per minute (21.8×5000).

The relationship between oxygen attached to arterial haemoglobin (SaO_2) and oxygen dissolved in plasma (PaO_2) is described by the oxyhaemoglobin dissociation curve (see Figure 11.14). As PaO_2 falls SaO_2 decreases in an S-shaped curve. If PaO_2 falls as low as 8 kPa (60 mmHg) SaO_2 will remain around 90%. Therefore natural fluctuations in oxygenation, such as occur when singing, laughing and talking, will not result in dramatic reductions in oxygen saturations. The release of oxygen from haemoglobin can be increased by 2,3-diphosphoglycerate (2,3-DPG), which is released during hypoxia and high temperatures.

Hypoxia and hypoxaemia

Hypoxia is defined as a lack of oxygen within body tissues. Hypoxaemia is defined as a lack of oxygen within arterial blood. Naturally hypoxaemia will lead to hypoxia as the tissues are receiving less oxygen. However as respiration also relies on a fully functioning cardiovascular system hypoxia can also occur even when arterial blood is fully oxygenated – see Table 11.5.

Transport of carbon dioxide (CO_2)

Just like oxygen (O_2) a small amount of carbon dioxide (CO_2), around 10%, is transported in plasma. Carbon dioxide is also transported attached to haemoglobin (Hb), although only around 30% is transported that way. Nevertheless haemoglobin has a greater affinity for carbon dioxide than oxygen. Within the tissues this facilitates the release of oxygen as carbon dioxide is being created. However as carbon dioxide levels increase (hypercapnia), the amount of oxygen binding to haemoglobin will be reduced. Any buildup of carbon dioxide will affect the oxyhaemoglobin dissociation curve by pulling the natural curve to the right, resulting in a greater risk of hypoxaemia. Conversely, a fall in carbon dioxide (hypocapnia) has the opposite effect (see Figure 11.14).

Clinical considerations

Sputum

Often the nurse has the responsibility to examine and observe the sputum (sometimes this is called phlegm, secretions or expectorate) that a person may produce. At times the nurse is required to obtain a specimen of the person's sputum for microbiological analysis. The nurse must be able to carry out these important tasks safely and effectively. The skills required to do this include the ability to determine what is sputum and what are oral secretions (spit), the application of infection control activities and the ability to document findings accurately and report any concerns.

The production of sputum is an important part of a person's immune system. You may be required to ask the person you are caring for about their sputum production. The following questions can help generate important information:

- Is there anything that causes (provokes) you to produce sputum?
- When do you produce it?
- How often do you produce it?
- Can you describe it – what does it look like?
- Does your sputum have any particular smell?
- How much do you produce?
- The sputum you are producing at the moment, has this changed recently? If so, tell me about that

It can be difficult for the person to provide you with answers concerning their sputum production. You can help them by asking them to measure it in relation to teaspoons, tablespoons or an egg cup. Understanding the sputum produced and describing and reporting its characteristics – for example, the consistency, the amount produced, the odour and its colour – can provide you with much information about the person you are caring for. Also note if the person producing the sputum did this with ease or difficulty, and if, after the specimen was produced, whether he/she became breathless or cyanotic.

If the person you are caring for needs to use a sputum pot, must make sure that it is placed within their reach and that you offer them tissues and a receptacle to dispose of the used tissues. Disposing safely of sputum can help prevent and control infection; sputum is potentially an infectious body fluid. Care interventions include ensuring that the sputum pot is changed daily and that the lid is firmly closed when it is not in use. Used tissues and sputum pots must be carefully disposed of regardless of the care setting. Disposable, one-use-only sputum pots must be provided. Incineration is needed if sputum is infectious. Local policy and procedure must be adhered to.

Clinical considerations

Measuring oxygen levels

Pulse oximeters gauge the percentage of haemoglobin carrying oxygen. This reading is called 'oxygen saturation' (SpO_2). In health SpO_2 should be between 95 and 99%, however tremors, anaemia, polycythaemia, cold extremities and nail varnish can all jeopardise an accurate reading. For this reason SpO_2 should only be used in conjunction with other nursing observations (Clark *et al.* 2006).

For a more accurate measure practitioners use an **arterial blood gas** reading. In such instances a sample of the patient's arterial blood is placed into a blood gas analyser. A printed or visual result is produced within seconds. Arterial blood gas readings provide information on pH, carbon dioxide and bicarbonate as well as oxygen. An oxygen saturation produced via blood gas analysis is referred to as SaO_2. In addition to an oxygen saturation blood gas analysis measures the pressure exerted by the oxygen dissolved in plasma. In health arterial oxygen should be around 11–13.5 kPa (82–101 mmHg) and is expressed as PaO_2 (partial pressure of arterial oxygen).

Acid base balance

The majority of carbon dioxide is transported as bicarbonate ions (HCO_3^-). As carbon dioxide enters the erythrocyte it combines with water to form carbonic acid (H_2CO_3). Carbonic acid then quickly dissociates into hydrogen ions (H^+) and bicarbonate ions (HCO_3^-). The formation of carbonic acid is very slow in plasma, in the red blood cell this reaction is speeded up by the presence of the enzyme carbonic anhydrase. The newly produced hydrogen ions (H^+) combine with haemoglobin, whereas bicarbonate leaves the erythrocyte and enters blood plasma. For this

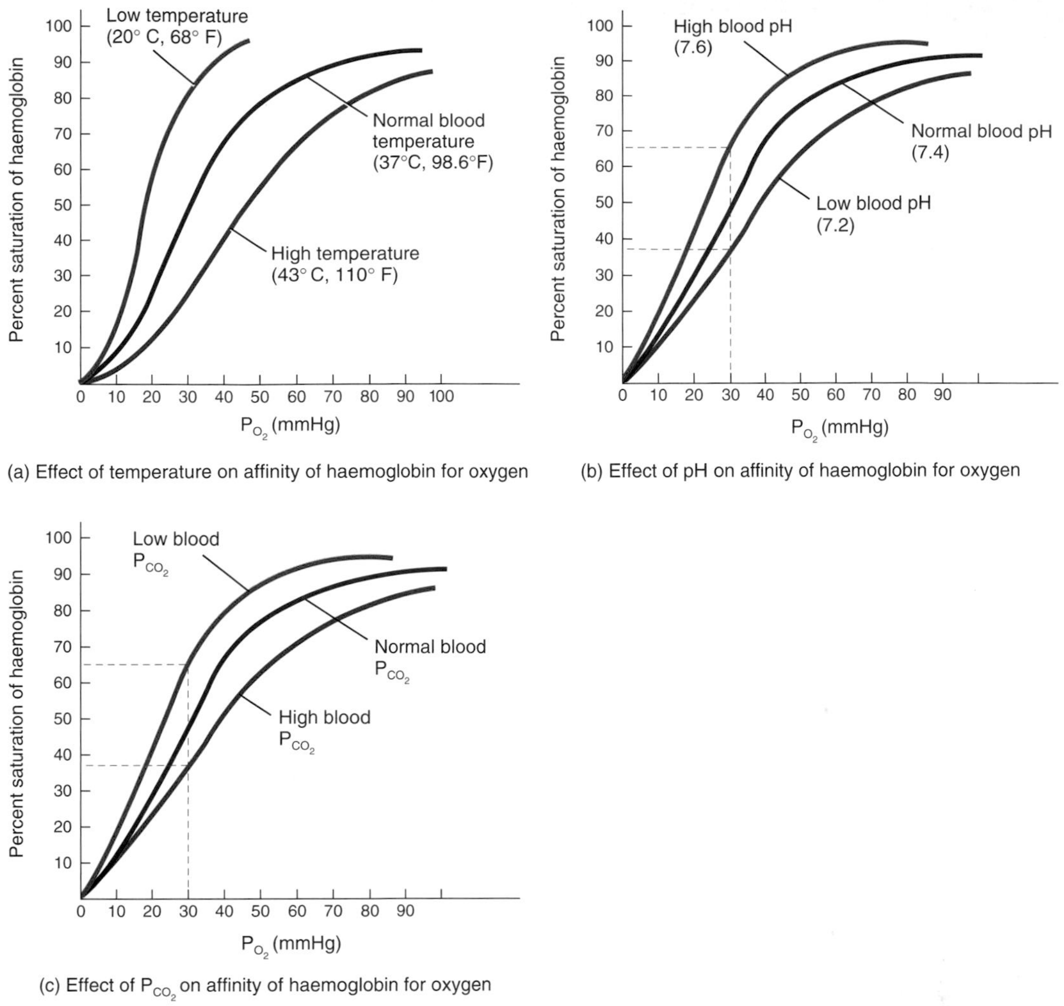
Low temperature (20° C, 68° F)
Normal blood temperature (37°C, 98.6°F)
High temperature (43° C, 110° F)
Percent saturation of haemoglobin
P_{O_2} (mmHg)
(a) Effect of temperature on affinity of haemoglobin for oxygen
High blood pH (7.6)
Normal blood pH (7.4)
Low blood pH (7.2)
(b) Effect of pH on affinity of haemoglobin for oxygen
Low blood P_{CO_2}
Normal blood P_{CO_2}
High blood P_{CO_2}
(c) Effect of P_{CO_2} on affinity of haemoglobin for oxygen

Figure 11.14 The oxyhaemoglobin dissociation curve: (a) at normal body temperature, arterial carbon dioxide levels and normal arterial blood pH, (b) with high or low arterial blood pH, and (c) with high or low arterial carbon dioxide levels (Tortora and Derrickson 2009)

Table 11.5 The major types of hypoxia and their causes

Type of hypoxia	Cause
Stagnant or circulatory hypoxia	Heart failure, lack of cardiac output, leads to hypoxia
Haemic hypoxia	Lack of blood or haemoglobin (haemorrhage for example)
Histotoxic hypoxia	Poisoning (e.g. carbon monoxide inhalation)
Demand hypoxia	May occur when the demand for oxygen is high (e.g. during fever)
Hypoxic hypoxia	Hypoxia as a result of hypoxaemia

reason increased and decreased levels of hydrogen ions can also influence the oxyhaemoglobin dissociation curve (see Figure 11.14). Within the lungs as carbon dioxide leaves pulmonary circulation and enters the alveoli this process is reversed. The transport of carbon dioxide as bicarbonate is summarised by the following equation. Note that the arrow symbols indicate that the equation moves both ways. For example at a tissue level the equation moves from left to right, whereas within the lungs it moves in the opposite direction.

$$\underset{\text{Carbon dioxide}}{CO_2} + \underset{\text{Water}}{H_2O} \leftrightarrow \underset{\text{Carbonic acid}}{H_2CO_3} \leftrightarrow \underset{\text{Hydrogen ions}}{H^+} + \underset{\text{Bicarbonate ions}}{HCO_3^-}$$

Arterial blood pH is mainly influenced by the levels of hydrogen ions (H^+). If blood pH falls out of its optimum range of 7.35 and 7.45 an acid base imbalance may occur. The respiratory system can help to maintain acid base balance by controlling the expulsion and retention of carbon dioxide (CO_2). When pH falls (acidosis), the respiration rate increases and more carbon dioxide is expelled. This results in greater amounts of hydrogen ions (H^+) and bicarbonate ions (HCO_3^-) combining to form carbonic acid (H_2CO_3). In other words, the above equation moves from right to left. There are now fewer hydrogen ions (H^+) and pH increases as a result. Carbonic acid is a weak acid and only has a minimal affect on blood pH. If blood pH rises, the opposite will occur. Respiration rate and depth may fall and carbon dioxide will be retained. The above equation will now move from left to right and more hydrogen ions (H^+) will be created.

Internal respiration

Internal respiration describes the exchange of oxygen and carbon dioxide between blood and tissue cells, a phenomenon governed by the same principles as external respiration. Cells utilise oxygen when manufacturing the cells' prime energy source, adenosine tri-phosphate (ATP). In addition to ATP the cells produce water and carbon dioxide. Because cells are continually using oxygen, its concentration within tissues is always lower than within blood. Likewise the continual use of oxygen ensures that the level of carbon dioxide within tissue is always higher than within blood. As blood flows through the capillaries oxygen and carbon dioxide follow their pressure gradients and continually diffuse between blood and tissue (see Figure 11.15). The concentration of oxygen in blood flowing away from the tissues back towards the heart is described as being deoxygenated. In reality, if measured, the oxygen saturation of venous blood would probably be around 75%. This means that only around 25% of oxygen content (CaO_2) leaves the bloodstream, leaving a plentiful supply. The actual amount of oxygen used by the tissues every minute is referred to as oxygen consumption (VO_2) or oxygen extraction ratio (OER) (see Table 11.4).

Conclusion

This chapter has examined the anatomy and physiology of the respiratory system. The respiratory system is divided into the upper and lower respiratory tracts. The lower respiratory tract consists of lung tissue and major airways. The structures within the lower respiratory tract are fragile and susceptible to infection, the main function of the upper respiratory tract therefore is the protection of the lower respiratory tract. The main function of the lower respiratory tract is the re-oxygenation of arterial blood and the expulsion of excess carbon dioxide – a process called respiration. Respiration involves four distinct physiological processes, pulmonary ventilation (breathing), external respiration (gaseous exchange), transport of gases and internal respiration. Only the first two processes are the sole responsibility of the respiratory system and effective respiration is also reliant upon a fully functioning cardiovascular system.

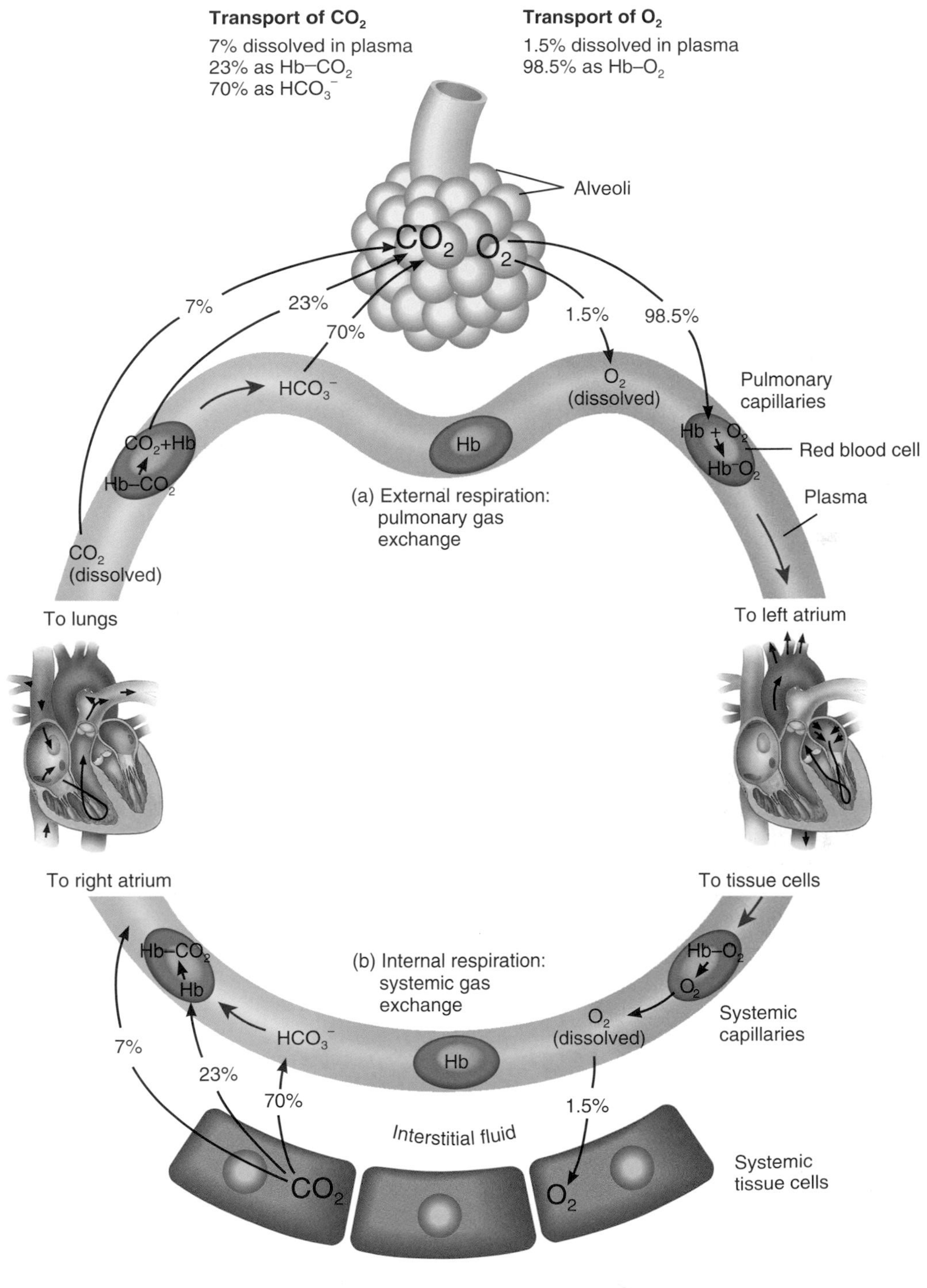
Transport of CO_2
7% dissolved in plasma
23% as Hb–CO_2
70% as HCO_3^-
Transport of O_2
1.5% dissolved in plasma
98.5% as Hb–O_2
Alveoli
CO_2
O_2
7%
23%
70%
1.5%
98.5%
HCO_3^-
O_2 (dissolved)
Pulmonary capillaries
CO_2+Hb
Hb–CO_2
Hb
Hb + O_2
Hb–O_2
Red blood cell
Plasma
(a) External respiration: pulmonary gas exchange
CO_2 (dissolved)
To lungs
To left atrium
To right atrium
To tissue cells
Hb–CO_2
Hb
Hb–O_2
O_2
(b) Internal respiration: systemic gas exchange
HCO_3^-
O_2 (dissolved)
Systemic capillaries
7%
23%
70%
Hb
1.5%
Interstitial fluid
CO_2
O_2
Systemic tissue cells

Figure 11.15 External and internal respiration – oxygen and carbon dioxide follow their pressure gradients (Tortora and Derrickson 2009)

Glossary

Accessory muscles: Muscles not normally involved in respiration that can be utilised to increase inspiration.

Acid base balance: The mechanisms by which the body maintains arterial blood pH between 7.35 and 7.45.

Alveolar minute ventilation: The amount of air reaching the respiratory portion of the lungs each minute.

Anatomical deadspace: The portion of the airway not involved in the exchange of oxygen and carbon dioxide (also referred to as the conducting zone).

Aorta: First major blood vessel of arterial circulation. Emerges from the left ventricle of the heart.

Apex: The tip or highest point of a structure.

Apneustic centre: Area of the pons (brain stem), which influences inspiration.

Arytenoid cartilage: Cartilage tissue involved in the production of the voice.

Aspiration: The inhalation of solid or liquid substances.

Asthma: A chronic inflammatory disorder of the lungs. It causes the bronchi and bronchioles to become inflamed and constricted. As a result airflow becomes obstructed, often resulting in a characteristic wheeze.

Auditory: Pertaining to the sense of hearing.

Bronchial artery: Artery which delivers oxygenated blood from the aorta to the bronchi and bronchioles.

Bronchial tree: The lower respiratory tract.

Bronchial veins: Veins which carry de-oxygenated blood from the bronchi and bronchioles to the superior vena cava.

Bronchiole: Section of the lower respiratory tract found beyond the tertiary bronchus.

Cardiac notch: The space between the right and left lung occupied by the heart and its major blood vessels.

Carotid artery: Major artery supplying the brain stems from the aorta.

Cartilage: Type of connective tissue which contains collagen and elastic fibres. Cartilage can stand up to both tension and compression.

Cilia: Hair-like extensions to the plasma membrane.

Cerebrospinal fluid (CSF): Fluid found within the brain and spinal cord.

Chemoreceptors:	Sensory cells sensitive to specific chemicals.
Chronic obstructive pulmonary disease (COPD):	An umbrella term that encompasses chronic bronchitis, emphysema and chronic asthma – respiratory diseases which obstruct airflow.
Clavicle:	Anatomical term for the collar bone.
Conducting zone:	Section of the airways which plays no part in the exchange of oxygen and carbon dioxide (also referred to as anatomical deadspace).
Corniculate cartilage:	Cartilage tissue involved in the production of the voice.
Cricoid cartilage:	Ring of cartilage that forms the lower part of the larynx (voice box).
Cricothyroid ligament:	Tissue that connects the thyroid cartilage and the cricoid cartilage, the main structures found in the larynx (voice box).
Cuneiform cartilage:	Cartilage tissue involved in the production of the voice.
Diaphragm:	Concave respiratory muscle that separates the lungs and the abdomen.
Diffusion:	The passive movement of molecules or ions from a region of high concentration to low concentration until a state of equilibrium is achieved.
Embolism:	Blockage of a blood vessel by a foreign substance or blood clot.
Epiglottis:	Leaf-shaped piece of cartilage that sits atop the larynx.
Ethmoid bone:	Sponge-like bone found in the skull. Forms part of the nasal septum.
Expectorate:	To cough up and spit out mucus or sputum.
Expiratory reserve volume:	The potential capacity for exhalation beyond a normal breath out.
External respiration:	The process by which oxygen and carbon dioxide are exchanged between the lungs and blood.
Fauces:	The opening into the pharynx from the oral cavity.
Glossopharyngeal nerve:	Cranial nerve IV – nerve that communicates with tongue and pharynx. Also transmits information on oxygen and carbon dioxide levels.
Goblet cells:	Mucus-secreting cells found in epithelial tissue.
Hypothalamus:	Region of the diencephalon area of the brain. Responsible for the maintenance of homeostasis.
Hypoxaemia:	A reduced amount of oxygen within arterial blood.
Hypoxia:	A reduced amount of oxygen within the tissues.
Hypoventilation:	Decreased ventilation – lack of air entering the alveoli.

Inspiratory reserve volume (IRV):	The potential capacity for inspiration beyond a normal breath in.
Intercostal nerves:	Nerves which link the respiratory centre in the brain stem with the intercostal muscles.
Intercostal spaces:	The anatomical spaces found between the ribs.
Internal respiration:	The process by which oxygen is exchanged for carbon dioxide within the tissues.
Intrapulmonary pressure:	The pressure exerted by all the gases present within the lungs.
Laryngopharynx:	The lower section of the pharynx (throat).
Larynx:	The physiological term for the voice box.
Limbic system:	Part of the functional brain, which processes emotion.
Lingual tonsils:	Tonsils found underneath the tongue.
Lobes:	Distinct regions of the lungs. There are three lobes in the right lung and two in the left lung.
Lobule:	Minute portion of lung tissue served by its own capillary.
Lower respiratory tract:	All respiratory passages found below the larynx.
Lung compliance:	The ease with which the lungs can be inflated.
Lymph nodules:	Egg-shaped masses of lymph tissues that provide an immune response.
Lymph vessel:	A vessel that carries lymphatic fluid. Part of the lymphatic system which forms part of the immune system.
Meatuses:	Three passageways found within the nasal cavity.
Medulla oblongata:	Area of the brain stem.
Minute volume (V_E):	The amount of air breathed in one minute.
Nasal cavity:	Anatomical space within the nose.
Nasal conchae:	Bones found within the nasal cavity.
Nasal septum:	Structure that divides the nose into two nostrils.
Nasopharynx:	The upper section of the pharynx (throat).

Non-keratinised stratified squamous epithelium: Cuboid or columnar-shaped cells that line and protect wet surfaces such as the mouth, oesophagus, epiglottis, tongue and vagina.

Oesophagus: Tubular vessel which carries food and liquid from the pharynx to the stomach.

Olfactory: Pertaining to the sense of smell.

Oropharynx: The middle section of the pharynx (throat).

Oxyhaemoglobin dissociation curve: An S-shaped curve that describes the relationship between the volume of oxygen attached to haemoglobin and the amount of oxygen dissolved in plasma.

Palatine tonsils: Tonsils found towards the rear of the oral cavity. Usually visible when the mouth is open.

Parietal pleura: Protective membrane which attaches the walls of the thorax to the lungs.

Pharyngeal tonsil: Tonsil that sits on the back wall of the pharynx. Also known as the adenoid.

Pharynx: Passageway for food and air, which links the nasal and oral cavity with the larynx. More commonly called the throat.

Phrenic nerve: Nerve which links the diaphragm to the respiratory centre in the brain stem.

Pleural space: The minute space between the visceral and parietal pleura.

Pneumotaxic centre: Portion of the medulla oblongata (brain stem) which influences inspiration.

Pons: Area of the brain stem.

Pseudostratified ciliated columnar epithelium: Covering or lining of internal body surface which contains cilia and mucus-secreting goblet cells.

Pulmonary artery: Artery which carries deoxygenated blood from the right-hand side of the heart towards the lungs.

Pulmonary ventilation: The process by which air enters and exits the lungs (breathing).

Pulmonary oedema: A condition characterised by the leakage of fluid into the alveoli.

Pulmonary veins: Veins which carry oxygenated blood from the lungs back to the left-hand side of the heart.

Pyrexia: Elevated temperature associated with fever.

Residual volume (RV): A small amount of air that permanently remains in the lungs.

Respiratory zone: The portion of lung tissue involved in the exchange of oxygen and carbon dioxide.

Sternum: Flat bone, which forms part of the thoracic cage. Protects the heart and lungs. Commonly referred to as the breastbone.

Surfactant: A detergent-like substance manufactured by cells of the alveoli, which reduces surface tension and increases lung compliance.

Systemic circulation: The flow of blood from the left ventricle and right atrium delivering oxygen to and collecting carbon dioxide from body tissues.

Thoracic cage: Framework of bones, which consists of the ribs, sternum (breast bone) and vertebrae (spine).

Thorax: The body trunk above the diaphragm and below the neck.

Thyroid cartilage: The outer wall of the larynx (voice box)

Tidal volume (T_v): The volume of air that passes in and out of the lungs during one breath.

Tonsils: Lymph nodules found within the upper respiratory tract. They form part of the body's defence.

Total lung capacity (TLC): The maximum amount of air that a person's lungs can accommodate.

Tracheostomy: A procedure in which an incision is made in the trachea to facilitate breathing.

Transport of gases: The process by which oxygen and carbon dioxide are delivered between the lungs and the tissues.

Upper respiratory tract: All structures of the respiratory system situated between the oral and nasal passageways and the larynx.

Vagus nerve: Cranial nerve X – major nerve in parasympathetic function. Also transmits information on oxygen and carbon dioxide levels.

Ventilation V_A: Perfusion Q ratio: The ratio of blood and air delivery to the lungs every minute. Ideally 4 litres of air to 5 litres of blood.

Vestibule: The space inside the nasal cavity, just inside the nostrils.

Visceral pleura: Protective membrane, which lines the lungs.

Vital capacity (VC): The maximum potential for inspiration and expiration, measured in litres.

Vomer: Triangular-shaped bone that forms the base of the nasal cavity.

References

Bassett, C. and Makin, L. (2000) *Caring For The Seriously Ill Patient.* London: Arnold.

Brimblecombe, P. (1986) *Air Composition and Chemistry*, 2nd edn. Cambridge: Cambridge University Press.

Clark, A.P., Giuliano, K. and Chen, H. (2006) Pulse oximetry revisited: 'but his O2 sat was normal!' *Clinical Nurse Specialist* 20(6):268–272.

Corbridge, S.J. and Corbridge, T.C. (2004) Severe exacerbations of asthma. *Critical Care Quarterly* 27(3):207–228.

Davies, A. and Moores, C. (2003) *The Respiratory System: Basic Science and Clinical Conditions.* Edinburgh: Churchill Livingstone.

Hogan, J. (2006) Why don't nurses monitor the respiratory rates of patients? *British Journal of Nursing* 15(9):489–492.

Levitzky, M.G., Cairo J.M. and Hall, S.M. (1990) *Introduction to Respiratory Care.* London: WB Saunders.

Lumb, A.B. (2005) *Nunn's Applied Respiratory Physiology*, 6th edn. Oxford: Butterworth-Heinemann.

Lutgens, F.K. and Tarbuck, E.J. (2001) *The Atmosphere: An Introduction to Meteorology*, 8th edn. Upper Saddle River, NJ: Prentice Hall.

Nair, M. and Peate, I. (2009). *Fundamentals of Applied Pathophysiology: An Essential Guide for Nursing Students.* Oxford: Wiley-Blackwell.

Margereson, C. (2001) Anatomy and physiology. In: Esmond, G. (ed.) *Respiratory Nursing.* Edinburgh: Baillière Tindall.

Martini, F.H. and Nath, J.L. (2009) *Fundamentals of Anatomy and Physiology*, 8th edn. San Francisco: Pearson Benjamin Cummings.

McGowan, P., Jeffries, A. and Turley, A. (2003) *Crash Course Respiratory System*, 2nd edn. London: Mosby.

Ochs, M., Nyengaard, A.J., Knudsen, L. Voigt *et al.* (2004) The number of alveoli in the human lung. *American Journal of Respiratory and Critical Care Medicine* 169:120–124.

Russell, C. and Matta, B. (2004) *Tracheostomy: A Multiprofessional Handbook.* Cambridge: Cambridge University Press.

Sheldon, R.L. (2005) Pulmonary function testing. In: Wilkins, R.L. and Krider, S.J. (Eds) *Clinical Assessment in Respiratory Care*, 5th edn. St Louis, MO: Elsevier Mosby.

Simpson, H. (2006) Respiratory assessment. *British Journal of Nursing* 15(9):484–488.

Talley, N.J. and O'Connor, S. (2001) *Clinical Examination: A Systematic Guide to Physical Diagnosis*, 4th edn. Oxford: Blackwell Science.

Tortora, G.J. and Grabowski, S.R. (2003) *Principles of Anatomy and Physiology*, 10th edn. New York: John Wiley & Sons.

Tortora, G.J. and Derrickson, B.H. (2009) *Principles of Anatomy and Physiology*, 12th edn. Hoboken, NJ: John Wiley & Sons.

Activities

www.wiley.com/go/peate

Multiple choice questions

1. Which of the following structures is not found in the upper respiratory tract?

   (a) palatine tonsils
   (b) turbinates
   (c) carina
   (d) fauces

2. Which of the following structures is found in the respiratory zone?
   (a) alveolar ducts
   (b) terminal bronchioles
   (c) tertiary bronchus
   (d) trachea

3. Which gas law states that each gas exerts a pressure that is inversely proportional to its volume?
   (a) Henry's law
   (b) Boyle's law
   (c) Dalton's law
   (d) Fick's law

4. Which of the following statements on pulmonary ventilation is true?
   (a) The diaphragm is responsible for 75% of thoracic expansion
   (b) Expiration is dependent upon external intercostal muscle activity
   (c) Intrapulmonary pressure is always greater than atmospheric pressure
   (d) The diaphragm and external intercostal muscles are two major accessory muscles

5. Which of the following lung volumes can only be estimated?
   (a) inspiratory reserve volume
   (b) total lung capacity
   (c) vital capacity
   (d) tidal volume

6. Tidal volume (V_T) – Anatomical dead space (V_D) × Respiratory Rate =
   (a) minute volume (V_E)
   (b) oxygen content (CaO_2)
   (c) alveolar minute ventilation (V_A)
   (d) vital capacity

7. Which of the following statements on work of breathing is true?
   (a) Increased airway diameter increases airway resistance
   (b) Surfactant increases alveolar surface tension
   (c) Lung disease can increase work of breathing
   (d) In health work of breathing accounts for 50% of total body energy expenditure

8. Where are the respiratory centres?

(a) the medulla oblongata and pons
(b) the hypothalamus
(c) the limbic system
(d) cerebral cortex

9. Which of the following could increase the rate of breathing?

(a) increased carbon dioxide (CO_2) levels
(b) decreased oxygen (O_2) levels
(c) pyrexia
(d) all of the above

10. Which of the following statements on external respiration is true?

(a) The concentration of oxygen is greater in pulmonary circulation than in the alveoli
(b) The concentration of carbon dioxide is greater in the alveoli than in pulmonary circulation
(c) Carbon dioxide diffuses from the alveoli into pulmonary circulation
(d) Oxygen diffuses from the alveoli into pulmonary circulation

11. Why does very little nitrogen diffuse into pulmonary circulation?

(a) because there is only a very small concentration difference
(b) because nitrogen is highly insoluble
(c) because nitrogen is 20 times more soluble than oxygen
(d) because there is insufficient surface area available

12. How much carbon dioxide is transported as bicarbonate ions (HCO_3^-)?

(a) 10%
(b) 30%
(c) 40%
(d) 60%

13. Reduced levels of oxygen in blood is called

(a) hypoxaemia
(b) hypercapnia
(c) hypocapnia
(d) hypoxia

14. Which of the following can be transported attached to haemoglobin (Hb)?

(a) oxygen (O_2)
(b) carbon dioxide (CO_2)
(c) hydrogen ions (H^+)
(d) all of the above

15. The amount of oxygen utilised by cells is referred to as

(a) oxygen content (CaO_2)
(b) oxygen delivery (DO_2)
(c) oxygen consumption (VO_2)
(d) oxygen capacity

Test your learning

1 What are the main functions of the upper respiratory tract?

2 Explain the main principle of pulmonary ventilation.

3 Describe the main lung capacities and volumes.

4 List the major factors that can increase respiration rate.

5 Explain why gaseous exchange occurs and what factors influence the rate of diffusion.

6 Explain how the respiratory system can help maintain acid base balance.

Label the diagram

From the lists of words, label the diagrams below:

Visceral pleura, Parietal pleura, Pleural cavity, Right primary bronchus, Right secondary bronchus, Right tertiary bronchus, Right bronchiole, Right terminal bronchiole, BRANCHING OF BRONCHIAL TREE, Trachea, Primary bronchi, Secondary bronchi, Tertiary bronchi, Bronchioles, Terminal bronchioles, Location of carina, Left primary bronchus, Left secondary bronchus, Left tertiary bronchus, Left bronchiole, Left terminal bronchiole, Diaphragm, Larynx, Trachea

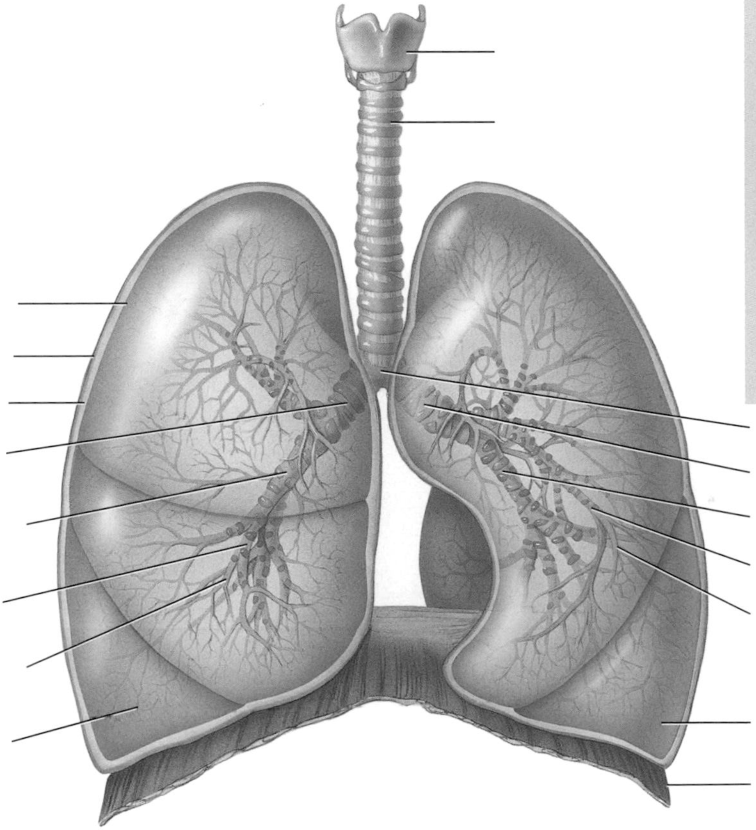

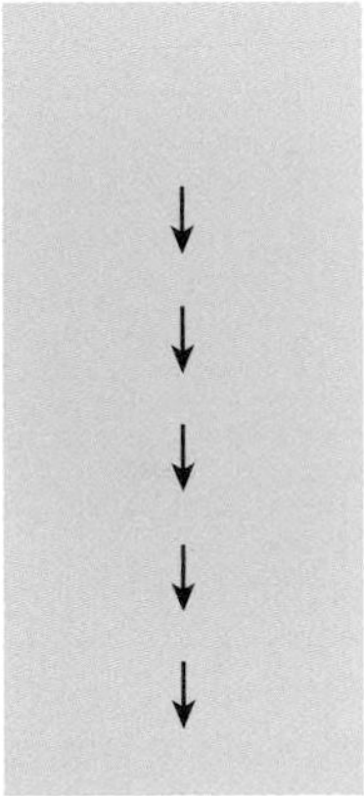

Pulmonary venule, Elastic connective tissue, Pulmonary capillary, Visceral pleura, Alveoli, Terminal bronchiole, Pulmonary arteriole, Lymphatic vessel, Respiratory bronchiole, Alveolar ducts, Alveolar sac

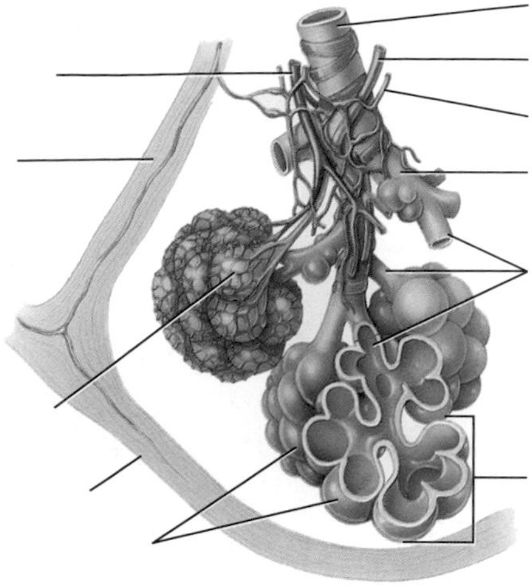

Sternocleidomastoids, Scalenes, External intercostals, Diaphragm, Internal intercostals, Abdominal muscles, Inspiration, Expiration

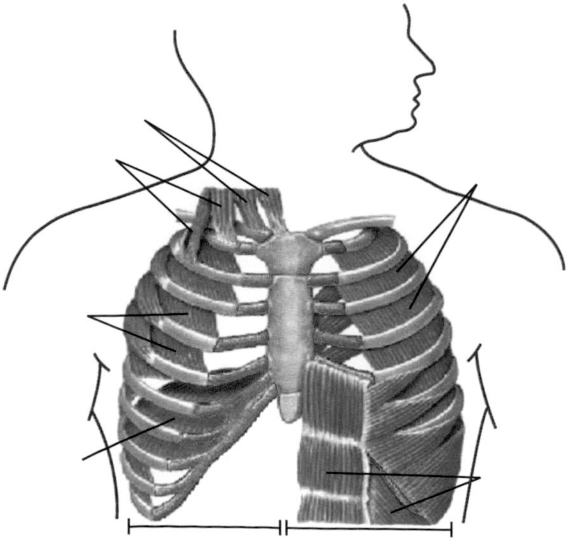

Crossword

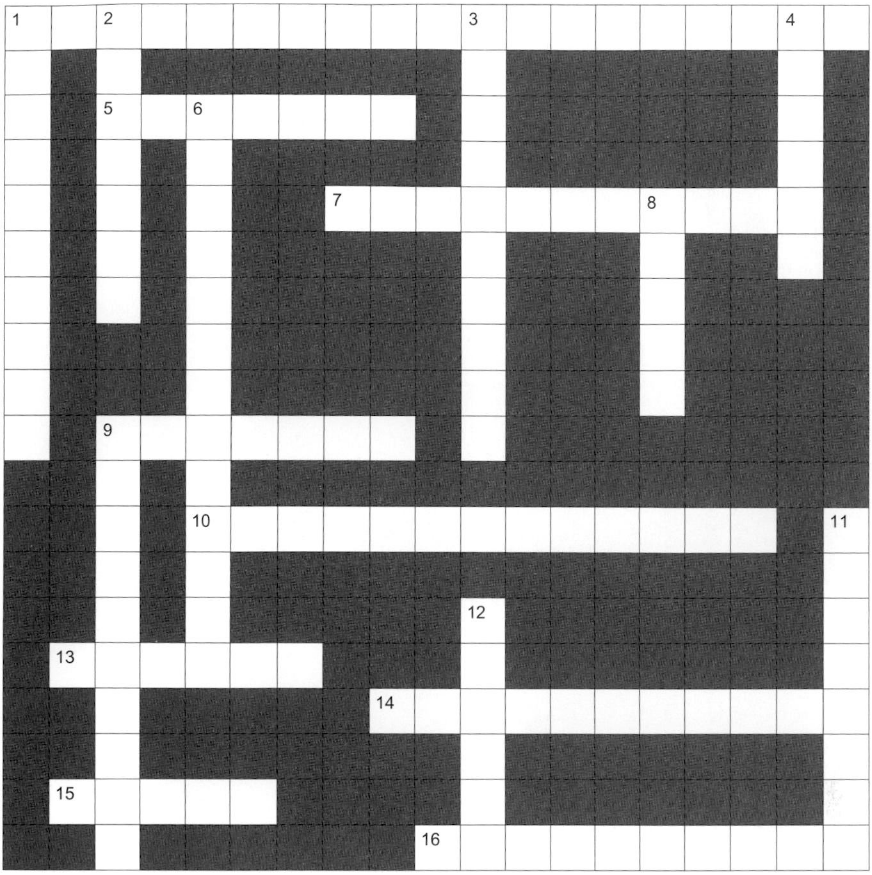
1
2
3
4
5
6
7
8
9
10
11
12
13
14
15
16

Across:

1. The process of gaseous exchange (8, 11).
5. Structure found in a lobule (7).
7. The amount of air inspired and expired during one breath (5, 6).
9. Diminished amount of oxygen in tissues (7).
10. Waste gas disposed by lungs (6, 7).
13. Voice box (6).
14. Main carrier of oxygen in blood (11).
15. ___________ law of diffusion (5).
16. Fast respiration rate (10).

Down:

1. Breathing out (10).
2. Connects the larynx to the bronchi (7).
3. Reduces surface tension in alveoli (10).
4. Gas essential for life (6).
6. Total lung volume minus residual volume (5, 8).
8. Your right lung has three, your left lung has two (5).
9. Diminished amount of oxygen in blood (10).
11. Difficulty in breathing (8).
12. Protective layer of the lungs (6).

Conditions

Below is a list of conditions that are associated with the respiratory system. Take some time and write notes about each of the conditions. You may make the notes taken from text books or other resources, for example, people you work with in a clinical area or you may make the notes as a result of people you have cared for. If you are making notes about people you have cared for you must ensure that you adhere to the rules of confidentiality.

Asthma	
Chronic obstructive pulmonary disease (emphysema and/or chronic bronchitis)	
Lung cancer	
Pneumonia	
Tuberculosis	
Bronchiectasis	

Answers

MCQs

1c; 2a; 3b; 4a; 5b; 6c; 7c; 8a; 9d; 10d; 11b; 12d; 13a; 14d; 15c

Crossword

Across:

1. External respiration
5. Alveoli
7. Tidal volume
9. Hypoxia
10. Carbon dioxide
13. Larynx
14. Haemoglobin
15. Fick's
16. Tachypnoea

Down:

1. Expiration
2. Trachea
3. Surfactant
4. Oxygen
6. Vital capacity
8. Lobes
9. Hypoxaemia
11. Dyspnoea
12. Pleura

12

The circulatory system

Muralitharan Nair

Contents

Introduction *368*
Composition of blood **368**
Properties of blood and plasma **369**
Blood plasma **370**
Water in plasma 371
Functions of blood **371**
Transportation 372
Formation of blood cells **374**
Red blood cells **374**
Haemoglobin 375
Formation of red blood cells 375
Life cycle of the red blood cell 376
Transport of respiratory gases 377
White blood cells **378**
Neutrophils 379
Eosinophils 379
Basophils 380
Monocytes 380
Lymphocytes 380
Platelets **382**
Haemostasis **382**
Vasoconstriction 382
Platelet aggregation 382
Coagulation 383
Blood groups **384**
Blood vessels **385**
Structure and function of arteries and veins 385
Capillaries 388
Blood pressure **389**
Physiological factors regulating blood pressure 389
Control of arterial blood pressure 390
Lymphatic system **391**
Lymph 391
Lymph capillaries and large lymph vessels 391
Lymph nodes 394
Lymphatic organs **394**
Spleen 394
The thymus gland 394
Functions of the lymphatic system **394**
Conclusion *396*
Glossary *397*
References *398*
Activities *398*

Fundamentals of Anatomy and Physiology for Student Nurses, First Edition. Edited by Ian Peate, Muralitharan Nair.

Test your knowledge

- List the differences between arteries and veins.
- How do elastic arteries differ from muscular arteries in structure?
- What is the function of the red blood cell?
- How many types of white blood cells are there? Name them.
- Describe how are the cells of arteries and veins nourished?
- What are the functions of the blood?
- What are components of blood plasma?
- Identify the major components of the lymphatic system.

Learning outcomes

By the end of this chapter the reader will be able to:

- Describe the normal composition of blood
- List the functions of the red blood cells, white blood cells and platelets
- Explain the life cycle of the red blood cells and the white blood cells
- Discuss factors affecting coagulation
- Explain the ABO and Rh systems of blood typing
- Describe the structures of the arteries, veins and capillaries
- List some of the difference between an artery and a vein
- Describe how venous valves function
- Describe the factors controlling blood vessel diameter
- Explain the microcirculation of the blood
- List the lymphatic organs of the body

Body map

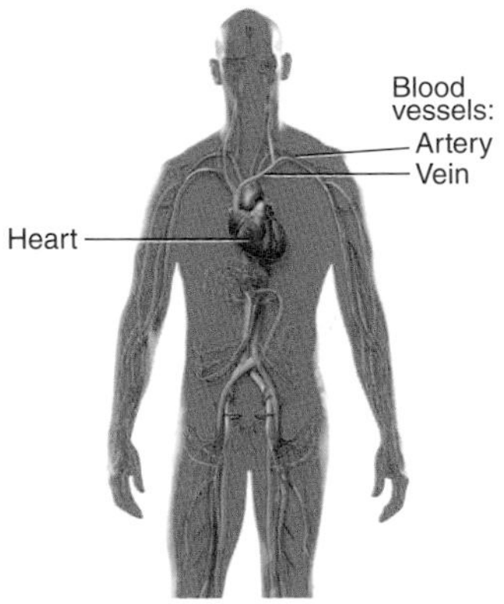
Blood vessels:
Artery
Vein
Heart

Introduction

The circulatory system is a complex system of distribution of nutrients, gases, electrolyte removal of waste products of metabolism and other substances. The circulatory system includes the heart (see Chapter 10), the blood, the blood vessels and the lymphatic system. The blood vessels transport blood throughout the body. Blood consists of formed elements and a fluid portion called plasma. The blood vessels form a network that allows blood to flow from the heart to all living cells and back to the heart. Blood has numerous functions, including transportation of nutrients, respiratory gases such as oxygen and carbon dioxide, nutrients, metabolic wastes such as urea and uric acid, hormones, electrolytes and antibodies. As the blood is circulating throughout the body, cells are constantly extracting nutrients, hormones, electrolytes, oxygen and other substances and excreting unwanted wastes into the blood. Blood is transported throughout the body by a network of blood vessels leading away and returning to the heart. The main types of blood vessels include arteries, arterioles, capillaries, venules and veins. Another important part of the circulatory system is the lymphatic system which drains the fluid called lymph. The lymphatic system consists of the lymph vessels, lymph nodes and lymph glands such as the spleen and the thymus gland. This chapter will focus on the composition, structure and functions of various blood cells, discuss the structure and functions of the blood vessels, factors affecting blood pressure and the structure and functions of the lymphatic system.

Composition of blood

Blood consists of formed elements such as red blood cells (erythrocytes), leucocytes (white blood cells) and platelets. The fluid portion of blood is called plasma which contains different types of proteins and other soluble molecules. When a blood sample is centrifuged, the formed elements accounts for 45% of the blood and plasma makes up 55% of the total blood volume. Between the plasma and erythrocytes lies the buffy coat which consists of white blood cells and platelets (see Figure 12.1). The percentage of the formed elements constitutes the haematocrit or packed cell volume. Haematocrit is a blood test that measures the percentage of red blood cells in whole

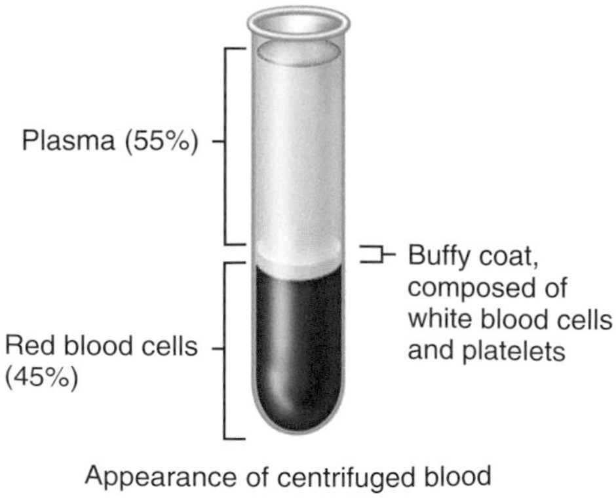
Plasma (55%)
Buffy coat, composed of white blood cells and platelets
Red blood cells (45%)
Appearance of centrifuged blood

Figure 12.1 Components of blood (Tortora and Derrickson 2009)

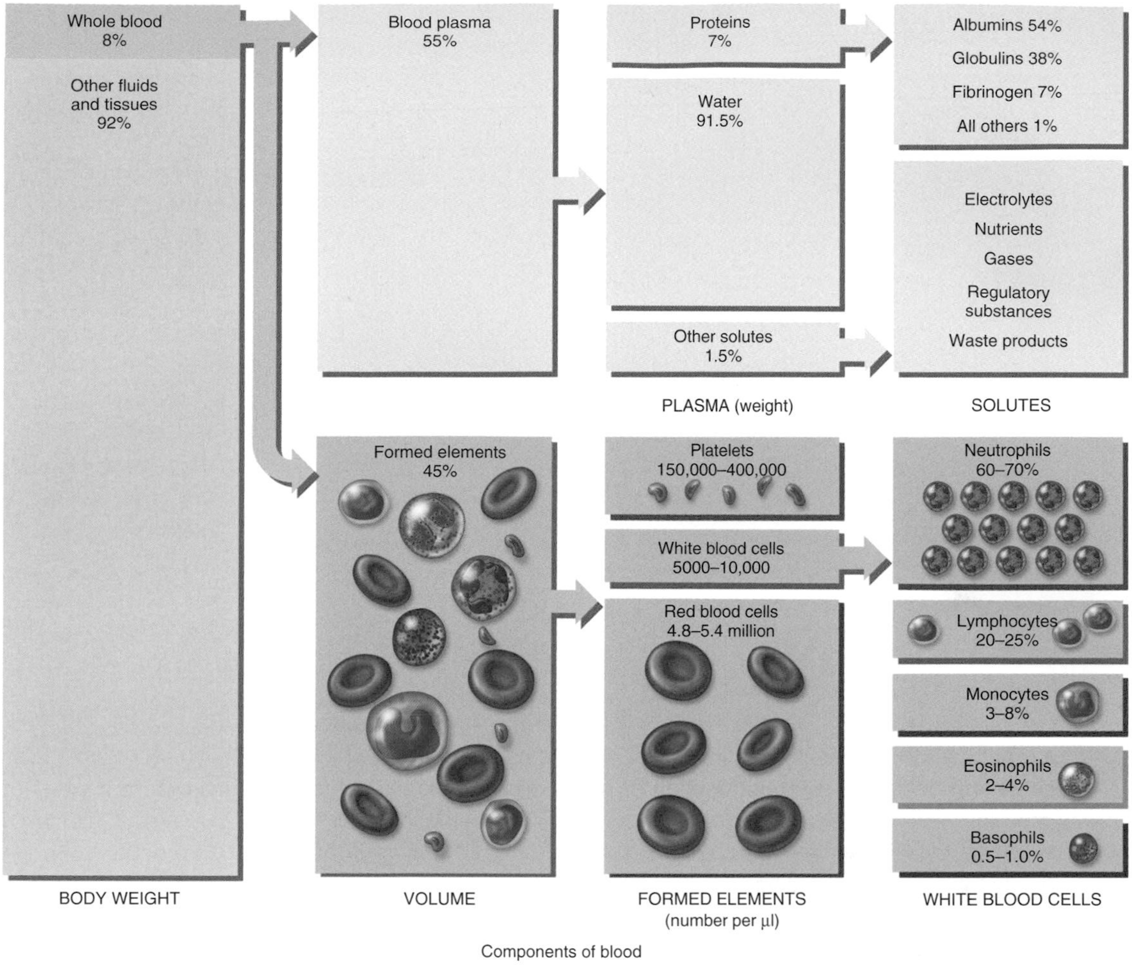
Whole blood
8%
Other fluids and tissues
92%
Blood plasma
55%
Proteins
7%
Water
91.5%
Other solutes
1.5%
Albumins 54%
Globulins 38%
Fibrinogen 7%
All others 1%
Electrolytes
Nutrients
Gases
Regulatory substances
Waste products
PLASMA (weight)
SOLUTES
Formed elements
45%
Platelets
150,000–400,000
White blood cells
5000–10,000
Red blood cells
4.8–5.4 million
Neutrophils
60–70%
Lymphocytes
20–25%
Monocytes
3–8%
Eosinophils
2–4%
Basophils
0.5–1.0%
BODY WEIGHT
VOLUME
FORMED ELEMENTS
(number per μl)
WHITE BLOOD CELLS
Components of blood

Figure 12.2 Cells of the blood (Tortora and Derrickson 2009)

blood. The volume of blood is constant unless a person has physiological problems such as haemorrhage.

Thus, blood is composed of plasma, a yellowish liquid containing nutrients, hormones, minerals and various cells, mainly red blood cells, white blood cells and platelets (see Figure 12.2). Both the formed elements and the plasma play an important role in homeostasis.

Properties of blood and plasma

The average adult has a blood volume of approximately 5 litres of blood, which comprises about 7–9 per cent of the body's weight. Men have 5–6 litres and women 4–5 litres. Blood is thicker, denser and flows much slower than water due to the red blood cells and plasma proteins such as albumin and fibrinogen. Plasma proteins, including albumin, fibrinogen, prothrombin and the gamma globulins, constitute about 8% of the blood plasma in the body. These proteins help maintain water balance which affects osmotic pressure, increase blood viscosity and help maintain blood pressure. All the plasma proteins except the gamma globulins are synthesised in the liver.

Normal human plasma has an osmolality in the range of 285–295 milliosmol/kg. The osmolality of the blood is important for the cells to survive. If the osmolality is approximately 600 milliosmol, the red blood cells could crenate (shrivel up) and die, and if the osmolality is below 150 milliosmol, haemolysis (rupture) of the red blood cells could occur. Thus in clinical practice, to avoid crenation or haemolysis of the red blood cell, intravenous infusion should have an osmolality close to plasma osmolality.

Blood has a high viscosity which offers resistance to blood flow. The red blood cells and proteins contribute to the viscosity of the blood which ranges from 3.5 to 5.5 compared with 1.000 for water. Viscosity means stickiness of blood and the normal viscosity of blood is low, allowing it to flow smoothly. However, the more red blood cells and plasma proteins in blood, the higher the viscosity and the slower the flow of blood. Normal blood varies in viscosity as it flows through the blood vessels but the viscosity decreases as it reaches the capillaries. The specific gravity (density) of blood is 1.045–1.065 compared with 1.000 for water and the pH of blood ranges from 7.35 to 7.45 (Nair 2009).

Blood plasma

Blood plasma is a pale yellow-coloured fluid and its total volume in an adult is approximately 2.5–3 litres. Blood plasma is approximately 91% water and 10% solutes, most of which are proteins. Plasma constitutes approximately 55% of blood's volume (see Figure 12.2).

- Plasma composition:
  - 91% water
  - 8% protein (albumin, globulin, prothrombin and fibrinogen)
  - 0.9% inorganic salts
- Sodium 135–145 mmol/l
- Potassium 3.5–5.0 mmol/l
- Calcium 2.1–2.7 mmol/l
- Hydrogen carbonate 23–31 mmol/l
- Phosphate 0.7–1.4 mmol/l
- Chloride 98–108 mmol/l
  - 0.1% organic substances such as fat, glucose, urea, uric acid and amino acids
  - It is estimated that plasma may contain as many as 40,000 different proteins from about 500 gene products. Approximately 1000 proteins have been identified
- Plasma contains 50–70 mg of protein per ml of which
  - Approximately 70% is albumin (35–50 mg/ml)
  - Approximately 10% is IgG (5–7 mg/ml)

Plasma proteins form three major groups:

- Albumin (60% of total plasma protein) is synthesised in the liver and its main function is to maintain plasma osmotic pressure. It also act as carrier molecules for other substances such as hormones and lipids. Albumin is the smallest plasma protein but the most abundant and

it is capable of passing through capillaries; hence the reason why some albumin is found in the interstitial fluid
- Fibrinogen (4% of total plasma protein) is essential for blood clotting and is synthesised in the liver
- Globulins (36% of total plasma protein) are synthesised in the liver. These proteins are divided into three groups based on their structure and function:
  - alpha globulin
  - beta globulin
  - gamma globulin.

The alpha and beta globulins are produced by the liver and transport lipids and fat-soluble vitamins. Gamma globulins are immunoglobulins which are complex proteins produced by lymphocytes and play a vital role in immunity. They help overcome diseases such as measles and tetanus.

Functions of the plasma proteins include:

- Providing intravascular osmotic effect which is important in maintaining fluid and electrolyte balance
- Contributing to the viscosity of the plasma
- Transport of insoluble substances by allowing them to bind to protein molecules
- Acting as a protein reserve for the body
- Aiding clotting and promoting wound healing
- Inflammatory response
- Protection from infection
- Maintenance of the acid base balance.

Other proteins that are present in plasma are immunoglobins and fibrinogen. Immunoglobins are also called antibodies and they function in the immune response. Antibodies attach to invading bacteria and other micro-organisms, preparing them for destruction by other immune cells. Fibrinogen is a protein that functions in a complex series of reactions that leads to the formation of blood clots.

Water in plasma

Water constitutes approximately 91% of plasma and is available to cells, tissues and extracellular fluid of the body to maintain homeostasis. It is considered the liquid portion of the blood. It is a solvent where chemical reactions between intracellular and extracellular reactions occur. Water contains solutes, for example, electrolytes whose concentrations change to meet body needs.

Functions of blood

The functions of the blood are:

- Transportation
- Maintaining body temperature
- Maintaining the acid base balance
- Regulation of fluid balance
- Removal of waste products.

Transportation

Blood transports many substances around the body and they include:

- Dissolved gases of respiration such as oxygen and carbon dioxide. Blood transports oxygen from the lungs to the cells of the body and the waste product carbon dioxide from the cells to the lungs to be exhaled. Oxygen is transported by haemoglobin in red blood cells and some are dissolved in plasma. Most of the carbon dioxide is transported by bicarbonate ions in plasma
- Waste products of metabolism, for example, urea and uric acid, are transported by blood for elimination
- Hormones are transported from the endocrine glands to other cells in the body
- Enzymes secreted by some organs are transported to other parts of the body for cellular function
- Nutrients such as glucose and amino acids from the gastrointestinal tract are transported to the cells for cellular function. They are vital for cellular function
- Blood cells such as red and white blood cells which have functions of their own, for example red blood cells transport oxygen while the white blood cells play a part in protection from infection.

Clinical considerations

Anaemia

Anaemia is a condition which occurs when there is an abnormally low number of red blood cells. Red blood cells contain haemoglobin, a red pigment which gives blood its colour. The role of haemoglobin is to transport oxygen around the body. When red blood cells and therefore haemoglobin are low the blood fails to supply the body's tissues with sufficient oxygen. Some people with anaemia do not have any symptoms for months but when symptoms do appear, they complain of lethargy, weakness, dizzy spells and feeling faint. As the anaemia becomes more severe, shortness of breath, palpitations, headaches, sore mouth and gums, and brittle nails may cause problems.

There are several different types of anaemia, and each one has a different cause. The most common form of the condition is iron-deficiency anaemia. Other forms of anaemia can be caused by a lack of vitamin B_{12} or folate in the body.

Maintaining body temperature

Heat is produced in great quantities by cellular metabolism and the blood is essential for the distribution and dispersal of the heat. Water in plasma helps to absorb heat and has coolant properties. An increased blood flow to the skin, by the dilatation of capillaries, aids excess heat loss through convection and radiation. When heat needs to be conserved, constriction of the capillaries reduces the blood flow to the skin thus reducing heat loss (see Figure 12.3).

Maintaining the acid base balance

The acid base balance can be defined as homeostasis of the body fluids at a normal arterial blood pH ranging between 7.35 and 7.45. Body fluid pH is significant because proteins are sensitive to pH, in terms of both their conformation and optimal range of function. pH affects membrane structure, enzyme activity and structural proteins. Blood helps to regulate the pH through the buffers in the blood such as bicarbonate ions.

Regulation of fluid balance

Fluid regulation is essential to maintain homeostasis. If the amount of fluid increases or falls beyond normal limits many bodily functions will be affected and cells in the body cannot function efficiently. Blood, with the help from other organs such as the kidneys and hormones, for example, antidiuretic hormone, ensures that the cells are supplied with the correct amount of fluid.

Removal of waste products

As a result of cellular metabolism, numerous waste products such urea, uric acid and carbon dioxide are produced. These wastes if not removed could disrupt cellular function and homeostasis. The blood transports these wastes to various organs such as the kidneys, lungs and skin for elimination.

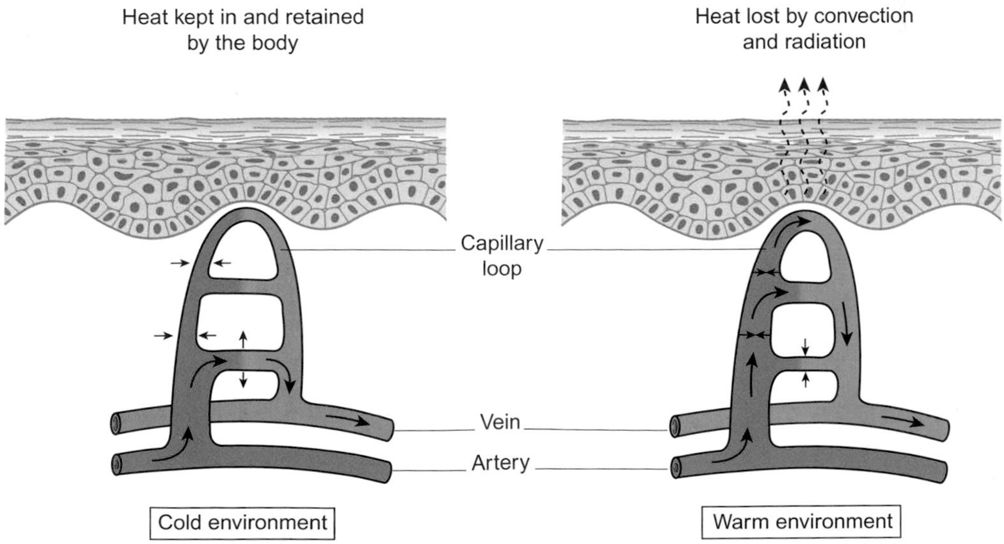
Heat kept in and retained by the body
Heat lost by convection and radiation
Capillary loop
Vein
Artery
Cold environment
Warm environment

Figure 12.3 Heat loss through the skin by conduction and radiation

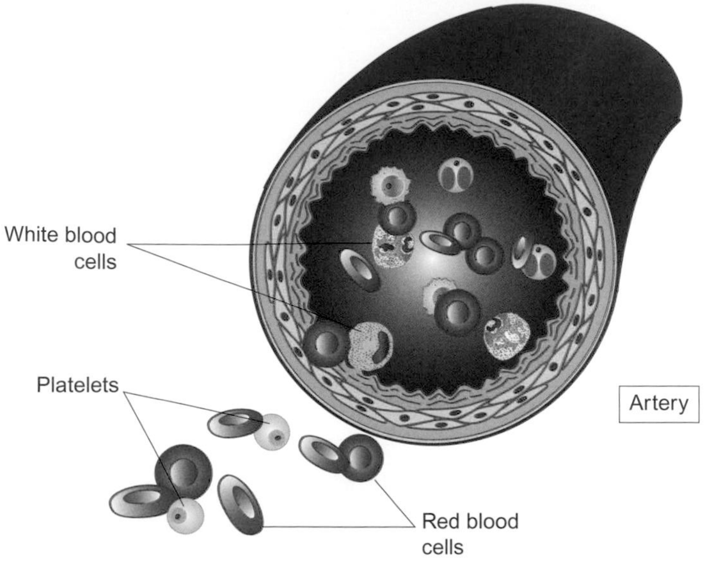
White blood cells
Platelets
Artery
Red blood cells

Figure 12.4 Formed elements of blood

Formation of blood cells

Red blood cells and most white blood cells and platelets are produced in the bone marrow. The red blood and white blood cells and the platelets are the formed elements of blood (see Figure 12.4). The bone marrow is the soft fatty substance found in bone cavities. Within the bone marrow, all blood cells originate from a single type of unspecialised cell called a stem cell. When a stem cell divides, it first becomes an immature red blood cell, white blood cell or platelet-producing cell. The immature cell then divides, matures further and ultimately becomes a mature red blood cell, white blood cell or platelet (see Figure 3.1, page 65).

In order to produce blood cells, multipotent (also called pluripotent) stem cells divide into myeloid and lymphoid stem cells in the bone marrow. The myeloid stem cells further subdivide in the bone marrow to produce red blood cells, platelets (thrombocytes), basophil, eosinophil, neutrophil and monocytes. The lymphoid stem cells begin the development in the bone marrow as B- and T-lymphocytes. B-lymphocytes continue development in bone marrow, before migrating to other lymph organs such as lymph nodes, spleen or tonsils. T-lymphocytes continue their development in the thymus, and may then migrate to other lymph tissues.

Red blood cells

Red blood cells (also known as erythrocytes) are the most abundant blood cells. They are biconcave discs (see Figure 12.5) and contain oxygen-carrying protein called haemoglobin. The biconcave shape is maintained by a network of proteins called spectrin. This network of protein allows the red blood cells to change shape as they are transported through the blood vessel. The plasma membrane of a red blood cell is strong and flexible. There are approximately 4–5.5 million

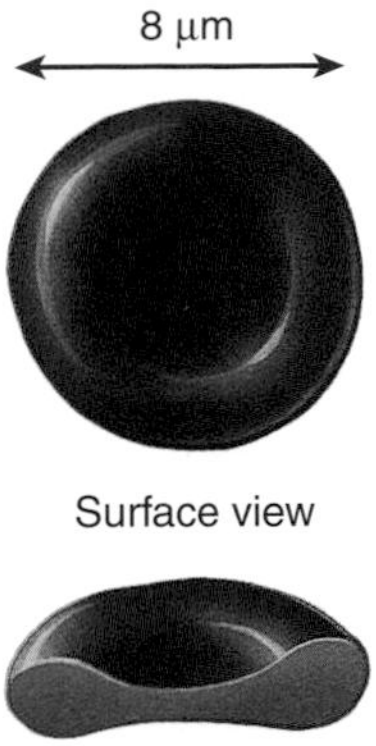
8 µm
Surface view
Sectioned view
RBC shape

Figure 12.5 Red blood cells (Tortora and Derrickson 2009)

red blood cells in each cubic millimetre of blood. They are a pale buff colour that appears lighter in the centre. Young red blood cells contain a nucleus, however, the nucleus is absent in a mature red blood cell and without any organelles such as mitochondria, thus increasing the oxygen-carrying capacity of the red blood cell.

The main function of haemoglobin in the red blood cell is to transport oxygen and carbon dioxide (approximately 20%). As the blood flows through the capillaries in the tissues, carbon dioxide is picked up by the haemoglobin and oxygen is released. As the blood reaches the lungs carbon dioxide is released and oxygen is picked up by the haemoglobin molecules. As red blood cells lack mitochondria to produce energy (adenosine triphosphate), they utilise anaerobic respiration to produce energy and do not use any of the oxygen they are transporting. Apart from transporting oxygen and carbon dioxide, the haemoglobin plays an important role in maintaining blood pressure and blood flow.

Haemoglobin

Haemoglobin is composed of a protein called globin bound to the iron-containing pigments called haem. Each globin molecule has four polypeptide chains consisting of two alpha and two beta chains (see Figure 12.6). Each haemoglobin molecule has four atoms of iron and each atom of iron transports one molecule of oxygen, therefore, one molecule of haemoglobin transports four molecules of oxygen. There are approximately 250 million haemoglobin molecules in one red blood cell and therefore one red blood cell transports 1 billion molecules of oxygen. At the capillary end the haemoglobin releases the oxygen molecule into the interstitial fluid, which is then transported into the cells.

Formation of red blood cells

Erythroblasts undergo development in the red bone marrow to form red blood cells (see Figure 3.1). During maturation red blood cells lose their nucleus and organelles and gain more

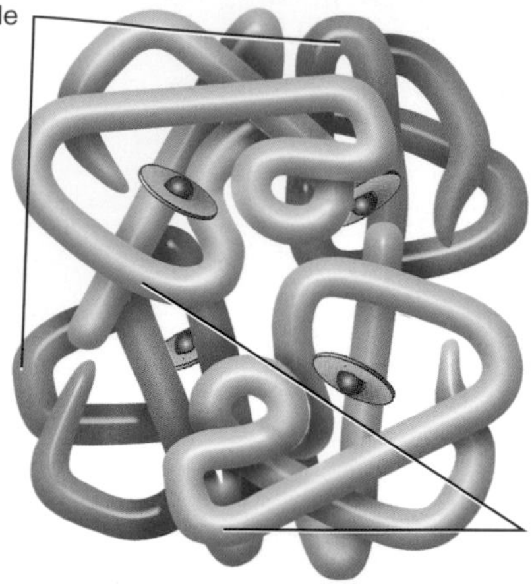
Beta polypeptide chains
Alpha polypeptide chains
Haemoglobin molecule

Figure 12.6 Haemoglobin molecule (Tortora and Derrickson 2009)

haemoglobin molecules thus increasing the amount of oxygen they transport. Mature red blood cells do not have a nucleus, their life span is approximately 120 days. It is estimated that approximately 2 million red blood cells are destroyed per second; however an equal number are replaced each time to maintain the balance. The production of red blood cells is controlled by the hormone erythropoietin. Other essential components for the synthesis of red blood cells include:

- Iron
- Folic acid
- Vitamin B_{12}

Erythropoietin is a hormone produced by the kidneys, which is then transported by the blood to the bone marrow. In the bone marrow erythropoietin stimulates the production of red blood cells, which then enter the bloodstream. The production and release of erythropoietin is through negative feedback system (see Figure 12.7).

Life cycle of the red blood cell

Without a nucleus and other organelles the red blood cell cannot synthesise new structures to replace the ones that are damaged; The breakdown (haemolysis) of the red blood cell is carried out by macrophages in the spleen, liver and the bone marrow (see Figure 12.8). The globin is broken down into amino acids and reused for protein synthesis. Iron is separated from haem and is stored in the muscles and the liver and reused in the bone marrow to manufacture new red blood cells. Haem is the portion of the haemoglobin that is converted to bilirubin and is transported by plasma albumin to the liver and eventually secreted in bile. In the large intestine bacteria convert bilirubin into urobilinogen, some of which is reabsorbed into the bloodstream where it is converted into a yellow pigment called urobilin, which is excreted in urine, giving the urine a

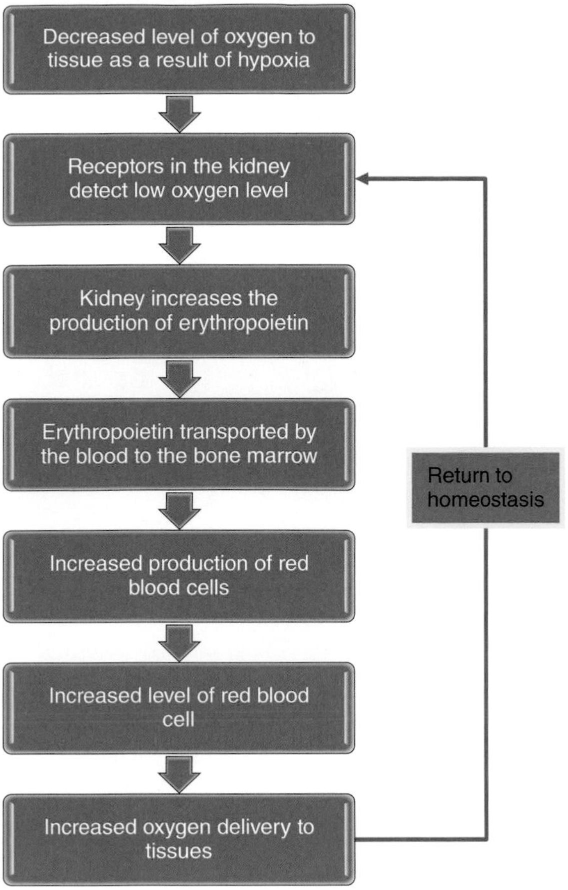
Decreased level of oxygen to tissue as a result of hypoxia
Receptors in the kidney detect low oxygen level
Kidney increases the production of erythropoietin
Erythropoietin transported by the blood to the bone marrow
Increased production of red blood cells
Increased level of red blood cell
Increased oxygen delivery to tissues
Return to homeostasis

Figure 12.7 Negative feedback for erythropoiesis

yellowish colour. The remainder of the urobilinogen is eliminated in faeces as a brown pigment called stercobilin.

Transport of respiratory gases

The major role of red blood cells is to transport oxygen from the lungs to the tissues. The oxygen in the alveoli (air sac) of the lungs combines with iron molecules in the haemoglobin to form oxyhaemoglobin. This is then transported by the blood to the tissues. As the oxygen level in the red blood cell increases, it becomes bright red and when the level of oxygen content drops the colour changes to dark bluish-red.

In addition to transporting oxygen from the lungs to the body tissues, red blood cells transport carbon dioxide from the tissues to the lungs. Carbon dioxide is transported in three ways:

- 10% of the carbon dioxide is dissolved in the plasma
- 20% of the carbon dioxide combines with haemoglobin of the red blood cell to form carbaminohaemoglobin

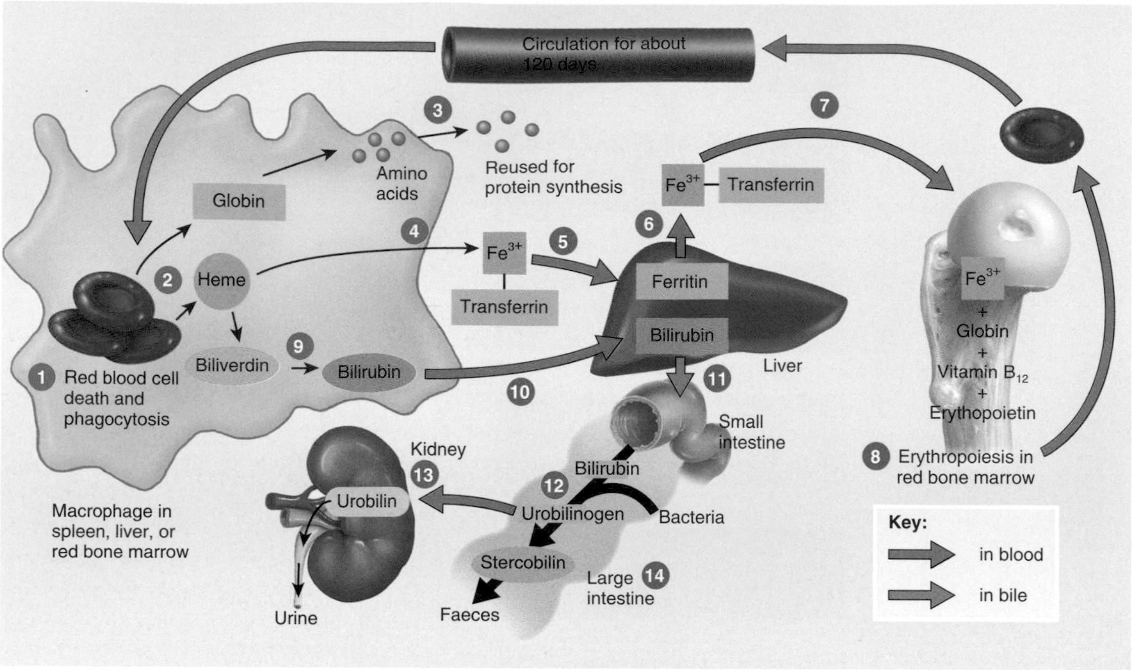

Circulation for about 120 days
1 Red blood cell death and phagocytosis
2 Heme
Globin
3
Amino acids
Reused for protein synthesis
4
Fe^{3+}
Transferrin
5
Ferritin
6
Fe^{3+} — Transferrin
7
Biliverdin
9
Bilirubin
10
Bilirubin
Liver
11
Small intestine
Fe3+
+
Globin
+
Vitamin B12
+
Erythropoietin
8 Erythropoiesis in red bone marrow
Macrophage in spleen, liver, or red bone marrow
Kidney
13
Urobilin
Urine
12
Bilirubin
Urobilinogen
Bacteria
Stercobilin
Faeces
Large intestine 14
Key:
in blood
in bile

Figure 12.8 Destruction of the red blood cell (Tortora and Derrickson 2009)

- 70% of the carbon dioxide reacts with water to form carbonic acid, which is converted to bicarbonate and hydrogen ions:

$$CO_2 + H_2O \xleftrightarrow{\text{carbonic anhydrase}} \underset{\text{carbonic acid}}{H_2CO_3} \longleftrightarrow \underset{\text{bicarbonate ion}}{HCO_3^-} + \underset{\text{hydrogen ion}}{H^+}$$

The reaction occurs primarily in red blood cells which contain large amounts of carbonic anhydrase (an enzyme that facilitates the reaction). Once the bicarbonate ions are formed, they move out of the red blood cells into the plasma.

White blood cells

White blood cells are also known as leucocytes. There are approximately 5,000–10,000 white blood cells in every cubic millimetre of blood. The number may increase in infections to approximately 25,000 per cubic millimetre of blood. An increase in white blood cells is called leucocytosis and an abnormally low level of white blood cell is called leucopenia. Unlike red blood cells, white blood cells have nuclei and they are able to move out of blood vessel walls into the tissues. White blood cells are able to produce a continuous supply of energy, unlike the red blood cells. They are able to synthesise proteins and thus their life span can be from a few days to years.

There are two main types of white blood cells:

- Granulocytes (contain granules in the cytoplasm)
  - neutrophils
  - eosinophils
  - basophils
- Agranulocytes (despite the name contain a few granules in the cytoplasm)
  - monocytes
  - lymphocytes.

Neutrophils

Neutrophils are the most abundant white blood cells and play an important role in the immune system. They form approximately 60–65% of granulocytes and are phagocytes. They are approximately 10–12 μm in diameter and capable of ingesting micro-organisms. They contain lysozymes and therefore their main function is to protect the body from any foreign material. They are capable of moving out of blood vessel walls by a process called diapedesis and are actively phagocytic. A non-active neutrophil lasts approximately 12 hours while an active neutrophil may last 1–2 days. Neutrophils are the first immune cells to arrive at a site of infection, through a process known as **chemotaxis**. A deficiency of neutrophils is called **neutropenia** and may be congenital or acquired, for example in certain kinds of anaemia and leukaemia, or as a side-effect of chemotherapy. Since neutrophils are such an important part of the immune response, a lowered neutrophil count results in a compromised immune system.

The nuclei of the neutrophils are multi-lobed (see Figure 12.9). The number of neutrophils increases in:

- Pregnancy
- Infection
- Leukaemia
- Metabolic disorders such as acute gout
- Inflammation
- Myocardial infarction.

Eosinophils

These form approximately 2–4% of granulocytes and have B-shaped nuclei (see Figure 12.10). Like neutrophils, they too migrate from blood vessels and they are 10–12 μm in diameter. They are

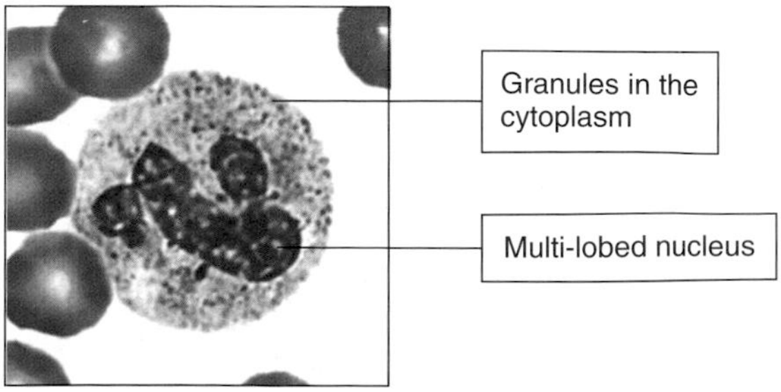
Granules in the cytoplasm
Multi-lobed nucleus

Figure 12.9 Neutrophil (Tortora and Derrickson 2009)

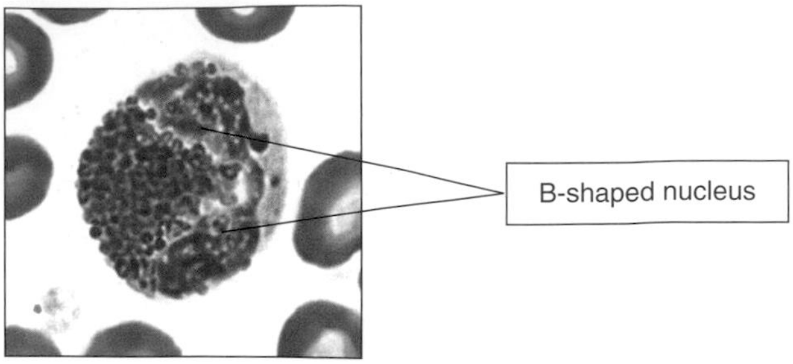
B-shaped nucleus

Figure 12.10 Eosinophil (Tortora and Derrickson 2009)

phagocytes; however, they are not as active as neutrophils. They contain lysosomal enzymes and peroxidase in their granules, which are toxic to parasites, resulting in the destruction of the organism. Numbers increase in allergy, such as hay fever and asthma, and parasitic infection, for example, tapeworm infection.

Basophils

Basophils are least abundant, accounting for approximately 1% of granulocytes, and contain elongated lobed nuclei (see Figure 12.11). Basophils are 8–10 µm in diameter. In inflamed tissue they become mast cells and secrete granules containing heparin, histamine and other proteins that promote inflammation. They also secrete lipid mediators like leucotrienes and several cytokines. Basophils play an important role in providing immunity against parasites and also in the allergic response as they have IgE on their surface and release chemical mediators causing allergic symptoms when the IgE binds to its specific allergen.

Monocytes

Monocytes account for 5% of the agranulocytes and are circulating leucocytes (see Figure 12.12). Monocytes develop in the bone marrow and spread through the body in 1–3 days. They are approximately 12–20 µm in diameter. The nucleus of the monocyte is kidney- or horseshoe-shaped. Some of the monocytes migrate into the tissue where they develop into macrophages and engulf pathogens or foreign proteins. Macrophages play a vital role in immunity and inflammation by destroying specific antigens.

Lymphocytes

Lymphocytes account for 25% of the leucocytes and most are found in the lymphatic tissue such as the lymph nodes and the spleen (see Figure 12.13). Small lymphocytes are approximately 6–9 µm in diameter while the larger ones are 10–14 µm in diameter. They get their name from the lymph, the fluid that transports them. They can leave and re-enter the circulatory system and their life span ranges from a few hours to years. The main difference between lymphocytes and other white blood cells is that lymphocytes are not phagocytes. Two types of lymphocytes are identified and they are T- and B-lymphocytes. T-lymphocytes originate from the thymus

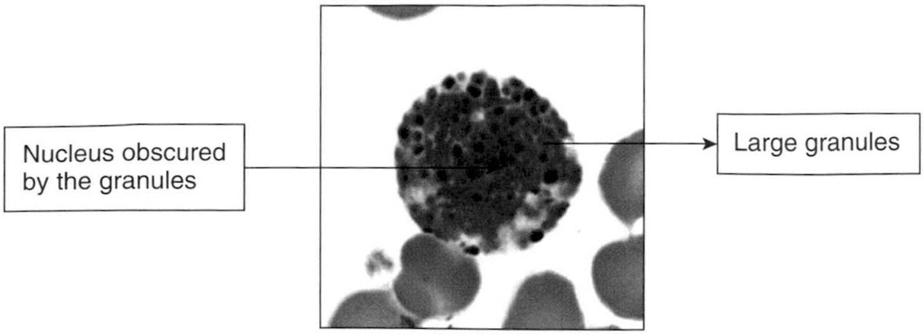
Nucleus obscured by the granules
Large granules

Figure 12.11 Basophil (Tortora and Derrickson 2009)

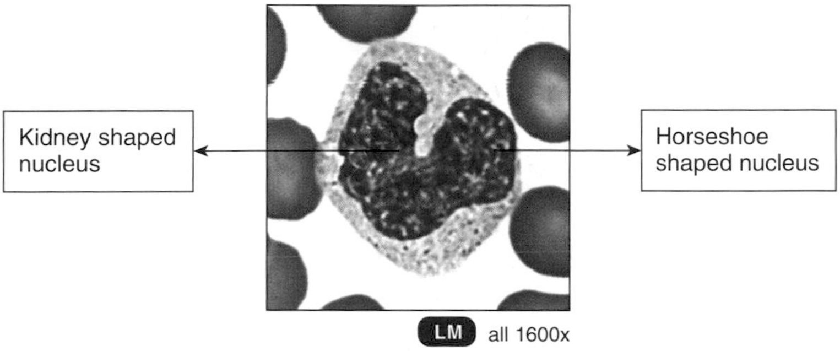
Kidney shaped nucleus
Horseshoe shaped nucleus
LM all 1600x

Figure 12.12 Monocytes (Tortora and Derrickson 2009)

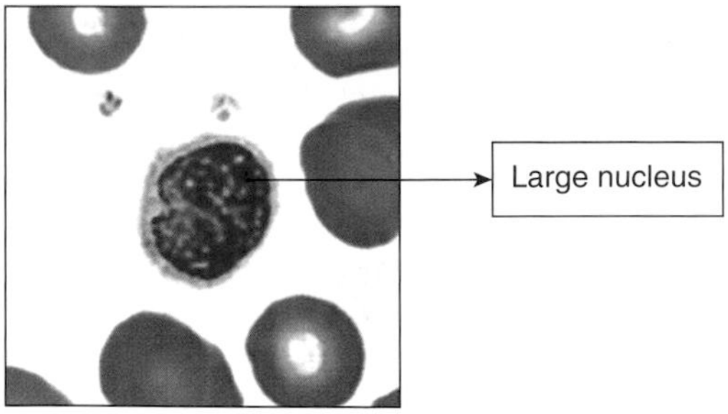
Large nucleus

Figure 12.13 Lymphocyte (Tortora and Derrickson 2009)

gland (hence the name), while B-lymphocytes originate in the bone marrow. T-lymphocytes mediate cellular immune response which is part of the body's own defence. The B-lymphocytes, on the other hand, become large plasma cells and produce antibodies which attach to antigen.

Platelets

Platelets are small blood cells consisting of some cytoplasm surrounded by a plasma membrane. They are produced in the bone marrow from megakaryocytes and fragments of megakaryocytes break off to form platelets. They are approximately 2–4 μm in diameter but have no nucleus and the life span is approximately 5–9 days. Old and dead platelets are removed by macrophages in the spleen and the Kupffer cells in the liver. The surface of platelets contains proteins and glycoproteins that allow them to adhere to other proteins such as collagen in the connective tissues. Platelets play a vital role in blood loss by the formation of platelet plugs which seal the holes in the blood vessels and release chemicals which aid blood clotting. If the platelet number is low excessive bleeding can occur, however if the number increases blood clots (thrombosis) can form leading to cerebrovascular accident, deep vein thrombosis, heart attack or pulmonary embolism.

Haemostasis

Haemostasis is a sequence of responses that stop bleeding and can prevent haemorrhage from smaller blood vessels. Haemostasis plays an important part in maintaining homeostasis and it consists of three main components. They are:

- Vasoconstriction
- Platelet aggregation
- Coagulation.

Vasoconstriction

- Results from contraction of the smooth muscle of the vessel wall, a reaction called vascular spasm
- Constriction blocks small blood vessels thus preventing blood flow through them
- The action of the sympathetic nervous system is to cause vasoconstriction which restricts blood flow for several minutes or several hours
- Platelets release thromboxanes which belong to the lipid group eicosanoids. Thromboxanes are vasoconstrictors and potent hypertensive agents; they facilitate platelet aggregation.

Platelet aggregation

- Platelets adhere to the exposed collagen fibres of the connective tissue of the damaged blood vessels
- Platelets release adenosine diphosphate, thromboxane and other chemicals which make other platelets in the area stick and they all clump together to form a platelet plug. Platelet plugs are very effective in preventing blood loss in small blood vessels and with fibrin threads form tight plugs.

Table 12.1 Blood clotting factors

Factor	Common Name
I	Fibrinogen
II	Prothrombin
V	Proaccelerin, labile factor
VII	Proconvertin
VIII	Antihaemophilic factor A
IX	Antihaemophilic factor B
X	Thrombokinase, Stuart–Prower factor
XI	Antihaemophilic factor C
XII	Hageman factor
XIII	Fibrin stabilising factor

Coagulation

Blood coagulation is an important process to maintain homeostasis. If blood vessel damage is so extensive that platelet aggregation and vasoconstriction cannot stop the bleeding, the complicated process of coagulation (blood clotting) will begin to take place with the aid of clotting factors (see Table 12.1). Coagulation factors are a group of proteins essential for clotting and most of the clotting factors are synthesised in the liver and some are obtained from our diet.

The simplified clotting stages involve the following:

(1) Thromboplastinogenase is an enzyme released by the blood platelets and combines with antihaemophilic factor to convert the plasma protein thromboplastinogen into thromboplastin.
(2) Thromboplastin combines with calcium ions to convert the inactive plasma protein prothrombin into thrombin.
(3) Thrombin acts as a catalyst to convert the soluble plasma protein fibrinogen into insoluble plasma protein fibrin.
(4) The fibrin threads trap blood cells to form a clot.
(5) Once the clot is formed, the healing of the damaged blood vessel takes place, which restores the integrity of the blood vessel.

Two pathways were identified in triggering a blood clot and they include the intrinsic and extrinsic pathways. The extrinsic pathway is a rapid clotting system activated when the blood vessels are ruptured and tissue damage takes place. The intrinsic pathway is slower than the extrinsic pathway and is activated when the inner walls of the blood vessels are damaged.

Blood groups

It is the red blood cells which define which blood group an individual belongs to. On the surface of the red cells there are markers called antigens; which are so small they cannot even be seen under a microscope. Apart from identical twins, each person has different antigens and these antigens are the key to identifying blood types and must be matched in transfusions to avoid serious complications. The structure for defining blood groups is known as the ABO system. If an individual has blood group A, then they have A antigens covering their red cells. Group B has B antigens on their red blood cell; while group O has neither antigens and group AB has both antigens (Tortora and Derrickson 2009).

The ABO system also covers antibodies in the plasma which are the body's natural defence against foreign antigens. So, for example, blood group A has anti-B in their plasma, B has anti-A, and so on. However, group AB has no antibodies and group O has both (see Figure 12.14). If these antibodies find the wrong red blood cells, they will attack them and destroy them. That is why transfusing the wrong blood to a patient can be fatal.

There is also another factor (factor D) to be considered – the rhesus factor (Rh) system. Rh antigens can be present in each of the blood groups. Not everyone has the Rh antigen on the red blood cell, however if a person has Rh antigen on their red blood cell then they are Rh positive and if they do not have the Rh antigen then they are Rh negative. A person with A blood group and Rh positive is known as A+, while if the Rh is negative, they are A–. The same applies for B, AB and O. In the UK, approximately 85% of the population are rhesus positive, that is they possess factor D on their red blood cell. The remaining 15% of the population are rhesus negative as their red blood cells do not have factor D. It is important to consider the rhesus factor when cross-matching and transfusing blood to patients to avoid unnecessary complications such as agglutination (see Table 12.2).

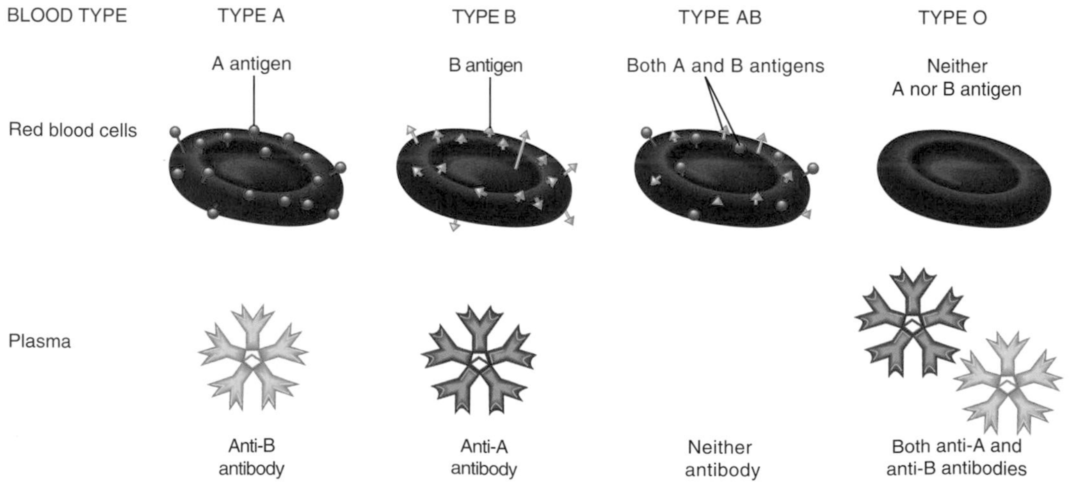
BLOOD TYPE
TYPE A
TYPE B
TYPE AB
TYPE O
A antigen
B antigen
Both A and B antigens
Neither
A nor B antigen
Red blood cells
Plasma
Anti-B
antibody
Anti-A
antibody
Neither
antibody
Both anti-A and
anti-B antibodies

Figure 12.14 ABO blood groups (Tortora and Derrickson 2009)

Table 12.2 Blood groups

Blood type	Antigens	Antibodies	Can donate blood to	Can receive blood from
A	Antigen A	Anti-B	A, AB	A, O
B	Antigen B	Anti-A	B, AB	B, O
AB	Antigen A Antigen B	None	AB	A, B, AB, O
O	None	Anti-A Anti-B	A, B, AB, O	O

Blood vessels

Blood vessels are part of the circulatory system that transports blood throughout the body. There are three major types of blood vessels: the arteries, which carry the blood away from the heart, the capillaries, which enable the actual exchange of water, nutrients and chemicals between the blood and the tissues; and the veins, which carry blood from the capillaries back towards the heart (see Figure 12.15). All arteries, with the exception of the pulmonary and umbilical arteries, carry oxygenated blood, while most veins carry deoxygenated blood from the tissues back to the heart; exceptions are pulmonary and umbilical veins, both of which carry oxygenated blood. The capillaries form the microcirculatory system and it is at this point that nutrients, gases, water and electrolytes are exchanged between the blood and the tissue fluid. Capillaries are tiny, extremely thin-walled vessels and act as a bridge between arteries and veins. The thin walls of the capillaries allow oxygen and nutrients to pass from the blood into tissue fluid and allow waste products to pass from tissue fluid into the blood.

Structure and function of arteries and veins

For most of the blood vessels, the walls consist of three layers and:

- The tunica interna
- The tunica media
- The tunica externa.

See Figure 12.16.

The tunica interna is a thin layer (only a few cells thick) of a vein and artery. It is sometimes referred to as the intima membrane. It is this layer that gives smoothness to the lining of the vessel, enhancing blood flow. It is lined by endothelial cells and elastic tissues; however it varies in thickness between the blood vessels:

- Arteries – most elastic tissue
- Veins – very little tissue
- Capillaries – no elastic layer.

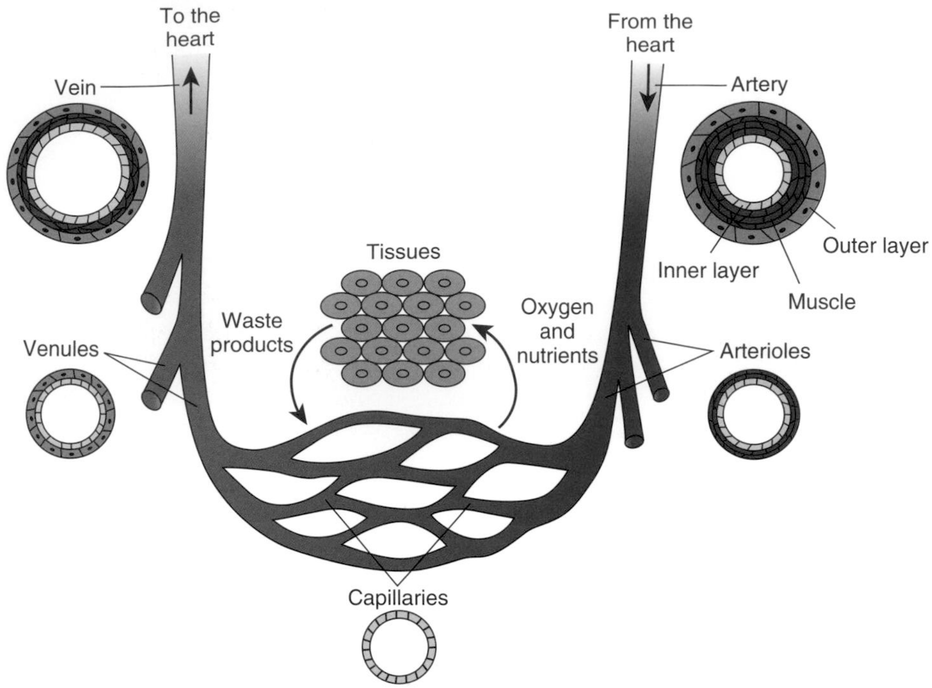
To the heart
From the heart
Vein
Artery
Outer layer
Tissues
Inner layer
Muscle
Waste products
Oxygen and nutrients
Venules
Arterioles
Capillaries

Figure 12.15 Blood vessels

The tunica media consist of elastic fibres and smooth muscle which allows for vasoconstriction, changing blood flow and pressure. The tunica media is supplied by the sympathetic branch of the autonomic nervous system. When stimulated, the walls contract narrowing the lumen and increasing pressure within the blood vessel:

- Arteries – varies by the size of the artery
- Veins – thin layer
- Capillaries – do not have tunica media.

The tunica externa (adventia) consist of collagen fibres and varies in thickness between the vessels. The collagen serves to anchor the blood vessel to nearby organs, giving it support and stability:

- Arteries – relatively thick
- Veins – relatively thick
- Capillaries – very delicate.

Although the arteries and veins have similar layers, there are some clear differences between these two vessels. For a summary see Table 12.3 and Figure 12.17.

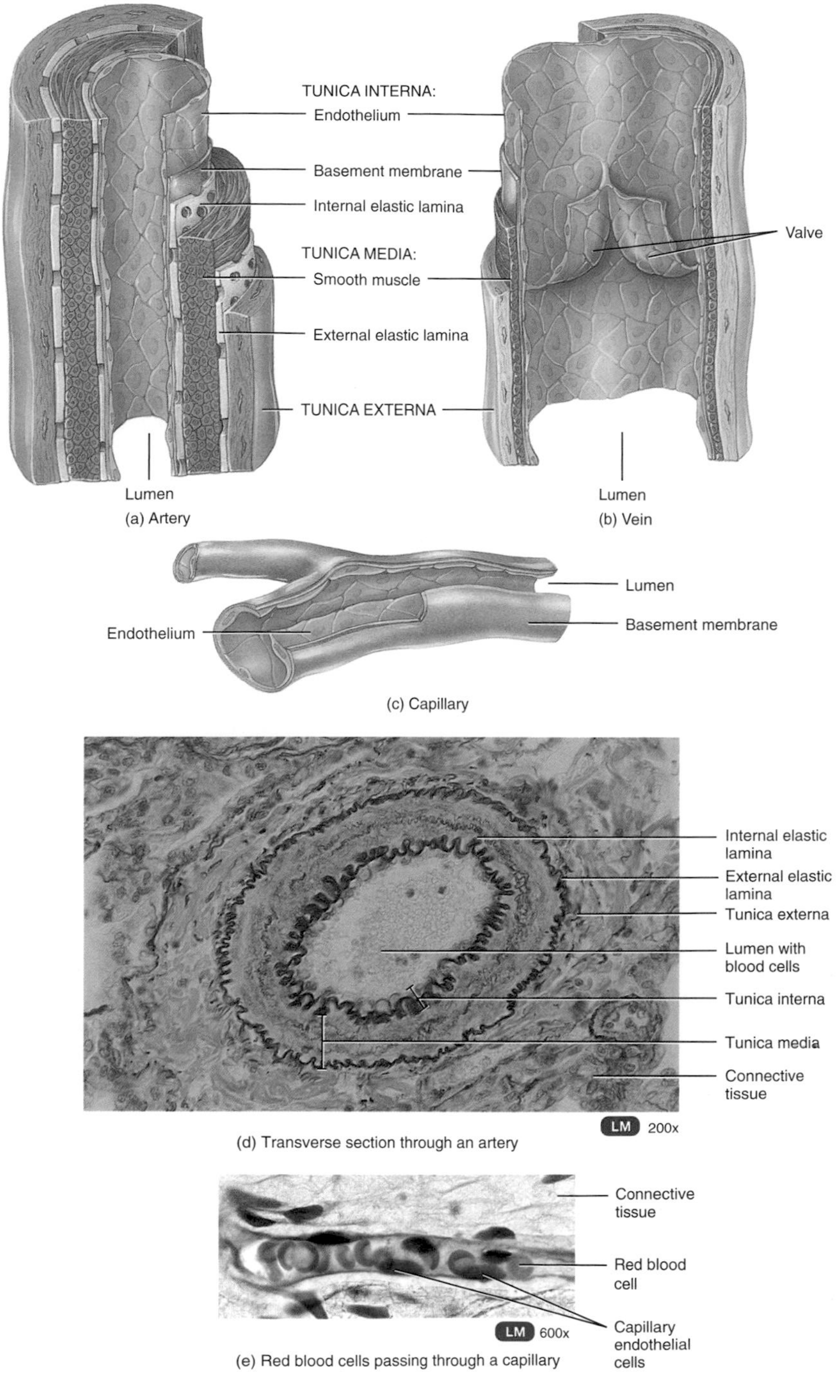

TUNICA INTERNA:
Endothelium
Basement membrane
Internal elastic lamina
TUNICA MEDIA:
Smooth muscle
External elastic lamina
TUNICA EXTERNA
Valve
Lumen
(a) Artery
Lumen
(b) Vein
Lumen
Basement membrane
Endothelium
(c) Capillary
Internal elastic lamina
External elastic lamina
Tunica externa
Lumen with blood cells
Tunica interna
Tunica media
Connective tissue
LM 200x
(d) Transverse section through an artery
Connective tissue
Red blood cell
Capillary endothelial cells
LM 600x
(e) Red blood cells passing through a capillary

Figure 12.16 Layers of a blood vessel (Tortora and Derrickson 2009)

Table 12.3 Differences between arteries and veins

Arteries	Veins
Transport blood away from the heart	Transport blood to the heart
Carry oxygenated blood except the pulmonary and umbilical arteries	Carry deoxygenated blood, except pulmonary and umbilical veins
Have a narrow lumen	Have a wider lumen
Have more elastic tissue	Have less elastic tissue
Do not have valves	Do have valves
Transports blood under pressure	Transports blood under low pressure

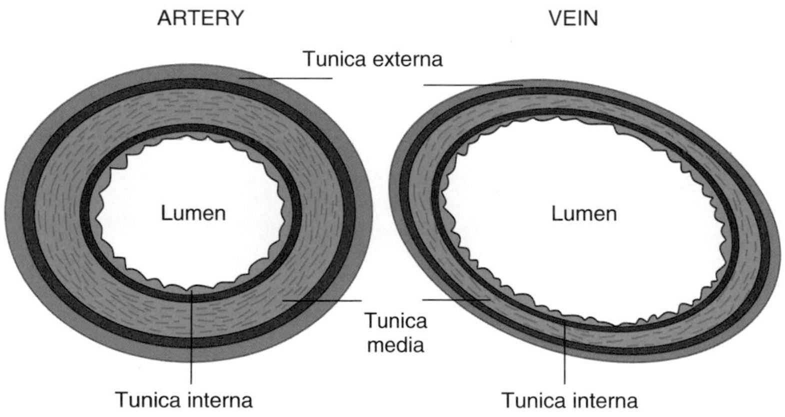
ARTERY
VEIN
Tunica externa
Lumen
Lumen
Tunica
media
Tunica interna
Tunica interna

Figure 12.17 Artery and vein

Capillaries

Capillaries are tiny blood vessels, approximately 5–20 µm in diameter. There are networks of capillaries (see Figure 12.18) in most of the organs and tissues of the body. Capillary walls are only one cell thick, which allows exchange of material between the contents of the capillary and the surrounding tissue fluid. The walls of capillaries are composed of a single layer of cells, the endothelium. This layer is so thin that molecules such as oxygen, water and lipids can pass through them by diffusion and enter the tissues. Waste products such as carbon dioxide and urea can diffuse back into the blood to be carried away for removal. Capillaries are so small the red blood cells need to change shape in order to pass through them in single file.

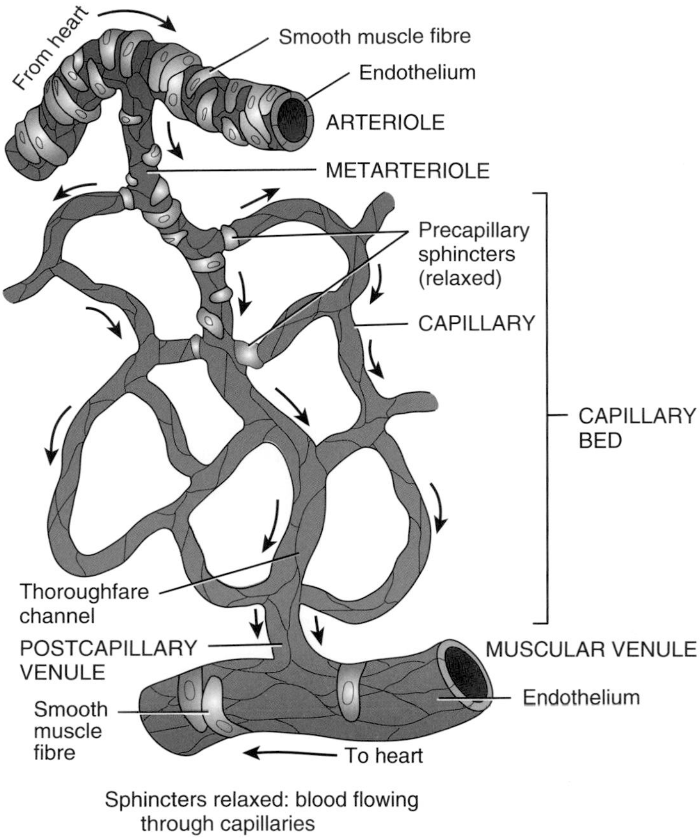
From heart
Smooth muscle fibre
Endothelium
ARTERIOLE
METARTERIOLE
Precapillary sphincters (relaxed)
CAPILLARY
CAPILLARY BED
Thoroughfare channel
POSTCAPILLARY VENULE
MUSCULAR VENULE
Endothelium
Smooth muscle fibre
To heart
Sphincters relaxed: blood flowing through capillaries

Figure 12.18 Capillary (Tortora and Derrickson 2009)

Blood pressure

Blood pressure is the pressure exerted by blood within the blood vessel. The pressure is at its greatest near the heart and decreases as the blood moves further from the heart. Three factors regulate blood pressure. They are:

- Neuronal regulation – through the autonomic nervous system
- Hormonal regulation – adrenaline, noradrenaline, renin and others
- Autoregulation – through the renin-angiotensin system.

Physiological factors regulating blood pressure

Several factors affect blood pressure and they include:

- Cardiac output, the volume of blood pumped out by the heart in one minute. Cardiac output is a function of heart rate and stroke volume. The heart rate is simply the number of heart

beats per minute. The stroke volume is the volume of blood, in millilitres (ml), pumped out of the heart with each beat
- Circulating volume, the volume of circulating blood perfusing tissues
- Peripheral resistance, the resistance provided by the blood vessels
- Blood viscosity, the measure of the resistance of blood flow. The resistance is provided by plasma proteins and other substances in the blood
- Hydrostatic pressure, the pressure exerted by the blood on the vessel wall.

Control of arterial blood pressure

Blood pressure within the large systemic arteries must be maintained to ensure adequate blood flow to the tissues. This is maintained by:

- Baroreceptors, situated in the arch of the aorta and the carotid sinus, are sensitive to pressure changes within the blood vessel. When blood pressure increases signals are sent to the cardio-regulatory centre (CRC) in the brain stem (medulla oblongata). The cardio-regulatory centre increases the parasympathetic activity to the heart reducing heart rate and inhibiting sympathetic activity to the blood vessels, causing vasodilatation. This reduces blood pressure. On the other hand, if the blood pressure falls, the CRC increases the sympathetic activity to the heart and the blood vessels thus increasing heart rate and vasoconstriction resulting in increased blood pressure.
- Chemoreceptors situated in carotid and aortic bodies help to regulate blood pressure by detecting changes in the levels of oxygen, carbon dioxide and hydrogen ions. Changes in the levels of carbon dioxide, oxygen and hydrogen ions can affect heart and respiration rates.
- Circulating hormones, such as antidiuretic and atrial natriuretic peptide hormones, help to regulate circulating blood volume thus affecting blood pressure.
- The renin – angiotensin system helps to maintain blood pressure though its action on vasoconstriction.
- The hypothalamus responds to stimuli such as emotion, pain and anger and stimulates sympathetic nervous activity affecting blood pressure.

Clinical considerations

Taking blood pressure

Blood pressure is the force exerted by the blood on the vessel wall as the blood flows through vessels. When we refer to blood pressure, we mean arterial blood pressure because arteries carry blood from the heart through the vessel with a great deal of pressure. How is blood pressure measured?

Blood pressure is measured using a sphygmomanometer (electronic, digital or aneroid) and is a non-invasive method of monitoring a patient's blood pressure. It may be used as a diagnostic test on patients with arterial blood pressure problems. It can be recorded with the patient sitting comfortably in a chair or lying in bed. Taking and recording blood pressure is a skill that all nurses need to be competent in.

How to record blood pressure

Using the proper cuff is important. Cuffs come in small, medium, large and paediatric sizes. Once the appropriate size is found, the cuff is placed over bare skin above the elbow. At this point the patient should be as relaxed as possible throughout the recording. The nurse should then feel for the radial pulse on the same arm. Once the radial pulse is felt, the cuff is inflated to a pressure at which the radial pulse cannot be palpated in the wrist. A stethoscope is then placed over the brachial artery in the region of the patient's elbow. The cuff is then slowly deflated and the blood pressure recorded. It is the nurse's responsibility to record the blood pressure accurately and to report changes to the person in charge.

Lymphatic system

The lymphatic system (see Figure 12.19) is part of the circulatory system and it transports a clear fluid called lymph. The lymphatic system begins with very small, closed-end vessels called lymphatic capillaries (see Figure 12.20), which are in contact with the surrounding tissues and the interstitial fluid. The lymphatic system consists of:

- Lymph
- Lymph vessels
- Lymph nodes
- Lymphatic organs such as spleen and the thymus.

Lymph

Lymph is a clear fluid found inside the lymphatic capillaries and has a similar composition to plasma. Lymph is the ultra-filtrate of the blood which occurs at the capillary ends of the blood vessels. Blood pressure in the blood vessel forces fluid and other substances such as small protein (albumin) from the capillaries into the tissue space as interstitial fluid, which then enters the lymphatic capillaries as lymph. The body contains approximately 1–2 litres of lymph which forms about 1–3 per cent of body weight. Lymph transports plasma proteins, bacteria, fat from the small intestine and damaged tissues to the lymph nodes for destruction. The lymph contains lymphocytes and macrophages, which play an important role in the immune system.

Lymph capillaries and large lymph vessels

Both the blood and the lymphatic capillaries have a similar structure in that they both consist of a single layered endothelial cell that allows movement of substances from the interstitial space into the lymphatic capillaries (see Figure 12.21). However, lymphatic capillaries are one-way vessels with a blind end (see Figure 12.20) in the interstitial space. Lymphatic vessels resemble veins in structure, however the lymphatic vessels have thinner walls and more valves in them. The larger lymphatic vessels have numerous valves within them to prevent backflow of lymph. The lymphatic vessels combine to form two large ducts, the right lymphatic and thoracic ducts, which then empty into the subclavian veins.

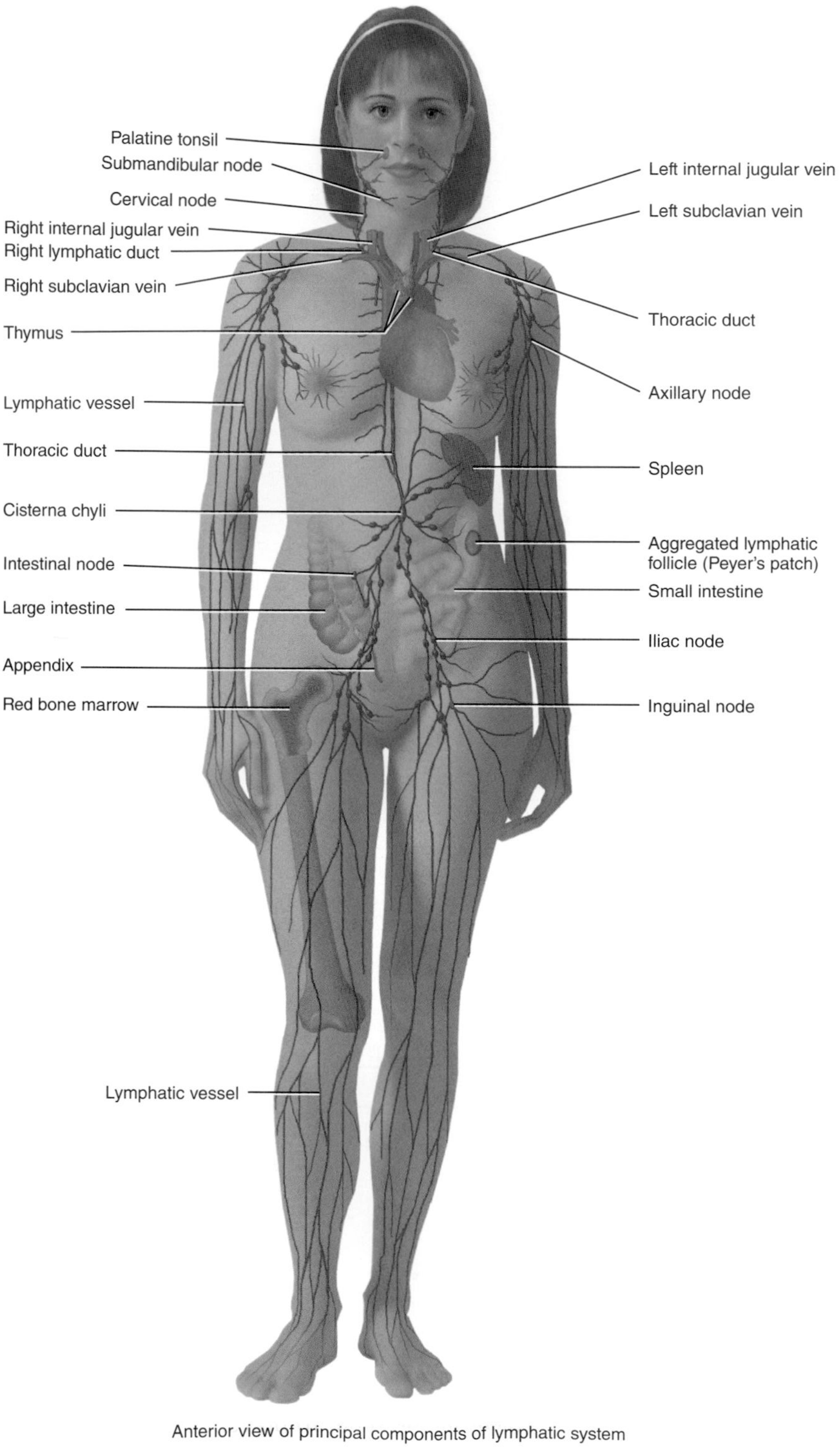
Palatine tonsil
Submandibular node
Cervical node
Right internal jugular vein
Right lymphatic duct
Right subclavian vein
Thymus
Lymphatic vessel
Thoracic duct
Cisterna chyli
Intestinal node
Large intestine
Appendix
Red bone marrow
Lymphatic vessel
Left internal jugular vein
Left subclavian vein
Thoracic duct
Axillary node
Spleen
Aggregated lymphatic follicle (Peyer's patch)
Small intestine
Iliac node
Inguinal node
Anterior view of principal components of lymphatic system

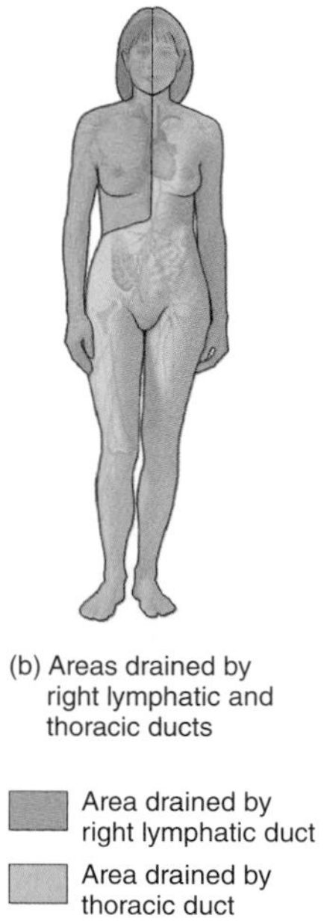
(b) Areas drained by right lymphatic and thoracic ducts
Area drained by right lymphatic duct
Area drained by thoracic duct

Figure 12.19 Lymphatic system (Tortora and Derrickson 2009)

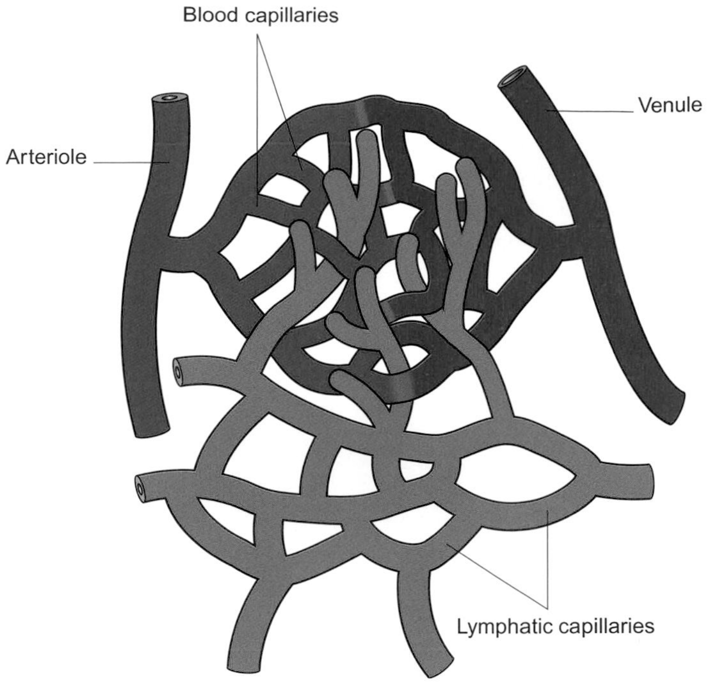
Blood capillaries
Venule
Arteriole
Lymphatic capillaries

Figure 12.20 Lymphatic capillaries

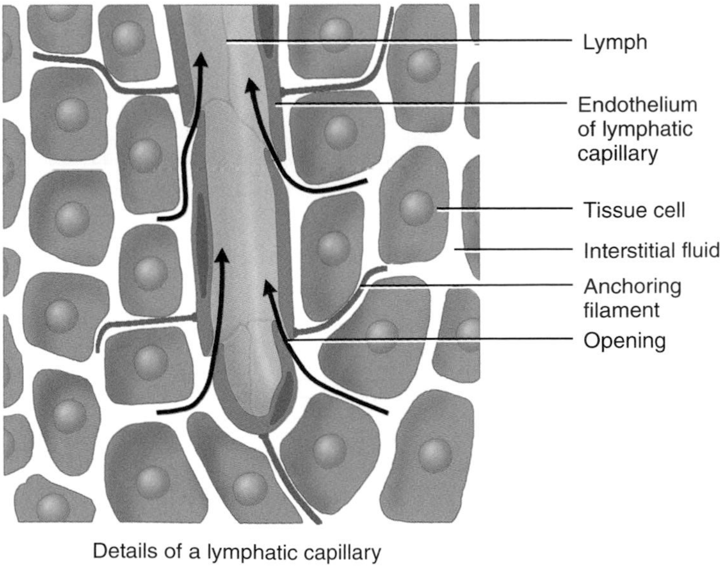
Lymph
Endothelium of lymphatic capillary
Tissue cell
Interstitial fluid
Anchoring filament
Opening
Details of a lymphatic capillary

Figure 12.21 Lymphatic circulation (Tortora and Derrickson 2009)

Lymph nodes

Lymph nodes are bean-shaped organs located along the lymphatic vessels. These nodes are found in the largest concentrations in the neck, armpit, thorax, abdomen and the groin; lesser concentrations are found behind the elbows and knees. The lymphocytes in the lymph nodes filter out harmful substances from the lymph and are sites for specific defences of the immune system. The lymph node is made up of an outer fibrous capsule which dips down into the node to form partitions (trabeculae), thus dividing the node into compartments (see Figure 12.22). Approximately four or five afferent vessels may enter a lymph node; however, only one efferent vessel will transport the lymph out of the node.

Lymphatic organs

Spleen

The two main organs of the lymphatic system are the spleen and the thymus gland. The spleen is the largest lymphoid organ and is approximately 12 cm in length, 7 cm wide and 2.5 cm thick. It weighs about 200 g and is purplish in colour. The main functions of the spleen are:

- Filtering the blood – the destruction of old red blood cells and the remnants of manufacturing phagocytic lymphocytes and monocytes
- Storage of blood – approximately 350 ml.

The structure of the spleen is similar to the lymph node. It is surrounded by a capsule of connective tissue and, like the lymph nodes, the spleen is divided into compartments by trabeculae. The two main functional sections of the spleen are the red and the white pulp. It is in contact with the stomach, the left kidney and the diaphragm. The blood supply to the spleen derives from the splenic artery and the splenic vein transports the blood out of the spleen.

The thymus gland

The thymus gland is a ductless, pinkish-grey mass of lymphoid tissue located in the thorax. At birth it is about 5 cm in length, 4 cm in breadth and about 6 mm in thickness. The organ enlarges during childhood and atrophies at puberty. The thymus gland consists of two lobes joined by a connective tissue and each lobe is covered by an outer cortex and an inner portion called the medulla. Each lobe is divided into lobules by trabeculae and each lobule has an outer cortex and inner medulla. The cortex contains many immature lymphocytes which migrate from the bone marrow to the thymus gland to become specialised T-lymphocytes (T-cells). Mature T-cells then migrate to the medulla and it is from the medulla the mature T-cells enter the general circulation where they are transported by the blood to the spleen and the lymph nodes.

Functions of the lymphatic system

- The lymphatic system aids the immune system in destroying pathogens and filtering waste so that the lymph can be safely returned to the circulatory system

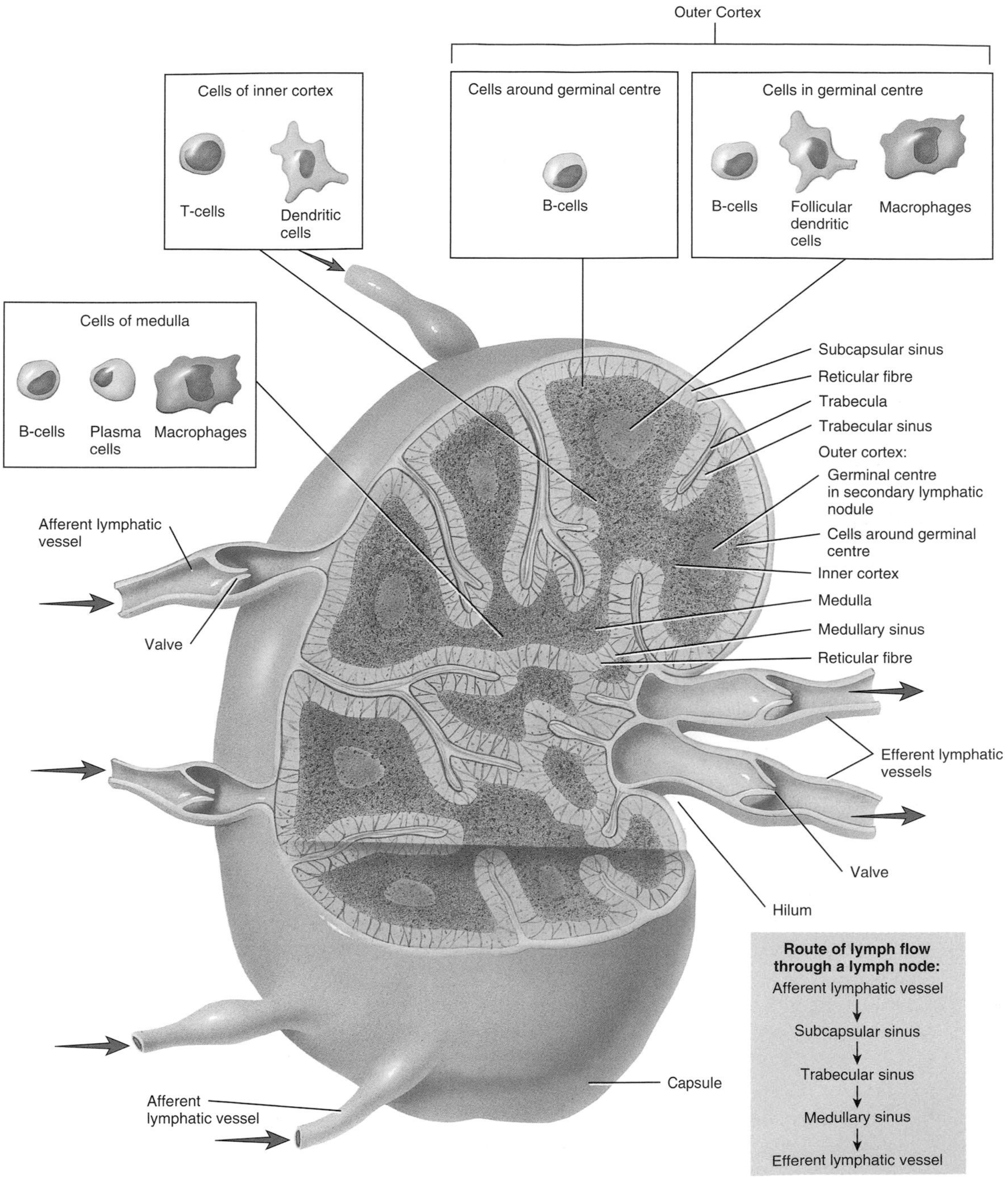

Outer Cortex
Cells of inner cortex
T-cells
Dendritic cells
Cells around germinal centre
B-cells
Cells in germinal centre
B-cells
Follicular dendritic cells
Macrophages
Cells of medulla
B-cells
Plasma cells
Macrophages
Subcapsular sinus
Reticular fibre
Trabecula
Trabecular sinus
Outer cortex:
Germinal centre in secondary lymphatic nodule
Cells around germinal centre
Inner cortex
Medulla
Medullary sinus
Reticular fibre
Afferent lymphatic vessel
Valve
Efferent lymphatic vessels
Valve
Hilum
Capsule
Afferent lymphatic vessel
Route of lymph flow through a lymph node:
Afferent lymphatic vessel
Subcapsular sinus
Trabecular sinus
Medullary sinus
Efferent lymphatic vessel

Figure 12.22 A lymph node (Tortora and Derrickson 2009)

- The lymphatic system removes excess fluid, waste, debris, dead blood cells, pathogens, cancer cells and toxins from these cells and the tissue spaces between them
- The lymphatic system also works with the circulatory system to deliver nutrients, oxygen and hormones from the blood to the cells that make up the tissues of the body
- Important protein molecules are created by cells in the tissues. These molecules are too large to enter the capillaries of the circulatory system, thus these protein molecules are transported by the lymph to the bloodstream.

Clinical considerations

Tonsillitis

Tonsillitis is a very common condition, most frequent in children aged 5–10 years and young adults between 15 and 25 years. Tonsillitis occurs when the tonsils, the collections of lymphoid tissue in the back of the mouth at the top of the throat, are involved in a bacterial or viral infection that causes them to become swollen and inflamed. The tonsils normally help to filter out bacteria and other micro-organisms to aid the body in fighting infection. Symptoms include sore throat, high fever and difficulty swallowing. The infection may also spread to the throat and surrounding areas, causing pain and inflammation (pharyngitis). The treatment of tonsillitis includes antibiotics to treat the infection, antipyretic therapy or surgery (tonsillectomy).

Conclusion

The circulatory system is a very efficient and complex system. It ensures that all the cells and tissues of the body receive all they need, including oxygen, nutrients and electrolytes to ensure that all systems are functioning efficiently. The blood transports many substances such as red blood cells, white blood cells, hormones and electrolytes essential for cellular function. It also plays a major role in the body's defence against bacteria and other organism through the action of the white blood cells. The blood also transports waste products of metabolism, for example urea, carbon dioxide and uric acid.

Blood that is pumped out of the left ventricle of the heart is transported by a network of vessels called arteries and the blood is returned to the heart by the veins. There are three types of blood vessels: arteries, veins and capillaries. Arteries carry blood away from the heart while the veins transport blood to the heart. The blood vessels of the circulatory system are a closed system in that blood does not leave or leak out of the blood vessels unless they are damaged. It is at the capillary end that nutrients and other products essential for cellular function leave the blood vessels. White blood cells may also leave the blood vessels at the capillary end; however, red blood cells are contained within the circulatory system.

The lymphatic system is also known as the secondary circulation. It transports fluid called lymph which is an ultrafiltrate of the blood. It plays an important part in the immune system. The fluid lymph is transported by the lymphatic system from all parts of the body and returned to the circulatory system via the right lymphatic and thoracic ducts, which then empty into the subclavian veins.

Glossary

Adenosine triphosphate:	Organic molecule that stores and releases chemical energy for use in body cells.
Agglutination:	Process by which red blood cells adhere to one another.
Aggregation:	Clumping together.
Antibodies:	Protein produced in response to the presence of some foreign substances.
Antigens:	Foreign proteins against which antibodies are produced.
Aorta:	The biggest artery that emerges from the left ventricle.
Arteries:	Blood vessels that carry blood away from the heart.
Arterioles:	Small arteries.
Baroreceptor:	Neurone sensing changes in fluid, air and blood pressures.
B-lymphocytes:	A type of lymphocytes that produces specific antibodies.
Blood pressure:	Force exerted by the blood against the walls of the blood vessel due to the contraction of the heart.
Bilirubin:	A pigment found in bile resulting from the destruction of red blood cells.
Blood groups:	Classification of blood based on the type of antigen found on the surface of the red blood cell.
Coagulation:	Changing from liquid to solid; formation of a blood clot.
Erythrocytes:	Another name for red blood cells.
Haemoglobin:	An iron-containing protein found in red blood cells which transports oxygen.
Homeostasis:	A state of inner balance in the body which remains relatively constant despite external environment changes.
Lymph:	Fluid found in the lymphatic system.
Lymph nodes:	Small masses of lymphoid tissue.
Plasma:	Fluid portion of blood.
Platelet:	A type of blood cell important in blood clotting.
Polypeptide:	A chain of amino acids.
Tunica externa:	Membranous outer layer of the blood vessel.
Tunica intima:	The inner lining of a blood vessel.

Tunica media: Middle muscle layer of the blood vessel.

White blood cells: Leucocytes.

Urobilinogen: A product of bilirubin breakdown.

References

Nair, M. (2009) The blood and associated disorders. In: Nair, M. and Peate, I. (eds) *Fundamentals of Pathophysiology*. Chichester: John Wiley & Sons.

Tortora, G.J. and Derrickson, B.H. (2009) *Principles of Anatomy and Physiology*, 12th edn. Hoboken, NJ: John Wiley & Sons.

Activities

www.wiley.com/go/peate

Multiple choice questions

1. The smallest blood cells are?

   (a) basophils
   (b) erythrocytes
   (c) monocytes
   (d) esinophils

2. Haemotocrit is a measure of:

   (a) blood volume
   (b) total number of blood cells
   (c) number of white blood cells
   (d) volume percentage of red blood cells

3. The blood cell that can attack a specific antigen is a:

   (a) lymphocyte
   (b) monocyte
   (c) neutrophil
   (d) basophil

4. The protein threads that trap blood cells and form a clot are:

(a) fibrinogen
(b) thrombin
(c) fibrin
(d) prothrombin

5. Blood vessels that carry blood away from the heart are the:

(a) veins
(b) venules
(c) capillaries
(d) arteries

6. Which of the following layers contain connective tissue and smooth muscle?

(a) tunica media
(b) tunica interna
(c) tunica externa
(d) both b and c

7. Veins that transport deoxygenated blood are the:

(a) pulmonary
(b) umbilical
(c) hepatic portal
(d) both a and b

8. Blood vessels that supply the walls of the arteries and veins with blood are:

(a) coronary vessels
(b) vasa vasorum
(c) capillaries
(d) venules

9. Excess interstitial fluid drains directly from the body tissues into:

(a) the right lymphatic duct
(b) the thoracic duct
(c) the subclavian veins
(d) lymphatic capillaries

10. The body's largest collection of lymphoid tissue is in the:

(a) thymus gland
(b) spleen
(c) bone marrow
(d) tonsils

True or false

1. Red blood cells are also known as leucocytes.
2. Monocytes contain haemoglobin.
3. All mature red blood cells have no nucleus.
4. White blood cells are produced in the tonsils.
5. The normal pH of blood is 7.35–7.45.
6. Platelets play an important role in clotting.
7. Arteries do not have valves.
8. Arteries and veins have similar thickness of tunica media.
9. The thymus gland is the largest lymphoid organ.
10. Both the blood and lymphatic capillaries have similar structure.

Test your learning

1. Describe the composition of blood.
2. What is the function of the red blood cell?
3. Explain what would happen if type A blood was transfused into a patient with type B.
4. Discuss the formation of red blood cells.
5. What role do the white blood cells play in the immune system?
6. List the layers of the blood vessels.
7. List the differences between an artery and a vein.
8. Discuss the factors affecting blood pressure.
9. What is the function of valves in the veins?
10. List the organs of the lymphatic system.
11. Into which blood vessel does the lymphatic system drain?
12. Describe the structure of a lymph node.
13. What are the differences between blood and lymph?

Label the diagram

From the lists of words, label the diagrams below:

Decreased level of oxygen to tissue as a result of hypoxia, Receptors in the kidney detect low oxygen level, Kidney increases the production of erythropoietin, Erythropoietin transported by the blood to the bone marrow, Increased production of red blood cells, Increased level of red blood cell, Increased oxygen delivery to tissues, Return to homeostasis

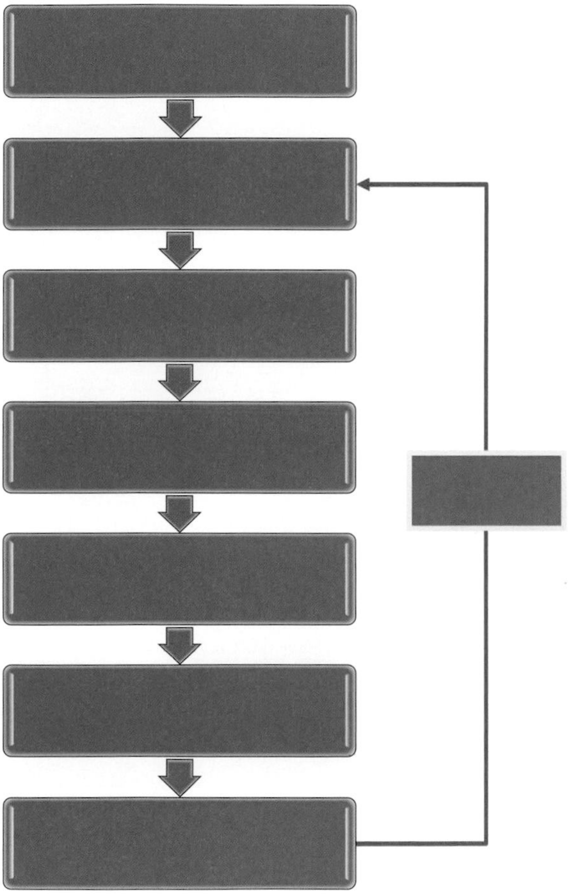

TUNICA INTERNA:, Endothelium, Basement membrane, Valve, Internal elastic lamina, TUNICA MEDIA:, Smooth muscle, External elastic lamina, TUNICA EXTERNA, Lumen, Lumen, Lumen, Basement membrane, Endothelium, Internal elastic lamina, External elastic lamina, Tunica externa, Lumen with blood cells, Tunica interna, Tunica media, Connective tissue, Connective tissue, Red blood cell, Capillary endothelial cells

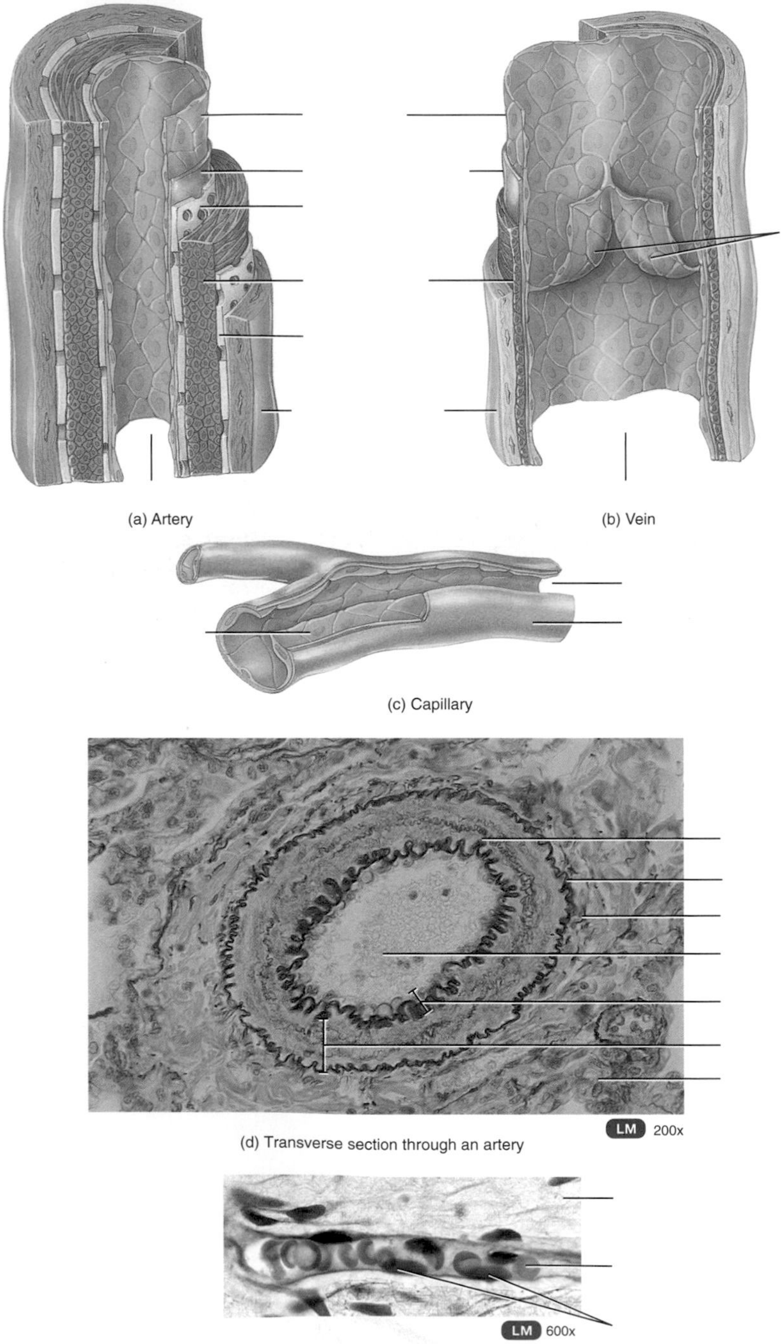
LM 200x
LM 600x

(a) Artery

(b) Vein

(c) Capillary

(d) Transverse section through an artery

(e) Red blood cells passing through a capillary

Blood groups

Complete the table for the ABO blood groups

Blood type	Antigens	Agglutinins	Can donate to	Can receive from
Type A	Antigen A			
Type B		Anti-A		
Type AB			AB	
Type O	None			

Matching words

Which of the following words best describe the following statements:

1. Tunica intima 2. Tunica media 3. Tunica externa

1. Single thin layer of endothelium
2. Contains smooth muscle and elastin
3. Also called adventitia
4. The only layer that plays a role in blood pressure regulation
5. Support and protective coat of blood vessels

Fill in the blanks

Excess ____________________is drained from the _______by the _________________. Once inside the _______________________, the fluid is called _____. The composition of lymph is similar to _____, except the _____ does not have ________________ and most of the _____________. Leucocytes in the lymph include __________, which develop into __________ and two types ____________, that is ______________________. Lymphatic capillaries are __________________. They join together to form _________________, which drain into the ______________________ and the ______________. These ducts then return the lymph to the blood via the _________________________________.

Conditions

Below is a list of conditions that are associated with the circulatory system. Take some time and write notes about each of the conditions. You may make the notes taken from text books or other resources, for example, people you work with in a clinical area, or you may make the notes as a result of people you have cared for. If you are making notes about people you have cared for you must ensure that you adhere to the rules of confidentiality.

Hypertension	
Oedema	
Atherosclerosis/ arteriosclerosis	
Peripheral vascular diseases	
Anaemias	
Deep vein thrombosis	
Leukaemia	
Disseminated intravascular coagulation	
Lymphomas	
Splenomegaly	

Answers

MCQs

1b; 2d; 3a; 4c; 5d; 6a; 7c; 8b; 9d; 10b

True or false

1F; 2F; 3T; 4F; 5T; 6T; 7T; 8F; 9F; 10T

Fill in the blanks

Excess interstitial fluid is drained from the tissues by the lymphatic system. Once inside the lymphatic capillaries, the fluid is called lymph. The composition of lymph is similar to blood, except the lymph does not have red blood cells and most of the blood proteins. Leucocytes in the lymph include monocytes, which develop into macrophages and two types lymphocytes, that is B and T lymphocytes. Lymphatic capillaries are closed-end vessels. They join together to form lymphatic vessels, which drain into the right lymphatic duct and the thoracic duct. These ducts then return the lymph to the blood via the right and left subclavian veins.

Blood groups

Blood type	Antigens	Agglutinins	Can donate to	Can receive from
Type A	Antigen A	Anti-B	A, AB	A, O
Type B	Antigen B	Anti-A	B, AB	B, O
Type AB	Antigen A Antigen B	None	AB	A, B, AB, O
Type O	None	Anti-A Anti-B	A, B, AB, O	O

Matching words

Which of the following words best describe the following statements:

1. Tunica intima 2. Tunica media 3. Tunica externa

1. Single thin layer of endothelium
2. Contains smooth muscle and elastin
3. Also called adventitia
4. The only layer that plays a role in blood pressure regulation
5. Support and protective coat of blood vessels

13 The digestive system and nutrition

Louise McErlean

Contents

Introduction	*408*
The activity of the digestive system	**408**
The mouth (oral cavity)	409
Tongue	409
Palate	409
Teeth	409
Salivary glands	410
Pharynx	413
Swallowing (deglutition)	413
Oesophagus	414
The structure of the digestive system	**414**
Stomach	416
Small intestine	418
The pancreas	**421**
The liver and production of bile	**423**
The functions of the liver	424
The gall bladder	**425**
The large intestine	**425**
Digestive tract hormones	**427**
Nutrition, chemical digestion and metabolism	**427**
Nutrients	428
Balanced diet	428
Nutrient groups	429
Conclusion	*431*
Glossary	*435*
References	*439*
Activities	*439*

Test your knowledge

- What is the function of the digestive system?
- List the structures of the digestive system.
- Name the food groups.
- Differentiate between macronutrients and micronutrients.

Fundamentals of Anatomy and Physiology for Student Nurses, First Edition. Edited by Ian Peate, Muralitharan Nair.

Learning outcomes

On completion of this chapter the reader will be able to:

- Describe the structures of the digestive system
- Describe the functions of each of these structures
- Explain the action of the enzymes and hormones associated with the digestion of proteins, carbohydrates and fats
- Describe what proteins, carbohydrates and fats are broken down into and how the body uses these constituent parts
- Describe the structure and function of the accessory organ of the digestive system
- List the common vitamins and minerals and the problems associated with a deficit or excess

Body map

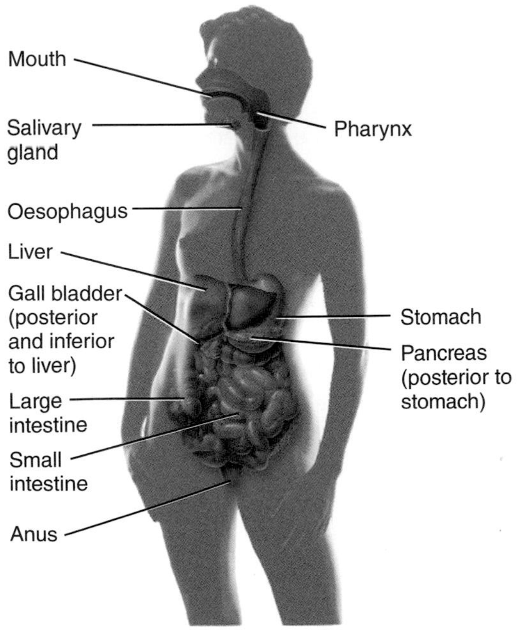
Mouth
Salivary gland
Oesophagus
Liver
Gall bladder (posterior and inferior to liver)
Large intestine
Small intestine
Anus
Pharynx
Stomach
Pancreas (posterior to stomach)

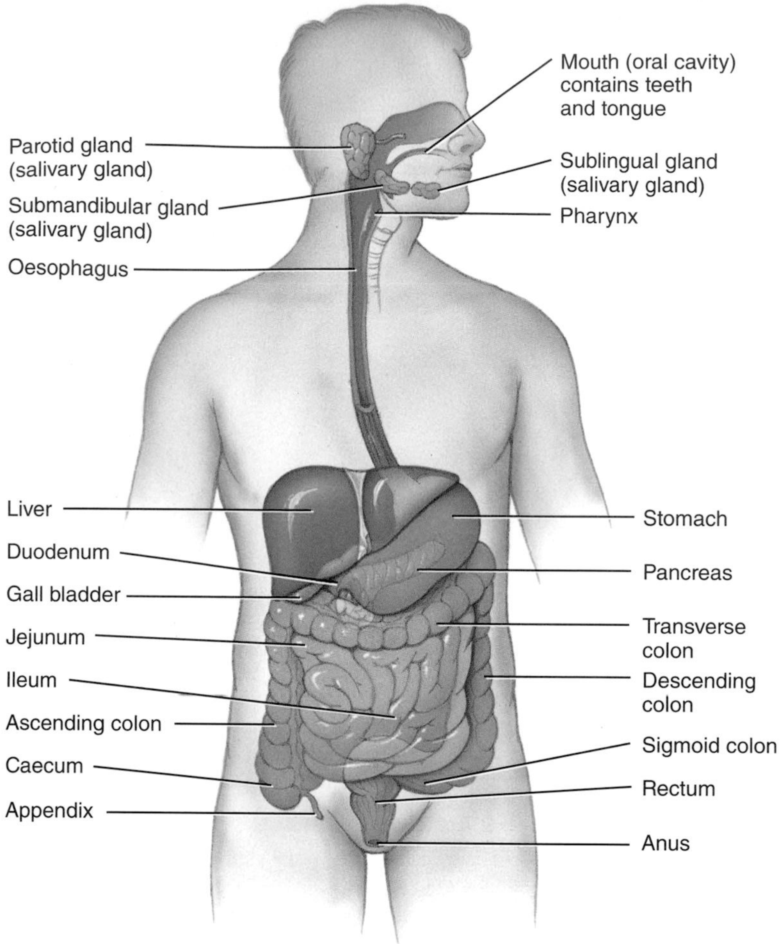
Mouth (oral cavity) contains teeth and tongue
Parotid gland (salivary gland)
Sublingual gland (salivary gland)
Submandibular gland (salivary gland)
Pharynx
Oesophagus
Liver
Stomach
Duodenum
Pancreas
Gall bladder
Jejunum
Transverse colon
Ileum
Descending colon
Ascending colon
Sigmoid colon
Caecum
Rectum
Appendix
Anus

Figure 13.1 The digestive system (Tortora and Derrickson 2009)

Introduction

The digestive system is also known as the gastrointestinal system or the alimentary canal. This vast system is approximately 10 metres long. It travels the length of the body from the mouth through the thoracic, abdominal and pelvic cavities where it ends at the anus (see Figure 13.1). The digestive system has one major function: to convert food from the diet into a form that can be utilised by the cells of the body in order to carry out their specific functions. This chapter discusses the structure and function of the digestive system. It also discusses how dietary nutrients are broken down and used by the body.

The activity of the digestive system

The activity of the digestive system can be categorised into five processes:

- **Ingestion:** the process of taking food into the digestive system
- **Propulsion:** the process of moving the food along the length of the digestive system
- **Digestion:** the process of breaking down food. This can be achieved *mechanically* as food is chewed or moved through the digestive system, or *chemically* by the action of *enzymes* mixed with the food as it moves through the digestive system
- **Absorption:** during this process the products of digestion exit the digestive system and enter the blood or lymph capillaries for distribution
- **Elimination:** the waste products of digestion are excreted from the body as faeces.

The digestive system consists of the mouth, pharynx, oesophagus, stomach, small intestine and large intestine. Accessory organs also contribute to the function of the digestive system. The accessory organs are the salivary glands, the liver, the gall bladder and the pancreas.

The mouth (oral cavity)

The mouth or oral cavity is where the process of digestion begins. The oral cavity consists of several structures (see Figure 13.2).

The **lips** and **cheeks** are muscular and connective tissue structures, lined with mucus-secreting, stratified, squamous epithelial cells, which provides protection against abrasion caused by wear and tear.

The lips and cheeks help to move and hold food in the mouth while the teeth tear and grind the food. This process is called **mastication** (chewing). The lips and cheeks are also involved in speech and facial expression.

Tongue

The tongue is a large, voluntary muscular structure which occupies much of the oral cavity. It is attached posteriorly to the *hyoid* bone and inferiorly by the *frenulum*.

The superior surface of the tongue is covered in stratified squamous epithelium for protection against wear and tear. This surface also contains many little projections called papillae. The papillae (or taste buds) contain the nerve endings responsible for the sense of taste. As well as taste, other functions of the tongue include swallowing (deglutition), holding and moving food around and speech.

Palate

The palate forms the roof of the mouth and consists of two parts: the hard palate and the soft palate. The hard palate is located anteriorly and is bony. The soft palate lies posteriorly and consists of skeletal muscle and connective tissue. The palate plays a part in swallowing. The *palatine tonsils* lie laterally and are lymphoid tissue. The *uvula* is a fold of tissue that hangs down from the centre of the soft palate.

Teeth

Temporary teeth also known as deciduous or milk teeth begin to appear at about 6 months old. There are 20 temporary teeth and these are replaced by permanent teeth from about the age of 6 (Nair and Peate 2009). There are 32 permanent teeth. Sixteen are located in the maxilla arch (upper) and 16 are located in the mandible (lower) (see Figure 13.3).

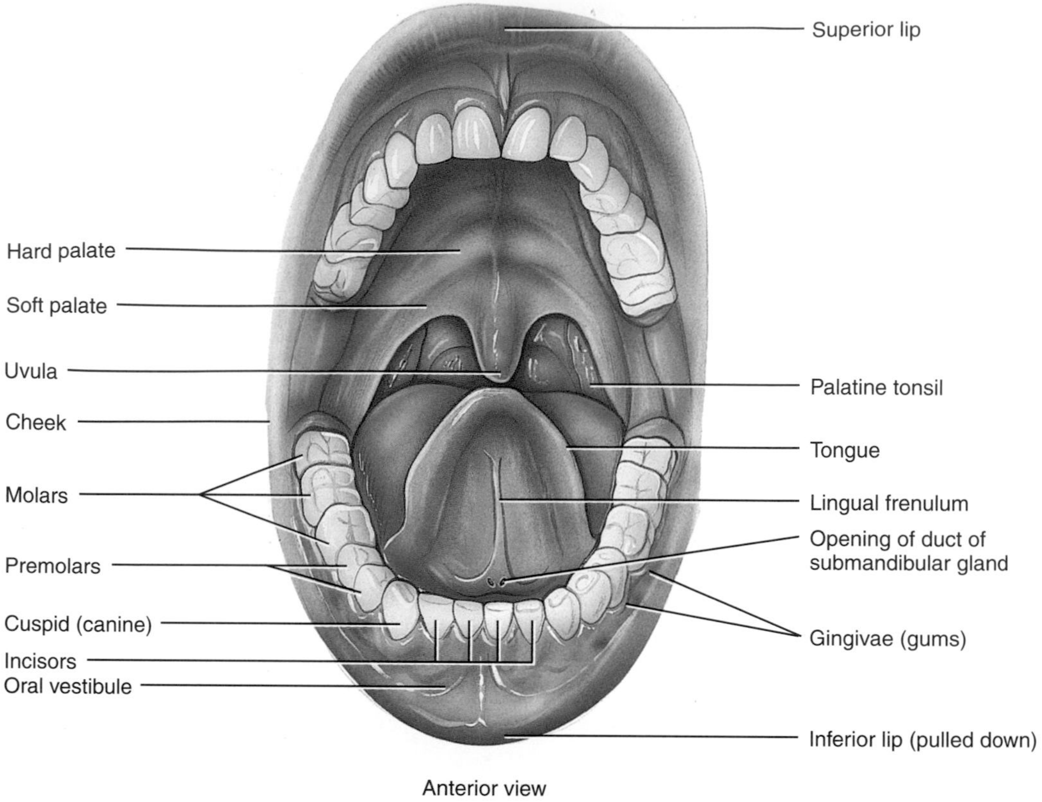
Superior lip
Hard palate
Soft palate
Uvula
Cheek
Molars
Premolars
Cuspid (canine)
Incisors
Oral vestibule
Palatine tonsil
Tongue
Lingual frenulum
Opening of duct of submandibular gland
Gingivae (gums)
Inferior lip (pulled down)
Anterior view

Figure 13.2 The oral cavity (Tortora and Derrickson 2009)

Canines and incisors are cutting and tearing teeth. Premolars and molars are used for the grinding and chewing of food. Despite their different functions and shape the structure of each tooth is the same. The visible part of the tooth is called the *crown.* The centre of the tooth is called the *pulp cavity*. Blood and lymph vessels and nerves enter and leave the tooth here. Surrounding this is a calcified matrix called the *dentine*. Surrounding the dentine is a very hard, protective material called *enamel*. The neck of the tooth is where the crown meets the root. The teeth are anchored in a socket with a bone-like material called *cementum* and the function of the teeth is to chew (masticate) food.

Salivary glands

There are three pairs of salivary glands (see Figure 13.4).

The *parotid glands* are the largest and they are located anterior to the ears. Saliva from the parotid glands enters the oral cavity close to the level of the second upper molar tooth. The submandibular glands are located below the jaw on each side of the face. Saliva from these glands enters the oral cavity from beside the frenulum of the tongue. The sublingual glands are the smallest. They are located in the floor of the mouth.

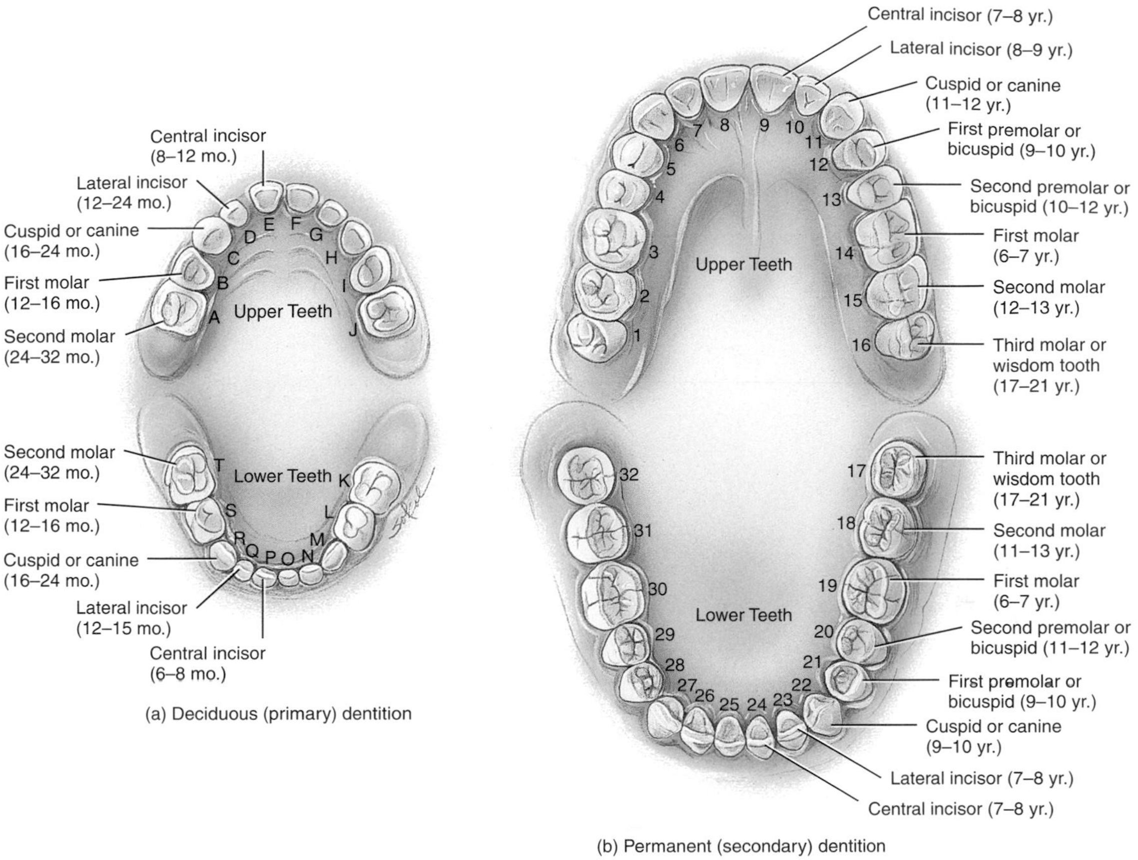
Central incisor
(8–12 mo.)
Lateral incisor
(12–24 mo.)
Cuspid or canine
(16–24 mo.)
First molar
(12–16 mo.)
Second molar
(24–32 mo.)
Upper Teeth
Lower Teeth
Second molar
(24–32 mo.)
First molar
(12–16 mo.)
Cuspid or canine
(16–24 mo.)
Lateral incisor
(12–15 mo.)
Central incisor
(6–8 mo.)
(a) Deciduous (primary) dentition
Central incisor (7–8 yr.)
Lateral incisor (8–9 yr.)
Cuspid or canine
(11–12 yr.)
First premolar or
bicuspid (9–10 yr.)
Second premolar or
bicuspid (10–12 yr.)
First molar
(6–7 yr.)
Second molar
(12–13 yr.)
Third molar or
wisdom tooth
(17–21 yr.)
Third molar or
wisdom tooth
(17–21 yr.)
Second molar
(11–13 yr.)
First molar
(6–7 yr.)
Second premolar or
bicuspid (11–12 yr.)
First premolar or
bicuspid (9–10 yr.)
Cuspid or canine
(9–10 yr.)
Lateral incisor (7–8 yr.)
Central incisor (7–8 yr.)
(b) Permanent (secondary) dentition

Figure 13.3 Teeth (Tortora and Derrickson 2009)

The salivary glands are innervated with parasympathetic fibres which stimulate increased secretion of saliva and sympathetic fibres which decrease secretion of saliva.

Approximately 1–1.5 l of saliva are secreted daily. Saliva consists of:

- Water
- Salivary amylase
- Mucus
- Mineral salts
- Lysozyme
- Immunoglobulins
- Blood clotting factors.

Saliva has several important functions:

- Salivary amylase is a digestive enzyme responsible for beginning the breakdown of carbohydrate molecules from complex polysaccharides to the disaccharide maltase.

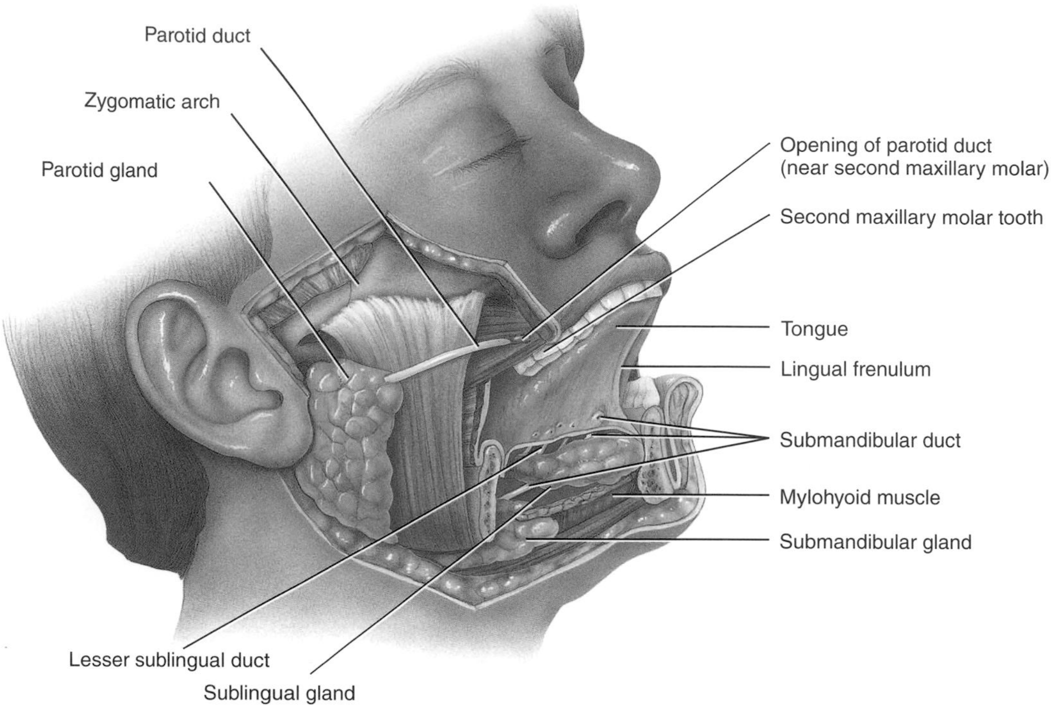
Parotid duct
Zygomatic arch
Parotid gland
Opening of parotid duct
(near second maxillary molar)
Second maxillary molar tooth
Tongue
Lingual frenulum
Submandibular duct
Mylohyoid muscle
Submandibular gland
Lesser sublingual duct
Sublingual gland

Figure 13.4 Salivary glands (Tortora and Derrickson 2009)

- The fluid nature of saliva helps to moisten and lubricate food that enters the mouth. This makes it easier to hold the food in the mouth and also assists in forming the food into a bolus in preparation for swallowing.
- The continuous secretion of saliva is cleansing and helps to maintain moisture in the oral cavity. A lack of moisture can lead to oral mucosal infections and formation of mouth ulcers.
- The oral cavity is an entry route for pathogens from the external environment. Lysozyme, a constituent of saliva, has an antibacterial action. Immunoglobulin and clotting factors also prevents infection.
- Taste is only possible when food substances are moist. Saliva is required to moisten food.

Clinical considerations

Salivary gland calculi

The mineral salt content in saliva can cause problems for some people. In susceptible individuals the mineral salts can crystallise and form stones (calculi) which completely or partially obstruct the ducts preventing saliva from entering the mouth. The patient can complain of pain and swelling at the site of the gland, dryness of the mouth and a predisposition to oral infections.

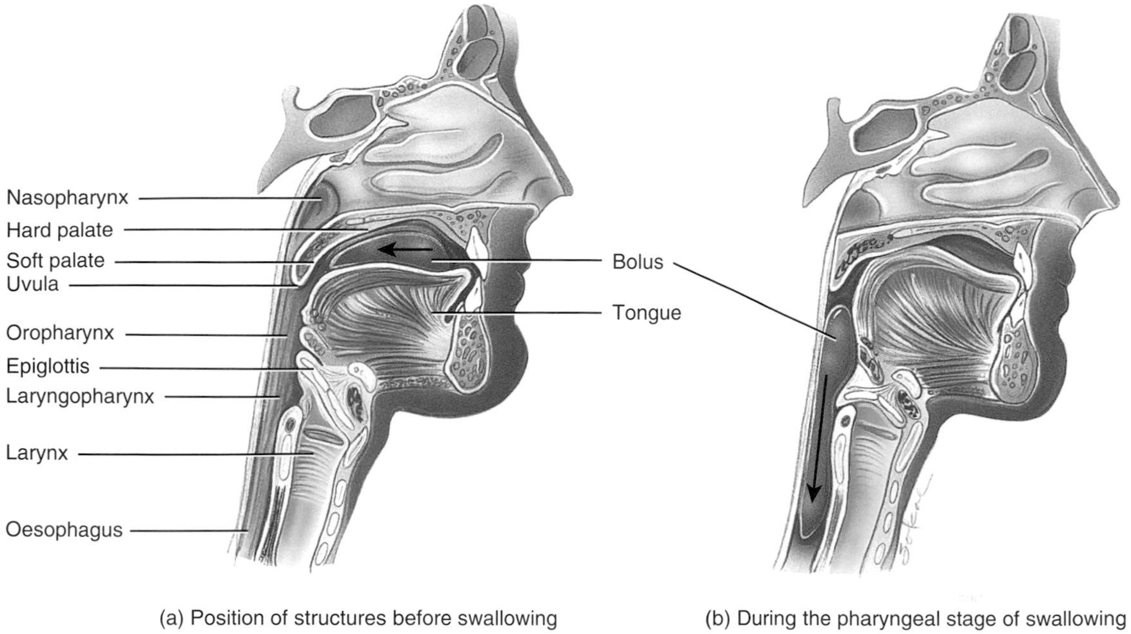
Nasopharynx
Hard palate
Soft palate
Uvula
Oropharynx
Epiglottis
Laryngopharynx
Larynx
Oesophagus
Bolus
Tongue
(a) Position of structures before swallowing
(b) During the pharyngeal stage of swallowing

Figure 13.5 Swallowing (Tortora and Derrickson 2009)

Pharynx

The pharynx consists of three parts: the *oropharynx*, the *nasopharynx* and the *laryngopharynx*. The nasopharynx is considered a structure of the respiratory system. The oropharynx and the laryngopharynx are passages for both food and respiratory gases (see Figure 13.5). The *epiglottis* is responsible for closing the entrance to the larynx during swallowing and this action prevents food from entering the larynx and obstructing the respiratory passages.

Swallowing (deglutition)

Once the food has been adequately chewed and formed into a bolus, it is ready to be swallowed. Swallowing (deglutition) occurs in three phases:

1. Voluntary phase: during this phase the action of the voluntary muscles serving the oral cavity manipulates the food bolus into the oropharynx. The tongue is pressed against the palate and this prevents the food from moving forward again.
2. Pharyngeal phase: during this phase a reflex action is initiated in response to the sensation of the food bolus in the oropharynx. This reflex is coordinated by the swallowing centre in the medulla oblongata and the motor response is contraction of the muscles of the pharynx. The soft palate elevates, closing off the nasopharynx and preventing the food bolus from using this route. The larynx moves up and moves forward, allowing the epiglottis to cover the entrance to the larynx so the food bolus cannot move into the respiratory passages.

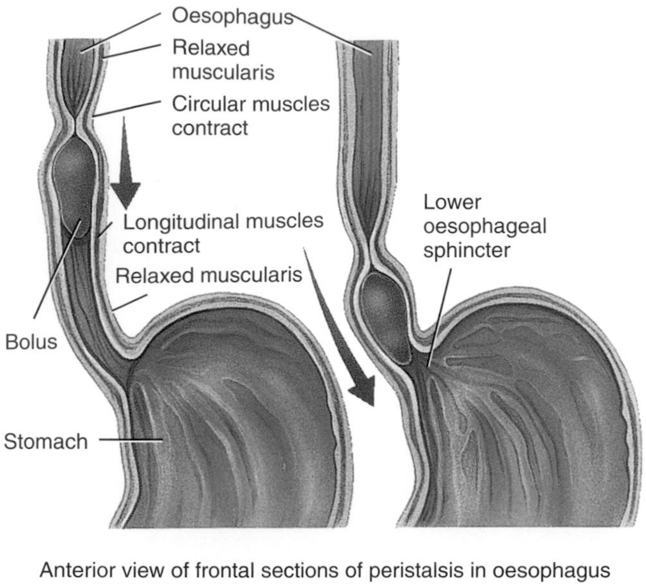
Oesophagus
Relaxed muscularis
Circular muscles contract
Longitudinal muscles contract
Relaxed muscularis
Bolus
Stomach
Lower oesophageal sphincter
Anterior view of frontal sections of peristalsis in oesophagus

Figure 13.6 Peristalsis in the oesophagus (Tortora and Derrickson 2009)

3. Oesophageal phase: the food bolus moves from the pharynx into the oesophagus. Waves of oesophageal muscle contractions move the food bolus down the length of the oesophagus and into the stomach. This wave of muscle contraction is known as peristalsis (see Figure 13.6).

Oesophagus

When food exits the oropharynx it enters the oesophagus. The oesophagus extends from the laryngopharynx to the stomach. It is a thick-walled structure, measures about 25 cm in length and lies in the thoracic cavity, posterior to the trachea. The function of the oesophagus is to transport substances (the food bolus) from the mouth to the stomach. Thick mucus is secreted by the mucosa of the oesophagus and this aids the passage of the food bolus and protects the oesophagus from abrasion.

The upper oesophageal sphincter regulates the movement of substances into the oesophagus and the lower oesophageal sphincter (also known as the cardiac sphincter) regulates the movement of substances from the oesophagus to the stomach. The muscle layer of the oesophagus differs from the rest of the digestive tract as the superior portion consists of skeletal (voluntary) muscle and the inferior portion consists of smooth (involuntary) muscle. Breathing and swallowing cannot occur at the same time (Nair and Peate 2009).

The structure of the digestive system

There are four layers of tissue or tunicas which exist throughout the length of the digestive tract from oesophagus to anus (see Figure 13.7).

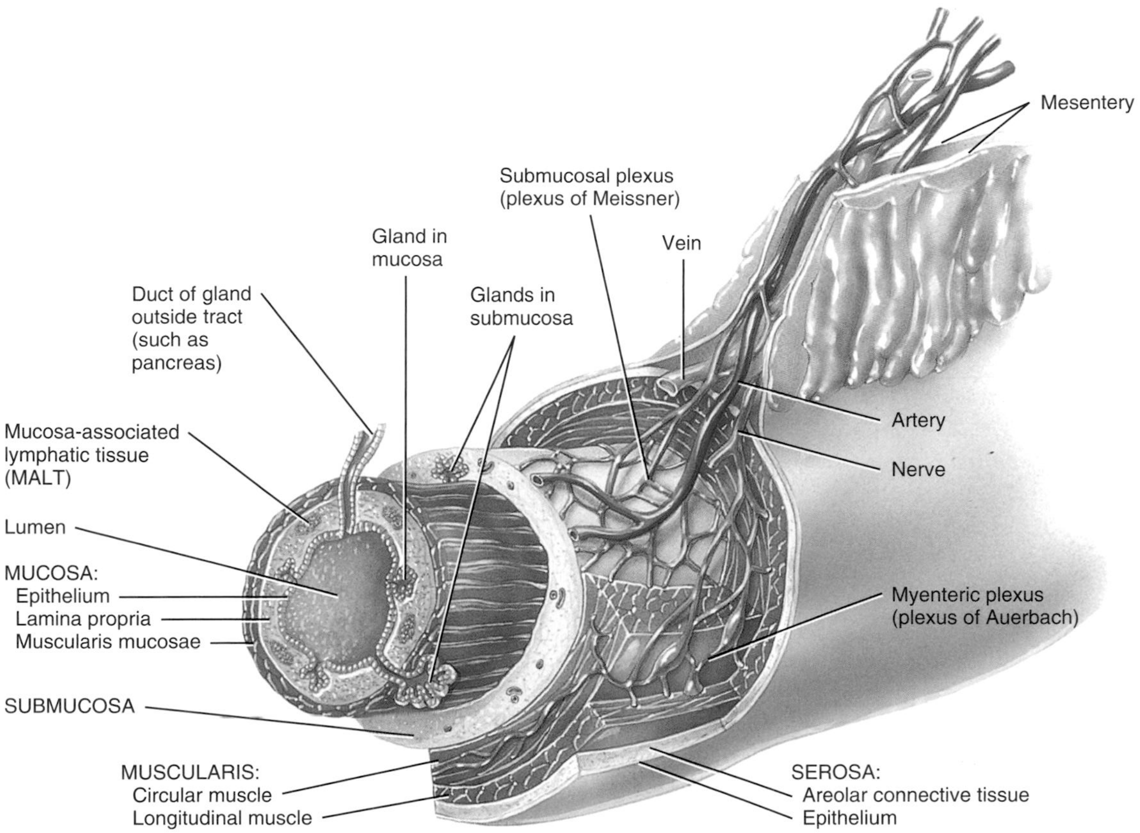
Mesentery
Submucosal plexus
(plexus of Meissner)
Gland in
mucosa
Vein
Glands in
submucosa
Duct of gland
outside tract
(such as
pancreas)
Mucosa-associated
lymphatic tissue
(MALT)
Artery
Nerve
Lumen
MUCOSA:
Epithelium
Lamina propria
Muscularis mucosae
Myenteric plexus
(plexus of Auerbach)
SUBMUCOSA
MUSCULARIS:
Circular muscle
Longitudinal muscle
SEROSA:
Areolar connective tissue
Epithelium

Figure 13.7 Structure of the digestive tract (Tortora and Derrickson 2009)

The **mucosa** is the innermost layer. The products of digestion are in contact with this layer as they pass through the digestive tract. The mucosa consists of three layers: the mucous epithelium (mucous membrane), which is involved in the *secretion* of mucus and other digestive system secretions such as saliva or gastric juice. This layer helps to *protect* the digestive system from the continuous wear and tear it endures. In the small intestine this layer is involved in *absorption* of the products of digestion. The next layer is the *lamina propria* which consists of loose connective tissue which has a role in supporting the blood vessels and lymphatic tissue of the mucosa. The outermost layer is called the *muscularis mucosa* and consists of a thin smooth muscle layer which helps to form the gastric pits or the microvilli of the digestive system.

The **submucosa** is a thick layer of connective tissue. It contains blood and lymphatic vessels and some small glands. It also contains *Meissner's plexus* – nerves that stimulate the intestinal glands to secrete their products.

The **muscularis** consists of an inner layer of circular smooth muscle and an outer layer of longitudinal smooth muscle. The stomach has three layers of smooth muscle and the upper oesophagus has skeletal muscle. Blood and lymph vessels and the *myenteric plexus* (a network of sympathetic and parasympathetic nerves) are located between the two layers of smooth muscle.

The wavelike contraction and relaxation of this muscle layer are responsible for moving food along the digestive tract – a process known as *peristalsis* (see Figure 13.7). Peristalsis helps to churn and mechanically digest food.

The outer layer of the digestive tract is the **serosa (adventitia)**. The largest area of serosa is found in the abdominal and pelvic cavities and is known as the *peritoneum*. The peritoneum is a closed sac. The visceral peritoneum covers the organs of the abdominal and pelvic cavity and the parietal peritoneum lines the abdominal wall. A small amount of serous fluid lies between the two layers. The peritoneum has a good blood supply and contains many lymph nodes and lymphatic vessels. It acts as a barrier, protecting the structures it encloses and can act to isolate areas of infection to prevent damage to neighbouring structures.

Stomach

The stomach lies in the abdominal cavity. It is continuous with the oesophagus superiorly and the duodenum of the small intestine inferiorly. It is divided into regions (see Figure 13.8).

The entrance to the stomach from the oesophagus is via the lower oesophageal sphincter or cardiac sphincter. This leads to a small area within the stomach called the *cardiac region*. The *fundus* is the dome-shaped region in the superior part of the stomach. The *body region* occupies the space between the lesser and greater curvature of the stomach and the *pyloric region* narrows

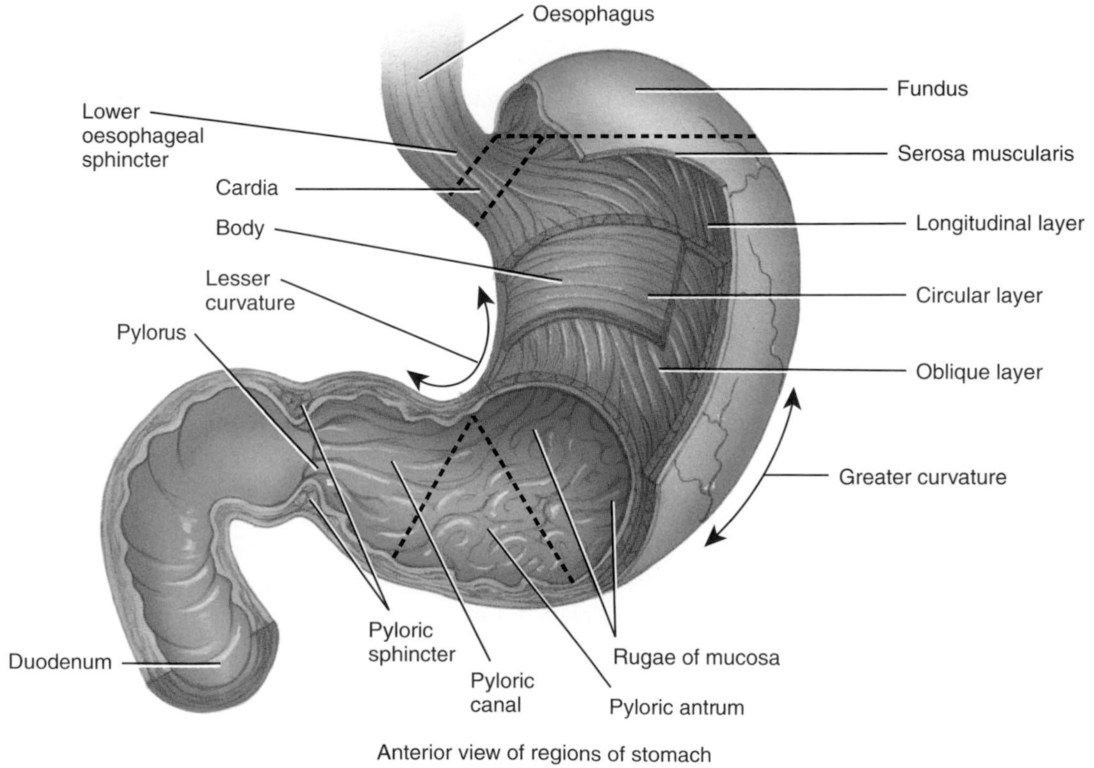
Oesophagus
Fundus
Lower oesophageal sphincter
Serosa muscularis
Cardia
Body
Longitudinal layer
Lesser curvature
Circular layer
Pylorus
Oblique layer
Greater curvature
Duodenum
Pyloric sphincter
Rugae of mucosa
Pyloric canal
Pyloric antrum
Anterior view of regions of stomach

Figure 13.8 Stomach (Tortora and Derrickson 2009)

into the *pyloric canal*. The *pyloric sphincter* controls the exit of *chyme* from the stomach into the small intestine. The food bolus is converted to chyme within the stomach as the chemical digestion of protein begins.

The stomach is supplied with arterial blood from a branch of the celiac artery and venous blood leaves the stomach via the hepatic vein. The vagus nerve innervates the stomach with parasympathetic fibres which stimulate gastric motility and the secretion of gastric juice. Sympathetic fibres from the celiac plexus reduce gastric activity.

The stomach has the same four layers of tissue as the digestive tract but with some differences. The muscularis contains three layers of smooth muscle instead of two. It has longitudinal, circular and oblique muscle fibres. The extra muscle layer facilitates the churning, mixing and mechanical breakdown of food that occurs within the stomach as well as supporting the onward journey of the food by peristalsis.

The mucosa within the stomach is also different from the rest of the digestive tract. When the stomach is empty, the mucosal epithelia falls into long folds known as *rugae*. The rugae fill out when the stomach is full. A very full stomach can contain approximately 4 l while an empty stomach contains only about 50 ml (Marieb and Hoehn 2007). The shape and size of the stomach varies from person to person and depending on the quantity of food stored within it.

The mucosa also contains many gastric glands (see Figure 13.9):

- *Surface mucous cells* produce thick bicarbonate-coated mucus. This thick layer of mucus protects the stomach from corrosion by acidic gastric juice. The mucosal epithelia have tight junctions preventing leakage of gastric juice into the underlying tissues. Any epithelial cells that do become damaged are quickly shed and replaced
- *Mucous neck cells* also secrete mucus – this mucus is different from surface neck cell mucus
- *Parietal cells* produce *hydrochloric acid* and *intrinsic factor*. Intrinsic factor is necessary for the absorption of vitamin B_{12}. This vitamin is essential for the production of mature erythrocytes. Hydrochloric acid creates the acidic environment of the stomach (pH 1–3)
- *Chief cells* produce *pepsinogen* which is converted to *pepsin* in the presence of hydrochloric acid and other pepsin. Pepsin is necessary for the breakdown of protein into smaller peptide chains
- *Enteroendocrine cells* produce a variety of hormones including *gastrin* (from the G cell). These hormones help regulate gastric motility.

This concoction of secretions plus water and mineral salts is more commonly called gastric juice. About 2 litres of gastric juice is produced daily.

Regulation of gastric juice secretion is divided into three phases (see Figure 13.10):

- The cephalic phase: The sight, taste or smell of food stimulates the secretion of gastric juice
- The gastric phase: When food enters the stomach, the hormone gastrin is secreted into the bloodstream and this stimulates the secretion of gastric juice. The secretion of hydrochloric acid reduces the pH of the stomach contents and when the pH drops below 2, the secretion of gastrin is inhibited
- The intestinal phase: As the acidic contents of the stomach enter the duodenum of the small intestine the hormones secretin and cholecystokinin (CKK) are secreted. These hormones also act to reduce the secretion of gastric juice and gastric motility.

The rate of gastric emptying depends on the size and content of the meal. A large meal takes longer than a small meal. Liquids quickly pass through the stomach while solids require longer to

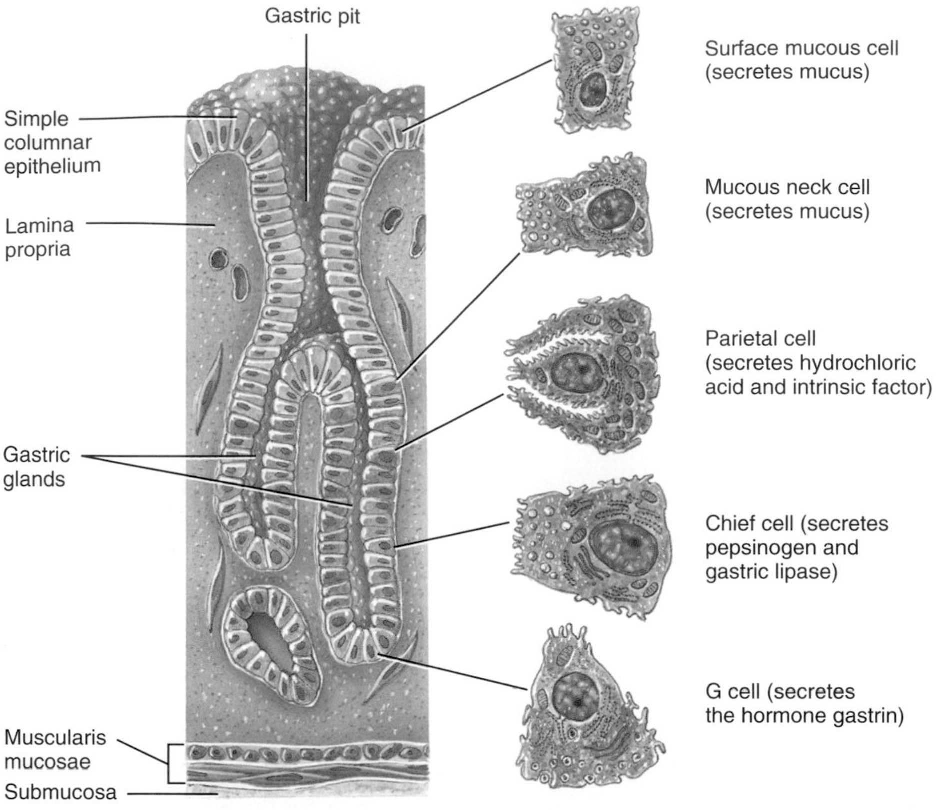
Gastric pit
Simple columnar epithelium
Lamina propria
Gastric glands
Muscularis mucosae
Submucosa
Surface mucous cell (secretes mucus)
Mucous neck cell (secretes mucus)
Parietal cell (secretes hydrochloric acid and intrinsic factor)
Chief cell (secretes pepsinogen and gastric lipase)
G cell (secretes the hormone gastrin)

Figure 13.9 Gastric glands and cells (Tortora and Derrickson 2009)

be thoroughly mixed with gastric juice. Most meals will have left the stomach 4 hours after ingestion.

Small intestine

The small intestine is approximately 6 metres long. It is divided into three parts (see Figure 13.11):

(1) The duodenum is approximately 25 cm long. The pancreas secretes *pancreatic juice* along the *pancreatic duct* into the duodenum. *Bile* is delivered to the duodenum via the *common bile duct*. These ducts meet and enter the duodenum at the *hepatopancreatic ampulla*. The entry of bile and pancreatic juice is controlled by the *sphincter of Oddi*.
(2) The jejunum measures 2.5 m and is the middle part of the small intestine.
(3) The ileum measures 3.5 m. It meets the large intestine at the *ileocaecal valve*. This valve prevents the backflow of the products of digestion from the large intestine back into the small intestine.

The small intestine is innervated with both parasympathetic and sympathetic nerves. It receives its arterial blood supply from the *superior mesenteric artery* and nutrient rich venous blood drains into the *superior mesenteric vein* and eventually into the *hepatic portal vein* towards the liver.

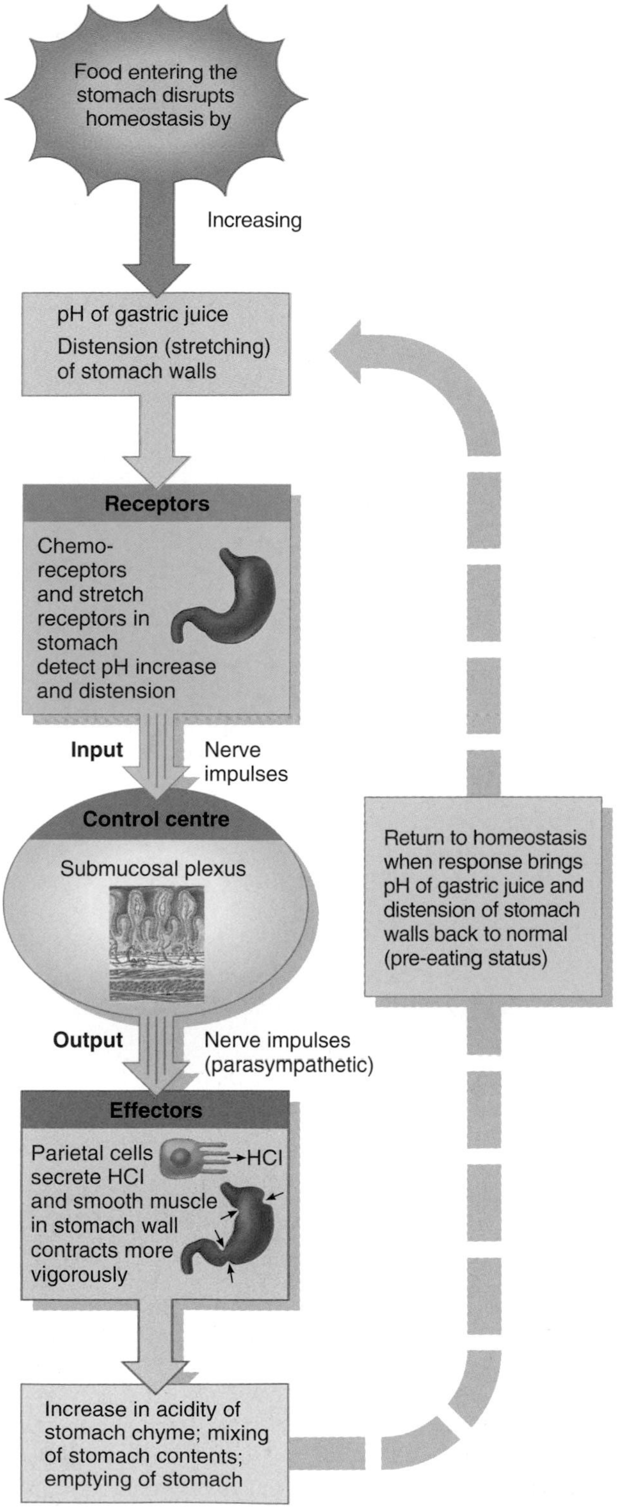

Food entering the stomach disrupts homeostasis by
Increasing
pH of gastric juice
Distension (stretching) of stomach walls
Receptors
Chemo-receptors and stretch receptors in stomach detect pH increase and distension
Input
Nerve impulses
Control centre
Submucosal plexus
Output
Nerve impulses (parasympathetic)
Effectors
Parietal cells secrete HCl and smooth muscle in stomach wall contracts more vigorously
HCl
Increase in acidity of stomach chyme; mixing of stomach contents; emptying of stomach
Return to homeostasis when response brings pH of gastric juice and distension of stomach walls back to normal (pre-eating status)

Figure 13.10 Phases of gastric juice secretion (Tortora and Derrickson 2010)

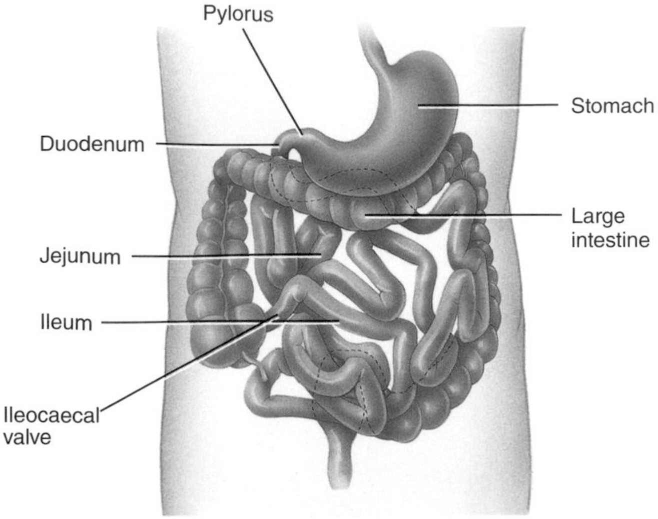
Pylorus
Stomach
Duodenum
Large
intestine
Jejunum
Ileum
Ileocaecal
valve

Figure 13.11 Small intestine (Tortora and Derrickson 2009)

The primary function of the small intestine is absorption of nutrlents and it has several adaptations to facilitate this:

- Permanent circular folds, called *plicae circulars*, within the mucosa and submucosa slow down the movement of the products of digestion, allowing time for absorption of nutrients
- On the surface of the mucosa are tiny, finger-like projections called *villi*. The walls of the villi are columnar epithelial cells. At the centre of the villi is a capillary bed and a *lacteal* (lymph capillary). This allows nutrients to be absorbed directly into the blood or the lymph
- On the surface of the villi are cytoplasmic extensions called *microvilli*. The presence of the microvilli greatly increases the surface area available for absorption. The appearance of the microvilli resembles the surface of a brush hence it is called the *brush border*.

There are four types of cell present in the mucosa of the small intestine (see Figure 13.12):

- The absorptive cell produces digestive enzymes and absorbs digested foods
- Goblet cells secrete mucus to protect the intestine from abrasion
- Enteroendocrine cells produce regulatory hormones such as secretin and cholecystokinin
- Paneth cells produce lysozyme, which protects the small intestine from pathogens which have survived the acid conditions of the stomach. The Peyer's patches (lymphatic tissue of the small intestine) also protect the small intestine.

In the pits between villi are glands called the intestinal crypts or the *crypts of Lieberkühn*. Intestinal juice is secreted from the cells of the crypts in response either to acidic chyme irritating the intestinal mucosa or distension from the presence of chyme in the small intestine. Between 1 and 2 l of intestinal juice is secreted daily. It is slightly alkaline (pH 7.4–8.4) and contains water, mucus, mineral salts and enterokinase.

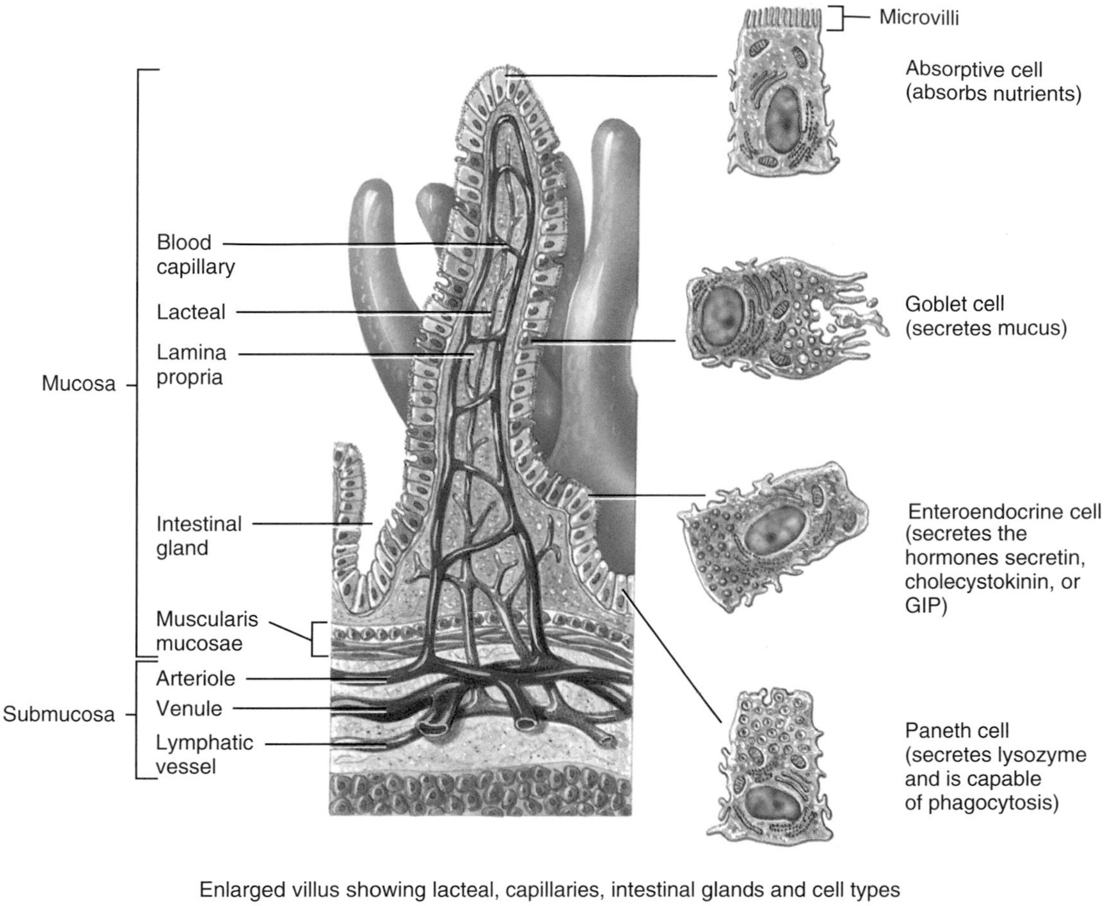
Microvilli
Absorptive cell
(absorbs nutrients)
Blood
capillary
Lacteal
Lamina
propria
Mucosa
Goblet cell
(secretes mucus)
Intestinal
gland
Enteroendocrine cell
(secretes the
hormones secretin,
cholecystokinin, or
GIP)
Muscularis
mucosae
Arteriole
Submucosa
Venule
Lymphatic
vessel
Paneth cell
(secretes lysozyme
and is capable
of phagocytosis)
Enlarged villus showing lacteal, capillaries, intestinal glands and cell types

Figure 13.12 Cells within the villi of the small intestine (Tortora and Derrickson 2009)

Partially digested food enters the small intestine and spends from 3–6 hours moving through its 6 m length. Here it mixes with intestinal juice secreted by the cells of the small intestine. However, intestinal juice alone cannot complete the final breakdown of fats, carbohydrate and protein. Two accessory organs of digestion, the pancreas and the liver (with some assistance from the gall bladder, provide the secretions necessary for this.

The pancreas

The pancreas is composed of exocrine and endocrine tissue. It consists of a head, body and tail (see Figure 13.13). The cells of the pancreas are responsible for making the endocrine and exocrine products.

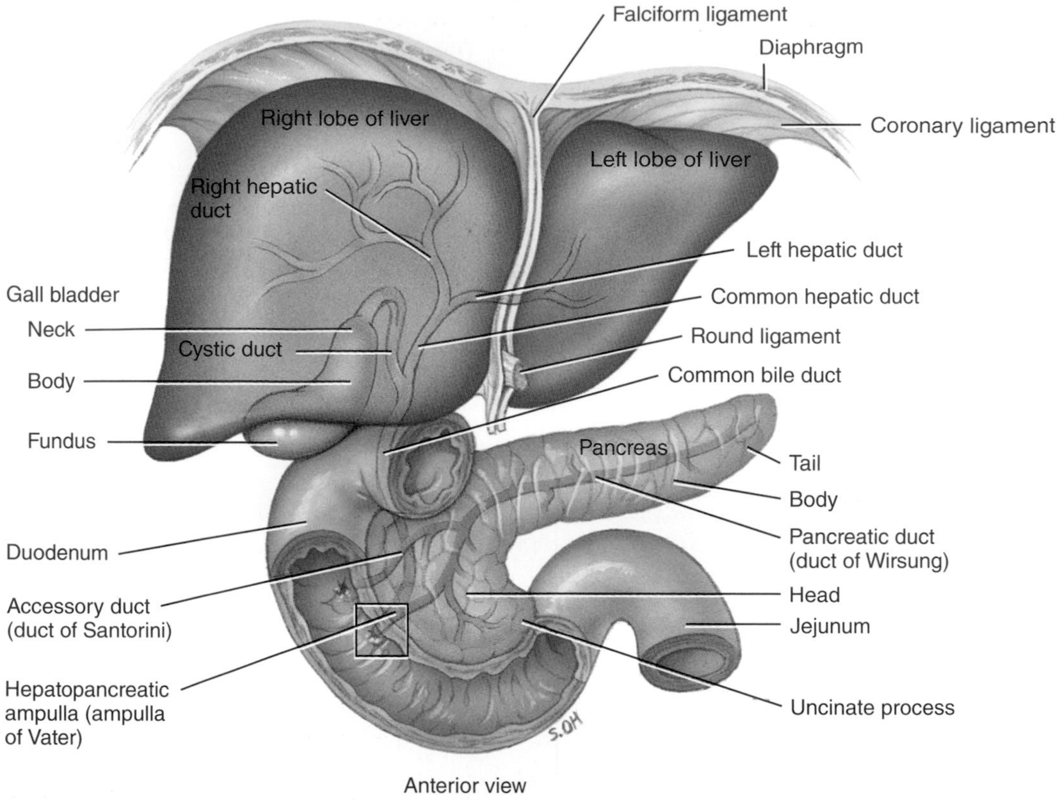
Falciform ligament
Diaphragm
Coronary ligament
Right lobe of liver
Left lobe of liver
Right hepatic duct
Left hepatic duct
Gall bladder
Common hepatic duct
Neck
Cystic duct
Round ligament
Body
Common bile duct
Fundus
Pancreas
Tail
Body
Pancreatic duct (duct of Wirsung)
Duodenum
Accessory duct (duct of Santorini)
Head
Jejunum
Hepatopancreatic ampulla (ampulla of Vater)
Uncinate process
Anterior view

Figure 13.13 View of the liver, gall bladder and pancreas (Tortora and Derrickson 2009)

- The islet cells of the *islets of Langerhans* produce the endocrine hormones *insulin* and *glucagon*. These hormones control carbohydrate metabolism.
- The *acini glands* of the exocrine pancreas produce 1.2–.5 l of *pancreatic juice* daily. Pancreatic juice consists of water, mineral salts, the enzymes *amylase* and *lipase* and the inactive enzyme precursors *trypsinogen, chymotrypsinogen* and *procarboxypeptidase.* Pancreatic juice travels from the pancreas via the pancreatic duct into the duodenum at the hepatopancreatic ampulla.
- The cells of the pancreatic ducts secrete bicarbonate ions which gives pancreatic juice its high pH (pH 8). This helps to neutralise acidic chyme from the stomach, thus protecting the small intestine from damage by the acidity. The action of amylase and lipase are most effective at the higher pH (pH 6–8).

Pancreatic juice consists of:

- Water
- Mineral salts
- Pancreatic amylase used to complete the digestion of carbohydrates
- Lipase used in the digestion of fat

- *Trypsinogen, chymotrypsinogen* and *procarboxypeptidase* are released in this inactive form to protect the pancreas from autodigestion. Once they enter the duodenum they are activated by enterokinase from intestinal juice, and become trypsin, chymotrypsin and carboxypeptidase respectively. They are then used in the digestion of protein.

Pancreatic juice travels from the pancreas via the pancreatic duct into the duodenum at the hepatopancreatic ampulla.

Two hormones regulate the secretion of pancreatic juice. *Secretin*, produced in response to the presence of hydrochloric acid in the duodenum, promotes the secretion of bicarbonate ions. *Cholecystokinin*, secreted in response to the intake of protein and fat, promotes the secretion of the enzymes present in pancreatic juice. Parasympathetic vagus nerve stimulation also promotes the release of pancreatic juice.

The liver and production of bile

The liver is the body's largest gland. It weighs between 1 and 2 kg. It lies under the diaphragm protected by the ribs. The liver occupies most of the right hypochondriac region and extends through part of the epigastric region into the left hypochondriac region. The right lobe is the largest of the four liver lobes. On the posterior surface of the liver there is an entry and exit to the organ called the portal fissure. Blood, lymph vessels, nerves and bile ducts enter and leave the liver through the portal fissure.

The liver is composed of tiny hexagonal-shaped lobules which contain hepatocytes (see Figure 13.14). The hepatocytes are protected by Kupffer cells (hepatic macrophages). The Kupffer cells deal with any foreign particles and worn out blood cells.

Each corner of the hexagonal-shaped lobule has a portal triad. A branch of the hepatic artery, a branch of hepatic portal vein and a bile duct are present here. The hepatic artery supplies the hepatocytes with oxygenated arterial blood. The hepatic portal vein delives nutrient-rich deoxygenated blood from the digestive tract to the hepatocytes. The hepatocytes' function is to filter, detoxify and process the nutrients from the digestive tract. Nutrients can be used for energy, stored or used to make new molecules. The liver sinusoids are large, leaky capillaries that drain the blood from the hepatic artery and hepatic portal vein into the central vein. This processed blood is then drained into the hepatic vein and on to the inferior vena cava.

As the blood flows towards the centre of the triad to exit at the central vein, the bile produced by the hepatocyte as a metabolic by-product moves in the opposite direction towards the bile canaliculi and on to the bile ducts. Bile then leaves the liver via the common hepatic duct towards the duodenum of the small intestine.

The liver produces and secretes up to 1 litre of yellow/green, alkaline bile per day.

Bile is composed of:

- Bile salts such as bilirubin from the breakdown of haemoglobin
- Cholesterol
- Fat-soluble hormones
- Fat
- Mineral salts
- Mucus.

The role of bile is to emulsify fats, giving the fat-digesting enzymes a larger surface area to work on.

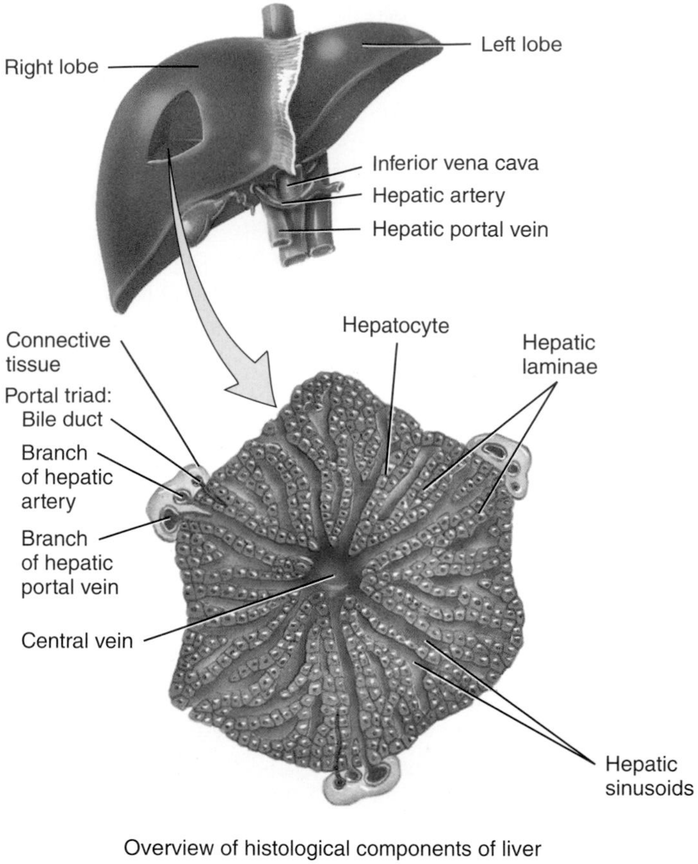
Right lobe
Left lobe
Inferior vena cava
Hepatic artery
Hepatic portal vein
Connective tissue
Portal triad:
Bile duct
Branch of hepatic artery
Branch of hepatic portal vein
Central vein
Hepatocyte
Hepatic laminae
Hepatic sinusoids
Overview of histological components of liver

Figure 13.14 Liver lobule (Tortora and Derrickson 2009)

When the duodenum is exposed to chyme containing fat, secretin is released and this stimulates liver cells to secrete bile. Bile is stored and concentrated in the gall bladder.

The functions of the liver

Apart from the production of bile and the metabolism of carbohydrate, fat and protein (discussed further on in this chapter) the liver has many additional functions:

- Detoxification of drugs – the liver deals with medication, alcohol, ingested toxins and the toxins produced by the action of microbes
- Recycling of erythrocytes
- Deactivation of many hormones, including the sex hormones, thyroxine, insulin, glucagon, cortisol and aldosterone
- Production of clotting proteins
- Storage of vitamins, minerals and glycogen
- Synthesis of vitamin A
- Heat production.

The gall bladder

The gall bladder is a small, green, muscular sac which lies posterior to the liver. It functions as a reservoir for bile until it is needed for digestion. It also concentrates bile by absorbing water. The mucosa of the gall bladder, like the rugae of the stomach, contains folds that allow the gall bladder to stretch in order to accommodate varying volumes of bile. When the smooth muscle walls of the gall bladder contract, bile is expelled into the cystic duct and down into the common bile duct before entering the duodenum via the hepatopancreatic ampulla.

The stimulus for gall bladder contraction is the hormone cholecystokinin (CKK). This enteroendocrine hormone, secreted from the small intestine into the blood, is produced in response to the presence of fatty chyme in the duodenum. Cholecystokinin also stimulates the secretion of pancreatic juice and the relaxation of the hepatopancreatic sphincter. When the sphincter is relaxed both bile and pancreatic juice can enter the duodenum. Figure 13.15 summarises the production and release of bile.

The large intestine

The contents of the small intestine move slowly through the small intestine by a process called segmentation. This allows time to complete digestion and absorption. Entry to the large intestine is controlled by the ileocaecal sphincter. The sphincter opens in response to the increased activity of the stomach and the action of the hormone gastrin. Once food residue has reached the large intestine it cannot backflow into the ileum (see Figure 13.15).

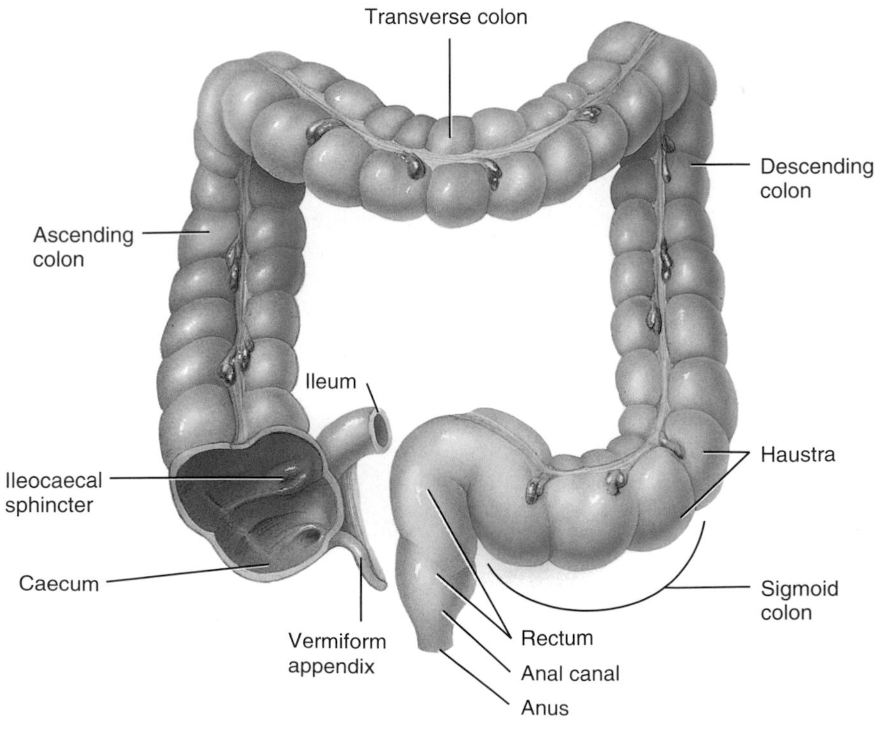
Transverse colon
Descending colon
Ascending colon
Ileum
Haustra
Ileocaecal sphincter
Caecum
Sigmoid colon
Vermiform appendix
Rectum
Anal canal
Anus

Figure 13.15 Large intestine (Tortora and Derrickson 2009)

The large intestine measures 1.5 m in length and 7 cm in diameter. It is continuous with the small intestine from the ileocaecal valve and ends at the anus.

Food residue enters the caecum and has to pass up the ascending colon along the transverse colon, down the descending colon and out of the body via the rectum, anal canal and anus. The caecum is a descending, sac-like opening into the large intestine. The vermiform appendix is a narrow, tube-like structure which leaves the caecum but is closed at its distal end. It is composed of lymphoid tissue and has a role in immunity. Two sphincter muscles control exit from the anus. The internal anal sphincter is smooth muscle and is under the control of the parasympathetic nervous system, whereas the external anal sphincter is composed of skeletal muscle and is under voluntary control.

The large intestine mucosa contains large numbers of goblet cells that secrete mucus to ease the passage of faeces and protect the walls of the large intestine. The simple columnar epithelium changes to stratified squamous epithelium at the anal canal. Anal sinuses secrete mucus in response to faecal compression. This protects the anal canal from the abrasion associated with defaecation.

The longitudinal muscle layer of the large intestine is formed into bands called the taeniae coli. These give the large intestine its gathered appearance. The sac created by this gathering is called haustrum.

The food residue from the ileum is fluid when in enters the caecum and contains few nutrients. The small intestine is responsible for some of the absorption of water but the primary function of the large intestine is to absorb water and turn the food residue into semi-solid faeces. The large intestine also absorbs some vitamins, minerals, electrolytes and drugs. Food residue usually takes 24–48 hours to pass through the large intestine. 500 ml of food residue enters the large intestine daily and approximately 150 ml leaves as faeces.

As faeces enters the rectum, the stretching of the walls of rectum initiates the *defaecation reflex*. Acquired, voluntary control of the defaecation reflex occurs between the ages of 2 and 3 years. The external anal sphincter is under voluntary control and, if it is appropriate to do so, defaecation can occur. Contraction of the abdominal muscles and diaphragm (the Valsalva manoeuvre) creates intra-abdominal pressure and assists in the process of defaecation. If it is not appropriate to defaecate, as it is under voluntary control, it can be postponed. After a few minutes the urge to go will subside and will only be felt again when the next mass movement through the large intestine occurs.

Faeces is a brown, semi-solid material. It contains fibre, stercobilin (from the breakdown of bilirubin), water, fatty acids, shed epithelial cells and microbes. Stercobilin gives faeces its brown colour. An excess of water in faeces results in *diarrhoea*. This occurs when food residue passes too quickly through the large intestine, the absorption of water cannot occur. Conversely, *constipation* occurs if food residue spends too long in the large intestine.

Clinical considerations

Appendicitis

The narrow lumen of the appendix does not allow much room for inflammation. If it becomes blocked by faecoliths (hard faecal material) or becomes twisted and kinked, this results in inflammation of the appendix. The swelling associated with this can lead to ulceration of the mucosal lining. This presents initially as central abdominal pain which eventually localises at the region of the appendix. Appendicitis can subside but often it results in abscess formation and even rupture.

Table 13.1 Summary of the role of the digestive system hormones

Hormone	Origin	Target	Action	Stimulus
Gastrin	Stomach	Stomach	Increases gastric gland secretion of hydrochloric acid Gastric emptying	Presence of protein in the stomach
Secretin	Duodenum	Stomach	Inhibits gastric gland secretion Inhibits gastric motility	Acidic and fatty chyme in the duodenum
		Pancreas	Increases pancreatic juice secretion Promotes cholecystokinin action	
		Liver	Increase bile secretion	
Cholecystokinin	Duodenum	Pancreas	Increases pancreatic juice secretion	Chyme in the duodenum
		Gall bladder	Stimulate contraction	
		Hepatopancreatic sphincter	Relaxes – entry to duodenum open	

Digestive tract hormones

Many hormones are responsible for the activity of the digestive system. A summary of their role is contained in Table 13.1.

This chapter has concentrated on how the digestive tract deals with food ingested in order to break it down into its constituent parts for use by the cells of the body.

The next section will look at nutrition and the role of a balanced diet in health.

Nutrition, chemical digestion and metabolism

An adequate intake of nutrients is essential for health. Nutrition also has an important role in social and psychological wellbeing. If managed inappropriately, nutrition can lead to many physical and psychological illnesses. Therefore it is important to have an understanding of the role of nutrients within the body in order to understand how a lack or excess of nutrients will lead to ill health.

The remainder of this chapter will identify the macro- and the micronutrients and the food groups that provide the source of macro- and micronutrients. It will examine what the nutrients are broken down into and how the body uses these constituent parts.

Nutrients

A nutrient is a substance that is ingested and processed by the gastrointestinal system. It is digested and absorbed and can be used by the body to produce energy or become the building block for a new molecule or to participate in essential chemical reactions. Nutrients are required for body growth, repair and maintenance of cell function. Not all of food ingested can be classed as nutrients. Some non-digestible plant fibres are not nutrients but are required for healthy functioning of the digestive system.

Balanced diet

The body has the ability to break down some nutrients in order to create new molecules, but this ability is finite and there remains a group of essential nutrients that the body cannot make but are required to be ingested in the diet for homeostasis to be maintained. A balanced diet is therefore essential for health (Department of Health 2003). The daily recommended portions of food groups required for a balanced diet are shown in the food pyramid (see Figure 13.16). Lack of a balanced diet can lead to malnourishment and overindulgence can lead to obesity.

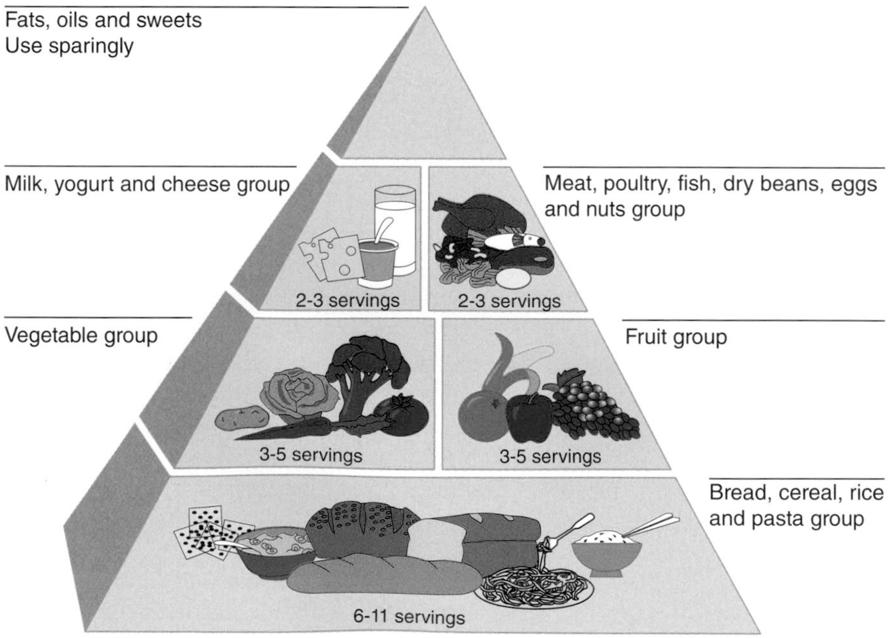
Fats, oils and sweets
Use sparingly
Milk, yogurt and cheese group
Meat, poultry, fish, dry beans, eggs and nuts group
2-3 servings
2-3 servings
Vegetable group
Fruit group
3-5 servings
3-5 servings
Bread, cereal, rice and pasta group
6-11 servings

Figure 13.16 The food pyramid (Nair and Peate 2009)

Clinical considerations

Obesity

Obesity is on the increase in Western society. Obesity occurs when more calories are taken in than used by the body. Lack of exercise, a sedentary lifestyle, generous diet all contribute to weight gain. Obesity has serious health consequences as it predisposes people to indigestion, gallstone, hernias, cardiovascular disease, varicose veins, osteoarthritis and type 2 diabetes mellitus.

Dietary nutrients begin life as large food molecules. They enter the digestive tract and are broken down into smaller molecules. This process is called catabolism. Digestive enzymes facilitate the breakdown of foods by a process called hydrolysis. Hydrolysis is the addition of water to break down the chemical bonds of the food molecules.Each of the three different types of food is broken down (lysed) by different enzymes.

Nutrient groups

Carbohydrates, proteins and lipids are known as the major nutrients or macronutrients. They are required in quite large quantities. Vitamins and minerals are required in much smaller quantities but they also are crucial for the maintenance of health. They are also known as the micronutrients. There are therefore six classes of nutrients:

- Water
- Carbohydrates
- Proteins
- Lipids (fats)
- Vitamins
- Minerals.

Water

The importance of water is discussed in Chapter 14.

Carbohydrates

Monosaccharides, disaccharides and polysaccharides are all carbohydrates. The dietary source of carbohydrates is plants. However, the milk sugar lactose is a form of carbohydrate found in cow and human milk. Carbohydrates are found in many foods, such as bread, pasta, cereal, biscuits, vegetables and fruit.

Carbohydrates consist of carbon, hydrogen and oxygen. They can be complex, such as the polysaccharides: starch and glycogen; or simple, such as the disaccharides: sucrose (table sugar) and lactose (milk sugar) and the monosaccharides: glucose, fructose and galactose.

Digestion of carbohydrates supplies the body with fructose, galactose and glucose. The liver converts fructose and galactose to glucose as glucose is the molecule used by the body cells.

Digested carbohydrates are absorbed into the blood via the villi of the small intestine. They enter the hepatic portal circulation and are transported to the liver for processing. The liver is a highly metabolic organ which requires a plentiful supply of glucose to carry out its metabolic activity.

Insufficient carbohydrate intake will lead to an inability to meet the cells, energy demands. If this happens, the body will break down amino acids and lipids to create new glucose, a process called gluconeogenesis.

Fats

Dietary sources of fat include butter, eggs, cheese, milk, oily fish and the fatty part of meat. These contain saturated fat which is mainly saturated fatty acids and glycerol. Vegetable oils and margarine are sources of unsaturated fats. The body can also create fat from excess carbohydrate and protein intake.

Fat also contains carbon, hydrogen and oxygen, but in a different combination from carbohydrates.

When fat enters the small intestine it mixes and is emulsified by bile. The action of pancreatic lipase completes the digestion of fat and it is broken down into monoglycerides, glycerol and fatty acids. The monoglycerides and some of the fatty acids enter the lacteals of the villi and are transported via the lymph to the thoracic duct and into the circulation, where they eventually reach the liver. Glycerol and the remaining fatty acids are absorbed more directly into the capillary blood and reach the liver via the hepatic portal vein.

The liver uses some of the fatty acids and glycerol to provide energy and heat. In fact, hepatocytes and skeletal muscle use triglycerides as their major energy source. It also converts fatty acids and glycerol into triglycerides which act as an energy store for when there is a lack of glucose available to both the liver and body cells. Excessive triglycerides can also be stored as adipose tissue and this can also be used as an energy store when glucose is not available.

Dietary fats make food seem tender and lead to a feeling of satisfaction with food. They are necessary for the absorption of fat-soluble vitamins. Adipose tissue protects, cushions and insulates vital organs in the body. Phospholipids are required to form the myelin sheath and cell membranes. Cholesterol is obtained from egg yolk and dairy produce but is also synthesised in the body to form steroid hormones and bile salts.

Excess fat in the diet can lead to obesity and cardiovascular disease. A lack of fat in the diet can lead to weight loss, poor growth and skin lesions.

Proteins

Dietary sources of protein include meat, eggs and milk. Beans and peas (legumes), nuts, cereals and leafy green vegetables are also sources of amino acids.

Protein digestion begins in the stomach and is completed in the small intestine. Proteins are broken down into amino acids. They are absorbed via the villi of the small intestine where they reach the capillaries and then the hepatic portal circulation to the liver or general circulation.

Proteins are used by the body for many purposes. They are used to form muscle, collagen, elastin, necessary for body structure and tissue repair. The hormones insulin and growth hormone are required for this. Amino acids are also used to form hormones and enzymes within the body. All of the amino acids required to form a required protein must be available within the cell in order for that protein to be made. This is called the all or nothing rule. Protein can also be used as a source of energy for the body. The amino acid is broken down mainly at the liver where the nitrogenous part of the amino acid is removed and converted first to ammonia and then to urea. Urea is excreted as a waste product in urine. The remainder of the amino acid is used to produce energy. Protein cannot be stored by the body. Any excess amino acids are converted to carbohydrate or fat to be stored as adipose tissue.

Too much protein in the diet can lead to obesity. A lack of dietary protein can lead to muscle/ tissue wasting and weight loss. A lack of plasma proteins can lead to oedema.

Vitamins

Vitamins are organic molecules that are required in small amounts for healthy metabolism. Essential vitamins cannot be manufactured by the body and must come from the diet, highlighting again the importance of a balanced diet. Some vitamins can be manufactured. Vitamin K is synthesised by intestinal bacteria; the skin makes vitamin D; and vitamin A is made from beta-carotene found for example in carrots.

Many vitamins act as *coenzymes* (Seeley *et al.* 2006). These vitamins combine with enzymes to make them functional. For example, the formation of clotting proteins requires the presence of vitamin K.

During metabolism a reaction takes place involving oxygen. Potentially harmful free radicals are formed as part of this process. Vitamins A, C and E are antioxidants that disarm free radicals and protect tissue from their potentially dangerous effects.

Vitamins are either fat-soluble or water-soluble. The fat-soluble vitamins combine with lipids from the diet and are absorbed in this way. Apart from vitamin K, the fat-soluble vitamins can be stored in the body and therefore there can be problems associated with toxicity when these vitamins accumulate.

The water-soluble vitamins are absorbed with water along the digestive tract. They cannot be stored and any excess ingested will be excreted in urine. A summary of vitamins and their functions is contained in Table 13.2.

Minerals

Small quantities of inorganic compounds called minerals are required by the body for many purposes. They give structure and strength to tissues, such as calcium, or form ions essential for maintaining osmotic pressure, such as sodium. They also form approximately 5% of the body weight (Nair and Peate 2009).

There are minerals that are required in moderate amounts, such as calcium and magnesium, and many other known where trace amounts are required, such as cobalt and copper. A summary of some of the minerals and their function is available in Table 13.3.

Conclusion

Digestion and nutrition play a vital role in the maintenance of health. The digestive tract processes ingested nutrients by breaking them down chemically and mechanically. Accessory structures such as the pancreas, liver and gall bladder have an essential role in providing the digestive tract with bile and pancreatic juice to facilitate the digestion of the macronutrients protein, carbohydrate and fat. The small intestine provides the large surface area available for the absorption of nutrients and the liver processes the products of digestion. The large intestine plays an excretory role,

Table 13.2 Vitamins summary

Vitamin	Source	Function	Deficiency
Fat-soluble			
A retinol	Manufactured from beta-carotene. Egg yolk, cream, fish oil, cheese, liver	Skin, mucosa integrity; bone and tooth development during growth; photoreceptor pigment synthesis in the retina, normal reproduction, antioxidant	Night blindness, dry skin and hair, loss of skin integrity, increased infection particularly respiratory, GI and urinary
D	Manufactured by the skin. Cheese, eggs, fish oil, liver	Regulates calcium and phosphate metabolism	Rickets in children, osteomalacia in adults
E	Egg yolk, wheat germ, whole cereals, milk and butter	Antioxidant	In severe deficiency ataxia and visual disturbances, decreased life span of red blood cells
K	Synthesised by bacteria in the large intestine. Liver, fish, fruit and leafy green vegetables	Formation of clotting proteins at the liver	Prolonged clotting times, bruising, bleeding
Water-soluble			
B_1 thiamine	Egg yolk, liver, nuts, meat, legumes cereal germ	Coenzyme required for carbohydrate metabolism	Beriberi – muscle wasting, stunted growth polyneuritis and infection Vision disturbances, confusion, unsteadiness, memory loss, fatigue, tachycardia, heart enlargement
B_2 riboflavine	Milk, green vegetables, yeast, cheese, fish roe, liver	Coenzyme required for carbohydrate and protein metabolism	Skin-cracking, particularly around the corners of the mouth, blurred vision, corneal ulcers, intestinal mucosa lesions

Table 13.2 *Continued*

Vitamin	Source	Function	Deficiency
Folic acid	Liver, kidney, yeast, fresh leafy vegetables, eggs, whole grains	Coenzyme essential for DNA synthesis, red blood cell formation	Anaemia, spina bifida in newborn, increased risk of heart attack and stroke
Niacin Nicotinic acid	Liver, cheese, yeast, eggs, cereals, nuts, fish	Coenzyme involved in glycolysis, fat breakdown – assists with breakdown and inhibits cholesterol production	Pellagra – skin reddening to light, anorexia, nausea and dysphagia, delirium and dementia
B_6 pyridoxine	Meat, liver, fish, grains, bananas, yeast	Coenzyme involved in amino acid metabolism	Increased risk of heart disease, eye and mouth lesions. In children, nervous irritability, convulsions, abdominal pain and vomiting
B_{12} cyanocobalamin	Meat, fish, liver, eggs, milk	Coenzyme in all cells, involved in DNA synthesis. Formation and maintenance of myelin around nerves	Pernicious anaemia, peripheral neuropathy
B_5 pantothenic acid	Meat, grains, legumes, yeast, egg yolk	Coenzyme associated with amino acid metabolism and formation of steroids	Non-specific symptoms
Biotin	Egg yolk, liver, legumes, tomatoes	Coenzyme in carbohydrate metabolism	Pallor, anorexia, nausea, fatigue
C ascorbic acid	Fruit, particularly citrus fruit, vegetables	Antioxidant, enhances iron absorption and use, maturation of red blood cells	Poor wound healing, joint pain, anaemia, scurvy

Table 13.3 Mineral summary

Mineral	Source	Function	Deficiency(D)/excess(E)
Calcium	Milk, egg yolk, shell fish, cheese, green vegetables	Bones and teeth, cell membrane permeability, nerve impulse transmission, muscle contraction, heart rhythm, blood clotting	D: osteomalacia, osteoporosis, muscle tetany. In children – rickets and retarded growth E: lethargy and confusion, kidney stones
Chlorine	Table salt	Works with sodium to maintain osmotic pressure of extracellular fluid	D: alkalosis, muscle cramps E: vomiting
Magnesium	Nuts, milk, legumes, cereal	Constituent of coenzymes. Muscle and nerve irritability	D: neuromuscular problems, irregular heartbeat E: diarrhoea
Sodium	Table salt	Extracellular cation. Works with chloride to maintain osmotic pressure of extracellular fluid Muscle contraction, nerve impulse transmission electrolyte balance	D: rare – nausea E: hypertension, oedema
Potassium	Fruit and vegetables and many foods	Intracellular cation Muscle contraction, nerve impulse transmission electrolyte balance	D: Rare – muscle weakness, nausea, tachycardia E: cardiac abnormalities, muscular weakness
Iron	Liver, kidney, beef, green vegetables	Constituent of haemoglobin	D: anaemia E: haemochromatosis, liver damage
Iodine	Salt water fish, vegetables	Constituent of thyroid hormones	D: hypothyroidism E: thyroid hormone synthesis depressed

ridding the body of the waste products from digestion and absorbing any remaining water back into the body.

The maintenance of homeostasis is achieved through the ingestion of a balanced diet, containing a variety of elements from each of the food groups.

Without all of this activity normal cell functioning would be at risk, leading to ill health. Digestive health contributes greatly to physical, psychological and social wellbeing.

Glossary

Absorption: Process whereby the products of digestion move into the blood or lymph fluid.

Acini glands: Produce pancreatic juice.

Amylase: Carbohydrate-digesting enzyme.

Anus: End of the digestive tract.

Bile: Fluid produced by the liver and required for the digestion of fat.

Bile duct: Tube that carries bile from the liver.

Body region: Region of the stomach. Caecum: Beginning of the large intestine.

Canine: Type of tooth.

Carbohydrate: One of the major food groups.

Cardiac region: Region of the stomach closest to the oesophagus.

Catabolism: Process of breaking down substances into simpler substances.

Chief cells: Pepsinogen-producing cells.

Cholecystokinin: Digestive system hormone.

Chyme: Creamy, semi-fluid mass of partially digested food mixed with gastric secretions.

Deglutition: Swallowing.

Digestion: The chemical and mechanical breakdown of food for absorption.

Duodenum: First part of the small intestine.

Enamel: Covering of the tooth.

Epiglottis: Cartilage that covers the larynx during swallowing.

Faeces: Brown, semi-solid digestive system waste.

Fats: One of the major food groups.

Frenulum: Fold between the lip and gum.

Fundus: Anatomical base region of the stomach.

Gluconeogenesis: The creation of glucose from non-carbohydrate molecules.

Glycolysis: The anaerobic breakdown of glucose to form pyruvic acid.

Goblet cell: Mucus-producing cell.

Haustrum: Sac-like section of the large intestine.

Hepatocyte:	Liver cell.
Hepatic portal vein:	Vein that delivers dissolved nutrients to the liver.
Hepatopancreatic ampulla:	The site where the bile duct and pancreatic duct meet.
Hepatopancreatic sphincter:	Muscular valve that controls the entrance of pancreatic juice and bile to the duodenum.
Hyoid bone:	Bone that acts as the base of the tongue.
Hydrochloric acid:	Acid produced by the parietal cells of the stomach.
Hydrolysis:	Addition of water to breakdown food molecules.
Hypochondriac region:	Upper lateral divisions of the abdominopelvic cavity.
Ileum:	The end part of the small intestineIleocaecal valve: site where the small and large intestine meet.
Ingestion:	The process of taking food into the body via the mouth.
Incisors:	Type of tooth.
Intestinal crypts:	Also known as the crypts of Lieberkuhn – glands found in the villi of the small intestine.
Intrinsic factor:	Substance required for the absorption of vitamin B_{12}.
Jejunum:	The middle part of the small intestine between the duodenum and the ileum.
Kuppffer cell:	Hepatic macrophage.
Lacteal:	Lymphatic capillary of the small intestine.
Lamina propria:	Loose connective tissue layer of the digestive tract.
Laryngopharynx:	Where the larynx and pharynx meet.
Lipase:	Fat-digesting enzyme.
Liver:	Accessory organ located in the abdominal cavity that has many metabolic and regulatory functions.
Liver sinusoid:	Liver capillary.
Lower oesophageal sphincter:	Valve between the oesophagus and stomach.
Lysozyme:	Bactericidal enzyme.
Macronutrient:	Food consumed in large quantities.

Mastication:	Chewing.
Metabolism:	Sum total of the chemical reactions occurring in the body.
Meissner's plexus:	Nerves of the small intestine.
Micronutrient:	Nutrient required in small quantities.
Microvilli:	Cytoplasmic extensions of the villi.
Minerals:	Salts – inorganic compounds.
Molars:	Type of tooth.
Mucosa:	Layer of the digestive tract.
Mucous neck cells:	Mucus-secreting cells of the stomach.
Muscularis mucosa:	Muscular layer of the digestive tract.
Mesenteric plexus:	Digestive tract innervation.
Nutrient:	Product obtained from the digestion of food and used by the body.
Oesophagus:	Muscular tube from laryngopharynx to stomach.
Oral cavity:	The first part of the digestive system.
Oropharynx:	Part of the pharynx closest to the oral cavity.
Palate:	Roof of the mouth.
Pancreatic duct:	Duct that links the pancreas and common bile duct.
Paneth cell:	Cell that produces lysozyme.
Papillae:	Small mucosal projections.
Parasympathetic fibres:	Autonomic nervous system nerve fibre.
Parietal cells:	Hydrochloric acid-producing cell of the stomach.
Parotid glands:	Salivary glands located close to the ears.
Pepsin:	Enzyme required for the breakdown of protein.
Pepsinogen:	Enzyme precursor of pepsin.
Peristalsis:	Wave-like contractions that move food through the digestive tract.
Peritoneum:	Serous membrane that lines the abdominal cavity.
Peyer's patches:	Lymphatic tissue of the small intestine.
Pharyngeal phase:	Second phase of swallowing.
Pharynx:	Tube between the mouth and the oesophagus.

Plicae circulars: Permanent circular folds in the small intestine.

Portal fissure: Area where blood vessels and nerves enter and leave the liver.

Portal triad: Corner of liver lobule.

Premolars: Type of tooth located between the canine and molar teeth.

Propulsion: The process of moving the food along the length of the digestive system.

Proteins: Substance that contains carbon, hydrogen, oxygen and nitrogen.

Pulp cavity: Centre of the tooth.

Pyloric canal: Area where the stomach opens into the small intestine.

Pyloric region: Area of the stomach that occurs where the stomach meets the small intestine.

Pyloric sphincter: Valve that controls food movement from the stomach to the small intestine.

Rectum: Final portion of the large intestine.

Rugae: Folds or ridges found in the digestive tract.

Salivary amylase: Carbohydrate digesting enzyme found in saliva.

Secretin: Hormone that regulates secretion of pancreatic juice.

Segmentation: Movement of chyme in the small intestine.

Serosa: Outer layer of the digestive tract.

Sphincter of Oddi: Valve that controls the movement of bile and pancreatic juice into the small intestine.

Splanchnic circulation: Blood vessels of the digestive system.

Stercobilin: Waste product of bilirubin breakdown.

Stomach: Food reservoir where the digestion of protein begins.

Sublingual glands: Salivary gland located on the floor of the mouth.

Submandibular glands: Salivary glands located below the jaw bilaterally.

Submucosa: Thick connective tissue layer of the digestive tract.

Superior mesenteric artery: Vessel that supplies the small intestine with arterial blood.

Superior mesenteric vein: Blood vessel that drains venous blood from the small intestine.

Surface mucous cells: Mucus-secreting cells of the stomach.

Stomach: Reservoir for food involved in both chemical and mechanical digestion.

Taeniae coli: Muscle bands in the large intestine.

Upper oesophageal sphincter: Controls the movement of food into the oesophagus from the oropharynx.

Uvula: Small piece of tissue that protrudes from the soft palate.

Vermiform appendix: Blind-ended tube connected to the caecum and composed of lymphatic tissue.

Villi: Tiny, fingerlike projections found on the surface of the mucosa of the small intestine.

Visceral peritoneum: The innermost part of the peritoneum that is in contact with the abdominal organs.

Vitamins: Essential organic compounds require in small amounts.

Voluntary phase: The first phase of swallowing.

References

Department of Health (2003) *The Essence of Care: Patient-Focused Benchmarks for Clinical Governance.* London: The Stationery Office.

Marieb, E.N. and Hoehn K. (2007) *Human Anatomy and Physiology*, 7th edn. San Francisco: Pearson Benjamin Cummings.

Nair, M. and Peate, I. (2009) *Fundamentals of Applied Pathophysiology. An Essential Guide for Nursing Students.* Chichester: John Wiley & Sons.

Seeley R.R., Stephens T.D. and Tate P. (2006) *Anatomy and Physiology*, 7th edn. New York: McGraw-Hill.

Tortora G.J. and Derrickson B.H. (2009) *Principles of Anatomy and Physiology*, 12th edn. Hoboken, NJ: John Wiley & Sons.

Tortora, G.J. and Derrickson, B.H. (2010) *Essentials of Anatomy and Physiology*, 8th edn. New York: John Wiley & Sons.

Activities

www.wiley.com/go/peate.

Multiple choice questions

1. Which of these vitamins is essential for blood clotting?

   (a) vitamin A
   (b) vitamin B_{12}
   (c) vitamin E
   (d) vitamin K

2. Which mineral found in broccoli provides the body with an essential constituent of the thyroid hormone thyroxine?
   (a) iron
   (b) iodine
   (c) calcium
   (d) potassium

3. Which of these is true of fat?
   (a) used for the growth and repair of body cells
   (b) a constituent of myelin sheaths
   (c) essential for the transport of the water-soluble vitamins
   (d) all of the above

4. Which layer of the digestive tract is responsible for peristalsis?
   (a) mucosa
   (b) submucosa
   (c) muscularis
   (d) peritoneum

5. Which of these structures is considered an accessory organ?
   (a) salivary gland
   (b) pancreas
   (c) liver
   (d) all of them

6. Where does most of the absorption of nutrients occur?
   (a) small intestine
   (b) large intestine
   (c) stomach
   (d) oesophagus

7. Which of these is NOT a constituent of gastric juice?
   (a) hydrochloric acid
   (b) mucus
   (c) intrinsic factor
   (d) trypsinogen

8. Which enzyme is involved in the breakdown of protein?
   (a) chymotrypsin
   (b) lipase
   (c) amylase
   (d) bile

9. Where is bile produced?
   (a) the small intestine
   (b) the gall bladder
   (c) the pancreas
   (d) the liver

10. Which part of the large intestine is lymphoid tissue?
   (a) the appendix
   (b) the caecum
   (c) the ascending loop
   (d) the sigmoid colon

True or false

1. The large intestine is colonised with bacteria.
2. The first section of small intestine is called the jejunum.
3. Pancreatic juice reaches the duodenum through the cystic duct.
4. The function of bile is to emulsify fats.
5. There are 20 milk teeth.

Test your learning

1. Where does bile and pancreatic juice enter the duodenum?
2. Which teeth are used for grinding of food?
3. What is the exocrine pancreatic product essential for?
4. What are carbohydrates broken down into?
5. List the enzymes involved in the breakdown of protein.

Label the diagram

From the lists of words, label the diagrams below

Parotid gland (salivary gland), Submandibular gland (salivary gland), Oesophagus, Liver, Duodenum, Gall bladder, Jejunum, Ileum, Ascending colon, Caecum, Appendix, Mouth (oral cavity), Sublingual gland (salivary gland), Pharynx, Stomach, Pancreas, Transverse colon, Descending colon, Sigmoid colon, Rectum, Anus

Pylorus, Duodenum, Jejunum, Ileum, Ileocaecal value, Stomach, Large intestine

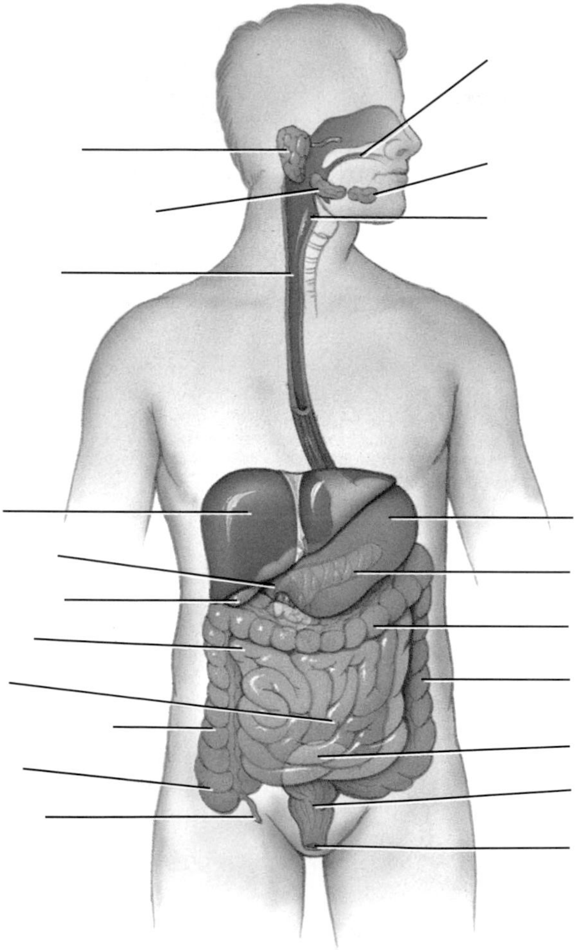

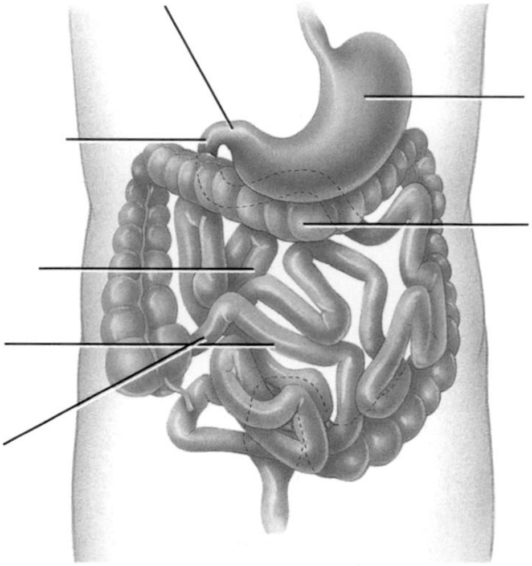

Crossword

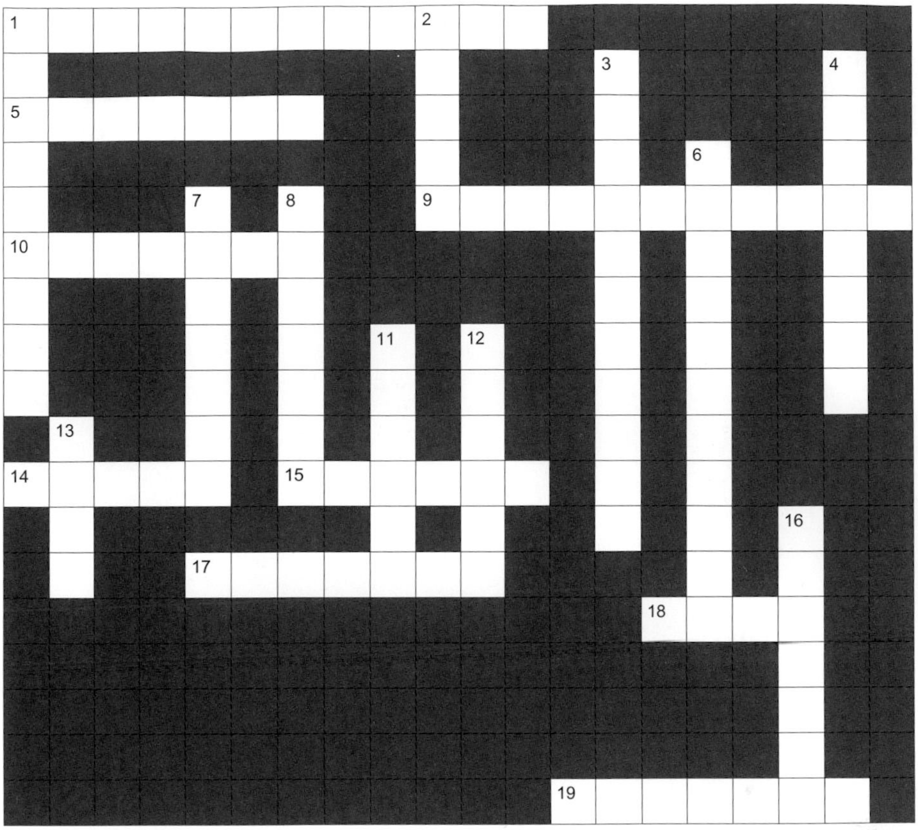
1
2
3
4
5
6
7
8
9
10
11
12
13
14
15
16
17
18
19

Across:

1. Another name for vitamin C (8, 4).
5. A cutting tooth (7).
9. Function of the large intestine (11).
10. Enzyme responsible for carbohydrate breakdown (7).
14. Another name for fat (5).
15. Innermost layer of the digestive tract (6).
17. Essential organic molecule (7).
18. End of the digestive system (4).
19. Passageway for air and food (7).

Down:

1. Protein is broken down into this (5, 4).
2. Food mixed with hydrochloric acid (5).
3. Describes the movement of the digestive tract (11).
4. Anti-bacterial constituent of saliva (8).
6. Another word for chewing (11).
7. Salivary gland (7).
8. Middle portion of the small intestine (7).
11. Entry to large intestine from the small intestine (6).
12. Enzyme responsible for the digestion of protein (6).
13. Made in the liver and required for the digestion of fat (4).
16. Hormone that stimulates the secretion of hydrochloric acid (7).

Conditions

Below is a list of conditions that are associated with the digestive system. Take some time and write notes about each of the conditions. You may make the notes taken from text books or other resources, for example, people you work with in a clinical area or you may make the notes as a result of people you have cared for. If you are making notes about people you have cared for you must ensure that you adhere to the rules of confidentiality.

Peptic ulcer	
Ulcerative colitis	
Peritonitis	
Paralytic ileus	
Obesity	
Malnutrition	
Dysphagia	

Answers

MCQs

1d; 2b; 3b; 4c; 5d; 6a; 7d; 8a; 9d; 10a

True or false

1T; 2F; 3F; 4T; 5T

Crossword

Across:

1. Ascorbic acid
5. Incisor
9. Elimination
10. Amylase
14. Lipid
15. Mucosa
17. Vitamin
18. Anus
19. Pharynx

Down:

1. Amino acid
2. Chyme
3. Peristalsis
4. Lysozyme
6. Mastication
7. Parotid
8. Jejunum
11. Caecum
12. Pepsin
13. Bile
16. Gastrin

14

The renal system

Muralitharan Nair

Contents

Introduction *448*

Renal system **448**

Kidneys – external structures **449**

Kidneys – internal structures **450**
Nephrons 451

Functions of the kidney **455**

Blood supply of the kidney **456**

Urine formation **457**
Filtration 457
Selective reabsorption 457
Secretion 459
Hormonal control of tubular reabsorption and secretion 460

Composition of urine 461
Characteristics of normal urine 462

Ureters **463**

Urinary bladder **464**

Urethra **466**
Male urethra 466
Female urethra 467

Micturition **467**

Conclusion *468*
Glossary *469*
References *470*
Activities *470*

Test your knowledge

- Name the functions of the kidneys.
- List the organs of the renal system.
- Describe the components of a nephron.
- List the composition of urine.
- What is the colour of urine? Think about the destruction of the red blood cells.

Fundamentals of Anatomy and Physiology for Student Nurses, First Edition. Edited by Ian Peate, Muralitharan Nair.

Learning outcomes

On completion of this section the reader will be able to:

- Describe the structure and functions of the kidney
- Describe the microscopic structures of the kidney
- Explain glomerular filtration
- List the chemical compositions of urine
- Discuss the structure and functions of the bladder

Body map

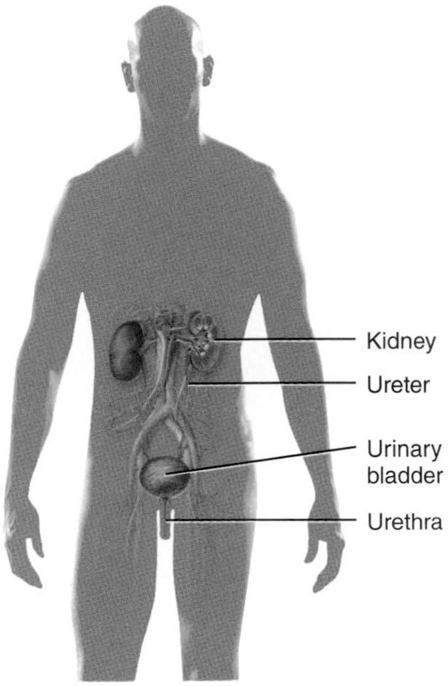
Kidney
Ureter
Urinary
bladder
Urethra

Introduction

The kidneys play an important role in maintaining homeostasis. They remove waste products through the production and excretion of urine and regulate fluid balance in the body. As part of their function, the kidneys filter essential substances, such as sodium and potassium from the blood, and selectively reabsorb substances essential to maintain homeostasis. Any substances not essential are excreted in the urine. The formation of urine is achieved through the processes of filtration, selective reabsorption and excretion. The kidneys also have an endocrine function, secreting hormones such as renin and erythropoietin. This chapter will discuss the structure and functions of the renal system. It will also include some common disorders and their related nursing management and treatment.

Renal system

The renal system, also known as the urinary system, consists of:

- Kidneys, which filter the blood to produce urine
- Ureters, which convey urine to the bladder
- Urinary bladder, a storage organ for urine until it is eliminated
- Urethra, which conveys urine to the exterior.

See Figure 14.1 for the organs of the renal system.

The organs of the renal system ensure that a stable internal environment is maintained for the survival of cells and tissues in the body – homeostasis.

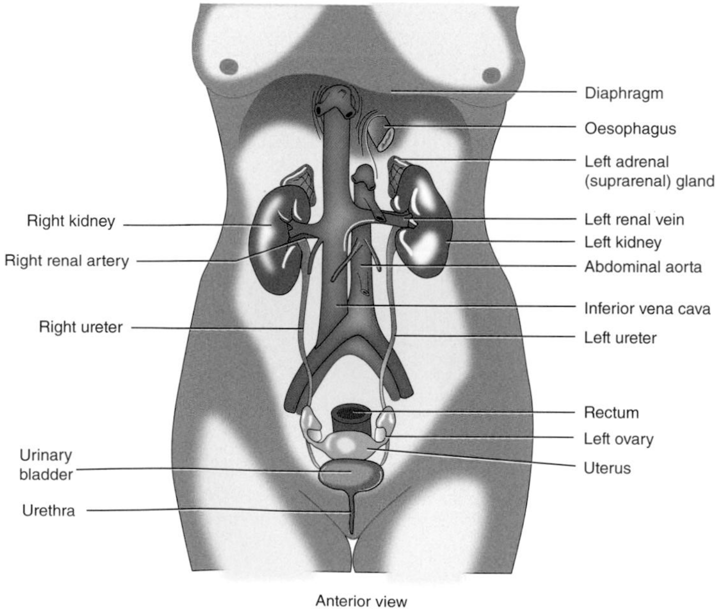
Diaphragm
Oesophagus
Left adrenal (suprarenal) gland
Right kidney
Left renal vein
Right renal artery
Left kidney
Abdominal aorta
Inferior vena cava
Right ureter
Left ureter
Rectum
Left ovary
Urinary bladder
Uterus
Urethra
Anterior view

Figure 14.1 Anterior view (Tortora and Derrickson 2009)

Kidneys – external structures

There are two kidneys, one on each side of the spinal column. They are approximately 11 cm long, 5–6 cm wide and 3–4 cm thick. They are said to be bean-shaped organs where the outer border is convex; the inner border is known as the hilum (also known as hilus), and it is here that the renal arteries, renal veins, nerves and the ureters enter and leave the kidneys. The renal artery carries blood to the kidneys and once the blood is filtered, the renal vein takes the blood away. The right kidney is in contact with the liver's large right lobe and hence the right kidney is approximately 2–4 cm lower than the left kidney.

Covering and supporting the kidneys are three layers:

- Renal fascia
- Adipose tissue
- Renal capsule.

The real fascia is the outer layer and it consists of a thin layer of connective tissue that anchors the kidneys to the abdominal wall and the surrounding tissues. The middle layer is called the adipose tissue and surrounds the capsule. It cushions the kidneys from trauma. The inner layer is called the renal capsule. It consists of a layer of smooth connective tissue which is continuous with the outer layer of the ureter. The renal capsule protects the kidneys from trauma and maintains their shape. See Figure 14.2 for the external layers.

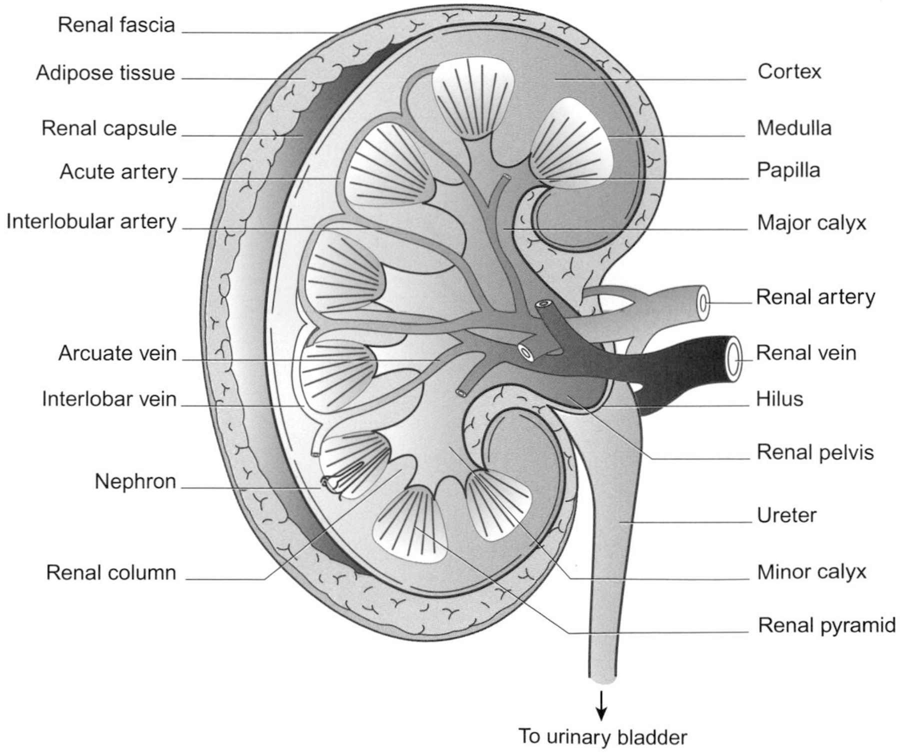
Renal fascia
Adipose tissue
Renal capsule
Acute artery
Interlobular artery
Arcuate vein
Interlobar vein
Nephron
Renal column
Cortex
Medulla
Papilla
Major calyx
Renal artery
Renal vein
Hilus
Renal pelvis
Ureter
Minor calyx
Renal pyramid
To urinary bladder

Figure 14.2 External layers of the kidney

Kidneys – internal structures

There are three distinct regions inside the kidney:

- Renal cortex
- Renal medulla
- Renal pelvis.

The renal cortex is the outermost part of the kidney. In adults, it forms a continuous, smooth outer portion of the kidney with a number of projections (renal column) that extend down between the pyramids. The renal column is the medullary extension of the renal cortex. The renal cortex is reddish in colour and has a granular appearance, which is due to the capillaries and the structures of the nephron. The medulla is lighter in colour and has an abundance of blood vessels and tubules of the nephrons (see Figure 14.3). The medulla consists of approximately 8–12 renal pyramids (see Figure 14.3). The renal pyramids, also called malpighian pyramids, are cone-shaped sections of the kidneys. The wider portion of the cone faces the renal cortex, while the narrow end points internally and this section is called the renal papilla. Urine formed by the nephrons

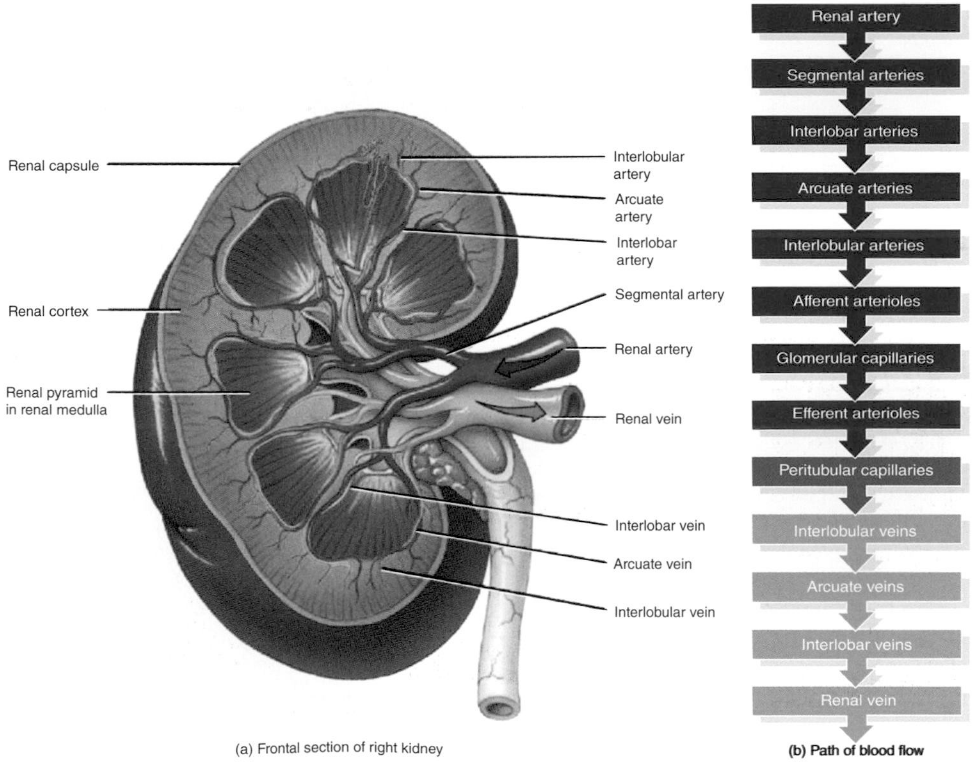
Renal capsule
Renal cortex
Renal pyramid in renal medulla
Interlobular artery
Arcuate artery
Interlobar artery
Segmental artery
Renal artery
Renal vein
Interlobar vein
Arcuate vein
Interlobular vein
(a) Frontal section of right kidney
Renal artery
Segmental arteries
Interlobar arteries
Arcuate arteries
Interlobular arteries
Afferent arterioles
Glomerular capillaries
Efferent arterioles
Peritubular capillaries
Interlobular veins
Arcuate veins
Interlobar veins
Renal vein
(b) Path of blood flow

Figure 14.3 Internal structures showing blood vessels (Tortora and Derrickson 2009)

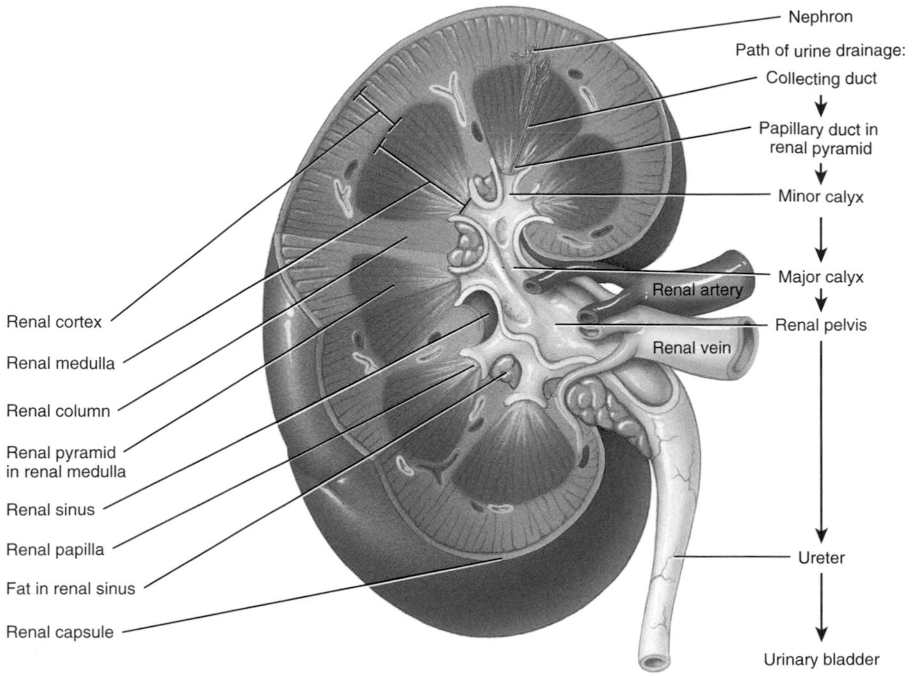
Nephron
Path of urine drainage:
Collecting duct
Papillary duct in renal pyramid
Minor calyx
Major calyx
Renal pelvis
Ureter
Urinary bladder
Renal artery
Renal vein
Renal cortex
Renal medulla
Renal column
Renal pyramid in renal medulla
Renal sinus
Renal papilla
Fat in renal sinus
Renal capsule

Figure 14.4 Internal structures (Tortora and Derrickson 2009)

flows into cup-like structures, called calyces, via papillary ducts. Each kidney contains approximately 8–18 minor calyces and 2–3 major calyces. The minor calyces receive urine from the renal papilla which conveys the urine to the major calyces. The major calyces unite to form the renal pelvis, which then conveys urine to the bladder (see Figure 14.4). The renal pelvis forms the expanded upper portion of the ureter which is funnel-shaped and it is the region where two or three calyces converge.

Nephrons

These are small structures and they form the functional units of the kidney. The nephron consists of a glomerulus and a renal tubule (see Figure 14.5). There are approximately over one million nephrons per kidney and it is in these structures where urine is formed. The nephrons:

- Filter blood
- Perform selective reabsorption
- Excrete unwanted waste products from the filtered blood.

The nephron is part of the homeostatic mechanism of the body. This system helps regulate the amount of water, salts, glucose, urea and other minerals in the body. The nephron is a filtration

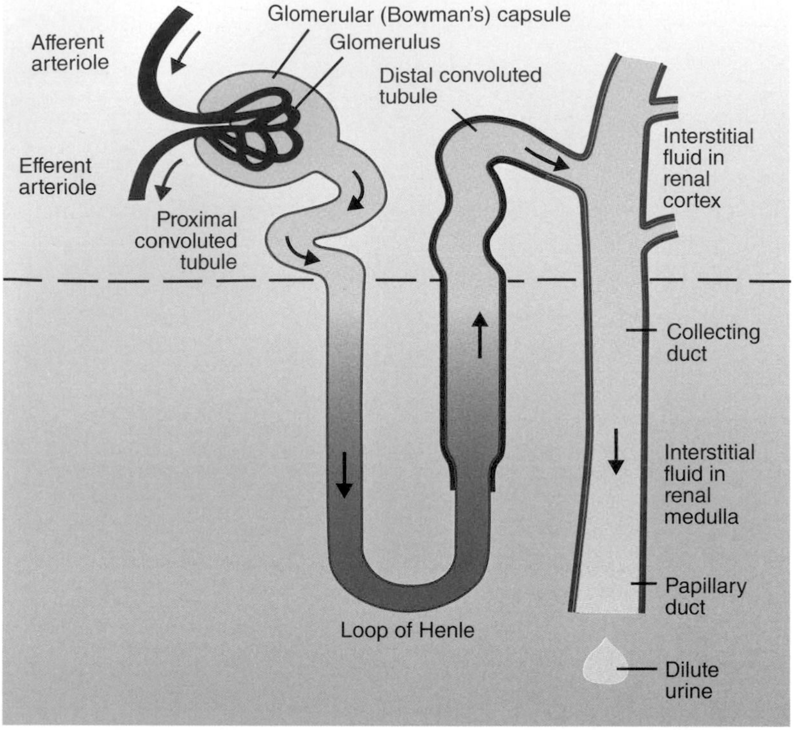
Glomerular (Bowman's) capsule
Glomerulus
Afferent arteriole
Distal convoluted tubule
Efferent arteriole
Interstitial fluid in renal cortex
Proximal convoluted tubule
Collecting duct
Interstitial fluid in renal medulla
Papillary duct
Loop of Henle
Dilute urine

Figure 14.5 Nephron (Tortora and Derrickson 2009)

system located in the kidney and is responsible for the reaborption of water, salts. The nephron is divided into several sections:

- Bowman's capsule
- Proximal convoluted tubule
- Loop of Henle
- Distal convoluted tubule.

Each section performs different function; these will be discussed in the following sections.

Bowman's capsule

Also known as glomerular capsule (see Figure 14.6), the Bowman's capsule is a cup-like sac and is the first portion of the nephron. The Bowman's capsule is part of the filtration system in the kidneys. When blood reaches the kidneys for filtration, it enters the Bowman's capsule first, with the capsule separating the blood into two components: a filtrated blood product and a filtrate which is moved through the nephron, another structure in the kidneys. The glomerular capsule consists of visceral and parietal layers (see Figure 14.6). The visceral layer is lined with epithelial cells called podocytes, while the parietal layer is lined with simple squamous epithelium and it is

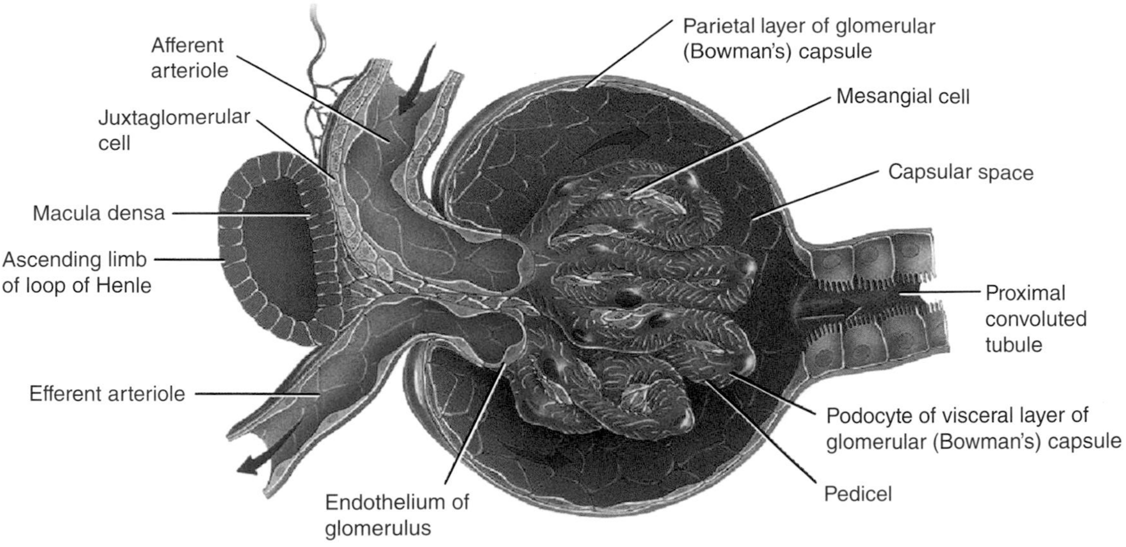
Afferent arteriole
Juxtaglomerular cell
Macula densa
Ascending limb of loop of Henle
Efferent arteriole
Endothelium of glomerulus
Parietal layer of glomerular (Bowman's) capsule
Mesangial cell
Capsular space
Proximal convoluted tubule
Podocyte of visceral layer of glomerular (Bowman's) capsule
Pedicel

Figure 14.6 Bowman's capsule (Tortora and Derrickson 2009)

in the Bowman's capsule that the network of capillaries called glomerulus (Marieb and Hoehn 2007) is found. Filtration of blood takes place in this portion of the nephron.

Proximal convoluted tubule

From the Bowman's capsule, the filtrate drains into the proximal convoluted tubule (see Figure 14.5). The surface of the epithelial cells of this segment of the nephron is covered with densely packed microvilli. The microvilli increase the surface area of the cells thus facilitating their resorptive function. The infolded membranes forming the microvilli are the site of numerous sodium pumps. Resorption of salt, water, and glucose from the glomerular filtrate occurs in this section of the tubule; at the same time certain substances, including uric acid and drug metabolites, are actively transferred from the blood capillaries into the tubule for excretion.

Loop of Henle

The proximal convoluted tubule then bends into a loop called the loop of Henle (see Figure 14.5). The loop of Henle is the part of the tubule which dips or 'loops' from the cortex into the medulla (descending limb), and then returns to the cortex (ascending limb). The loop of Henle is divided into the descending and ascending loops. The ascending loop of Henle is much thicker than the descending portion. The main function of the loop of Henle is to generate a concentration gradient which creates a region of a high concentration of sodium in the medulla of the kidney. The descending portion of the loop of Henle is highly permeable to water and has low permeability to ions and urea. The ascending loop of Henle is permeable to ions but not to water. When required, urine is concentrated in this portion of the nephron. This is possible because of the high concentration of solute in the substance or interstitium of the medulla. This high concentration of solutes is maintained by the counter-current multiplier. Different parts of the loop of Henle have different actions:

- The descending loop of Henle is relatively impermeable to solute but permeable to water so that water moves out by osmosis, and the fluid in the tubule becomes hypertonic.
- The thin section of the ascending loop of Henle is virtually impermeable to water, but permeable to solute, especially sodium and chloride ions. Thus sodium and chloride ions move out down the concentration gradient, the fluid within the tubule first becomes isotonic then hypotonic as more ions leave. Urea which was absorbed into the medullary interstitium from the collecting duct diffuses into the ascending limb. This keeps the urea within the interstitium of the medulla where it also has a role in concentrating urine.
- The thick section of the ascending loop of Henle and early distal tubule are virtually impermeable to water. However sodium and chloride ions are actively transported out of the tubule, making the tubular fluid very hypotonic.

Distal convoluted tubule

The thick ascending portion of the loop of Henle leads into the distal convoluted tubule (DCT) (see Figure 14.5). The DCT is lined with simple cuboidal cells and the lumen of the DCT is larger than the PCT lumen because the PCT has a brush border (microvilli). The DCT is an important site:

- Active secretion of ions and acids
- Plays a part in the regulation of calcium ions by excreting excess calcium ions in response to calcitonin hormone
- Selective reabsorption of water
- Arginine vasopressin receptor 2 proteins are also located in the distal convoluted tubule
- Plays a role in regulating pH by absorbing bicarbonate and secreting protons (H^+) into the filtrate.

The final concentration of urine, in this section, is dependent on a hormone called anti-diuretic hormone (ADH). If ADH is present, the distal tubule and the collecting duct become permeable to water. As the collecting duct passes through the medulla with a high solute concentration in the interstitium, the water moves out of the lumen of the duct and concentrated urine is formed. In the absence of ADH the tubule is minimally permeable to water so large quantities of dilute urine is formed.

Collecting ducts

The distal convoluted tubule then drains into the collecting ducts (see Figure 14.5). Several collecting ducts converge and drain into a larger system called the papillary ducts, which in turn empy into the minor calyx (plural – calices). From here the filtrate, now called urine, drains into the renal pelvis. It is the final stage where sodium and water are reabsorbed. When a person is dehydrated, approximately 25% of the water filtered is reabsorbed in the collecting duct. However, the cells of the collecting ducts are impermeable to water but with the aid of the ADH and aquaporins water is reabsorbed from the collecting ducts. Aquaporins are proteins embedded in the cell membrane that regulate the flow of water. Aquaporins selectively transport water molecules in and out of the cell, while preventing the passage of ions and other solutes.

Functions of the kidney

The kidneys maintain fluid balance, electrolyte balance and the acid base balance of the blood.

- The kidneys remove wastes and excess water (fluid) collected by, and carried in, the blood as it flows through the body. Approximately 190 l of blood enter the kidneys every day via the renal arteries. Millions of tiny filters, called glomeruli, inside the kidneys separate wastes and water from the blood. Most of these unwanted substances come from what we eat and drink. The kidneys automatically remove the right amount of salt and other minerals from the blood to leave just the quantities the body needs.
- By removing just the right amount of excess fluid, healthy kidneys maintain what is called the body's fluid balance. In women, fluid content stays at about 55% of total weight. In men, it stays at about 60% of total weight. The kidneys maintain these proportions by balancing the amount of fluid that leaves the body against the amount entering the body. When large volume of fluid is drunk, healthy kidneys remove the excess fluid and produce a lot of urine. On the other hand, if fluid intake is low, the kidneys retain fluid and the patient does not pass much urine. Fluid also leaves the body through sweat, breath and faeces. If the weather is hot and we lose a lot of fluid by sweating, then the kidneys will not pass much urine.
- Kidneys synthesise hormones such as renin and angiotensin. These hormones regulate how much sodium (salt) and fluid the body keeps, and how well the blood vessels can expand and contract. This in turn helps control blood pressure.
- Kidneys produce a hormone known as erythropoeitin (EPO), which is carried in the blood to the bone marrow where it stimulates the production of red blood cells. These cells carry oxygen throughout the body. Without enough healthy red blood cells anaemia develops a condition which causes weakness cold, tiredness and shortness of breath.
- Healthy kidneys keep bones strong by producing the hormone calcitriol. Calcitriol maintains the right levels of calcium and phosphate in the blood and bones. Calcium and phosphate balance are important to keep bones healthy. When the kidneys fail they may not produce enough calcitriol. This leads to abnormal levels of phosphate, calcium and vitamin D, causing renal bone disease. For the summary of the functions of the kidney see Table 14.1.

Table 14.1 Summary of the functions of the kidneys

• Filtration
• Regulation of blood volume
• Regulation of osmolarity
• Secretion of renin and erythropoietin
• Maintenance of acid base balance
• Synthesis of vitamin D
• Detoxification of free radicals and drugs
• Gluconeogenesis

Clinical considerations

Renal failure – acute and chronic

The kidney is a very vascular organ with numerous functions. The kidneys control the quantity and quality of fluids within the body. They also produce hormones and vitamins that direct cell activities in many organs; the hormone renin, for example, helps control blood pressure. When the kidneys are not working properly, waste products and fluid can build up to dangerous levels, creating a life-threatening situation. Among the important substances the kidneys help to control are sodium, potassium, chloride, bicarbonate (HCO_3^-), pH, calcium, phosphate and magnesium. The blood flow to the kidney depends on many physiological factors such as blood pressure, circulating volume and a healthy kidney. When blood flow to the kidneys is reduced as a result of haemorrhage from surgery or trauma, the functions of the kidneys are affected. The patient can go into renal failure.

Renal failure may occur with any serious illness or operation, particularly those complicated by severe infection. If the blood supply to the kidneys is reduced considerably from blood loss, a fall in blood pressure, severe dehydration or lack of salt, then the kidneys may be damaged. If this problem lasts long enough there can be permanent damage to the kidney tissue. Sudden blockage to the drainage of urine from the kidney can cause damage. A kidney stone is a possible cause of this. Acute kidney damage can occur as a rare side-effect of some medications and other rare conditions.

There are many causes of chronic renal failure, including inflammatory conditions affecting the kidney tissue, as a complication of long-standing diabetes mellitus (sugar diabetes), chronic blockage to the drainage of the kidneys and as a result of certain inherited conditions such as polycystic kidney disease. Often, the cause has occurred many years earlier and cannot be identified.

Blood supply of the kidney

The role of the kidney is to filter at least 20–25% of blood during the resting cardiac output. Approximately 1200 ml of blood flows through the kidney each minute. Each kidney receives its blood supply directly from the aorta via the renal artery (see Figure 14.4), which is divided into anterior and posterior renal arteries. There are several arteries that deliver blood to the kidneys and they include:

- Renal artery – arises from the abdominal aorta at the level of first lumbar vertebra
- Segmental artery – branch of the renal artery
- Interlobar artery – branch of the segmental artery
- Arcuate artery – renal columns leading to the corticomedullary junction
- Interlobular arteries – divisions of the arcuate arteries.

The branches of the interlobular artery enter the nephrons as afferent arterioles. Each nephron receives one afferent arteriole, which further subdivides into a tuft of capillaries called the glomerulus. The glomerular capillaries reunite and leave the Bowman's capsule as efferent arterioles. Efferent arterioles unite to form peritubular capillaries and then interlobular veins which unite to form the arcuate veins and finally into interlobar veins. Blood leave the kidneys through the renal vein, which then flows into the inferior vena cava. The diameter of the afferent arteriole is larger than the diameter of the efferent arteriole.

Urine formation

Three processes are involved in the formation of urine:

- Filtration
- Selective reabsorption
- Secretion.

Filtration

Urine formation begins with the process of filtration, which goes on continually in the renal corpuscles. Filtration takes place in the glomerulus which lies in the Bowman's capsule. The blood for filtration is supplied by the renal artery. In the kidney the renal artery divides into smaller arterioles. The arteriole entering the Bowman's capsule is called the afferent arteriole, which further subdivides into a cluster of capillaries called the glomerulus.

As blood passes through the glomeruli, much of its fluid, containing both useful chemicals and dissolved waste materials, soaks out of the blood through the membranes (by osmosis and diffusion) where it is filtered and then flows into the Bowman's capsule. This process is called glomerular filtration. The water, waste products, salt, glucose and other chemicals that have been filtered out of the blood are known collectively as glomerular filtrate.

The fluid from the filtered blood is protein-free but contains electrolytes such as sodium chloride, potassium and waste products of cellular metabolism, for example, urea, uric acid and creatinine (McCance and Huether 2006). The filtered blood then returns into circulation via the efferent arteriole and finally into the renal vein.

Selective reabsorption

Selective reabsorption processes ensure that any substances in the filtrate that are essential for body function are reabsorbed into the plasma. Substances such as sodium, calcium, potassium and chloride are reabsorbed to maintain fluid and electrolyte balance and the pH of blood. However, if these substances are in excess to body requirements, they are excreted in the urine. Only 1% of the glomerular filtrate actually leaves the body; 99% are reabsorbed into the bloodstream. The reabsorption occurs via three processes:

- Osmosis
- Diffusion
- Active transport.

For a summary see Tables 14.2a, 14.2b, 14.2c and 14.2d.

Blood glucose is entirely reabsorbed into the blood from the proximal tubules. In fact, it is actively transported out of the tubules and into the peritubular capillary blood. None of this valuable nutrient is wasted by being lost in the urine. Sodium (Na^+) and other ions are only

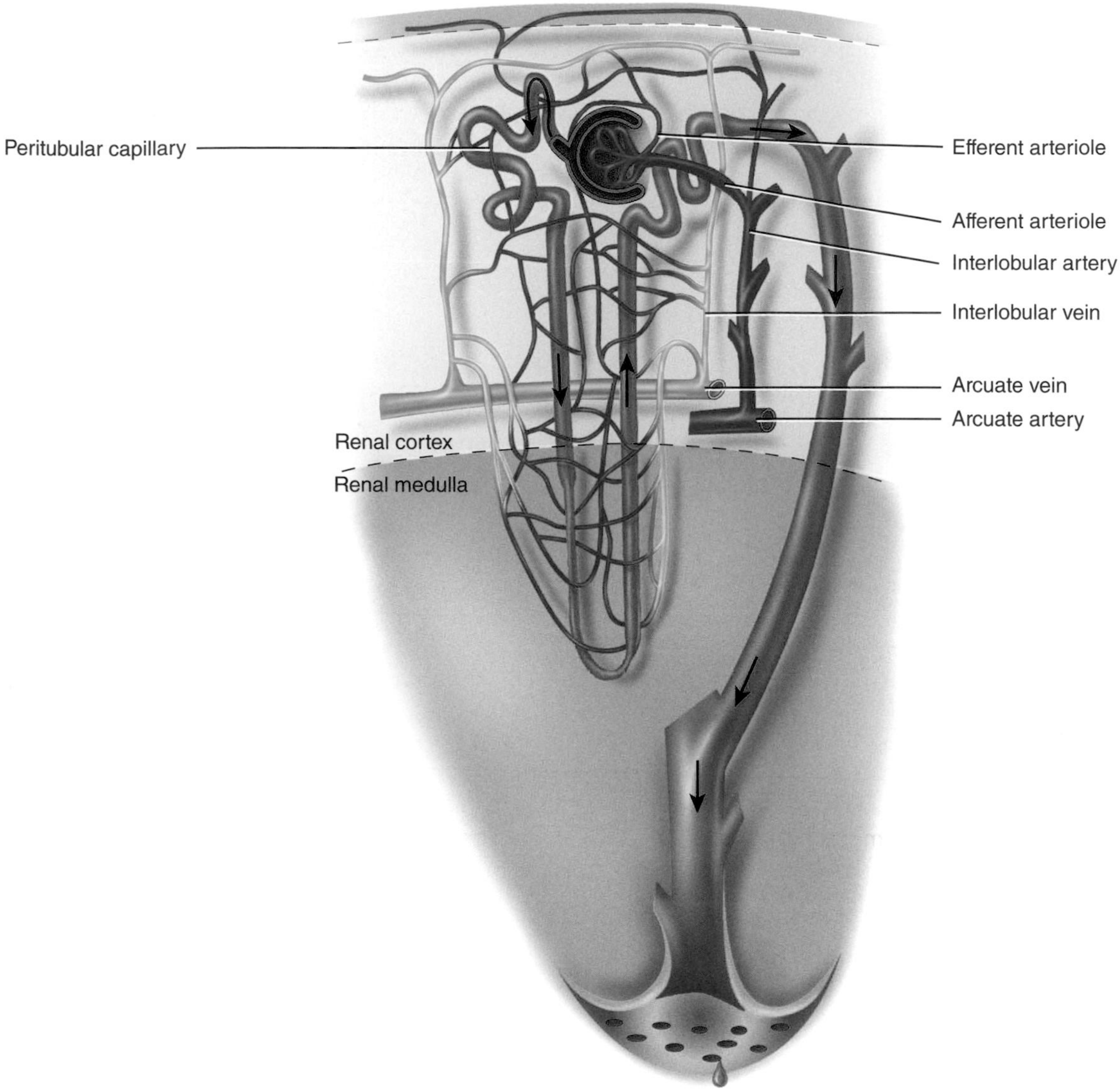
Peritubular capillary
Efferent arteriole
Afferent arteriole
Interlobular artery
Interlobular vein
Arcuate vein
Arcuate artery
Renal cortex
Renal medulla

Figure 14.7 Nephron with capillaries (Tortora and Derrickson 2009)

partially reabsorbed from the renal tubules into the blood. For the most part, however, sodium ions are actively transported back into blood from the tubular fluid. The amount of sodium reabsorbed varies; it depends largely on how much salt we take in from the foods that we eat.

As a person increases the amount of salt intake into the body, kidneys decrease the amount of sodium reabsorption into the blood. That is, more sodium is retained in the tubules. Therefore, the amount of salt excreted in the urine increases. The process works the other way as well. The less the salt intake, the greater the amount of sodium reabsorbed into the blood, and the amount of salt excreted in the urine decreases.

Secretion

Any substances not removed through filtration are secreted into the renal tubules from the peritubular capillaries (see Figure 14.7) of the nephron (Waugh and Grant 2006); these include drugs and hydrogen ions. Tubular secretion mainly takes place by active transport. Active transport is a process by which substances are moved across biological membrane. Tubular secretion occurs from epithelial cells lining the renal tubules and the collecting ducts. Substances secreted into the tubular fluid include:

- Potassium ions (K^+)
- Hydrogen ions (H^+)
- Ammonium ions (NH_4^+)
- Creatinine
- Urea
- Some hormones.

It is the tubular secretion of hydrogen and ammonium ions that helps to maintain the pH of blood. For a summary see Tables 14.2a, 14.2b, 14.2c and 14.2d.

Summary of filtration, reabsorption and excretion in the nephron and collecting ducts

Table 14.2a Proximal convoluted tubule

Reabsorption	Excretion
Water approximately 65%	Hydrogen ions
Sodium and potassium 65%	Urea
Glucose 100%	Creatinine
Amino acid 100%	Ammonium ions
Chloride approximately 50%	
Bicarbonate, calcium and magnesium	
Urea	

Table 14.2b Loop of Henle

Reabsorption	Excretion
Water	Urea
Sodium and potassium approximately 30%	
Chloride approximately 35%	
Bicarbonate approximately 20%	
Calcium and magnesium	

Table 14.2c Distal convoluted tubule

Reabsorption	Excretion
Water approximately 15%	Potassium, depending on serum values
Sodium and chloride approximately 5%	Hydrogen ions, depending on pH of blood
Calcium	
Some urea	

Table 14.2d Collecting duct

Reabsorption	Excretion
Bicarbonate, depending on serum values	Potassium, depending on serum values
Urea	Hydrogen ions, depending on pH of blood
Water approximately 9%	
Sodium approximately 4%	

Tables 14.2a, b, c and d adapted from Tortora and Derrickson (2007)

Hormonal control of tubular reabsorption and secretion

Four hormones play a role in the regulation of fluid and electrolytes:

- Angiotensin II
- Aldosterone
- Antidiuretic hormone
- Atrial natriuretic peptide.

Angiotensin and aldosterone

As the blood volume and blood pressure decrease, the juxtaglomerular cells secrete a hormone called renin. Juxtaglomerula cells are found near the glomerulus and these cells synthesise, store and secrete the hormone renin. Renin acts on a plasma protein called angiotensinogen and converts it into angiotensin I. Angiotensinogen is produced by the hepatocytes of the liver. Angiotensin I is transported by the blood to the lungs. In the lung capillaries there are enzymes called angiotensin-converting enzyme (ACE). ACE is predominately found in the lung capillaries but this enzyme is also found throughout the body. ACE converts angiotensin I into angiotensin II. Angiotensin II is a short-acting, powerful vasoconstrictor, thus increasing blood pressure. Angiotensin II promotes the reabsorption of sodium, chloride and water in the proximal convoluted tubule. It also stimulates the adrenal glands to release a hormone called aldosterone which stimulates the cells in the collecting duct to reabsorb sodium and chloride and secrete potassium.

Antidiuretic hormone (ADH)

The third principal hormone is anti-diuretic hormone (ADH). ADH is produced by the hypothalamus gland and is stored by the posterior pituitary gland. This hormone increases the permeability of the cells in the distal convoluted tubule and the collecting ducts. In the presence of ADH more water is reabsorbed from the renal tubules and therefore the patient will pass less urine. In the absence of ADH less water is reabsorbed and the patient will pass more urine. Thus ADH plays a major role in the regulation of fluid balance in the body.

Atrial natriuretic peptide (ANP)

The fourth hormone involved in tubular secretion and reabsorption is atrial natriuretic peptide hormone (ANP). ANP is a powerful vasodilator and is a protein produced by the myocytes of the atria of the heart in response to increased blood pressure. ANP stimulates the kidneys to excrete sodium and water from the renal tubules thus decreasing blood volume, which in turn lowers blood pressure. The hormone also inhibits the secretion of aldosterone and ADH.

ANP is involved in the long-term regulation of sodium and water balance, blood volume and arterial pressure. There are two major pathways of natriuretic peptide actions: vasodilator effects and renal effects, which lead to natriuresis and diuresis. ANP directly dilates veins (increases venous compliance) and thereby decreases central venous pressure, which reduces cardiac output by decreasing ventricular preload. ANP also dilates arteries, which decreases systemic vascular resistance and systemic arterial pressure.

Composition of urine

Urine is a sterile and clear fluid of nitrogenous wastes and salts. It is translucent with an amber or light-yellow colour. Its colour is due to the pigments from the breakdown of haemoglobin. Concentrated urine tends to be darker in colour than normal urine. However, other factors such as diet, medications and certain diseases may affect the colour of the urine. It is slightly acidic and the pH may range from 4.5–8. The pH is affected by an individual's dietary intake and state of health. Diet that is high in animal protein tends to make the urine more acidic, while a vegetarian diet may make the urine more alkaline. The volume of urine produced depends on the circulating volume of blood. ADH regulates the amount of urine passed by the individual. If the person is dehydrated, more ADH is released from the posterior pituitary gland resulting in water

Table 14.3 Solutes in the urine

***Inorganic solutes*:**
Sodium
Potassium
Calcium
Magnesium
Iron
Chloride
Sulphate
Phosphate
Bicarbonate
Ammonia
***Organic solutes*:**
Urea
Creatinine
Uric acid

Adapted from Mader 2005

reabsorption and less urine being produced. On the other hand, if the person has consumed a large amount of fluid which increases the circulating volume, less ADH is released and more water is passed as urine.

Urine is 96% water and approximately 4% solutes derived from cellular metabolism. The solutes include organic and inorganic waste products and unwanted substances such as drugs. Normally there is no protein or blood. If it is present then the person may be suffering from a disease. For a summary of solutes see Table 14.3.

Characteristics of normal urine

The volume produced is one of the physical characteristics of urine. Other physical characteristics that can apply to urine include colour, turbidity (transparency), smell (odour), pH (acidity/alkalinity) and density.

- Colour: Typically yellow-amber but varies according to recent diet, medication and the concentration of the urine. Drinking more water generally tends to reduce the concentration of urine and therefore causes it to have a lighter colour. However, if a person does not drink a large amount of fluid, this may increase the concentration and the urine will have a darker colour.
- Smell: The smell or odour, of urine may provide health information. For example, the urine of diabetics may have a sweet or fruity odour due to the presence of ketones (organic molecules of a particular structure). Generally, fresh urine has a mild smell but stale urine or infected urine has a stronger odour, similar to that of ammonia.
- Acidity: pH is a measure of the acidity (or alkalinity) of a solution. The pH of a substance (solution) is usually represented as a number in the range 0 (strong acid) to 14 (strong alkali, also known as a 'base'). Pure water is 'neutal' in the sense that it is neither neither acid nor alkali, it therefore has a pH of 7. The pH of normal urine is generally in the range 4.6–8, a typical average being around 6.0. Much of the variation is due to diet. For example, high-protein diets result in more acidic urine, but vegetarian diets generally result in more alkaline urine.

- Density: Density is also known as 'specific gravity'. This is the ratio of the weight of a volume of a substance compared with the weight of the same volume of distilled water. Given that urine is mostly water, but also contains some other substances dissolved in the water, its density is expected to be close to, but slightly greater than, 1.000.

Clinical considerations

Renal stones and renal colic

Kidney stones, one of the most painful of the urologic disorders, have beset humans for centuries. Unfortunately, kidney stones are one of the most common disorders of the urinary tract.

Normally kidney stones pass out of the body without any intervention, however, there are times when stones get lodged in the urinary tract and cause a severe health risk. Stones that cause lasting symptoms or other complications may be treated by various techniques, most of which do not involve major surgery. Also, research advances have led to a better understanding of the many factors that promote stone formation and thus better treatments for preventing stones.

Kidney stones often do not cause any symptoms. Usually, the first symptom of a kidney stone is extreme pain, which begins suddenly when a stone moves in the urinary tract and blocks the flow of urine in conditions such as renal colic. The patient feels a sharp, cramping pain in the back and side in the area of the kidney or in the lower abdomen. Sometimes nausea and vomiting occur. Later, pain may spread to the groin.

If the stone is too large to pass easily, pain continues as the muscles in the wall of the narrow ureter try to squeeze the stone into the bladder. As the stone moves, blood may appear in the urine as haematuria. As the stone moves down the ureter, the patient may feel the need to urinate more often or feel a burning sensation during urination.

Ureters

The ureters are tubular organs which run from the renal pelvis to the posterolateral base of the urinary bladder. The ureters are approximately 25–30 cm in length and 5 mm in diameter (Mader 2005) and extend from the kidney to the bladder. The ureters terminate at the bladder and enter obliquely through the muscle wall of the bladder. They pass over the pelvic brim at the bifurcation of the common iliac arteries (see Figure 14.8).

The ureters have three layers:

- Transitional epithelial mucosa (inner layer)
- Smooth muscle layer (middle layer)
- Fibrous connective tissue (outer layer).

Urine is transported through the ureters via muscular movements of the urinary tract's peristalic muscular waves. When the renal pelvis becomes laden with urine, the peristaltic wave action encourages urine to leave the body. The amount of urine in the renal pelvis determines the frequency of the peristaltic wave action, which can range from one to every few minutes to one to every few seconds. This action creates a pressure force that moves the urine through the ureters and into the bladder in small spurts.

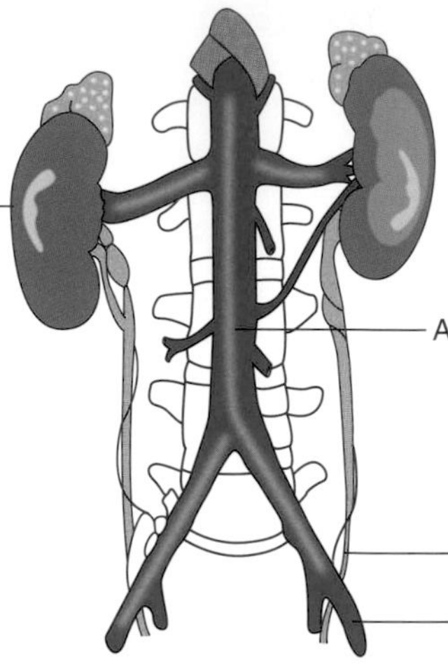
Right kidney
Aorta
Ureter
Common
iliac artery

Figure 14.8 Common iliac vessels and ureter (Nair and Peate 2009)

Urinary bladder

The urinary bladder is a hollow muscular organ and is located in the pelvic cavity posterior to the symphysis pubis. In the male the bladder lies anterior to the rectum and in the female it lies anterior to the vagina and inferior to the uterus (Mader 2005), it is a smooth muscular sac which stores urine. Although the shape of the bladder is spherical, the shape is altered from pressure of surrounding organs. When the bladder is empty, the inner section of the bladder forms folds but as the bladder fills with urine the walls of the bladder become smoother. As urine accumulates, the bladder expands without a significant rise in the internal pressure of the bladder. The bladder normally distends and holds approximately 350–750 ml of urine. In females the bladder is slightly smaller because the uterus occupies the space above the bladder.

The inner lining of the urinary bladder is a mucous membrane of transitional epithelium that is continuous with that in the ureters. When the bladder is empty, the mucosa has numerous folds called rugae. The rugae and transitional epithelium allow the bladder to expand as it fills. The second layer in the walls is the submucosa which supports the mucous membrane. It is composed of connective tissue with elastic fibres.

The inner floor of the bladder includes a triangular section called trigone. The trigone is formed by three openings in the floor of the urinary bladder. Two of the openings are from the ureters and form the base of the trigone. Small flaps of mucosa cover these openings and act as valves that allow urine to enter the bladder but prevent it from backing up from the bladder into the ureters. The third opening, at the apex of the trigone, is the opening into the urethra (see Figure 14.9). A band of the detrusor muscle encircles this opening to form the internal urethral sphincter.

The walls of the bladder consist of muscle fibres:

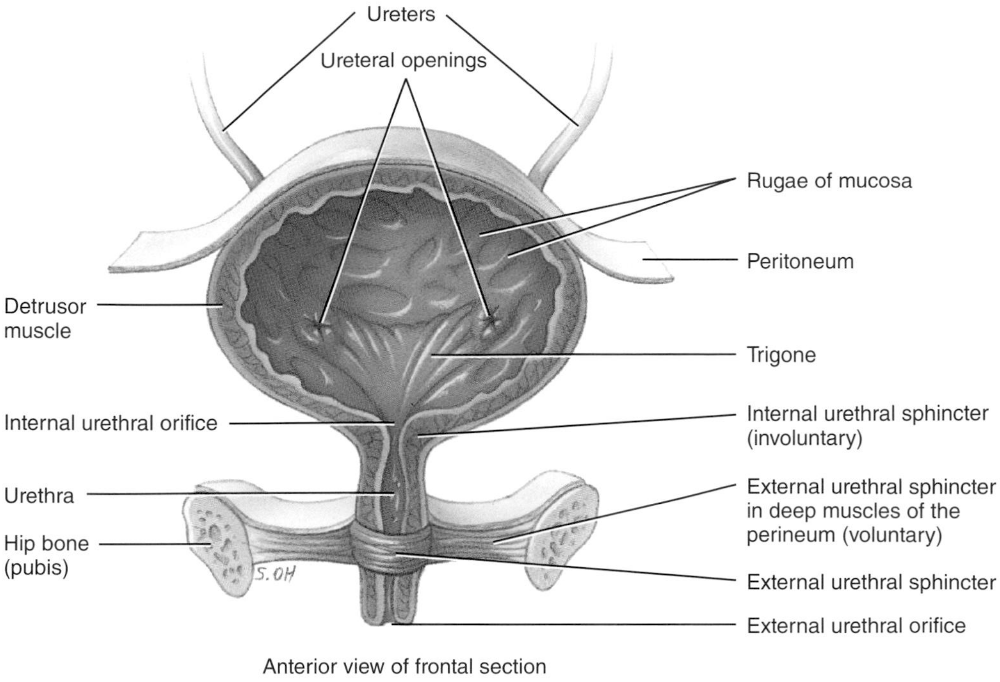
Ureters
Ureteral openings
Rugae of mucosa
Peritoneum
Detrusor muscle
Trigone
Internal urethral orifice
Internal urethral sphincter (involuntary)
Urethra
External urethral sphincter in deep muscles of the perineum (voluntary)
Hip bone (pubis)
External urethral sphincter
External urethral orifice
Anterior view of frontal section

Figure 14.9 Layers of the urinary bladder (Tortora and Derrickson 2009)

- Transitional epithelial mucosa
- A thick muscular layer
- A fibrous outer layer.

See Figure 8.9 for the layers of the urinary bladder.

Clinical considerations

Cystitis, urinary tract infection

Urinary tract infection is caused by organisms such as *E. coli* and *Proteus mirabilis*. Patients who suffer from urinary tract infection could present with the following signs and symptoms:

- Burning sensationon passing urine
- The need to urinate more often than usual
- Feeling the need to urinate urgently, even if passing very little or no urine
- Urine that is cloudy or dark, and may have a strong smell
- Haematuria
- Pain or tenderness in the lower back or lower abdomen
- A general feeling of being unwell.

Urinary tract infection and cystitis are more common in women than men. If untreated they can result in a more serious renal problem. Urinary tract infection can be prevented by ensuring adequate intake of fluid and good personal hygiene.

The urinary tract can become blocked or obstructed (for example, from a kidney stone, tumour, expanding uterus during pregnancy or enlarged prostate gland). The buildup of urine can lead to infection and injury of the kidney. With a kidney stone, often the blockage is painful. Other obstructions may produce no symptoms and be detected only when a blood or urine test is abnormal or an imaging procedure, such as an x-ray or ultrasound, detects it.

Urinary tract infections, such as cystitis (an infection of the bladder), can lead to more serious infections further up the urinary tract. Symptoms include fever, frequent urination, sudden and urgent need to urinate, and pain or a burning feeling during urination. There is often pressure or pain in the lower abdomen or back. Sometimes the urine has a strong or foul odour or is bloody. Pyelonephritis is an infection of kidney tissue; most often, it is the result of cystitis that has spread to the kidney. An obstruction in the urinary tract can make a kidney infection more likely. Infections elsewhere in the body, including, for example, streptococcal infections, the skin infection impetigo or a bacterial infection in the heart, can also be carried through the bloodstream to the kidney and cause a problem there.

Urethra

The urethra is a muscular tube that drains urine from the bladder and conveys it out of the body. It contains three coats and they are muscular, erectile and mucous; the muscular is the continuation of the bladder muscle layer. The urethra is encompassed by two separate urethral sphincter muscles. The internal urethral sphincter muscle is formed by involuntary smooth muscles while the lower voluntary muscles make up the external sphincter muscles. The internal sphincter is created by the detrusor muscle. The urethra is different in length in both males and females. Sphincters keep the urethra closed when urine is not being passed. The internal urethral sphincter is under involuntary control and lies at the bladder – urethra junction. The external urethral sphincter is under voluntary control.

Male urethra

The male urethra passes through three different regions:

- Prostatic region – passes through the prostate gland
- Membranous portion – passes through the pelvis diaphragm
- Penile region – extends the length of the penis.

In the male, the urethra not only excretes fluid wastes but is also part of the reproductive system. Rather than the straight tube found in the female body, the male urethra is S-shaped to follow the line of the penis. It is approximately 20 cm long. The male urethra can be segregated into three various portions, the spongy portion, the prostatic portion and the membranous portion. The proximal portion, which is also the prostatic portion, is only about 2.5 cm long and passes along the neck of the urinary bladder through the prostate gland. This section is designed to accept the drainage from the tiny ducts within the prostate and is equipped with two ejaculatory tubes (see Figure 14.10).

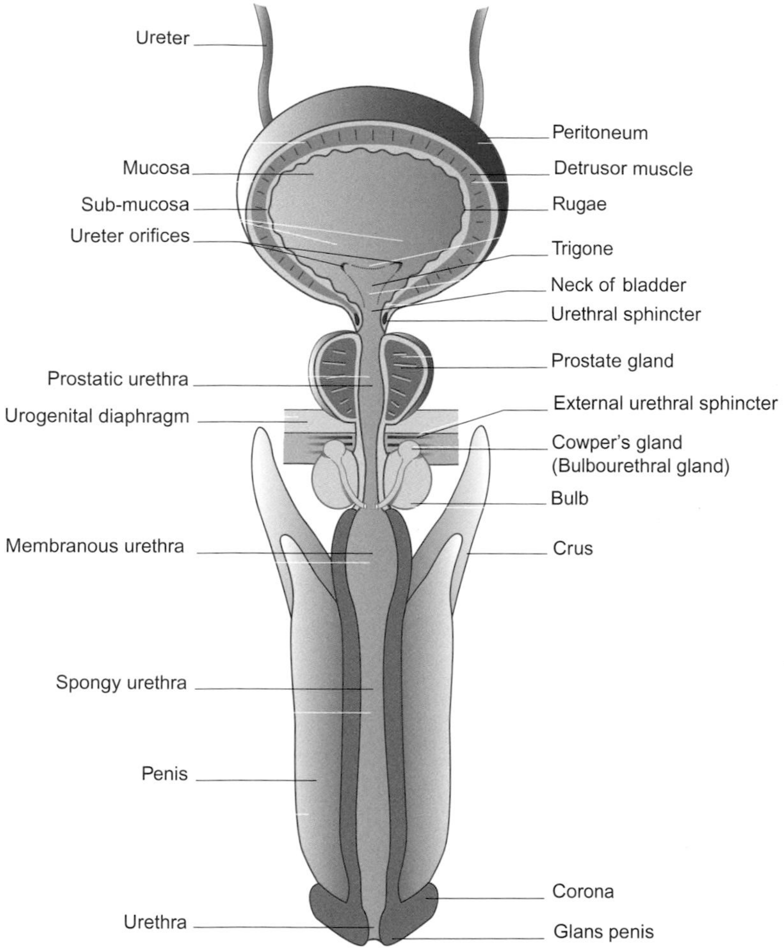
Ureter
Mucosa
Sub-mucosa
Ureter orifices
Prostatic urethra
Urogenital diaphragm
Membranous urethra
Spongy urethra
Penis
Urethra
Peritoneum
Detrusor muscle
Rugae
Trigone
Neck of bladder
Urethral sphincter
Prostate gland
External urethral sphincter
Cowper's gland
(Bulbourethral gland)
Bulb
Crus
Corona
Glans penis

Figure 14.10 Male urethra

Female urethra

The female urethra is bound to the anterior vaginal wall. The external opening of the urethra is anterior to the vagina and posterior to the clitoris. In the female, the urethra is approximately 4 cm long and leads out of the body via the urethral orifice. In the female, the urethral orifice is located in the vestibule in the labia minora. This can be found located in between the clitoris and the vaginal orifice. In the female body the urethra's only function is to transport urine out of the body (see Figure 14.11).

Micturition

When the volume of urine in the bladder reaches about 300 ml, stretch receptors in the bladder walls are stimulated and excite sensory parasympathetic fibres which relay information to the

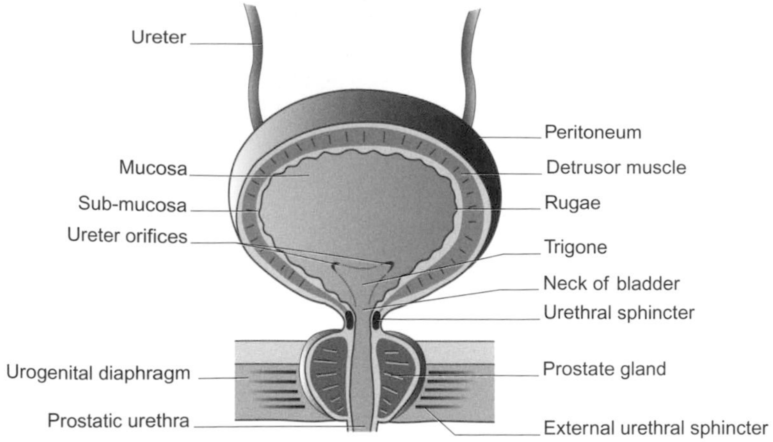
Ureter
Mucosa
Sub-mucosa
Ureter orifices
Urogenital diaphragm
Prostatic urethra
Peritoneum
Detrusor muscle
Rugae
Trigone
Neck of bladder
Urethral sphincter
Prostate gland
External urethral sphincter

Figure 14.11 Female urethra

sacral area of the spine. This information is integrated in the spine and relayed to two different sets of neurones. Parasympathetic motor neurones (in the pons) are excited and act to contract the detrusor muscles in the bladder so that bladder pressure increases and the internal sphincter opens. At the same time, somatic motor neurones supplying the external sphincter via the pudendal nerve are inhibited, allowing the external sphincter to open and urine to flow out, assisted by gravity.

A person has great control of the bladder. They can increase or decrease the rate of flow of urine, and stop and start at will (unless there are physiological problems), thus making micturition a simple reflex action.

Conclusion

The renal system consists of the kidneys, ureters, urinary bladder and the urethra. These systems collectively play an important role in maintaining homeostasis. They remove the waste products of metabolism, secrete hormones, regulate fluid balance and maintain homeostasis. Some of the functions it carries out include:

- Regulating blood volume through urine production and blood pressure by releasing renin
- Regulating the electrolyte balance in the body through hormones such as aldosterone
- Maintaining the acid base balance by regulating the secretion of hydrogen and bicarbonate ions
- Excreting waste products, for example, urea and uric acid and conserving valuable nutrients essential for the body.

Urine is formed by filtration, selective reabsorption and secretion. The selectivity of the glomerular filtrate is determined by the size of the opening of the filter and blood pressure. There are other factors that regulate urine production and electrolyte balance; they include hormone regulation such as antidiuretic hormone, aldosterone and atrial natriuretic peptide hormones and neuronal regulation through the autonomic nervous system.

The urinary bladder is a storage organ for urine and is located in the pelvic cavity. It contains three layers: the muscular, erectile and mucous layers. Urine is stored in the bladder until the person gets the urge to empty his/her bladder. The process of micturition is under the control of the sympathetic and parasympathetic system. During micturition, strong muscles in the bladder walls (the detrusor muscles) compress the bladder, pushing its contents into the urethra, thus voiding urine.

Glossary

Anterior:	Front.
Bifurcation:	Dividing into two branches.
Calyces:	Small, funnel-shaped cavities formed from the renal pelvis.
Diuresis:	Excess urine production.
Excretion:	The elimination of waste products of metabolism.
Erythropoietin:	Hormone produced by the kidneys that regulates red blood cell production.
Filtration:	A passive transport system.
Glomerulus:	A network of capillaries found in the Bowman's capsule.
Hilus:	A small, indented part of the kidney.
Kidneys:	Organs situated in the posterior wall of the abdominal cavity.
Nephron:	Functional unit of the kidney.
Posterior:	Behind.
Renal artery:	Blood vessel that takes blood to the kidney.
Renal cortex:	The outermost part of the kidney.
Renal medulla:	The middle layer of the kidney.
Renal pelvis:	The funnel-shaped section of the kidney.
Renal pyramids:	Cone-shaped structures of the medulla.
Renal vein:	Blood vessel that returns filtered blood into circulation.
Renin:	A renal hormone that alters systemic blood pressure.
Sphincter:	A ring-like muscle fibre that can constrict.
Ureter:	Membranous tube that drains urine from the kidneys to the bladder.
Urethra:	Muscular tube that drains urine from the bladder.

References

Mader, S.S. (2005) *Understanding Human Anatomy and Physiology*, 5th edn. Boston, MA: McGraw-Hill.

Marieb, E.N. and Hoehn, K. (2007) *Human Anatomy and Physiology*, 7th edn. San Francisco: Pearson Benjamin Cummings.

McCance, K.L. and Huether, S.E. (2006) *Pathophysiology: The Biological Basis for Disease in Adults and Children*. St Louis, MO: Mosby.

Nair, M. and Peate, I. (2009) *Fundamentals of Applied Pathophysiology: An Essential Guide for Nursing Students*. Oxford: Wiley-Blackwell.

Tortora, G.J. and Derrickson, B. (2007) *Principles of Anatomy and Physiology*, 11th edn. Hoboken, NJ: John Wiley & Sons.

Tortora, G.J. and Derrickson, B.H. (2009) *Principles of Anatomy and Physiology*, 12th edn. Hoboken, NJ: John Wiley & Sons.

Waugh, A. and Grant, A. (2006) *Ross and Wilson Anatomy and Physiology in Health and Illness*, 10th edn. Edinburgh: Churchill Livingstone.

Activities

www.wiley.com/go/peate

Multiple choice questions

1. Which of the following parts of the nephron is in the renal medulla?

   (a) loop of Henle
   (b) glomerulus
   (c) distal convoluted tubule
   (d) proximal convoluted tubule

2. Urine passes through the:

   (a) afferent artery → to the bladder → to the urethra
   (b) efferent artery → to the bladder → to the urethra
   (c) pelvis of the kidney → to the ureter → to the bladder → to the urethra
   (d) pelvis of the kidney → to the urethra → to the bladder → to the ureter

3. The functional units of the kidney are:

   (a) the nephron
   (b) glomerulus
   (c) collecting duct
   (d) loop of Henle

4. Which of the following statement is true of urine?

(a) urine is slightly alkaline
(b) haemoglobin colours the urine yellow
(c) urine contains nitrogenous waste
(d) urine has white blood cells

5. Sodium reabsorption in the DCT and the collecting duct is aided by the secreton of:

(a) ADH
(b) renin
(c) erythropoietin
(d) aldosterone

6. The glomerulus is located within the:

(a) renal pelvis
(b) renal tubule
(c) renal column
(d) renal corpuscle

7. Glucose:

(a) is in the filtrate and not in the urine
(b) is in the filtrate and in the urine
(c) undergoes tubular excretion and is in the urine
(d) undergoes tubular excretion and is not in the urine

8. Urine is:

(a) 90% water and 10% solutes
(b) 96% water and 4% solutes
(c) 99% water and 1% solutes
(d) 80% water and 20% solutes

9. When a large amount of ADH is secreted:

(a) the DCT becomes impermeable to water
(b) the amount of water reabsorbed decreases
(c) water reabsorption increases
(d) large amount of sodium ions are excreted

10. The removal of water and solutes from the filtrate in the renal tubule is:

(a) excretion
(b) filtration
(c) secretion
(d) reabsorption

Test your learning

1. What happens to the urine output in a patient who is hypovolaemic?
2. What happens to urine output if you eat large quantities of salty potato crisps?
3. List the functions of the kidney.
4. Explain the effect of alcohol on urine production?
5. What are the primary effects of angiotensin II on kidney function and regulation?
6. Discuss the role of renin in the regulation of blood pressure.
7. Discuss the role of the urinary bladder.
8. Are males or females more prone to cystitis? Explain.

Label the diagram

From the lists of words, label the diagrams below:

Renal cortex, Renal medulla, Renal column, Renal pyramid in renal medulla, Renal sinus, Renal papilla, Fat in renal sinus, Renal capsule, Nephron, Path of urine drainage: Collecting duct, Papillary duct in renal pyramid, Minor calyx, Major calyx, Renal pelvis, Ureter, Renal artery, Renal vein

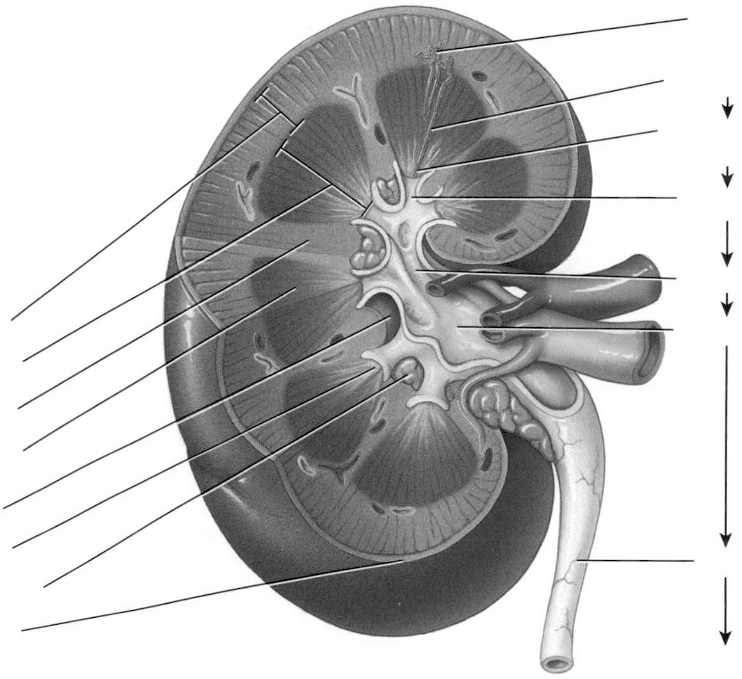

Afferent arteriole, Efferent arteriole, Proximal convoluted tubule, Glomerular Bowman's capsule, Glomerulus, Distal convoluted tubule, Interstitial fluid in renal cortex, Collecting duct, Interstitial fluid in renal medulla, Papillary duct, Dilute urine, Loop of Henle

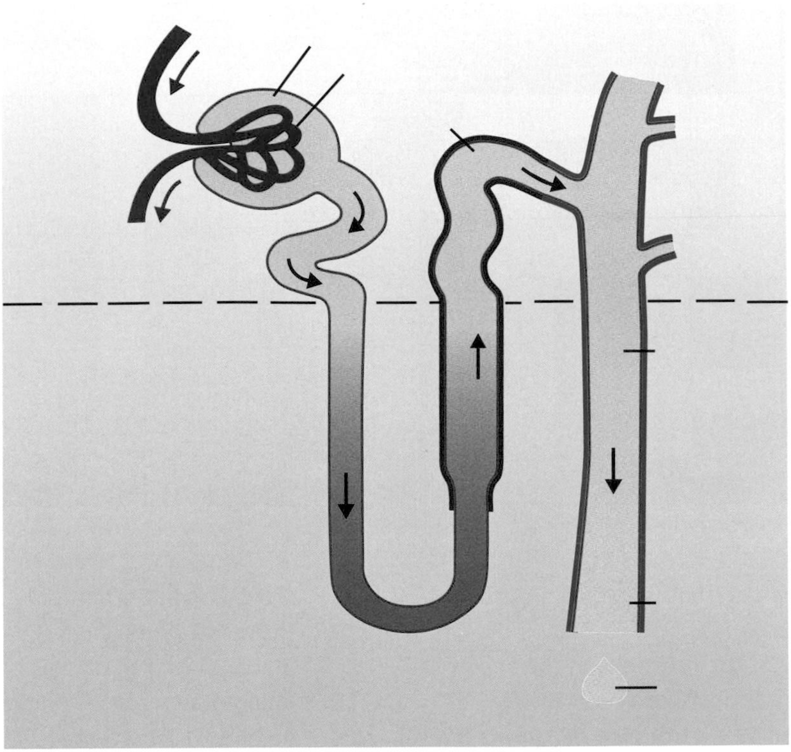

Crossword

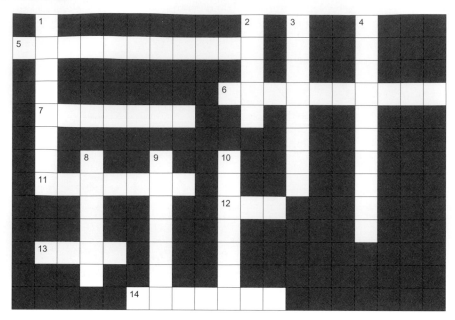
1
2
3
4
5
6
7
8
9
10
11
12
13
14

Across:

5. Hormone that regulates electrolyte balance (11).
6. One of the functions of the kidney (10).
7. Also carries sperm in man (7).
11. Gland that sits on top of each kidney (7).
12. Hormone that regulates fluid balance (3).
13. One of the waste products found in the urine (4).
14. Functional unit of the kidney (7).

Down:

1. Scanty urine output (8).
2. Hormone produced by the juxtaglomerular cells (5).
3. Inflammation of the bladder (8).
4. An invasive investigation of the bladder (10).
8. Conveys urine from the kidney to the bladder (6).
9. Outer protective layer of the kidney (7).
10. Storage organ for urine (7).

Conditions

Below is a list of conditions that are associated with the renal system. Take some time and write notes about each of the conditions. You may make the notes taken from text books or other resources, for example, people you work with in a clinical area or you may make the notes as a result of people you have cared for. If you are making notes about people you have cared for you must ensure that you adhere to the rules of confidentiality.

Acute and chronic renal failure	
Pyelonephritis	

Glomerulonephritis	
Cystitis	
Urinary tract infection	
Renal calculi	
Carcinoma of the kidney	
Bladder tumours	

Answers

MCQs

1a; 2c; 3a; 4c; 5d; 6b; 7a; 8b; 9c; 10d

Crossword

Across:		**Down:**	
5.	Aldosterone	**1.**	Oliguria
6.	Filtration	**2.**	Renin
7.	Urethra	**3.**	Cystitis
11.	Adrenal	**4.**	Cystoscopy
12.	ADH	**8.**	Ureter
13.	Urea	**9.**	Capsule
14.	Nephron	**10.**	Bladder

15 The reproductive systems

Ian Peate

Contents

Introduction	*478*
The male reproductive system	**478**
The testes	479
Spermatogenesis	482
Sperm	483
The testes and hormonal influences	484
The scrotum	484
The penis	486
Epididymis	487
The vas deferens, ejaculatory duct and spermatic cord	488
The prostate gland	488
The female reproductive system	**488**
The ovaries	489
The ovarian cortex	490
Graafian follicles	490
Corpus luteum	490
The ovarian medulla	490
Oogenesis	490
The role of the female sex hormones	490
The menstrual cycle	492
The internal organs	**494**
The uterus	494
The fallopian tubes	495
The vagina	496
The cervix	496
The external genitalia	497
The breasts	497
Conclusion	*497*
Glossary	*498*
References	*501*
Activities	*502*

Test your knowledge

- In which aspect of the female reproductive system are the eggs stored and released?
- Why do the contents of the scrotal sac sit outside of the abdominal cavity?
- Describe the role and function of the hormone testosterone.
- Describe the role and function of the hormone oestrogen.

Fundamentals of Anatomy and Physiology for Student Nurses, First Edition. Edited by Ian Peate, Muralitharan Nair.

- At what stage of the menstrual cycle is a woman likely to fall pregnant?
- What is the average number of spermatozoa produced on a daily basis?
- Why is the uterus a very muscular organ?
- List four forms of contraception.
- List four sex hormones.
- What does spermatogenesis mean?

Learning outcomes

After reading this chapter you will be able to:

- Name and locate the male reproductive organs
- Name and locate the female reproductive organs
- Describe and understand the role and the functions of the male reproductive system
- Describe and understand the role and the functions of the female reproductive system
- Understand the role and functions of the various hormones associated with the male and female reproductive systems
- Discuss the phases of the menstrual cycle

Body map

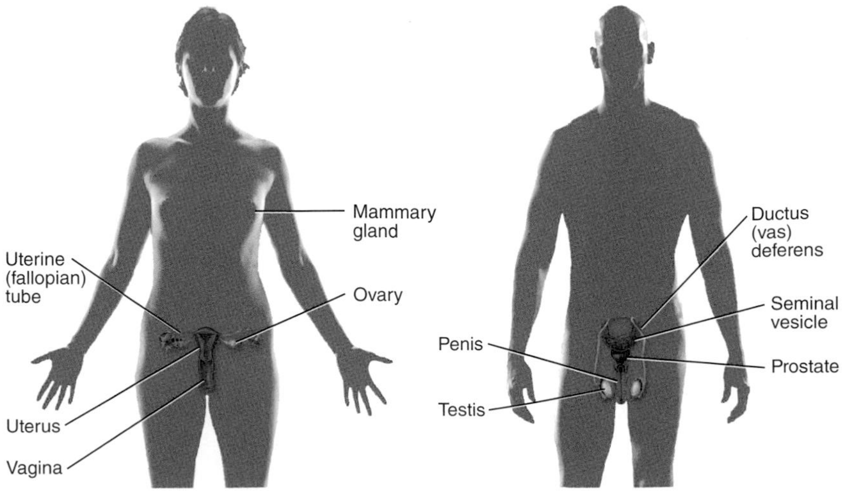
Mammary gland
Uterine (fallopian) tube
Ovary
Uterus
Vagina
Ductus (vas) deferens
Seminal vesicle
Penis
Prostate
Testis

Introduction

Reproduction is one of the most important and essential attributes of living organisms. Every sort of living organism multiplies to form new individuals of its own kind through reproduction. One generation of living organisms gives rise to the next generation as they reproduce. Reproduction is not critical to the life of any individual however; it is a function essential for the life of the species. In humans reproduction is sexual; this means that children are produced as a consequence of male and female mating (Stanfield 2011).

Fertilisation occurs inside the body of the female; the human sexual organs are dedicated to this. The reproductive systems work together to maintain homeostasis with other body systems.

Sexual reproduction usually concludes with the production of children for the continued existence of the species, as well as passing on hereditary characteristics from one generation to the next. It is the male and female reproductive systems that contribute to the events that lead to fertilisation. When this has occurred it is the female organs that take on the responsibility for developing the human and giving birth. The testes and ovaries produce sperm and ova as well as the hormones required for the development, upkeep and performance of the organs of reproduction and other organs and tissues.

This chapter provides an overview of the structure and functions of both male and female reproductive systems. The anatomical systems of the male and female, unlike any of the other anatomical systems in the body, differ in males and females (Tucker 2008).

The male and female reproductive systems consist of the reproductive organs. In the male the organs are the testes, accessory ducts, accessory glands and the penis. In the female the organs are the uterus, uterine tubes, ovaries, vagina and the vulva.

The male reproductive system

The male reproductive system is more obvious than the female reproductive system as most of the organs are outside of the body – but there are both internal and external structures. Male reproductive organs, working in tandem with other body systems, for example, the neuroendocrine system, make the hormones that are important in biological development and sexual behaviour, performance and actions. These organs also include and are central to the function of the urinary system. The male reproductive system is shown in Figure 15.1.

The male reproductive system has several functions:

- To produce, maintain and transport the sperm (the male reproductive cells) and the fluid semen
- To discharge sperm from the penis
- To produce and secrete the male sex hormones.

The major structures of the male reproductive system include the testes, the external genitalia, incorporating the penis, scrotum, reproductive tract and a number of ducts responsible for the transportation of the sperm from the testes to the penis and outside the body; there are also two seminal vesicles, bulbourethral glands and the prostate gland.

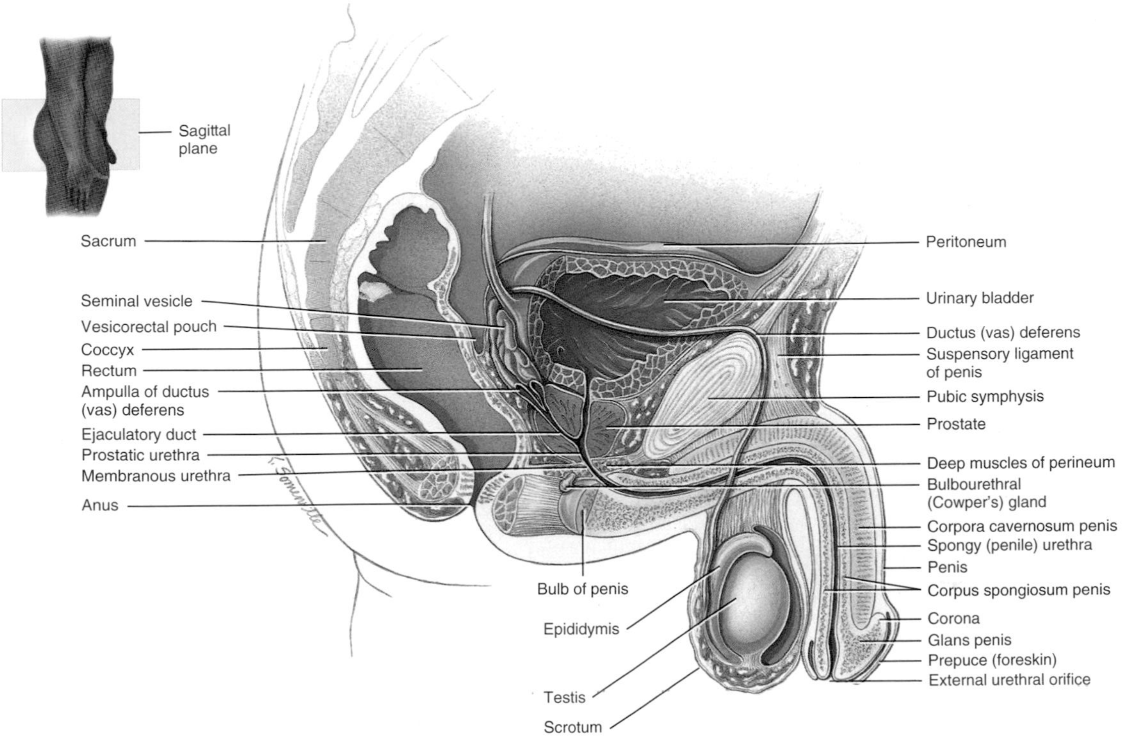
Sagittal plane
Sacrum
Seminal vesicle
Vesicorectal pouch
Coccyx
Rectum
Ampulla of ductus (vas) deferens
Ejaculatory duct
Prostatic urethra
Membranous urethra
Anus
Bulb of penis
Epididymis
Testis
Scrotum
Peritoneum
Urinary bladder
Ductus (vas) deferens
Suspensory ligament of penis
Pubic symphysis
Prostate
Deep muscles of perineum
Bulbourethral (Cowper's) gland
Corpora cavernosum penis
Spongy (penile) urethra
Penis
Corpus spongiosum penis
Corona
Glans penis
Prepuce (foreskin)
External urethral orifice

Figure 15.1 The male reproductive system (Tortora and Derrickson 2009)

The testes

In utero the testes develop within the abdominal cavity of the foetus and then move down through the inguinal canal into the scrotal sac. The testes are suspended in the scrotal sac, where they hang one on either side of the penis, and one often hangs lower than the other – this is a normal finding. For sperm to be viable it is essential that production is made at a temperature lower than the normal body temperature and for this reason the testes are external to the body.

The key functions of the testes are to:

- Produce sperm (spermatozoa)
- Produce the male sex hormones; testosterone is one of these hormones.

The testes are small, oval-shaped organs measuring approximately 5 cm long and 2.5 cm wide with a layer of serous fibrous connective tissue surrounding them. There are three layers that cover the testes:

- Tunica vaginalis
- Tunica albuginea
- Tunica vasculosa.

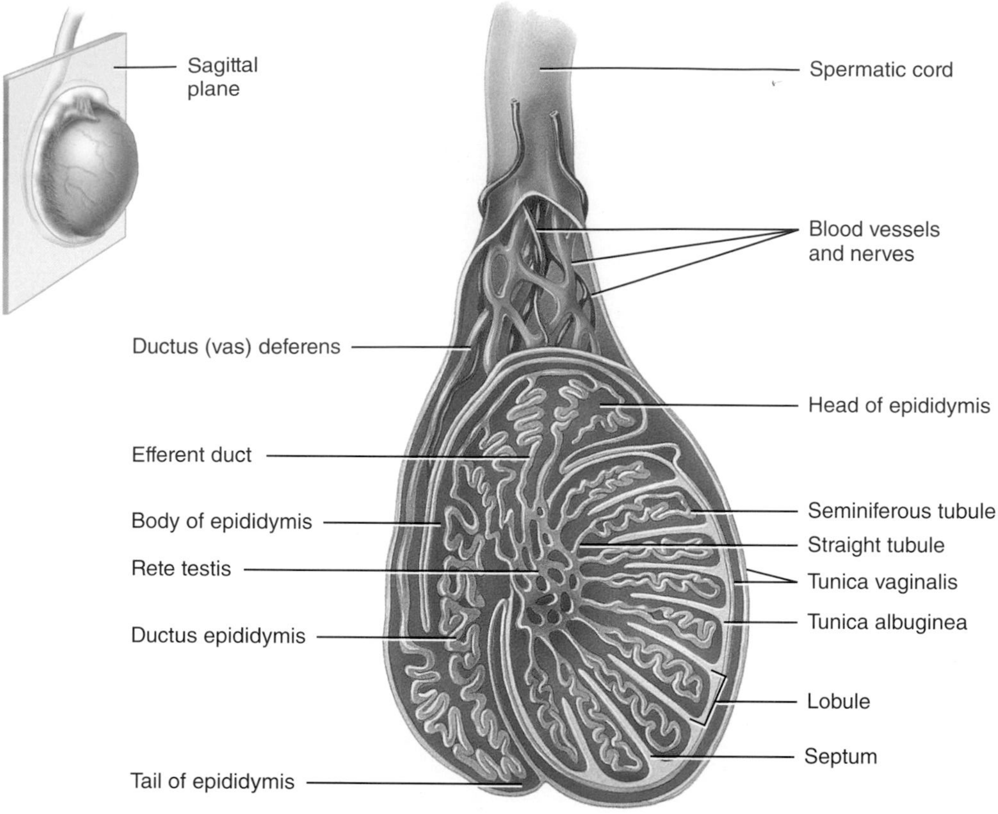
Sagittal plane
Spermatic cord
Blood vessels and nerves
Ductus (vas) deferens
Head of epididymis
Efferent duct
Seminiferous tubule
Body of epididymis
Straight tubule
Rete testis
Tunica vaginalis
Tunica albuginea
Ductus epididymis
Lobule
Septum
Tail of epididymis

Figure 15.2 A testicle demonstrating seminiferous tubules (Tortora and Derrickson 2009)

The testes are divided into approximately 250–300 compartments or lobules. Inside each compartment is a collection of tightly coiled hollow tubes called the seminiferous tubules; usually there are between one and four seminiferous tubules. Sperm is produced in these tubules in the form of sperm stem cells (see Figure 15.2). There are spaces between the tubules, and in these spaces is a cluster of cells called the Leydig cells; these cells synthesise and secrete the hormone testosterone as well as other androgens.

The seminiferous tubules have an outer and inner layer. The outer layer is composed of a smooth layer of muscle cells and an inner epithelial layer of cells known as the Sertoli cells. Sperm cells, in their various stages of development, are stored in the spaces between the Sertoli cells. Mature sperm are found in the lumen of the seminiferous tubules. The key function of the Sertoli cells is to nurture and control the developing sperm; these cells are sometimes referred to as the nurse or mother cells, and are sperm helper cells. The Sertoli cells have several functions, including phagocytosis, secretion of fluid that allows the sperm to develop and be transported, and providing a means whereby the developing sperm can be nourished.

Clinical considerations

The Tanner scale

The Tanner scale (Tanner 1966) can help to determine physical development in children, adolescents and adults. This scale can be used by nurses and other healthcare professionals to compare and measure physical characteristics based on development of external genitalia. In the male these include characteristics such as penis size, testicular growth and the appearance of pubic hair; there are five stages (see below).

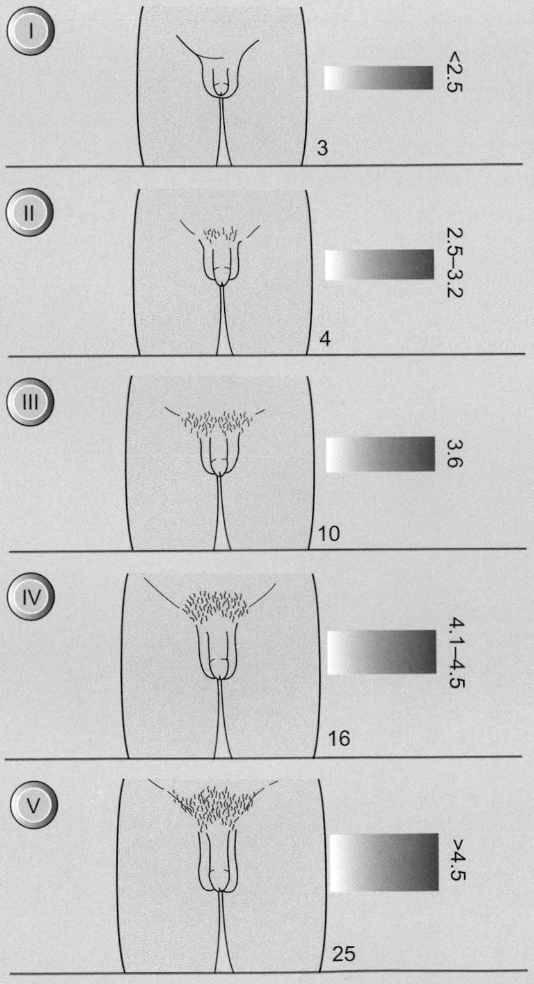
I
<2.5
3
II
2.5–3.2
4
III
3.6
10
IV
4.1–4.5
16
V
>4.5
25

It must be remembered that the Tanner scale is only one method of assessing physical development in the male. There are many other ways of determining whether developmental milestones have been met.

Spermatogenesis

Sperm production occurs in the seminiferous tubules of the testes and is termed spermatogenesis (see Figure 15.3). Spermatogenesis usually commences around puberty and persists for the rest of a man's life. A young healthy man will produce many hundred million sperm daily.

Spermatogenesis is a complex activity and it is estimated that it takes approximately 65–75 days to occur. Figure 15.3 highlights that spermatogenesis (the life of a single sperm) begins with the spermatogonia that contains the diploid (2n) number of chromosomes.

The spermatogonia divide continually as a result of mitotic division to produce cells that are called primary spermatocytes with 46 chromosomes. Some spermatogonia stay close to the basement membrane of the seminiferous tubule acting as a pool of cells ready to take part in future sperm production.

Division occurs again as a result of some spermatogonia breaking away from the basement membrane developing, differentiating and changing. Primary spermatocytes are produced with 46 chromosomes, then meiosis occurs with the emergence of secondary spermatocytes which now have 23 chromosomes each.

Spermatids are produced with the next stage of cell division; these then become spermatozoa or sperm cells; this is the final stage of spermatogenesis. The formed sperm cells have 23 chromosomes each, this is half the number required to begin human development. The other 23

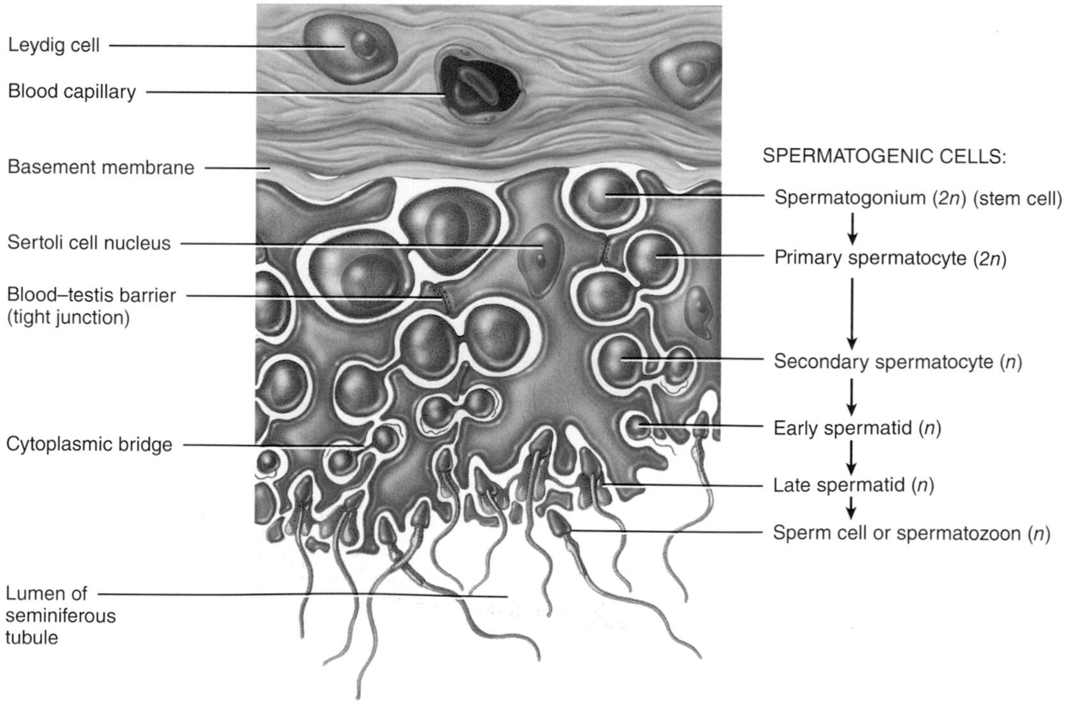
Leydig cell
Blood capillary
Basement membrane
Sertoli cell nucleus
Blood–testis barrier (tight junction)
Cytoplasmic bridge
Lumen of seminiferous tubule
SPERMATOGENIC CELLS:
Spermatogonium (2*n*) (stem cell)
Primary spermatocyte (2*n*)
Secondary spermatocyte (*n*)
Early spermatid (*n*)
Late spermatid (*n*)
Sperm cell or spermatozoon (*n*)

Figure 15.3 Stages of spermatogenesis (Tortora and Derrickson 2009)

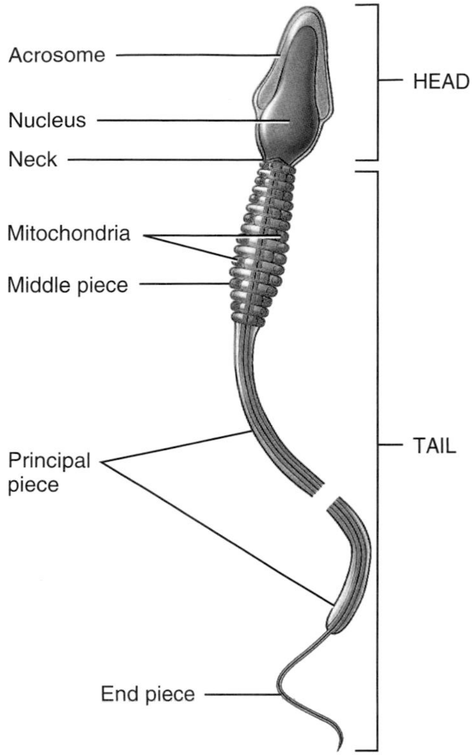
Acrosome
Nucleus
Neck
Mitochondria
Middle piece
Principal piece
End piece
HEAD
TAIL

Figure 15.4 Components of a sperm (Tortora and Derrickson 2009)

chromosomes are provided by the egg (ova) of a woman. When the sperm and ovum join, the result of conception (conceptus) will have the required 46 chromosomes.

The sperm are released from the Sertoli cells entering the lumen of the seminiferous tubules. The sperm are pushed along the various ducts located within the testes.

Sperm

Approximately 300 million sperm mature each day (Tortora and Derrickson 2010). Each sperm cell is usually equipped with a number of structures that allow it to penetrate the ova. The head of the sperm cell contains a fluid composed of enzymes which assists the sperm with its job of penetration which results in fertilisation (see Figure 15.4).

Once formed, the sperm travel up into the epididymis via a system of very small ducts known as the rete testes. These small ducts are C-shaped structures that unite from the back of the epididymis, which is positioned on the upper aspect of the testes. The crescent-shaped coiled epididymis is likened to a holding place that matures the sperm, taking on nutrients and growing for a number of weeks prior to travelling further. As the sperm mature further they develop motility.

Arrival at the vas deferens is the final stage for the sperm. The vas deferens emerges at the epididymis and twists up beyond the symphysis pubis and urinary bladder. There are two vas deferens, one arising from each testicle, and they join at the back of the bladder. Each vas deferens merges with one seminal vesicle; this seminal vesicle contains the fluids required at the time of ejaculation. The fluids from the vas deferens and seminal vesicles are released into the ejaculatory ducts, situated within the prostate gland.

The prostate gland also secretes fluids that are found in the ejaculate. The fluid secreted is a milky alkaline offering a friendly environment for sperm to survive, preparing them for survival in the acidity of the vagina. The ejaculatory ducts connect to the urethra where the sperm will be ejaculated during orgasm by sexual intercourse or masturbation. Once ejaculated it is unusual for sperm to survive longer than 48 hours within the female reproductive tract.

The testes and hormonal influences

The performance of the testes and their ability to function effectively are also under the influence of several hormones, the male sex hormones.

The male sex hormones are known as androgens. The majority of androgens are produced in the testes, although the adrenal cortex (located in the adrenal gland) is also responsible for producing a small amount. Testosterone is the main androgen that is produced by the testes; this hormone is essential for the growth and maintenance of the male sexual organs as well as the secondary sex characteristics (for example, pitch of voice, musculature and body hair) and for effective spermatogenesis. It also encourages metabolism, growth of muscles and bone, as well as sexual desire (libido).

There is a small amount of testosterone secreted by the testes *in utero*; after birth little testosterone is secreted until puberty. With the onset of puberty the hypothalamus intensifies its secretion of gonadotrophin-releasing hormone (GnRH). As GnRH is released this stimulates the anterior pituitary gland to release and increase its discharge of luteinising hormone (LH). These hormones work on the negative feedback system, controlling the secretion of testosterone in the blood and the production of sperm (spermatogenesis) (see Figure 15.5).

The scrotum

The scrotal sac is likened to a loose bag of skin that hangs between the thighs, anterior to the anus. This is a supporting structure suspended from the root of the penis. On the outside the scrotum usually appears as a single sac of skin separated into two portions by a ridge in the middle known as the raphe. From the inside the scrotum is divided into two sacs separated by a scrotal septum with a testicle in each (see Figure 15.6).

The scrotum helps to control the temperature of the testes. The most favourable temperature for sperm production is approximately 2 to 3 degrees below core body temperature; however too low a temperature can also impact on spermatogenesis.

Several mechanisms come into play when adjusting the position of the testes in the scrotum in relation to the body. When the temperature of the testes is too low (if the ambient temperature falls), the scrotum reacts in such a way that it contracts, bringing the testes up closer to the body. Conversely, if the testicular temperature is too high, then the scrotum relaxes; this enables the testes to descend moving them further away from the body, exposing surface area providing a faster dispersion of heat.

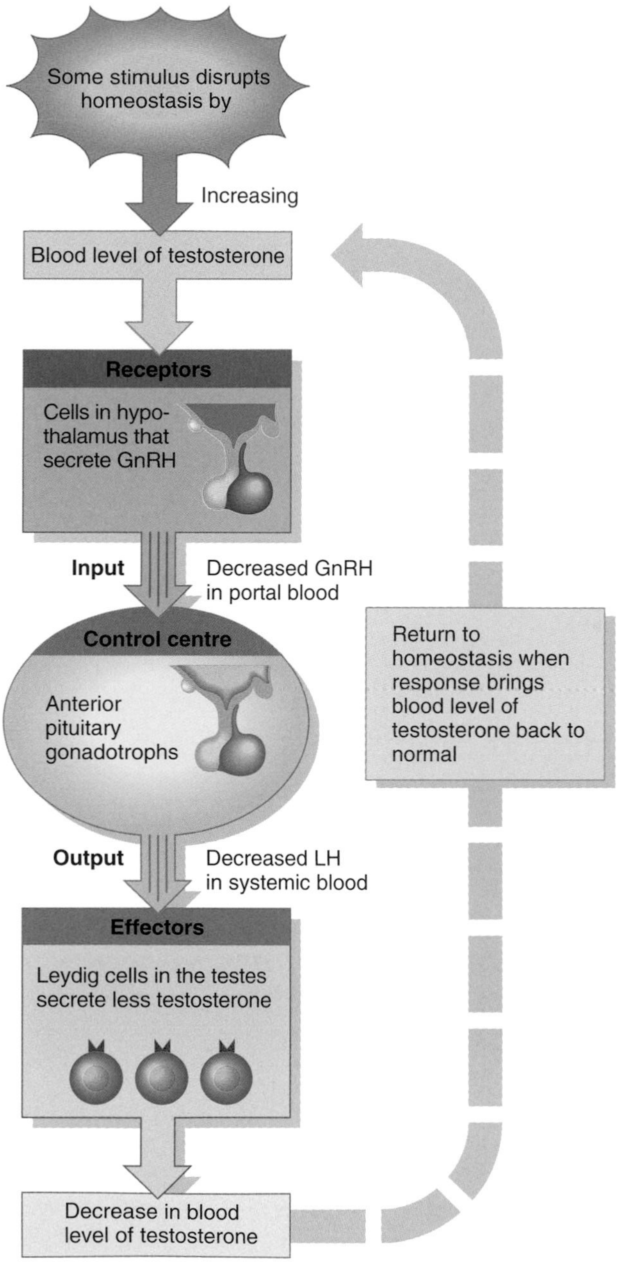
Some stimulus disrupts homeostasis by
Increasing
Blood level of testosterone
Receptors
Cells in hypothalamus that secrete GnRH
Input
Decreased GnRH in portal blood
Control centre
Anterior pituitary gonadotrophs
Output
Decreased LH in systemic blood
Effectors
Leydig cells in the testes secrete less testosterone
Decrease in blood level of testosterone
Return to homeostasis when response brings blood level of testosterone back to normal

Figure 15.5 Negative feedback system associated with the control of testosterone in the blood (Tortora and Derrickson 2009)

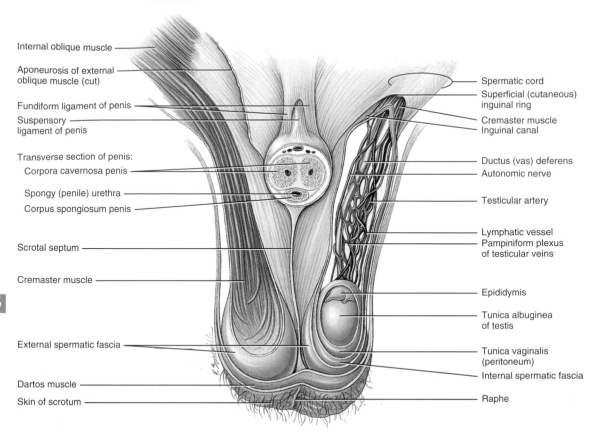

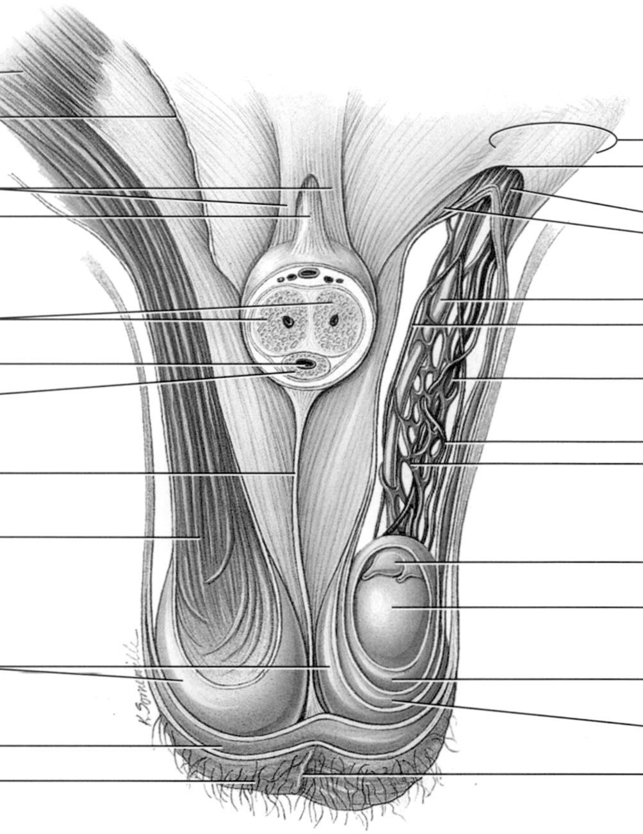
Internal oblique muscle
Aponeurosis of external oblique muscle (cut)
Fundiform ligament of penis
Suspensory ligament of penis
Transverse section of penis:
Corpora cavernosa penis
Spongy (penile) urethra
Corpus spongiosum penis
Scrotal septum
Cremaster muscle
External spermatic fascia
Dartos muscle
Skin of scrotum
Spermatic cord
Superficial (cutaneous) inguinal ring
Cremaster muscle
Inguinal canal
Ductus (vas) deferens
Autonomic nerve
Testicular artery
Lymphatic vessel
Pampiniform plexus of testicular veins
Epididymis
Tunica albuginea of testis
Tunica vaginalis (peritoneum)
Internal spermatic fascia
Raphe

Anterior view of scrotum and testes and transverse section of penis

Figure 15.6 The scrotum and testes (Tortora and Derrickson 2009)

The cremasteric reflex

The cremasteric reflex is a phenomenon that occurs when the body wants to lower or raise the position of the testes. The cremaster muscle is part of the spermatic cord and when this muscle contracts, the spermatic cord becomes shorter and the testicle is moved upwards toward the body. The result is that this will provide slightly more heat to ensure the most favourable testicular temperature. When cooling is needed, the cremaster muscle loosens up and the testicle is moved away from the heat of the body and cools down. It is the contraction of the dartos muscle (located in the subcutaneous layer of the scrotum) that causes the scrotum to appear wrinkled when it is tightened up.

The penis

The penis is the male copulatory organ. The penis encloses the urethra and is a highly vascular organ. This organ is the passageway for excretion of urine and the ejaculation of semen. The penis

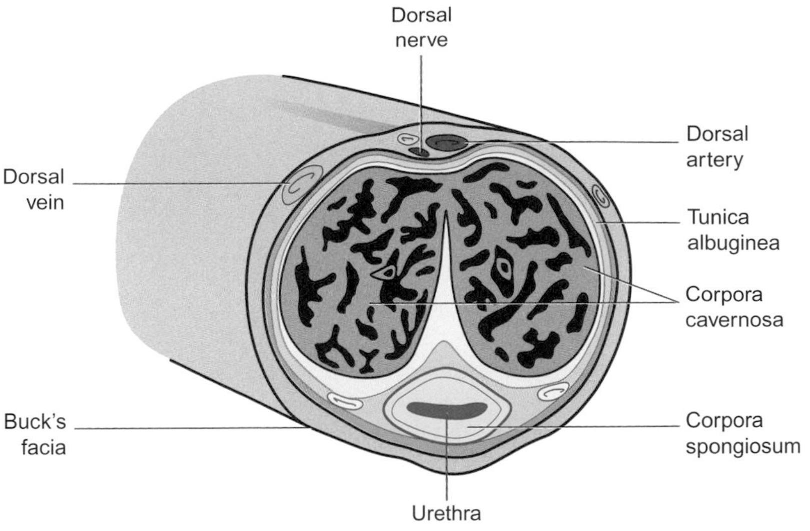
Dorsal
nerve
Dorsal
artery
Dorsal
vein
Tunica
albuginea
Corpora
cavernosa
Buck's
facia
Corpora
spongiosum
Urethra

Figure 15.7 The anatomy of the penis (Peate 2009a)

has a shaft and a tip known as the glans, and in the uncircumcised male this is covered by prepuce (also called the foreskin).

The penis is cylindrical in shape with three cylindrical masses of tissues. The three columns of erectile tissue in the penis are the shaft, the corpora cavernosa and the corpus spongiosum (see Figure 15.7). The attached portion of the penis is known as the root and the freer-moving aspect called the shaft or body.

The penis is usually flaccid and hangs down; during sexual excitation it becomes erect (an erection), swollen, engorged with blood, firmer and straighter. These changes occur as a result of blood filling the erectile tissue allowing the penis to penetrate the vagina and deposit sperm (ejaculation) as close to the site of fertilisation as possible.

Usually, when the penile compartments become filled with blood in response to a reaction or impulse that stimulates the parasympathetic nervous system arteriolar vasodilation erection takes place. The erection reflex can be prompted by sight, touch, pressure, sounds, smells or visions of a sexual encounter. When ejaculation has occurred the arterioles vasoconstrict and the penis becomes flaccid.

Epididymis

The epididymis (plural epididymides) is a comma-shaped duct. It lies on the posterior lateral aspect of the testes; the epididymis is approximately 4 cm long. The organ is composed of a highly coiled duct. This duct leads to a larger and more muscular tube called the vas deferens; the vas deferens enters the pelvic cavity.

Within the epididymis the sperm are matured further, being prepared to become more motile so that they can eventually fertilise the ova. It takes approximately 14 days for full maturation to occur (Jenkins *et al.* 2010). Sperm is stored in the epididymis and is released via peristaltic activity as the smooth muscle contracts during sexual arousal moving the sperm along the epididymis into the vas deferens. Sperm stored in the epididymis can stay there for several months; sperm not ejaculated are eventually reabsorbed.

The vas deferens, ejaculatory duct and spermatic cord

The vas deferens (plural vasa deferentia) or the ductus deferens as it enters the pelvic cavity is less convoluted than the epididymis, the diameter is also larger and the length of the vas deferens is about 45 cm (Tortora and Derrickson 2009). This tube contains ciliated epithelium with a thick muscle layer. The vas deferens runs from the anterior aspect of the scrotal sac as a pair of tubes via the inguinal canal into the pelvic cavity. Between the scrotal sac and the inguinal canal is a tube that the vas deferens runs through, this tube contains blood vessels and nerves and is called the spermatic cord (Colbert *et al.* 2007).

The vas deferens then joins the seminal vesicle to become the ejaculatory duct. This duct passes into the prostate gland discharging its fluid into the urethra.

The prostate gland

Laws (2006) notes that the function of the prostate gland is not well understood. The prostate is a single doughnut-shaped gland, measuring about 4 cm. It goes around the urethra under the urinary bladder and is made of 20–30 glands enclosed in smooth muscle (Marieb 2010).

The prostate consists of three distinct zones:

- The central zone
- The peripheral zone
- The transition zone.

Secretions of the prostate gland compose approximately one-third of the volume of the semen; the fluid helps sperm motility and maintain viability. Prostatic fluid is slightly acidic in nature (pH 6.5). These secretions enter the urethra via a number of ducts during ejaculation.

The female reproductive system

As with the male reproductive organs the female reproductive organs, along with the neuroendocrine system, manufacture hormones that are essential in biological development and sexual activity. The primary genitalia in the female are the ovaries, the secondary genitalia are the fallopian tubes, uterus and vagina; the vulva is the external genitalia. There are aspects of the female reproductive organs that are enclosed and integral to the function of the urinary system.

LeMone and Burke (2009) point out that the female reproductive system consists of the external genitalia: mons pubis, labia, clitoris and vaginal and urethral openings. The internal organs are: the vagina, cervix, uterus, fallopian tubes and ovaries.

The breasts are also a part of a women's reproductive organs. In women, the urethra and urinary meatus are not a part of the reproductive organs; nevertheless they are very close in proximity and as such health problems that affect one often affect the other. Figure 15.8 demonstrates the location and function of the female reproductive organs.

The female reproductive system is designed to produce eggs, receive the penis during intercourse and the sperm ejaculated, store, contain and nourish the foetus and feed the newborn after birth with breast milk. Usually, each month, a woman's body (from puberty to menopause)

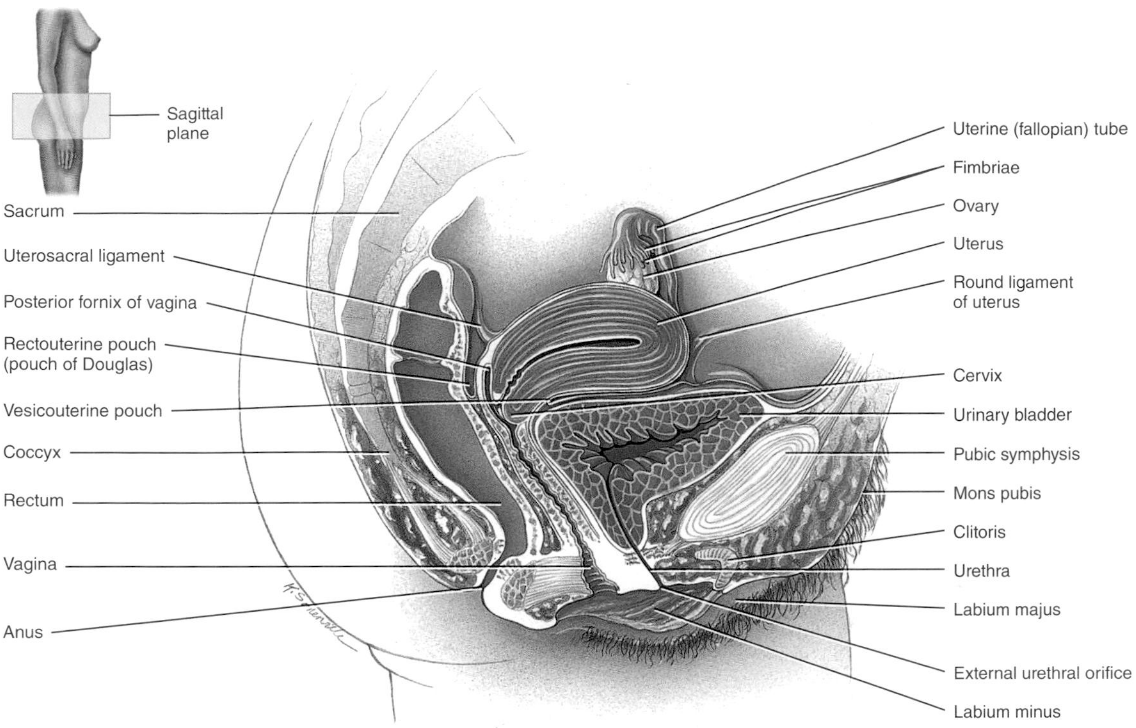
Sagittal plane
Sacrum
Uterosacral ligament
Posterior fornix of vagina
Rectouterine pouch (pouch of Douglas)
Vesicouterine pouch
Coccyx
Rectum
Vagina
Anus
Uterine (fallopian) tube
Fimbriae
Ovary
Uterus
Round ligament of uterus
Cervix
Urinary bladder
Pubic symphysis
Mons pubis
Clitoris
Urethra
Labium majus
External urethral orifice
Labium minus

Figure 15.8 The female reproductive system (Tortora and Derrickson 2009)

prepares itself to become pregnant. If pregnancy does not happen a menstrual period occurs and the cycle recommences.

The ovaries

The ovaries are flat, almond-shaped glands situated on each side of the uterus beneath the ends of the fallopian tubes. These glands in the female are compared to the testes in the male; the ovaries are internal organs. A collection of ligaments holds them in position, attaching the ovaries to the uterus; they are also attached to the broad ligament, which attaches them to the pelvic wall. The ovaries provide a space of storage for the female germ cells and produce the female hormones oestrogen and progesterone. A woman's total number of ova is present at her birth; when a girl reaches puberty she usually ovulates each month.

The ovary contains a number of small structures, called ovarian follicles. Each follicle contains an immature ovum, called an oocyte. Monthly, follicles are stimulated by two hormones – the follicle-stimulating hormone (FSH) and luteinising hormone (LH); these hormones stimulate the follicles to mature. The developing follicles are enclosed in layers of follicle cells, the mature follicles are called graafian follicles.

The ovarian cortex

This region lies deep and close to the tunica albuginea. The cortex contains the ovarian follicles surrounded by dense irregular connective tissue. These follicles contain oocytes in different stages of development as well as a number of cells that feed the developing oocyte. As the follicle grows it secretes oestrogen.

Graafian follicles

The graafian follicles manufacture oestrogen, which stimulates the growth of endometrium. Every month, one or two of the mature follicles (the graafian follicles) release an oocyte in what is called ovulation. The large ruptured follicle becomes a new structure called the corpus luteum composed of the remnants of a mature follicle.

Corpus luteum

The corpus luteum produces two hormones, oestrogen and progesterone, with the aim of supporting the endometrium until conception takes place or the cycle begins again. The corpus luteum gradually disintegrates and a scar is left on the outside of the ovary; this is called the corpus albicans.

The outer aspect of the ovary is enveloped in a fibrous capsule known as the tunica albuginea, and is composed of cuboidal epithelium. The inner aspect of the ovary is divided into parts.

The ovarian medulla

The ovarian medulla contains blood vessels, nerves and lymphatic tissues surrounded by loose connective tissue. There is an unclear border between the ovarian cortex and medulla.

Figure 15.9 demonstrates the ovary during the development of an oocyte.

Oogenesis

The term oogenesis relates to the development of relatively undifferentiated germ cells called oogonia (singular oogonium). Oogonia are fixed in number – between 2 and 4 million diploid (2n) stem cells (Stanfield 2011) before birth, during foetal development, whereas spermatogonia are continuously regenerated at puberty. All ova are ultimately derived from these clones. These oogonia develop into larger primary oocytes, the meiotic phase is not completed until the girl reaches puberty (see Figure 15.10).

Every month from puberty until menopause FSH and LH (two hormones) are released by the anterior aspect of the pituitary gland and stimulate the primordial follicles, however, usually only one will reach the maturity required for ovulation.

The role of the female sex hormones

Oestrogens, progesterone and androgens are produced by the ovaries in a recurring pattern. Although oestrogens are secreted throughout the menstrual cycle, they are at a higher level during this particular stage of the cycle.

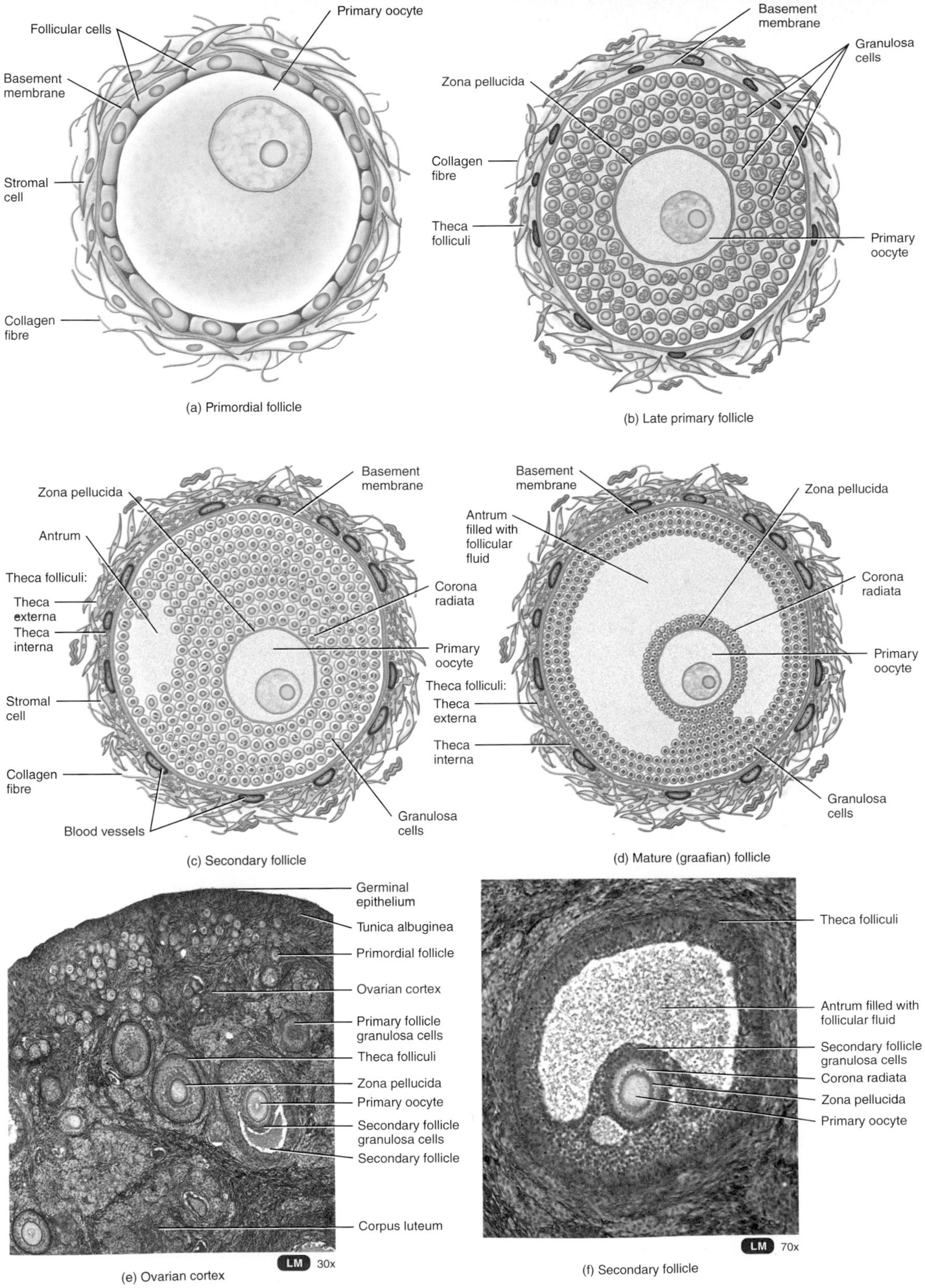
Follicular cells
Primary oocyte
Basement membrane
Stromal cell
Collagen fibre
(a) Primordial follicle
Basement membrane
Granulosa cells
Zona pellucida
Collagen fibre
Theca folliculi
Primary oocyte
(b) Late primary follicle
Zona pellucida
Basement membrane
Antrum
Theca folliculi:
Theca externa
Theca interna
Corona radiata
Primary oocyte
Stromal cell
Collagen fibre
Blood vessels
Granulosa cells
(c) Secondary follicle
Basement membrane
Zona pellucida
Antrum filled with follicular fluid
Corona radiata
Primary oocyte
Theca folliculi:
Theca externa
Theca interna
Granulosa cells
(d) Mature (graafian) follicle
Germinal epithelium
Tunica albuginea
Primordial follicle
Ovarian cortex
Primary follicle granulosa cells
Theca folliculi
Zona pellucida
Primary oocyte
Secondary follicle granulosa cells
Secondary follicle
Corpus luteum
LM 30x
(e) Ovarian cortex
Theca folliculi
Antrum filled with follicular fluid
Secondary follicle granulosa cells
Corona radiata
Zona pellucida
Primary oocyte
LM 70x
(f) Secondary follicle

Figure 15.9 The developmental sequences associated with maturation of an ovum (Tortora and Derrickson 2009)

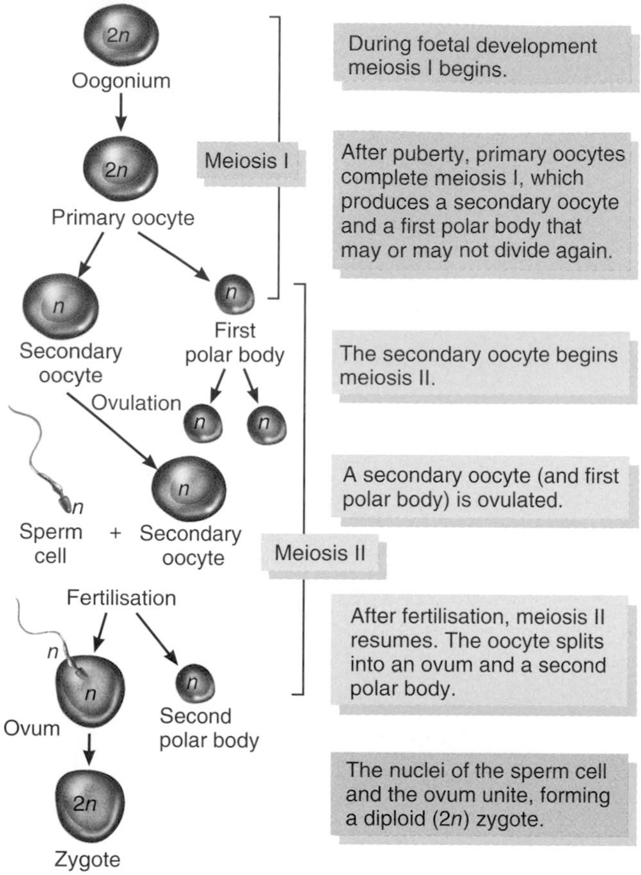

2n
Oogonium
2n
Primary oocyte
Meiosis I
n
Secondary oocyte
n
First polar body
Ovulation
n
n
n
Sperm cell
+
Secondary oocyte
Meiosis II
Fertilisation
n
n
Ovum
n
Second polar body
2n
Zygote
During foetal development meiosis I begins.
After puberty, primary oocytes complete meiosis I, which produces a secondary oocyte and a first polar body that may or may not divide again.
The secondary oocyte begins meiosis II.
A secondary oocyte (and first polar body) is ovulated.
After fertilisation, meiosis II resumes. The oocyte splits into an ovum and a second polar body.
The nuclei of the sperm cell and the ovum unite, forming a diploid (2n) zygote.

Figure 15.10 Oogenesis and follicular development (Tortora and Derrickson 2009)

For the development and maintenance of secondary sex characteristics oestrogens are essential; and, in combination with a number of other hormones, they stimulate the female reproductive organ to prepare for growth of a foetus (LeMone and Burke 2009). Oestrogens have a key role to play in the structure of the skin and blood vessels. They also help to reduce the rate of bone resorption (bone breakdown), enhance increased high-density lipoproteins, decrease cholesterol levels and increase blood clotting.

The menstrual cycle

The endometrium of the uterus responds to changes in oestrogen and progesterone during the ovarian cycle to prepare for implantation of the fertilised embryo. The endometrium is receptive to implantation of the embryo for only a brief period each month, coinciding with the time when the embryo would normally reach the uterus from the uterine tube (usually 7 days).

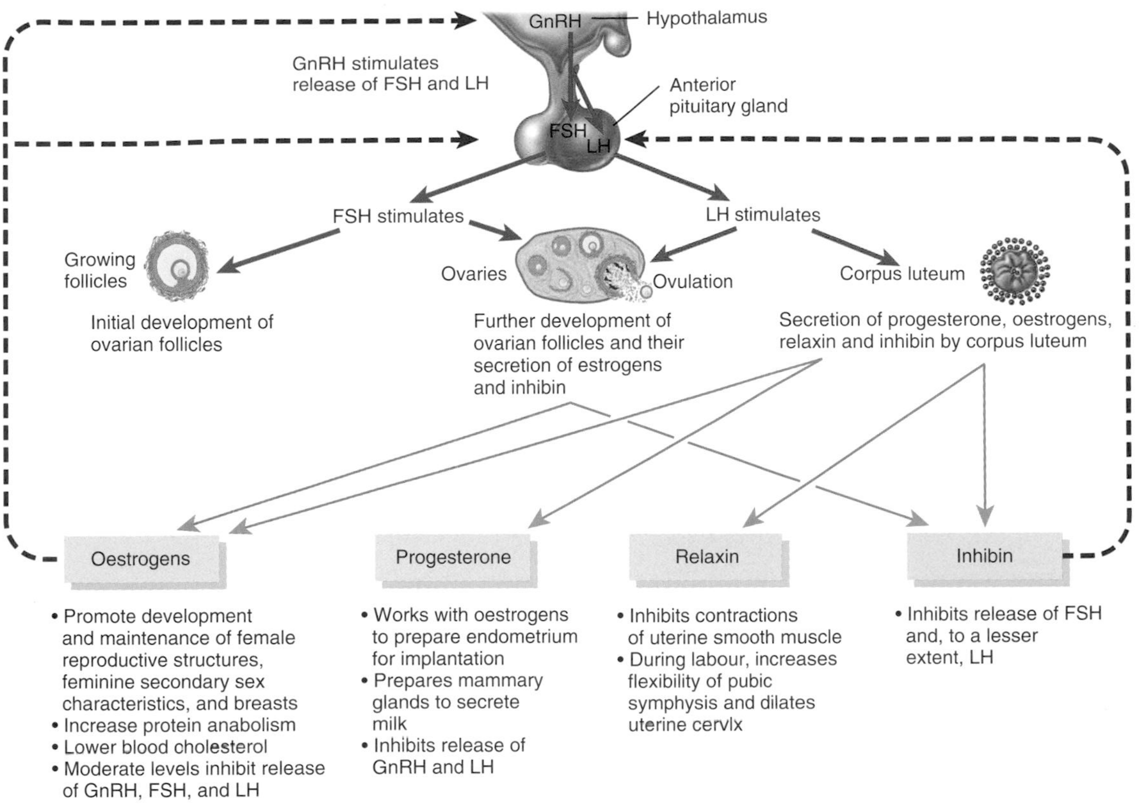
GnRH
Hypothalamus
GnRH stimulates release of FSH and LH
Anterior pituitary gland
FSH
LH
FSH stimulates
LH stimulates
Growing follicles
Ovaries
Ovulation
Corpus luteum
Initial development of ovarian follicles
Further development of ovarian follicles and their secretion of estrogens and inhibin
Secretion of progesterone, oestrogens, relaxin and inhibin by corpus luteum
Oestrogens
Progesterone
Relaxin
Inhibin
• Promote development and maintenance of female reproductive structures, feminine secondary sex characteristics, and breasts
• Increase protein anabolism
• Lower blood cholesterol
• Moderate levels inhibit release of GnRH, FSH, and LH
• Works with oestrogens to prepare endometrium for implantation
• Prepares mammary glands to secrete milk
• Inhibits release of GnRH and LH
• Inhibits contractions of uterine smooth muscle
• During labour, increases flexibility of pubic symphysis and dilates uterine cervix
• Inhibits release of FSH and, to a lesser extent, LH

Figure 15.11 The ovarian and uterine cycles (Tortora and Derrickson 2009)

The menstrual cycle starts with the menstrual phase and lasts from days 1 to 5. The inner endometrial layer (also called the functionalis) separates and this is then released as menstrual fluid lasting for 3–5 days. As the growing follicle begins to produce the hormone oestrogen (days 6 to 14), the next stage, the proliferative phase, commences. As a result of this the functionalis layer repairs and thickens while at the same time spiral arteries multiply and tubular glands form (LeMone and Burke 2009). Cervical mucus alters, becoming a thin, crystalline substance, forming channels enabling the sperm to travel up into the uterus.

The final phase, lasting from days 14 to 28, is the secretory phase. As the corpus luteum produces progesterone, the rising levels act on the endometrium, causing increased vascularity, changing the inner layer to secretory mucosa, stimulating the secretion of glycogen into the uterine cavity and causing the cervical mucus again to become thick and block the internal os (an os is a mouth or mouth-like opening). If fertilisation does not occur, hormone levels fall. Spasm of the spiral arteries causes hypoxia (lack of oxygen) of the endometrial cells, which begin to degenerate and slough off. As with the ovarian cycle, the process begins again with the sloughing of the functionalis layer. Figure 15.11 demonstrates the ovarian and uterine cycles.

Clinical considerations

Insertion of pessaries

Medicines that are inserted into the vagina are known as pessaries; these medicines, like all other medicines, must be prescribed. The medication is slowly released into the vagina at body temperature.

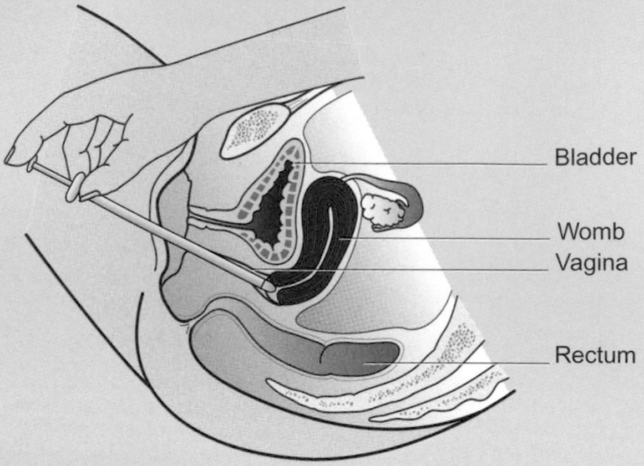
Bladder
Womb
Vagina
Rectum

Pessaries are hard, bullet-shaped preparations, and have been designed in such a way that insertion into the vagina is easy. Pessaries can be introduced with the fingers or with the use of a manufacturer's applicator. As the pessary dissolves (in response to body temperature) the medication can leak from its position in the vagina; because of this you may wish to encourage the woman to put it in place at night prior to going to bed. If the pessary is inserted during the day then the woman may be advised to use a sanitary towel to avoid any staining or soiling of her clothing.

The internal organs

The internal organs of the female reproductive system are the vagina, cervix, uterus, fallopian tubes and ovaries. The ovaries (discussed earlier) are the primary reproductive organs in women as well as producing female sex hormones. The vagina, uterus and fallopian tubes act as an accessory channel for the ovaries and a growing foetus.

The uterus

This hollow organ is also known as the womb. It is a very muscular organ lying in the pelvic cavity posterior and superior to the urinary bladder, it lies anterior to the rectum (Figure 15.12 outlines the uterus and associated structures).

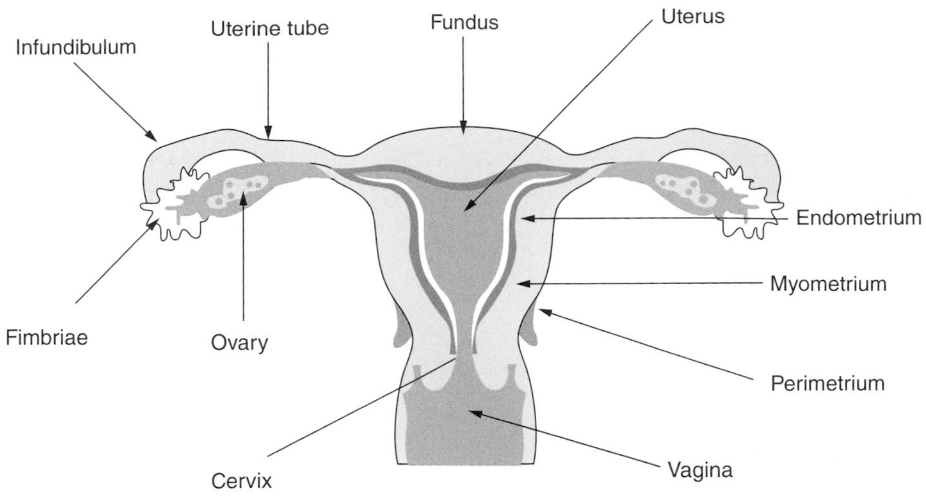
Infundibulum
Uterine tube
Fundus
Uterus
Endometrium
Myometrium
Perimetrium
Fimbriae
Ovary
Cervix
Vagina

Figure 15.12 The uterus and associated structures (Nair and Peate 2009)

The uterus is approximately 7.5 cm long. There are three main parts associated with uterus:

- The fundus is a thick muscular region situated above the fallopian tubes
- The body is the main portion of the uterus joined to the cervix by the isthmus
- The cervix is the narrowest part of the uterus opening out into the vagina.

As well as having three aspects or parts the uterus also has three layers. The perimetrium is the outer serous layer merging with the peritoneum. The middle layer is the myometrium and comprises most of the uterine wall, there are a number of muscle fibres in this layer running in a number of various directions, this arrangement allows contractions to occur during menstruation or childbirth and an increase in size as the foetus grows. The endometrium, the outermost layer, lines the uterus and this layer is shed during menstruation (the three layers are summarised in Table 15.1).

The fallopian tubes

The paired fallopian tubes (also called the salpinges) are delicate, thin, cylindrical structures approximately 8–14 cm long (Marieb 2010). They are affixed to the uterus on one end and are supported by the broad ligaments. The lateral ends of the fallopian tubes are open and made of projections called fimbriae that drape over the ovary. The fimbriae pick up the ovum after it is discharged from the ovary.

The fallopian tubes are composed of smooth muscle and are lined with ciliated, mucus-producing epithelial cells. The actions of the cilia and contractions of the smooth muscle transport the ovum along the tubes onwards to the uterus. It is in the outer portion of the fallopian tube where the fertilisation of the ovum by the sperm usually occurs.

The term adnex is used collectively when discussing the fallopian tubes, ovaries and supporting tissues.

Table 15.1 The layers of the uterus

Layer	Comments
The perimetrium	A serous membrane enveloping the uterus, this is the outer layer; it provides supports to the uterus located within the pelvis. This may also be known the parietal peritoneum
The myometrium	This is the middle layer and is composed of smooth muscle. During pregnancy and childbirth the uterus is required to stretch and the muscular layer allows this to happen. The muscle will contract during labour and postnatally this muscular layer contracts forcefully to force out the placenta. The contractions also help to control potential blood loss after birth.
The endometrium	The inner layer of the uterus with a mucous lining. The exterior is continuous with the vagina and the fallopian tubes. When the woman is menstruating the layers of the endometrium are shed and they slough away from the inner layer, this is the menstrual period and occurs as a result of the hormonal changes taking place. The endometrium thickens during the menstrual period and it becomes rich with blood vessels and glandular tissue until the next period occurs and the cycle happens again

The vagina

The vagina is a tubular, fibromuscular structure approximately 8–10 cm in length (Jenkins *et al.* 2011). It is the receptacle for the penis during sexual intercourse, an organ of sexual response, the canal that allows the menstrual flow to leave the body and the passage for the birth of the child. The vagina is situated posterior to the urinary bladder and urethra, it is anterior to the rectum. The upper element houses the uterine cervix in an area called the fornix. The vaginal walls are made of membranous folds of tissue known as rugae. These membranes are made up of mucous-secreting stratified squamous epithelial cells.

Usually the walls of the vagina are moist and have a pH ranging from 3.8 to 4.2. This pH inhibits the growth of bacteria (it is bacteriostatic) and is maintained by the action of the hormone oestrogen and healthy vaginal micro-organisms (the normal vaginal flora). Oestrogen causes the growth of vaginal mucosal cells, making them thicken and develop and increase glycogen content. The glycogen is fermented to lactic acid by lactobacilli (these are organisms that produce lactic acid) that usually live in the vagina causing slight acidifying of the vaginal fluid (LeMone and Burke 2009).

The cervix

Into the vagina projects the cervix and this forms a pathway between the uterus and the vagina. The uterine opening of the cervix is known as the internal os and the vaginal opening is called the external os. The space between these openings, the endocervical canal, acts as a conduit for the discharge of menstrual fluid, the opening for sperm and delivery of the infant during birth.

The cervix is a rigid structure, protected by mucus that alters consistency and quantity for the duration of the menstrual cycle and during pregnancy.

The external genitalia

Collectively, the external genitalia are known as the vulva. They include the mons pubis, labia, clitoris, vaginal and urethral openings, and glands (LeMone and Burke 2009).

The mons pubis is a pad of adipose tissue covered with skin. It lies anteriorly to the symphysis pubis, cushioning it. After puberty, the mons is covered with coarse pubic hair.

The labia are divided into two structures. The labia majora which are folds of skin and an abundance of adipose tissue covered with pubic hair are outermost; they begin at the base of the mons pubis and terminate at the anus. The labia minora, situated between the clitoris and the base of the vagina, are enclosed by the labia majora. They are made of skin, adipose tissue and some erectile tissues with a number of sebaceous glands. They are usually light pink and are devoid of pubic hair.

The clitoris is composed of two small erectile bodies, the corposa cavernosa, and several nerves and blood vessels. The glans clitoris is the exposed portion of the clitoris and is likened to the glans penis in the male. This aspect of the external genitalia is capable of enlargement; it has a role to play in sexual excitement in the woman.

The breasts

The breasts are dome-shaped protrusions differing in size between individuals; they are also sometimes called the mammary glands, these are external accessory sexual organs in the female. There are several milk-producing glands located within the breast. Milk production is controlled by a hormone called prolactin.

The breasts are located between the third and seventh ribs on the anterior aspect chest wall. The breasts are supported by the pectoral muscles and are provided with a rich supply of nerves, blood vessels and lymph (see Figure 15.13). A pigmented area known as the areola is situated a little below the centre of each breast and contains glands that secrete sebum, a thick substance composed of fat and cell debris (sebaceous glands) and a nipple. The nipple is usually protruding, becoming erect in response to cold and stimulation.

The breasts are made of adipose (fat) tissue, fibrous connective tissue and glandular tissue. There are bands of fibrous tissue that support the breast and extend from the outer breast tissue to the nipple, dividing the breast into 15 to 25 lobes. The lobe is comprised of alveolar glands joined by ducts that open out onto the nipple.

Conclusion

The male and female reproductive systems are complex. All living things reproduce; fundamentally, organisms make more organisms akin to themselves. Without these reproductive systems human life would end; they are essential for life. These systems have a number of functions, for example, the function of reproduction producing and transporting sex cells. In the human reproductive process, two types of sex cells, or gametes, are required. The male gamete, or sperm, and the female gamete, the egg or ovum, meet in the female's reproductive system to begin the creation of a new individual. Anatomical and physiological processes are required to ensure this marvel works effectively.

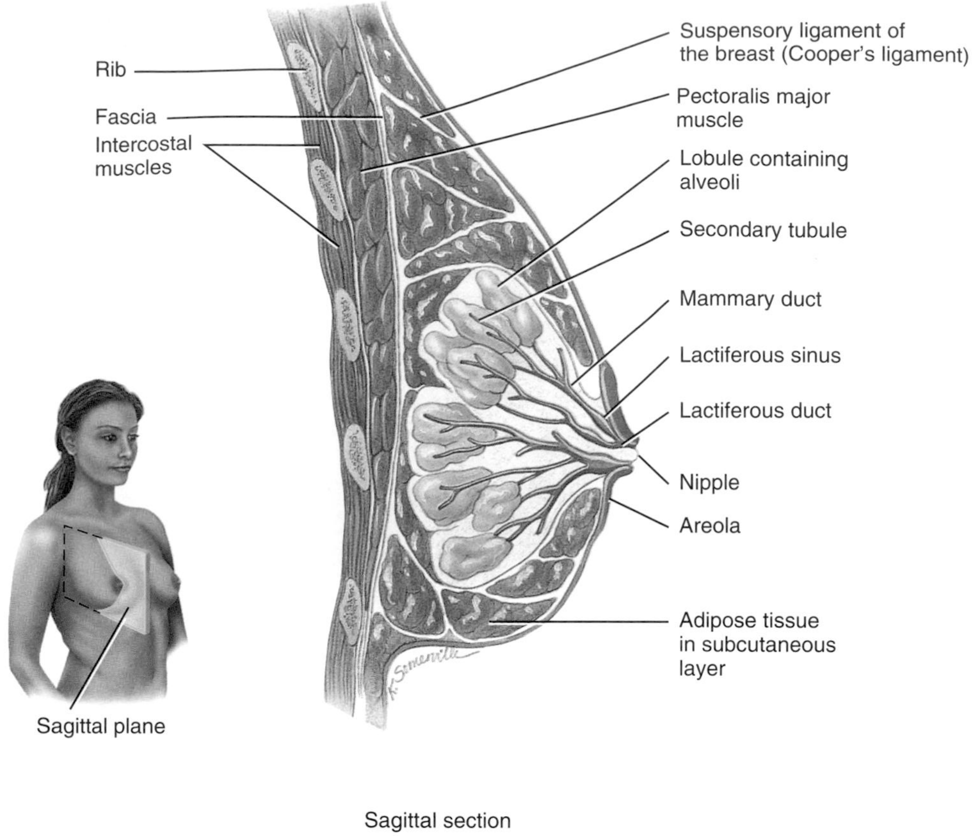
Rib
Fascia
Intercostal muscles
Suspensory ligament of the breast (Cooper's ligament)
Pectoralis major muscle
Lobule containing alveoli
Secondary tubule
Mammary duct
Lactiferous sinus
Lactiferous duct
Nipple
Areola
Adipose tissue in subcutaneous layer
Sagittal plane
Sagittal section

Figure 15.13 The breast (Tortora and Derrickson 2009)

Sexual reproduction, the process of producing offspring for the survival of the species and passing on hereditary traits from one generation to the next, is the key function of the male and reproductive systems. The male and female reproductive systems contribute to the events leading to fertilisation. The female organs take on responsibility for the developing human, birth and nourishment. The systems also provide pleasure, sexual pleasure and sexual excitement. For a number of people this is an important aspect of their being.

Glossary

Adrenal cortex: The outer portion of an adrenal gland.

Androgens: Masculinising male sex hormones produced by the testes in the male and the adrenal cortex in both sexes.

Anterior: Near to the front.

Bilateral: Related to both sides of the body.

Broad ligament: A double fold of parietal peritoneum attaching the uterus to the side of the pelvic cavity.

Canal: A channel or passageway, a narrow tube.

Connective tissue: The most prominent type of tissue in the body; this tissue provides support.

Corpus albicans: A whitish fibrous patch in the ovary formed after the corpus luteum regresses.

Corpus luteum: A yellowish body found in the ovary when a follicle has discharged its secondary oocyte.

Distal: Further away from the attachment of a limb to the trunk of the body.

Endometrium: The mucous membrane lining the uterus.

Foetus: The developing organism *in utero*.

Fimbriae: Finger-like structures found at the end of the fallopian tubes.

Follicle: A secretory sac or cavity containing a group of cells that contains a developing oocyte in the ovary.

Follicle stimulating hormone: Secreted by the anterior pituitary gland initiates the development of an ova.

Gamete: A male or female sex cell.

Glans penis: The enlarged region at the end of the penis.

Gonad: A gland that produces hormones and gametes – in men the testes; in females the ovaries.

Gonadatrophic hormone: Anterior pituitary hormone affecting the gonads.

Haploid: Having half the number of chromosomes.

Hormone: A secretion of endocrine cells that alters the physiological activity of target cells.

Human chorionic gonadotrophin: A hormone produced by the developing placenta.

Inferior: Away from the head or towards the lower part of a structure.

Inguinal canal: Passage in the lower abdominal wall in the male.

Inhibin: A hormone secreted by the gonads inhibiting the release of FSH by the anterior pituitary.

In utero: Within the uterus.

Isthmus: A narrow strip of tissue or a narrow passage connecting to bigger parts.

Lateral: Furthest from the midline of the body.

Leygid cell: A type of cell that secretes testosterone.

Ligament: Dense, regular connective tissue.

Luteinising hormone: A hormone secreted by the anterior pituitary stimulates ovulation and readies glands in the breast to produce milk; stimulates testosterone secretion in the testes.

Meatus: A passage or opening.

Medial: Near the midline of the body.

Meiosis: A kind of cell division occurring during the production of gametes.

Menopause: The termination of the menstrual cycle.

Myometrium: The smooth muscle layer of the uterus.

Oestrogens: Feminising sex hormones produced by the ovaries.

Oocyte: An immature egg cell.

Oogenesis: Formation and development of the female gametes.

Ovarian cycle: A series of events in the ovaries that occur during and after the maturation of the oocyte.

Ovarian follicle: A general name for immature oocytes.

Ovary: The female gonad.

Ovulation: The rupture of a mature graafian follicle with discharge of a secondary oocyte after penetration by sperm.

Ovum: The female egg cell.

Penis: The organ of urination and copulation.

Peristalsis: Consecutive muscular contractions along the walls of a hollow muscular organ.

pH: A measure of acidity and alkalinity.

Phagocytosis: The process by which phagocytes ingest and destroy microbes, cell debris and other foreign matter.

Placenta: An organ attached to the lining of the uterus during pregnancy.

Progesterone: A female sex hormone produced by the ovaries.

Prolactin: A hormone secreted by the anterior pituitary that initiates and maintains milk production.

Rete: The network of ducts in the testes.

Scrotum: The skin-covered pouch containing the testes.

Semen: Fluid discharged by ejaculation.

Spermatogenesis: The maturation of spermatids into sperm.

Testes: The male gonads.

Testosterone: Male sex hormone.

Urethra: The tube from the urinary bladder to the exterior of the body conveys urine in females and urine and semen in males.

Uterus: Hollow muscular organ in the female, also called the womb.

Vagina: A muscular tubular organ in the female leading from the uterus to the vestibule.

Vas deferens: The main secretory duct of the testicle, through which semen is carried from the epididymis to the prostatic urethra, where it ends as the ejaculatory duct.

Vulva: The female external genitalia.

References

Colbert, B.J., Ankney, J. and Lee, K.T. (2007) *Anatomy and Physiology for Health Professionals. An Interactive Journey.* Upper Saddle River, NJ: Pearson.

Jenkins, G.W., Kemnitz, C.P. and Tortora, G.J. (2010) *Anatomy and Physiology. From Science to Life*, 2nd edn. Hoboken, NJ: John Wiley & Sons.

Laws, T. (2006) *A Handbook of Men's Health*. Edinburgh: Elsevier.

LeMone, P. and Burke, K. (2009) *Medical–Surgical Nursing. Critical Thinking in Client Care*, 4th edn. Upper Saddle River, NJ: Pearson.

Marieb, E.N. (2010) *Human Anatomy and Physiology*, 8th edn. San Francisco: Pearson Benjamin Cummings.

Nair, M. and Peate, I. (2009) *Fundamentals of Applied Pathophysiology: An Essential Guide for Nursing Students.* Oxford: Wiley-Blackwell.

Peate, I. (2009a) *Men's Health.* Oxford: Wiley-Blackwell.

Peate, I. (2009b) Principles of medicines management. In: Lawson, L. and Peate, I. (eds) *Essential Nursing Care. A Workbook for Clinical Practice*, Ch 2, pp 31–77. Chichester: Wiley-Blackwell.

Stanfield, C.L. (2011) *Principles of Human Physiology*, 4th edn. Boston, MA: Pearson.

Tanner, J.M. (1966) *Growth at Adolescence.* New York: Appleton.

Tortora, G.J. and Derrickson, B. (2009) *Principles of Anatomy and Physiology*, 12th edn. Hoboken, NJ: John Wiley & Sons.

Tortora, G.J. and Derrickson, B. (2010) *Essentials of Anatomy and Physiology*, 8th edn. New York: John Wiley & Sons.

Tucker, L. (2008) *An Introductory Guide to Anatomy and Physiology*, 3rd edn. London: EMS Publishing.

Activities

www.wiley.com/go/peate

Multiple choice questions

1. Which of the following is not a function of the reproductive system?
   (a) to produce hormones
   (b) to produce ova and sperms
   (c) to nurture the developing foetus
   (d) to produce cholesterol

2. Out of all of the body systems what one functions for the survival of the species?
   (a) the skeletal system
   (b) the reproductive system
   (c) the renal system
   (d) the respiratory system

3. The final stage in the development of sperm is called
   (a) spermiogenesis
   (b) spermatogenesis
   (c) oogenesis
   (d) angiogenesis

4. When sperm are complete and as they become fertile they move through the
   (a) vas deferens
   (b) urethra
   (c) epididymis
   (d) ejaculatory duct

5. Which part of the female reproductive system contains thousands of eggs?
   (a) the vulva
   (b) the vagina
   (c) the uterus
   (d) the ovaries

6. When the lining of the uterus breaks down and flows slowly from the vagina over a period of 3 to 8 days this is known as
   (a) dehydration
   (b) menstruation
   (c) ovulation
   (d) fertilisation

7. What is another name for the womb?
   (a) the prostate gland
   (b) the vagina
   (c) the uterus
   (d) the cervix

8. Where is the hormone testosterone made?
   (a) the penis
   (b) the bladder
   (c) the kidney
   (d) the testes

9. What is the name of the tube that transports the egg cell to the uterus
   (a) the vein
   (b) the vagina
   (c) the fallopian
   (d) the ureter

10. What is the approximate number of sperm cells that are ejaculated during ejaculation?
   (a) only one or two
   (b) thousands
   (c) millions
   (d) billions

True or false

1. Menopause brings on the termination of menstruation and ovulation.
2. Secondary sex characteristics are said to be sexual attractants.
3. Another word for the uterus is the vagina.
4. The clitoris is analogous to the penis as it has an exposed glans and prepuce.
5. Only women can develop breast cancer.
6. An example of a female secondary sex characteristic is the vulva.
7. The ampulla is an area of the vagina.
8. Females are more likely to experience dysfunctions of the reproductive organs than males.
9. Dysmenorrhoea describes the absence of menstruation.
10. The prostate gland is located in the abdomen.

Label the diagram

From the lists of words, label the diagrams below:

Sagittal plane, Sacrum, Seminal vesicle, Vesicorectal pouch, Coccyx, Rectum, Ampulla of ductus (vas) deferens, Ejaculatory duct, Prostatic urethra, Membranous urethra, Anus, Bulb of penis, Epididymis, Testis, Scrotum, Peritoneum, Urinary bladder, Ductus (vas) deferens, Suspensory ligament of penis, Public symphysis, Prostate, Deep muscles of perineum, Bulbourethral (Cowper's) gland, Corpora cavernosum penis, Spongy (penile) urethra, Penis, Corpus spongiosum penis, Corona, Glans penis, Prepuce (foreskin), External urethral orifice

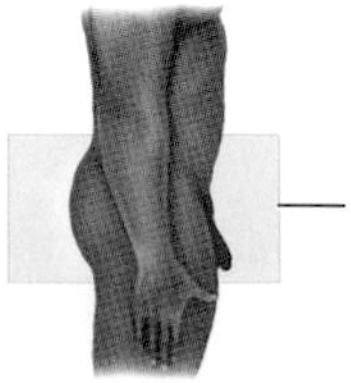

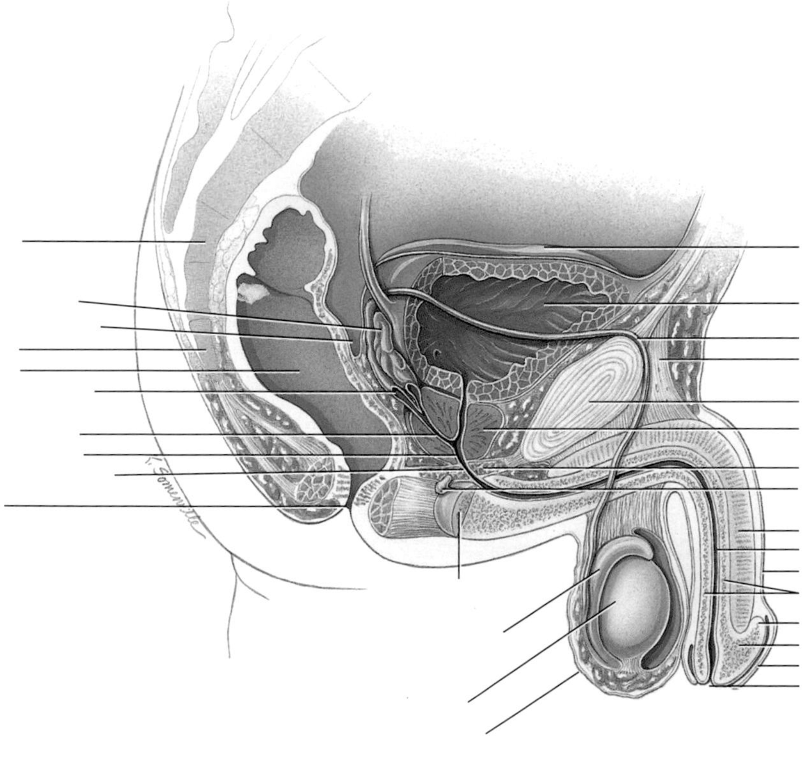

Sagittal plane, Sacrum, Uterosacral ligament, Posterior fornix of vagina, Rectouterine pouch (pouch of Douglas), Vesicouterine pouch, Coccyx, Rectum, Vagina, Anus, Uterine (fallopian) tube, Fimbriae, Ovary, Uterus, Round ligament of uterus, Cervix, Urinary bladder, Pubic symphysis, Mons pubis, Clitoris, Urethra, Labium majus, External urethral orifice, Labium minus

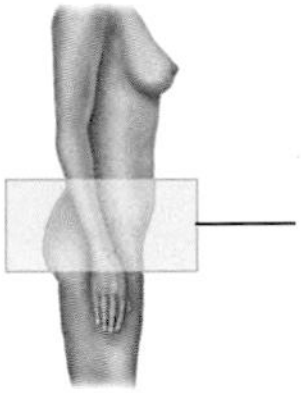

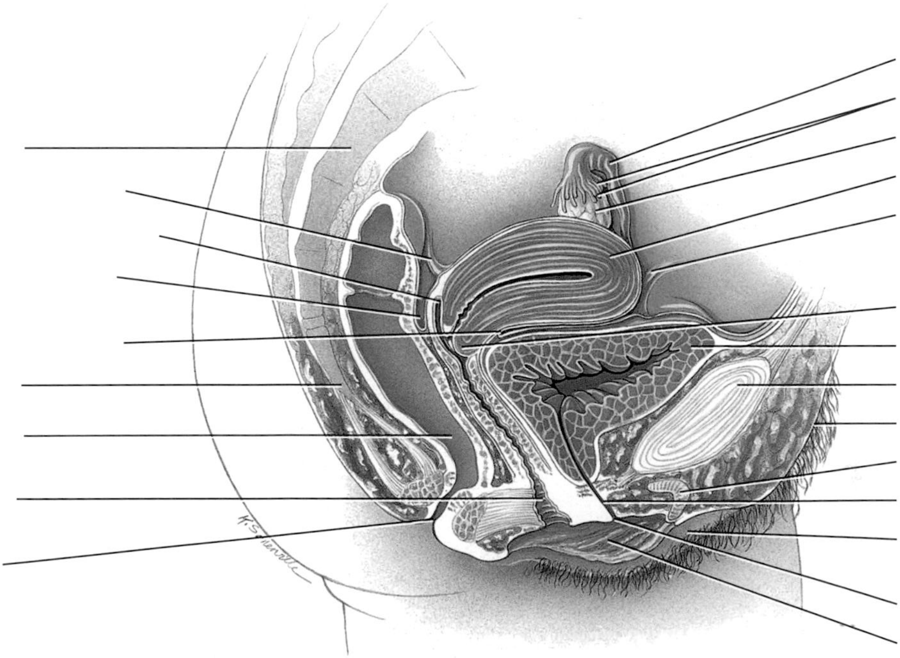

Word Search

In the grid below there are 14 words that you will have seen in this chapter. Can you find them all?

F	N	E	G	O	R	D	N	A	L	C
J	N	E	G	O	R	T	S	E	O	T
C	E	R	V	I	X	S	A	V	H	T
S	U	R	E	T	U	J	A	G	S	E
E	I	T	E	S	T	E	S	E	K	S
M	O	M	Q	E	W	A	M	T	S	T
E	V	W	Y	M	T	E	R	A	S	O
N	A	U	Q	D	N	Y	Q	T	U	S
K	I	R	G	S	I	M	C	S	P	T
P	N	E	T	C	U	D	X	O	R	E
S	O	T	K	B	L	H	I	R	O	R
H	G	H	P	Z	C	M	D	P	C	O
I	O	R	S	U	T	E	O	F	E	N
P	O	A	E	T	W	Y	R	L	K	E

Fill in the blanks

Each month women of reproductive age who are not pregnant go through a ______________ of fertility that results in either ____________ or ___________. The average menstrual cycle is __________ days but can vary. The menstrual cycle prepares a woman's body for the possibility of ____________. The cycle takes approximately a _________ to complete. The lining of the _________ grows and ___________ each month during the ___________ cycle in order for it to be ready in case ____________ occurs. The cell from a male a ___________ must join with the ___________ from a ________ ______ for a woman to become _________. Each _________ eggs are _________ from the ____________, this is called ____________. Sperm meets with the _________ if it is in the ______________ tube. If the woman does not become ____________ then the ______________ tissue in the ___________ as well as ___________ will flow out through the ___________. This is known as ______________.

Find out more

1. What does the surgical procedure vasectomy entail?
2. Discuss the various methods of intrauterine contraception.
3. What advice should be given to a woman who is considering going on the contraceptive pill?
4. What is the role and function of the nurse in respect to promoting sexual health?
5. How can the nurse ensure that the information provided to the people they care for in respect to the various methods of contraception is up to date and correct?
6. Describe the best way to conduct an assessment of a person's sexual health.
7. Discuss the changes that occur in the normal ageing process in relation to the reproductive systems.
8. List the changes a woman may experiences during the menopause.
9. Where is your nearest sexual health clinic located?
10. Discuss the issues that might be associated with female genital mutilation in contemporary society.

Conditions

Below is a list of conditions that are associated with the reproductive systems. Take some time and write notes about each of the conditions. You may make the notes taken from text books or other resources, for example, people you work with in a clinical area, or you may make the notes as a result of people you have cared for. If you are making notes about people you have cared for you must ensure that you adhere to the rules of confidentiality.

Balanitis	
Chlamydia	
Cervical cancer	
Mastitis	
Erectile dysfunction	

Answers

MCQs

1d; 2b; 3a; 4c; 5d; 6b; 7c; 8d; 9c; 10c

True or false

1. True
2. True
3. False
4. True
5. False
6. False
7. False
8. True
9. False
10. False

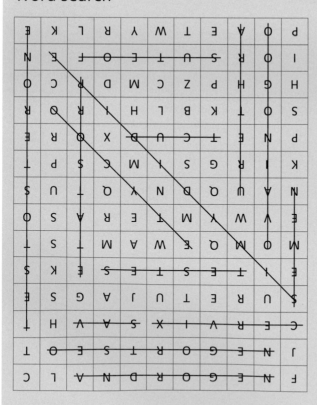

Word search

F	N	E	G	O	R	D	N	A	L	C
J	N	E	G	O	R	T	S	E	O	T
C	E	R	V	I	X	S	A	V	H	T
S	U	R	E	T	U	J	A	G	S	E
E	I	T	E	S	T	E	S	E	K	S
M	O	M	Q	E	W	A	M	T	S	T
E	V	W	Y	M	T	E	R	A	S	O
N	A	U	Q	D	N	Y	Q	T	U	S
K	I	R	G	S	I	M	C	S	P	T
P	N	E	T	C	U	D	X	O	R	E
S	O	T	K	B	L	H	I	R	O	R
H	G	H	P	Z	C	M	D	R	C	O
I	O	R	S	U	T	E	O	F	E	N
P	O	A	E	T	W	Y	R	L	K	E

Fill in the blanks

Each month women of reproductive age who are not pregnant go through a **cycle** of fertility that results in either **pregnancy** or **menstruation**. The average menstrual cycle is **28** days but can vary. The menstrual cycle prepares a woman's body for the possibility of **pregnancy**. The cycle takes approximately a **month** to complete. The lining of the uterus grows and **thickens** each month during the **menstrual** cycle in order for it to be ready in case **ovulation** occurs. The cell from a male a **sperm** must join with the **cell** from a **female egg** for a woman to become **pregnant**. Each **month** eggs are **released** from the **ovary**, this is called **ovulation**. Sperm meets with the **egg** if it is in the **fallopian** tube. If the woman does not become **pregnant** then the **thickened** tissue in the **uterus** as well as **blood** will flow out through the **vagina**. This is known as **menstruation**.

16

The special senses

Carl Clare

Contents

Introduction 512

The chemical senses 512

The sense of smell (olfaction) 512
Olfactory receptors 513
The olfactory pathway 514
Olfactory discrimination 514

The sense of taste 516
Taste buds 516
The taste receptor 517
The gustatory pathway 519

The special senses of equilibrium and hearing 520
The structure of the ear 520
Equilibrium 523
Pathways for the equilibrium sensations 526

Hearing 527
The hearing process 529

The special sense of sight 530
Lacrimal apparatus 531

The eye 531
The wall of the eye 531
Neural tunic (retina) 533
The chambers of the eye 535

Focusing images onto the retina 536
Refraction 536
Myopia, hyperopia and presbyopia 538

The processing of visual information 539
Central processing of visual information 540

Conclusion 540
Glossary 540
References 543
Activities 543

Fundamentals of Anatomy and Physiology for Student Nurses, First Edition. Edited by Ian Peate, Muralitharan Nair.

Test your knowledge

- Which cranial nerve is responsible for conveying information about perceived smells to the brain?
- Name the main parts of the ear involved in the sense of balance.
- What part of the tongue is involved in the sense of taste?
- Name the two substances that fill the eye chambers and help to maintain the shape of the eye.

Learning outcomes

By the end of this chapter the student will be able to:

- Describe the process by which we perceive smell
- Explain the mechanisms responsible for the perception of different tastes
- Describe the way in which human beings maintain a sense of balance
- Explore the mechanisms that lead to sound information being converted into action potentials to be relayed to the brain
- Describe the difference between rods and cones in the eye
- Explain how a visual image is focused on the retina

Introduction

The senses are usually thought of as the five senses of smell, taste, hearing, vision and touch. However, in physiology the sense of touch is excluded from the special senses as it is considered a somatic sense. Thus the 'special senses' is a term used to refer to the senses of:

- Smell
- Taste
- Hearing
- Sight.

Also included in this list of special senses is the sense of:

- Equilibrium.

This chapter will explore these five special senses in three sections:

- The 'chemical' senses of smell and taste
- The senses associated with the ear: those of equilibrium and hearing
- The sense of sight.

In all these sections there will be a review of the anatomy of the particular organs involved in these senses, followed by a discussion of the physiology of how these senses are monitored and create action potentials to be transmitted to the brain. Finally, the pathways of these action potentials take to the brain will be reviewed, along with a brief discussion of the processing of this information in the brain itself.

The chemical senses

With regard to the special senses the chemical senses are the senses of smell and taste which rely on chemoreceptors. There are two main types of chemoreceptor:

- Distance chemoreceptors – for instance, the olfactory (smell) receptors
- Direct chemoreceptors – for instance, the sense of taste, which relies on the taste buds.

The sense of smell (olfaction)

In evolutionary terms the sense of smell is one of the oldest senses. The sense of smell is useful to us for the identification of food that is safe to eat and that which has gone rotten; it helps us to identify dangers such as dangerous chemicals and gives us pleasure through the smell of flowers and perfume. Olfaction (the sense of smell) is dependent on receptors that respond to airborne particles. In the nasal cavity either side of the nasal septum there are paired olfactory organs made up of two layers (Figure 16.1):

- Olfactory epithelium – this layer contains the olfactory receptor cells, supporting cells and regenerative basal cells (stem cells) which mature into receptor cells to replace those that die

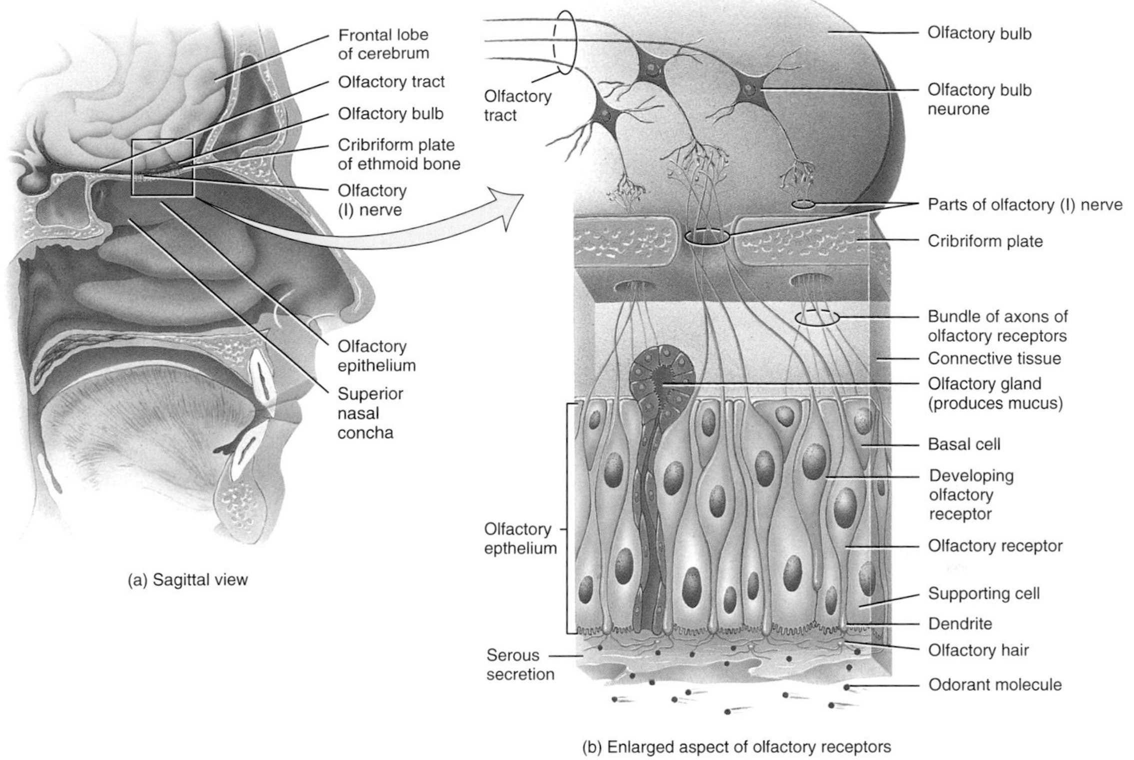
Frontal lobe
of cerebrum
Olfactory tract
Olfactory bulb
Cribriform plate
of ethmoid bone
Olfactory
(I) nerve
Olfactory
epithelium
Superior
nasal
concha
(a) Sagittal view
Olfactory
tract
Olfactory bulb
Olfactory bulb
neurone
Parts of olfactory (I) nerve
Cribriform plate
Bundle of axons of
olfactory receptors
Connective tissue
Olfactory gland
(produces mucus)
Basal cell
Developing
olfactory
receptor
Olfactory receptor
Supporting cell
Dendrite
Olfactory hair
Odorant molecule
Olfactory
epthelium
Serous
secretion
(b) Enlarged aspect of olfactory receptors

Figure 16.1 Gross and microscopic anatomy of olfaction (Tortora and Derrickson 2009)

- Lamina propria – a layer of areolar tissue containing numerous blood vessels and nerves. This layer also contains the olfactory glands which secrete a lipid-rich substance that absorbs water to form a thick mucus which covers the olfactory epithelium.

The olfactory region of each of the two nasal passages is about 2.5 square centimetres (Jenkins *et al.* 2007) and between them they contain approximately 50 million receptor cells.

When air is inhaled through the nose the air in the nasal cavity is subject to turbulent flow and this ensures that airborne smell particles (odorant molecules) are brought to the olfactory organs. Approximately 2% of the inhaled air in an average inspiration passes the olfactory organs, the act of sniffing increases this percentage by a large amount. The olfactory receptors can only be stimulated by compounds that are soluble in water or lipid and can therefore diffuse through the mucus that overlies the olfactory epithelium.

Olfactory receptors

The olfactory receptors are highly modified neurones contained within the olfactory epithelium. The tip of each receptor projects beyond the surface of the epithelium (Figure 16.1). This projection forms the base for up to 20 cilia (hair-like structures) that extend into the surrounding mucus.

These cilia lie laterally in the mucus (they lie relatively flat rather than upright) thus exposing a larger surface area to any compound that is dissolved into the mucus.

Dissolved chemicals interact with odorant-binding proteins on the surface of the cilia; a local depolarisation occurs by the opening of sodium channels in the cell membrane. If enough local depolarisations occur, then an action potential is generated within the receptor cell.

The olfactory pathway

The olfactory system is very sensitive and as little as four molecules can lead to the activation of a receptor. However, activation of a receptor cell does not mean there will be awareness of the smell. There is a significant amount of convergence along the olfactory nervous pathway and inhibition at intervening synapses can prevent the signal from reaching the olfactory cortex in the brain.

Axons leaving the olfactory epithelium receptor cells collect into 20 or more bundles that penetrate the cribiform plate of the ethmoid bone (Figure 16.2), continuing until they reach the olfactory bulb in the brain. At the olfactory bulb the axons converge to connect with post synaptic (mitral) cells in large synaptic structures called glomeruli. Efferent fibres of cells elsewhere in the brain also innervate the olfactory bulb, thus allowing for the potential inhibition of the signalling pathways for instance in central adaptation (Box 16.1).

Axons exiting from the olfactory bulb travel along the olfactory nerves (cranial nerve I, which is a paired nerve) to reach the olfactory cortex, the hypothalamus, and portions of the limbic system via the olfactory tracts. Olfactory stimulation is the only sensory information that reaches the cerebral cortex directly; all other senses are processed by the thalamus first (Martini and Nath 2009). The fact that the limbic system and hypothalamus receive olfactory input helps to explain the profound emotional response that can be triggered by certain smells.

Olfactory discrimination

The olfactory system can make distinctions among some 2,000–4,000 chemical stimuli; however, there are no reasons that can be found to explain this in the structure of the receptor cells themselves. However the epithelium is divided into areas of receptors with particular sensitivity for certain smells. It appears that the central nervous system interprets each smell by analysing the overall pattern of receptor activity (Tortora and Derrickson 2009). Smell appears to be perceived in primary odours, the exact number remains a source of contention and estimates vary from seven to 30 (Marieb and Hoehn 2007). Some of the smells that we perceive are not detected by

Box 16.1 Central adaptation

Have you ever noticed that when meeting someone during the day you will smell their perfume or aftershave, but having spent some time with them you will no longer be aware of that smell? Humans tend to 'habituate' to persistent smells to the point that they are no longer perceived. This is not due to the local receptors adapting to the persistent stimuli; it is a function of central adaptation. That is higher centres in the brain are responsible for our reduced perception of a persistent smell. The transmission of the sensory information for that particular smell is inhibited at the level of the olfactory bulb by nerve impulses from the centres in the brain.

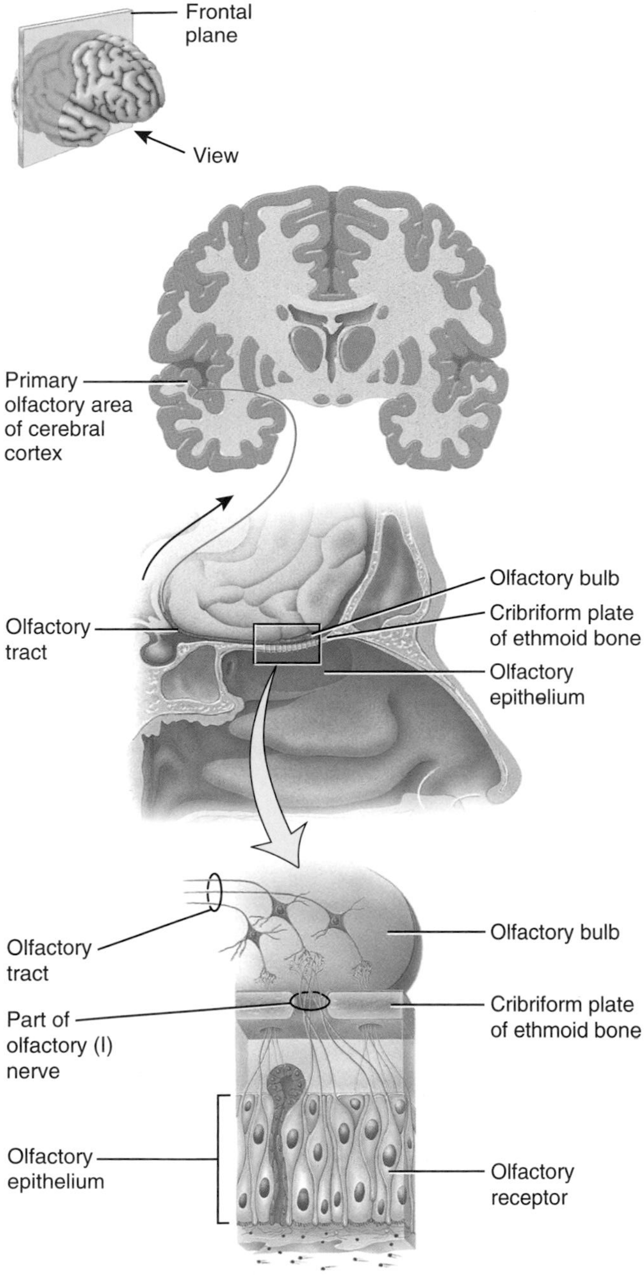
Frontal plane
View
Primary olfactory area of cerebral cortex
Olfactory bulb
Cribriform plate of ethmoid bone
Olfactory tract
Olfactory epithelium
Olfactory tract
Olfactory bulb
Cribriform plate of ethmoid bone
Part of olfactory (I) nerve
Olfactory epithelium
Olfactory receptor

Figure 16.2 Olfactory pathway (Tortora and Derrickson 2009)

the olfactory receptors at all; some of what we sense is actually pain. The nasal cavity contains pain receptors that respond to certain irritants such as ammonia, chillies and menthol. As we get older smell discrimination and sensitivity reduce as we lose receptors compared to the total number we had when younger and the receptors that remain become less sensitive.

The sense of taste

Like the sense of smell, the sense of taste helps to protect us from poisons but also drives our appetite. There are five basic tastes:

- Sweet
- Sour
- Bitter
- Salt
- Umami.

The first four tastes are already common knowledge, but the fifth was relatively unknown in the Western hemisphere until recently. Umami is the taste associated with the proteins found in meat and fish (Smith and Margolskee 2001) and has been known as a concept of taste to the Japanese for many years.

The sense of taste is associated with the taste buds, which are the sensory receptor for taste and are found primarily in the oral cavity. There are approximately 10,000 taste buds in the oral cavity, most are found on the tongue but a few are on the soft palate, the inner surface of the cheeks and the pharynx and epiglottis.

Most of the taste buds are found in peg-like projections of the tongue's mucosa. These projections are known as papillae and are what gives the tongue its slightly rough feel. The papillae (singular is papilla) are found in four major forms (Figure 16.3):

- Fungiform, mushroom-shaped papillae found scattered over the tongue surface but most abundant at the tip and sides. They usually contain five taste buds which are located on the top of these papillae
- Circumvallate (otherwise known as vallate), the largest of the papillae and found in the least number. Seven to 12 of them are found in an inverted 'V' shape at the back of the tongue. They contain approximately 100 taste buds which are located in the side walls of these papillae
- Foliate, 'leaf-like' papillae found on the sides of the rear of the tongue
- Filiform, thread-like structures that contain no taste buds. They provide friction to aid the movement of food by the tongue.

Taste buds

Each taste bud is globular in structure and consists of 40–60 epithelial cells of three major types (Figure 16.4):

- Supporting cells form the greatest part of the taste bud. They help to insulate the receptor cells from each other and the epithelium of the tongue

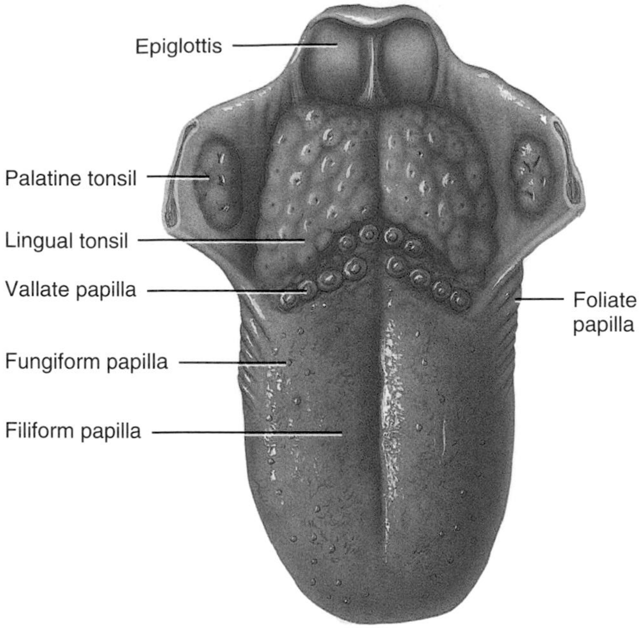
Epiglottis
Palatine tonsil
Lingual tonsil
Vallate papilla
Fungiform papilla
Filiform papilla
Foliate papilla

Figure 16.3 Tongue and the location of the papillae (Tortora and Derrickson 2009)

- Gustatory (or taste) cells – the chemoreceptor responsible for sensing taste
- Basal cells – stem cells that mature into new receptor cells to replace those that die.

Both the supporting cells and the gustatory cells have long microvilli (protrusions of the cell membrane that increases its surface area) called gustatory hairs. These gustatory hairs project from the tip of the cell and protrude through a 'taste pore' in the epithelium to allow them to be bathed in saliva. The gustatory hairs are the sensitive portion of the gustatory cell.

Coiling around the gustatory cells are the sensory dendrites which are the initial part of the gustatory pathway. Each afferent nerve fibre receives nerve signals from several receptor cells.

The taste receptor

The activation of the taste receptor requires the chemical compound (known as a tastant; Tortora and Derrickson 2009) that is to be tasted to dissolve in the saliva, then diffuse into the taste pore and come into contact with the gustatory hairs. Depending on the type of taste this has one of four potential effects (the exact mechanism that is involved in the sensing of umami is unknown):

- Salt – salty taste initiates an influx of sodium into the cell
- Sour – sour taste leads to a hydrogen ion blockade of sodium and potassium channels in the cell membrane
- Bitter – bitter taste leads to an influx of calcium ions into the cell
- Sweet – sweet taste leads to an inactivation of potassium channels.

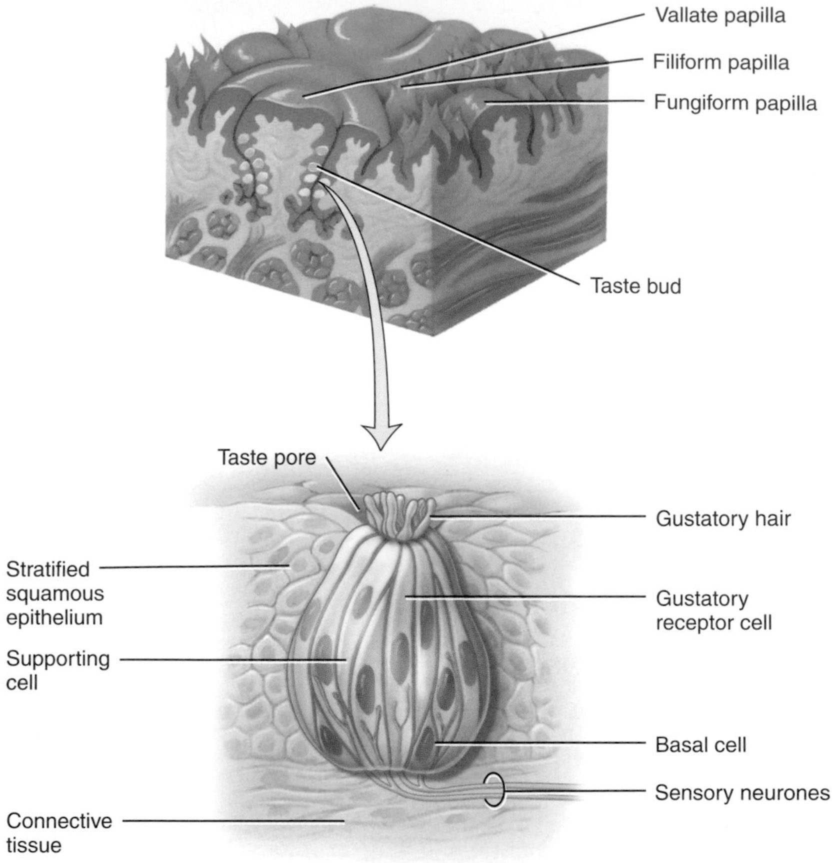
Vallate papilla
Filiform papilla
Fungiform papilla
Taste bud
Taste pore
Gustatory hair
Stratified squamous epithelium
Gustatory receptor cell
Supporting cell
Basal cell
Sensory neurones
Connective tissue

Figure 16.4 Cross-section of part of the tongue and microscopic view of a taste bud (Tortora and Derrickson 2009).

All these effects lead to the depolarisation of the cell and the release of neurotransmitters. Salt taste and sour taste have direct effects on the cell membrane. Bitter taste, sweet taste and umami exert their action on the cell by the use of messenger systems activated by G-protein coupled receptors.

It appears that we have various sensitivities for different tastes. We are most sensitive to bitter tastes, then sour and then sweet and salty. To an extent this makes evolutionary sense as poisons tend to taste bitter, whereas acids and food that has 'gone off' often taste sour. Thus we are most sensitive to those tastes that may indicate something that could harm us.

It should be noted that the taste buds are not the only methods by which we experience the taste of a food. It is clear that the sense of smell is also of vital importance to how we experience taste – just think of how food tastes when your nose is blocked due to a cold; 80% of the sense of taste is actually smell. As with the sense of smell there are also pain receptors involved with the sense of taste and certain tastes will elicit a pain stimulus as opposed to a gustatory one.

Box 16.2 Taste map of the tongue: a scientific myth

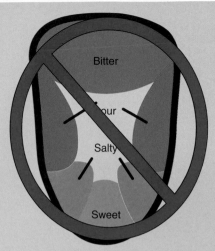
Bitter
Sweet

The taste map of the tongue is a common myth that is still seen in articles and textbooks to this day. In fact, the map is a misinterpretation of 19th-century German research (Smith and Margolskee 2001). The real truth of the matter is that while there may be very slight differences in the taste buds across the tongue there is no evidence to suggest that the variations are in any way as clear as the ones in the taste map; in fact, all tastes can be elicited from any taste bud regardless of its location, certain taste buds are just more sensitive to certain tastes.

The gustatory pathway

The release of neurotransmitters by the gustatory cells creates an action potential in related afferent nerve fibres. The sensory information from the tongue is transmitted along two cranial nerve pairs:

- Chorda tympani – a branch of the facial nerve (cranial nerve VII) relays impulses from the anterior two thirds of the tongue
- Lingual branch of the glossopharyngeal nerve (cranial nerve IX) – carries the sensory information of the posterior third of the tongue.

Sensory information from the taste buds in the epiglottis and pharynx are transmitted by the vagus nerve (cranial nerve X). All the afferent fibres terminate in the solitary nucleus of the medulla. The sensory messages are then transmitted, ultimately, to the thalamus and the gustatory cortex in the parietal lobes. Afferent fibres also project into the hypothalamus and limbic system. Ultimately, many of the branches of afferent nerves that divert to various parts of the brain, apart from the cortex, are involved in the triggering of reflexes involved with digestion (for instance, salivation).

The gustatory pathway is unique amongst the special senses because if the taste buds lose their afferent nerve fibres (for instance, they are cut) the taste bud then degenerates. As we get older we lose the sense of taste as there is a reduction in the number of taste buds; gustatory cells die and are not replaced at the same rate as they die and those cells that remain become less sensitive.

The special senses of equilibrium and hearing

The ear is divided into three sections: external, middle and inner (see Figure 16.5).

Each of these three sections is integral in the process of hearing and the inner ear is also essential in the maintenance of the sense of balance.

The structure of the ear

The outer ear

The outer ear consists of:

- Auricle (pinna)
- External auditory canal
- Tympanic membrane.

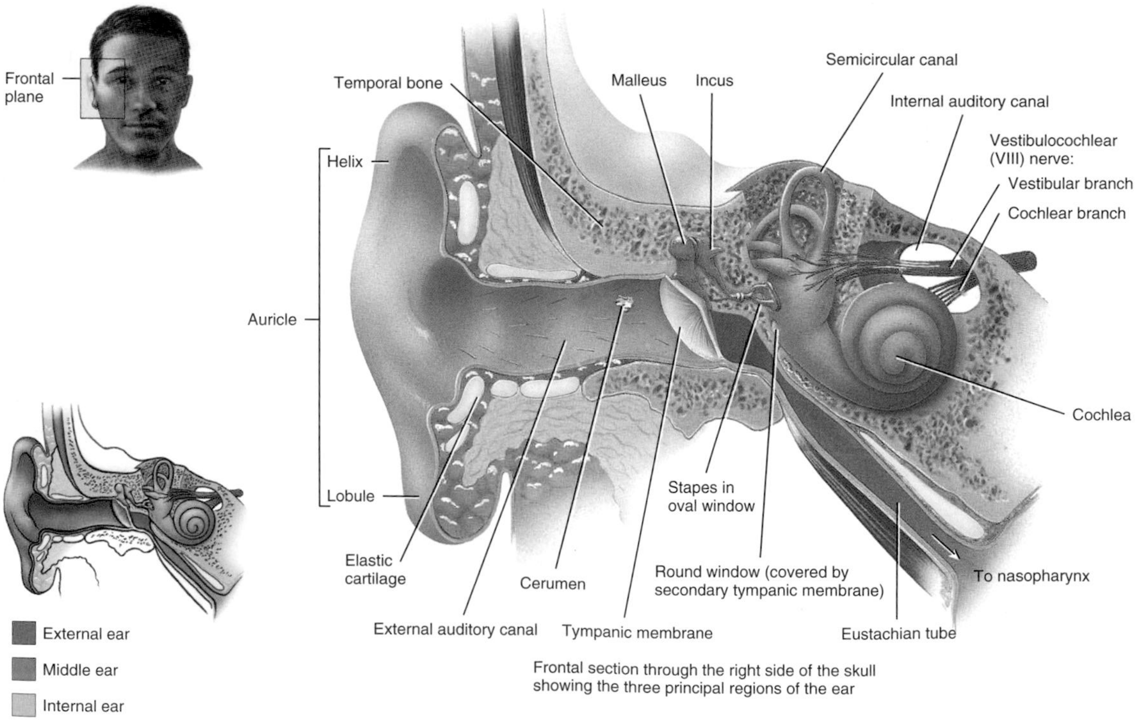
Frontal plane
Temporal bone
Malleus
Incus
Semicircular canal
Internal auditory canal
Vestibulocochlear (VIII) nerve:
Vestibular branch
Cochlear branch
Helix
Auricle
Cochlea
Lobule
Stapes in oval window
Elastic cartilage
Cerumen
Round window (covered by secondary tympanic membrane)
To nasopharynx
External auditory canal
Tympanic membrane
Eustachian tube
Frontal section through the right side of the skull showing the three principal regions of the ear
External ear
Middle ear
Internal ear

Figure 16.5 Structure of the ear (Tortora and Derrickson 2009)

The auricle is the shell-shaped projection surrounding the external auditory canal. It is made of elastic cartilage covered with skin. The auricle can be further broken down into the rim, known as the helix, and the earlobe, which lacks supporting cartilage and so is soft. The function of the auricle is to direct sound waves into the external auditory canal.

The external auditory canal (meatus) is a short, S-shaped, narrow passage about 2.5 cm long and 0.6 cm wide, which extends from the auricle to the tympanic membrane (Figure 16.5). At the end closest to the auricle the external auditory ear canal is made of elastic cartilage, the rest of the canal is a channel through the temporal bone and thus needs no supporting cartilage. The entire canal is lined with skin with associated hairs, sebaceous (oil) glands and modified sweat glands called ceruminous glands. The ceruminous glands secrete a yellow-brown waxy cerumen (ear wax). The purpose of the oils and the wax is to lubricate the ear canal, kill bacteria and, in conjunction with the hairs, keep the canal free of debris.

Sound waves entering the external auditory canal travel along until they reach the tympanic membrane (ear drum), a thin translucent connective tissue membrane covered by skin on its external surface and internally by mucosa, and shaped like a flattened cone protruding into the middle ear. Sound waves that reach the tympanic membrane make it vibrate and this vibration is transmitted to the bones of the middle ear.

Middle ear

Otherwise known as the tympanic cavity, this is a small, air-filled cavity lined with mucosa and contained within the temporal bone. It is enclosed at both ends, by the ear drum at the lateral end and medially by a bony wall with two openings:

- Oval (vestibular) window
- Round (cochlear) window.

The middle ear is connected to the nasopharynx by the eustachian (auditory) tube, a 4 cm long tube that consists of two portions:

- The section near the connection to the middle ear is relatively narrow and is supported by elastic cartilage.
- The section near the nasopharynx is relatively broad and funnel-shaped.

When open the eustachian tube allows the passage of air and thus ensures the equalisation of the pressures on both sides of the tympanic membrane so both are subject to the same atmospheric pressure. The eustachian tube is normally closed at the end nearest the nasopharynx but opens during yawning and swallowing (Jenkins *et al.* 2007). If equalisation of pressures does not happen, then the difference in pressures between the two sides can lead to reduced hearing as the tympanic membrane cannot move freely.

Within the inner ear there are three bones known as the ossicles or ossicular chain. These three bones connect the tympanic membrane with the receptor complexes of the inner ear:

- The malleus (hammer) attaches at three points to the inner surface of the tympanic membrane.
- The incus (anvil) attaches the malleus to the stapes.
- The stapes (stirrup) – the edges of the base of the stapes are bound to the edge of the oval window.

The joints between these three bones are the smallest synovial joints in the body and each has its own tiny capsule and supporting extra-capsular ligaments.

Vibration in the tympanic membrane is the first stage in the perception of sound, this vibration converts the sound waves into mechanical movement (the vibration). The ossicles act as levers and conduct the vibrations to the inner ear. They are connected in such a way that the in – out movement of tympanic vibration is converted into a rocking motion of the stapes. The ossicles collect the force applied to the tympanic membrane, amplify it and transmit it to the oval window. This amplification explains why humans can hear even very quiet noises, but can also be a problem in very noisy environments. In order to protect the tympanic membrane and the ossicular chain from violent movement resulting from extreme noises they are supported by two small muscles:

- The tensor tympani muscle is a short ribbon of muscle connected to the 'handle' of the malleus. When it contracts the malleus is pulled medially (towards the inner ear) stiffening the tympanic membrane
- The stapedius muscle is attached to the stapes and pulls it, reducing the movement against the oval window.

Clinical considerations

Noise exposure and ear damage

As noise levels increase the chance of damage to the ear increases the following table gives examples of the types of noise levels at certain decibel (dB) levels and the exposure time at which damage may occur.

dB level	Maximum exposure per day	Examples
10		Breathing
20		Rustling leaves
60		Conversation
75		Typical car interior on motorway
85	16 hours	City traffic (inside car)
90	9 hours	Power drill, food blender
97	3 hours	French horn at 10 feet
100	2 hours	Farm tractor, outboard motor, jet take-off at 1000 feet
110	0.5 hours	Chainsaw, pneumatic drill, car horn at 3 feet
120	0 hours	Typical rock concert, loud thunderclap

Continued

dB level	Maximum exposure per day	Examples
125	Hearing damage occurring	Pneumatic riveter at 4 feet
132–140	Permanent hearing damage	Gunshot, very loud rock concert 50 feet in front of speakers
150–160	Eardrum rupture	Jet take off at 75 feet, gunshot at one foot
190	Immediate death of tissue	Jet engine at one foot
194		Loudest sound in air, air particle distortion (sonic boom)

Inner ear

The senses of equilibrium (part of the sense of balance) and hearing are provided by the receptors in the inner ear.

The inner ear is also known as the labyrinth due to the complicated series of canals it contains (Jenkins *et al.* 2007). The inner ear is composed of two main, fluid-filled parts:

- Bony labyrinth – a series of cavities within the temporal bone that contain the main organs of balance (the semicircular canals and the vestibule) and the main organ of hearing (the cochlea)
- Membranous labyrinth – a series of fluid-filled sacs and tubes which are contained within the bony labyrinth.

Between the bony and membranous labyrinth flows perilymph, a liquid that is rather like cerebrospinal fluid, the fluid within the membranous labyrinth is known as endolymph.

As noted above, the bony labyrinth can be divided into three parts (Figure 16.6):

- The vestibule consists of a pair of membranous sacs: the saccule and the utricle. Receptors in these two sacs provide the sensations of gravity and linear acceleration
- The semicircular canals enclose slender semicircular ducts. Receptors in these ducts are stimulated by the rotation of the head. The combination of the vestibule and the semicircular canals is known as the vestibular complex
- The cochlea is a spiral-shaped, bony chamber which contains the cochlear duct of the membranous labyrinth. Receptors within this duct give us the sense of hearing.

Equilibrium

The sense of equilibrium is part of the sense of balance and is controlled by receptors in the semicircular ducts, the utricle and the saccule of the inner ear. The sensory receptors in the semicircular ducts are active during movement but inactive when the body is motionless. The sensory receptors in the ducts respond to rotational movements of the head. There are three of these ducts: lateral, posterior and anterior.

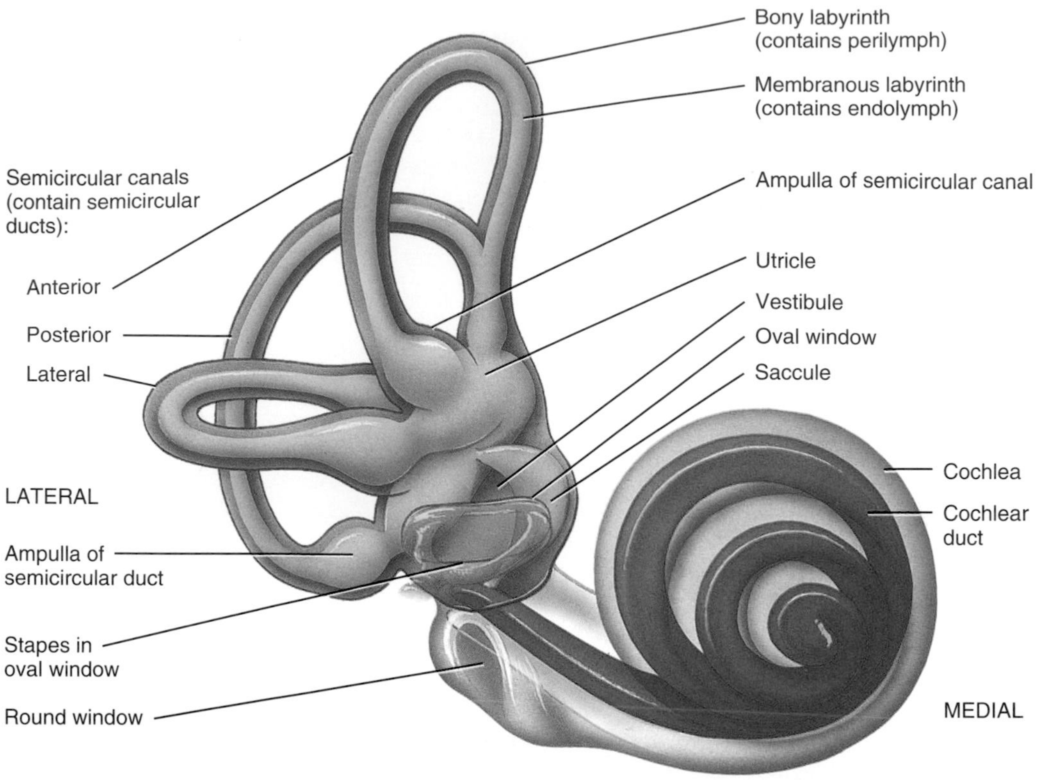
Bony labyrinth
(contains perilymph)
Membranous labyrinth
(contains endolymph)
Semicircular canals
(contain semicircular
ducts):
Anterior
Posterior
Lateral
Ampulla of semicircular canal
Utricle
Vestibule
Oval window
Saccule
Cochlea
Cochlear
duct
LATERAL
Ampulla of
semicircular duct
Stapes in
oval window
Round window
MEDIAL
Components of the right internal ear

Figure 16.6 Inner ear (Tortora and Derrickson 2009)

The ducts are continuous with the utricle. Each semicircular duct contains an ampulla, an expanded region that contains the majority of the receptors. The area in the wall of the ampulla that contains the receptors is known as the crista and each crista is bound to a cupula – a gelatinous structure that extends the full width of the ampulla. The hair cells (receptors) are surrounded by supporting cells and are monitored by the dendrites of sensory neurones.

The free surfaces of the hair cells are covered with stereocilia which resemble very long microvilli. Along with the fine stereocilia the hair cell will also have one kinocilium – a single large and thick cilium. When an external force pushes against the cilia the distortion of the plasma membrane of the hair cell alters the rate that the cell releases chemical transmitters. So, for instance, if a person moves their head to look to the left the cilia of the lateral semicircular canal are subject to pressure and thus the cell membranes are distorted, leading to an altered release of neurotransmitters and the perception of rotational movement (Figure 16.7). Any movement of the head can be perceived by varying combinations of stimulation of the three ducts and their receptors.

In contrast to the semicircular canals, the utricle and the saccule provide equilibrium information whether the body is moving or stationary. The two chambers are connected by a narrow

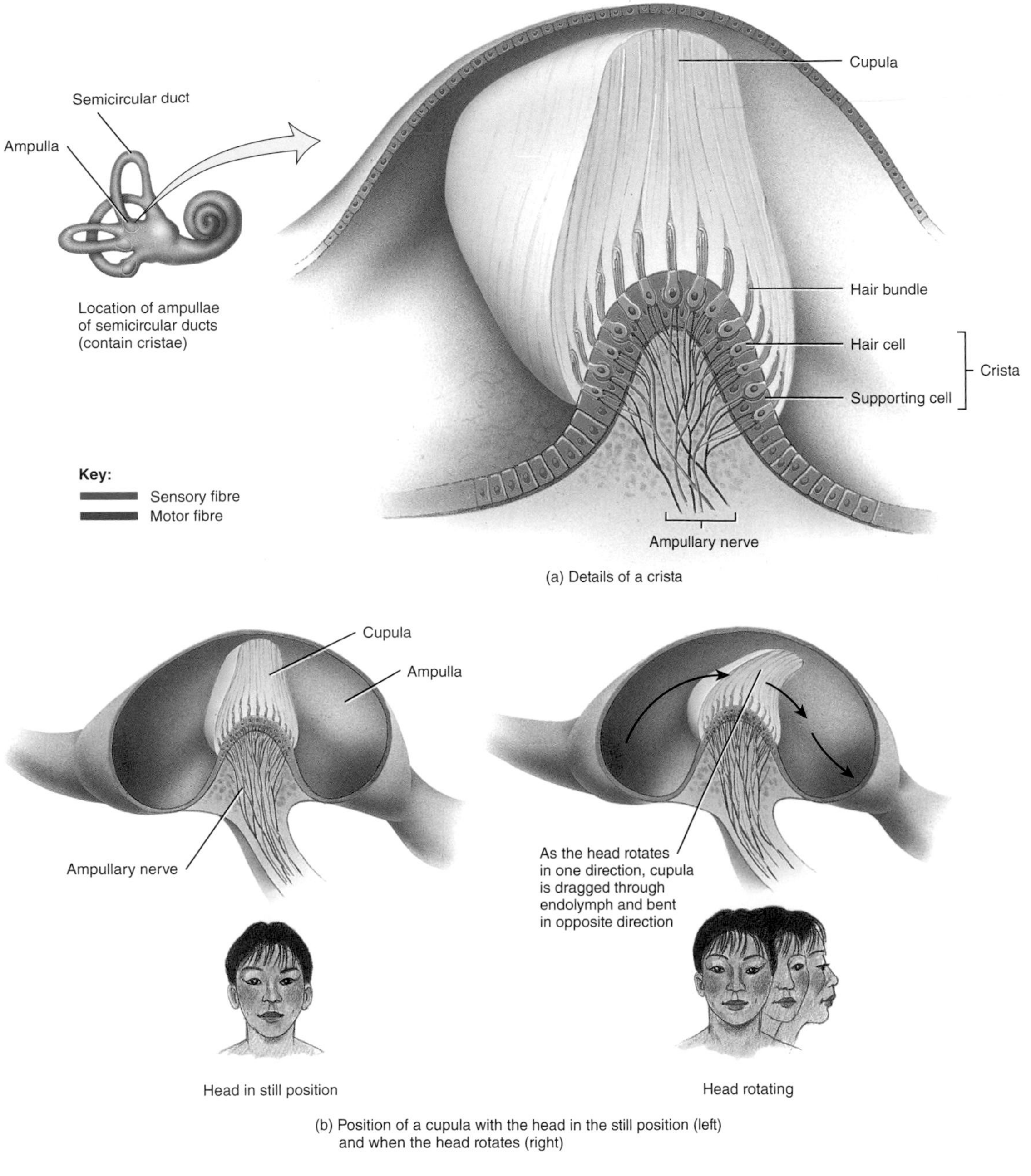

Semicircular duct
Ampulla
Location of ampullae of semicircular ducts (contain cristae)
Key:
Sensory fibre
Motor fibre
Cupula
Hair bundle
Hair cell
Supporting cell
Crista
Ampullary nerve
(a) Details of a crista
Cupula
Ampulla
Ampullary nerve
As the head rotates in one direction, cupula is dragged through endolymph and bent in opposite direction
Head in still position
Head rotating
(b) Position of a cupula with the head in the still position (left) and when the head rotates (right)

Figure 16.7 Ampulla at rest and in response to movement (Tortora and Derrickson 2009)

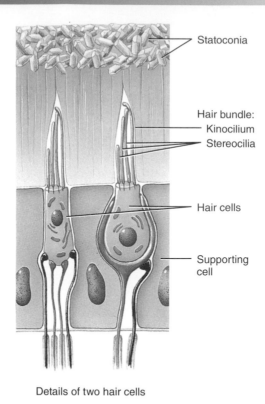

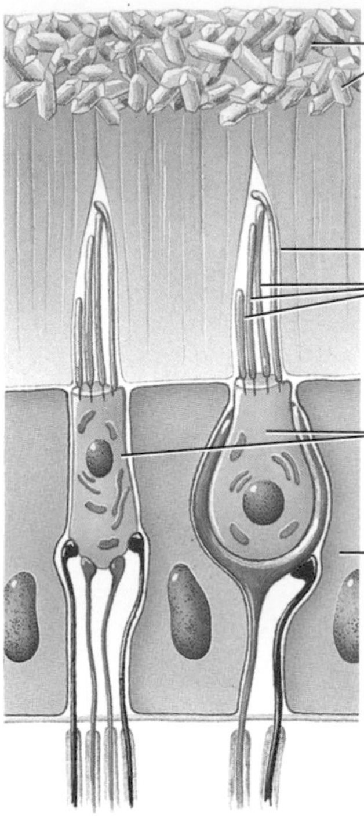
Statoconia
Hair bundle:
Kinocilium
Stereocilia
Hair cells
Supporting cell
Details of two hair cells

Figure 16.8 Hair cells and otolith (Tortora and Derrickson 2009)

passageway which is also connected to the endolymphatic duct. The hair cells of the utricle and saccule are clustered in oval structures called maculae. As with the hair cells of the ampullae the cilia of the hair cells in the utricle and saccule are embedded in a gelatine-like substance. However the surface of this substance contains densely packed calcium carbonate crystals called statoconia. This combination of gelatine-like substance and calcium carbonate crystals is known as an otolith (Figure 16.8).

When the head is in a neutral position the statoconia sit on top of the macula. The pressure they generate is therefore downwards and the hair cell microvilli are pushed down. When the head is tilted the pull of gravity on the statoconia shifts and the microvilli are moved to one side or the other. This distorts the cell membrane and triggers altered neurotransmitter release (Figure 16.9).

A similar type of activity happens when the body is subject to linear acceleration, as a car speeds up then the otolith lags behind due to inertia. The brain would normally differentiate between the action of gravity and the action of acceleration by integrating the information from the receptors with visual information.

Pathways for the equilibrium sensations

The hair cells in the semicircular canals, the vestibule and the saccule are monitored by sensory neurones located in the vestibular ganglia. Sensory fibres from these ganglia form the vestibular

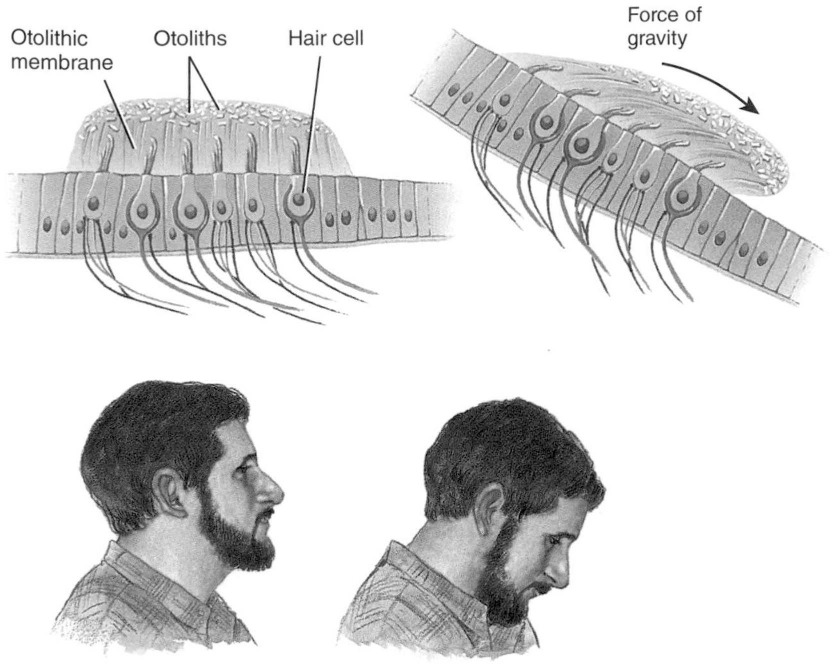
Otolithic membrane
Otoliths
Hair cell
Force of gravity
Head upright
Head tilted forward

Position of macula with head upright (left) and tilted forward (right)

Figure 16.9 Action of gravity on the otolith (Tortora and Derrickson 2009)

branch of the vestibulocochlear nerve (cranial nerve VIII). These fibres feed into neurones within the vestibular nuclei at the boundary of the pons and the medulla oblongata in the brain.

The vestibular nuclei have four functions:

- Integrating sensory information about equilibrium received from both sides of the head
- Relaying information to the cerebellum
- Relaying information to the cortex
- Sending commands to motor nuclei in the brain stem and the spinal cord. The motor commands are reflex-type commands for eye, head and neck movements, such as the movement of the eyes that occur in response to sensations of motion.

Hearing

The sense of hearing is provided by receptors in the cochlear duct, they are hair cells similar to those of the semicircular canals and vestibule. However, their positioning within the cochlear duct and the organisation of the surrounding structures protect them from stimuli generated by anything other than sound waves.

The ossicular chains transmit and amplify pressure waves from the air into pressure waves in the perilymph of the cochlea. These waves stimulate the hair cells along the cochlear spiral.

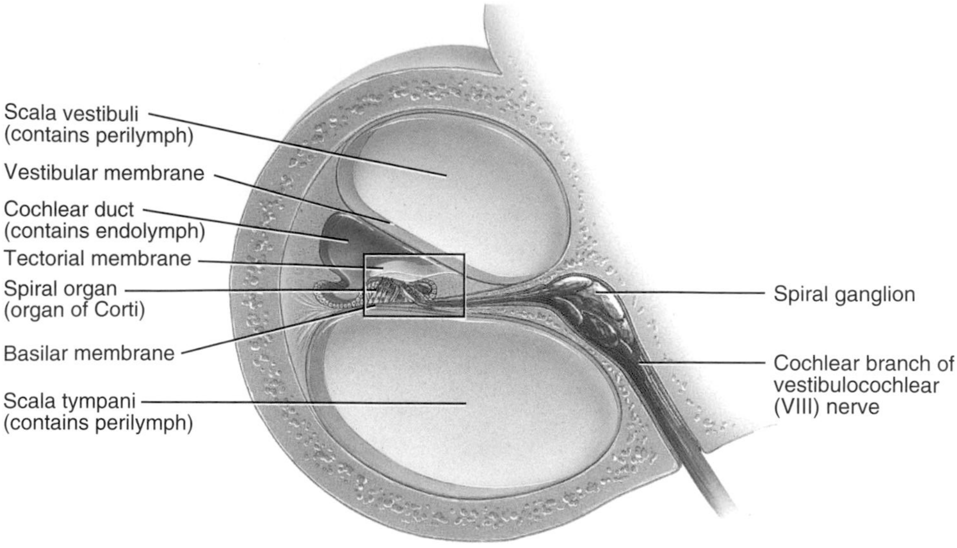
Scala vestibuli
(contains perilymph)
Vestibular membrane
Cochlear duct
(contains endolymph)
Tectorial membrane
Spiral organ
(organ of Corti)
Basilar membrane
Scala tympani
(contains perilymph)
Spiral ganglion
Cochlear branch of
vestibulocochlear
(VIII) nerve
Section through one turn of the cochlea

Figure 16.10 Cross-section of the cochlea, highlighted section is shown in detail in Figure 16.12 (Tortora and Derrickson 2009)

- Frequency of the perceived sound is detected by the part of the cochlear duct that is stimulated
- Intensity (volume) of the sound is detected by the number of hair cells that are stimulated at the particular point in the cochlea.

Within the bony labyrinth of the cochlea there are three ducts (Figure 16.10):

- The vestibular duct (scala vestibuli) connects to the oval window
- The tympanic duct (scala tympani) connects to the round window
- The cochlear duct (scala media) is separated from the tympanic duct by the basilar membrane.

Both the vestibular and the tympanic duct are connected at the tip of the cochlear spiral and therefore make up one continuous perilymphatic chamber (Figure 16.11).

Between the vestibular and the tympanic ducts is the cochlear duct, the hair cells of this duct are located in a structure called the organ of Corti (Figure 16.12). The organ of Corti sits on the basilar membrane and its hair cells are arranged in a series of longitudinal rows.

The hair cells of the organ of Corti do not have kinocilia and their stereocilia are in contact with the overlying tectorial membrane; this membrane is attached to the inner wall of the cochlear duct. When a portion of the basilar membrane bounces up and down in response to pressure waves in the perilymph the stereocilia of the hair cells are pressed against the tectorial membrane and become distorted.

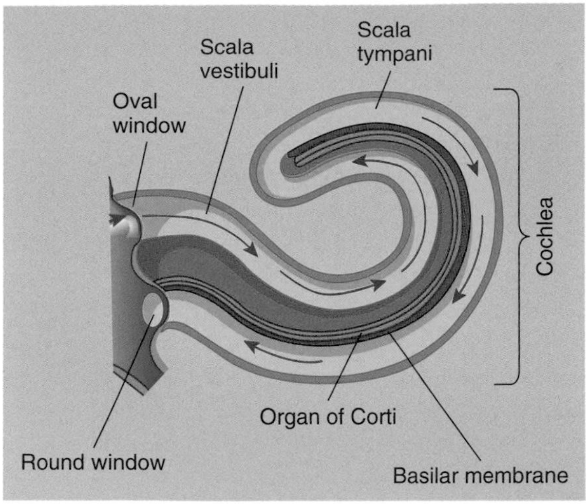
Scala vestibuli
Scala tympani
Oval window
Cochlea
Organ of Corti
Round window
Basilar membrane

Figure 16.11 Cochlea showing the continuous nature of the vestibular and tympanic ducts

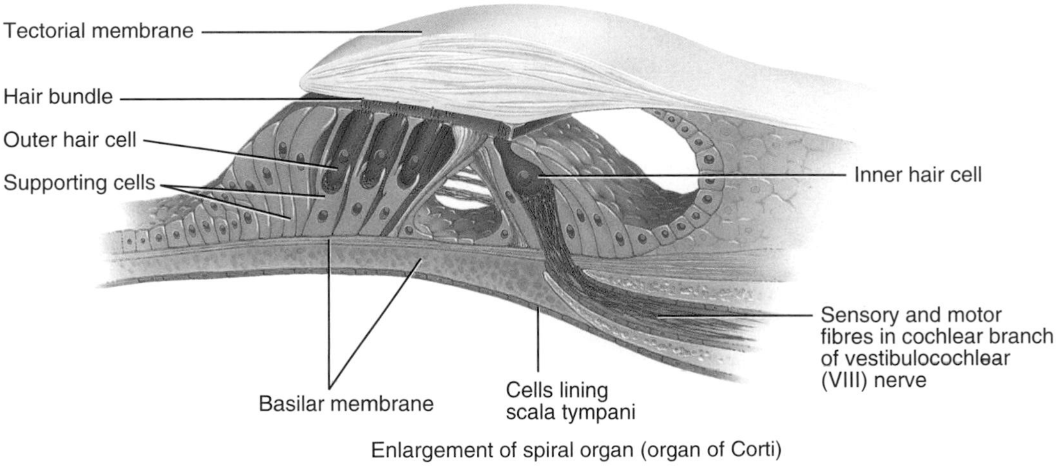
Tectorial membrane
Hair bundle
Outer hair cell
Supporting cells
Inner hair cell
Sensory and motor fibres in cochlear branch of vestibulocochlear (VIII) nerve
Basilar membrane
Cells lining scala tympani
Enlargement of spiral organ (organ of Corti)

Figure 16.12 Organ of Corti (Tortora and Derrickson 2009)

The hearing process

(1) Sound waves travel down the external auditory canal and arrive at the tympanic membrane.
(2) Movement is created in the tympanic membrane which leads to the movement of the ossicles and the amplification of the movement.
(3) Movement of the stapes at the oval window creates pressure waves in the perilymph of the vestibular duct.

(4) The pressure waves distort the basilar membrane. The location of the maximum distortion depends on the frequency of the sound as the basilar membrane varies in width and flexibility along its length. Higher pitch sounds create maximum distortion near to the oval window and lower pitch sounds further away from the window. The amount of distortion gives sensory information as to the volume of the sound.

(5) Vibration in the basilar membrane leads to vibration of the hair cell cilia against the tectorial membrane, leading to the release of neurotransmitters by the hair cells. As hair cells are arranged in rows, a soft sound may only distort a few hair cells in a single row but as the volume increases more cells in more rows will be stimulated.

(6) Information about the region of stimulation and the intensity of that stimulation are relayed to the brain via the cochlear branch of the vestibulocochlear nerve (cranial nerve VIII). The cell bodies of the neurones that monitor the hair cells of the cochlea are located in the spiral ganglia at the centre of the bony cochlea. The nerve impulses are then transmitted via the cochlear branch of cranial nerve VIII to the cochlear nuclei of the medulla oblongata and then to other centres in the brain.

The special sense of sight

Vision is perhaps the special sense that we value the most; we learn more about the world around us through sight than we do any of the other special senses. Without sight many of our daily tasks and pleasures would be impossible and many others would become more difficult. The sense of sight is based on the eyes, and around the eyes there are accessory structures that help to keep the eyes safe and working well (Figure 16.13):

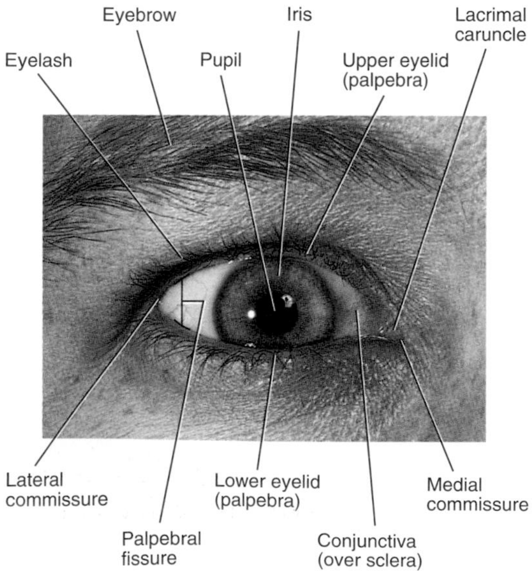
Eyebrow
Iris
Lacrimal caruncle
Eyelash
Pupil
Upper eyelid (palpebra)
Lateral commissure
Lower eyelid (palpebra)
Medial commissure
Palpebral fissure
Conjunctiva (over sclera)

Figure 16.13 Accessory structures of the eye (Tortora and Derrickson 2009)

- Eyelids (palpebra) – a continuation of the skin. Continual blinking keeps the surface of the eye lubricated and removes dirt. The gap between them is known as the palpebral fissure
- Eyelashes – robust hairs that help to keep foreign matter out of the eyes. They are associated with the tarsal glands which produce a lipid-rich secretion that helps to prevent the eyelids from sticking together
- Lacrimal caruncle – a mass of soft tissue that contains accessory glands
- Commissure – the point where the eyelids meet; there are two, the lateral and the medial
- Conjunctiva – the epithelial cell layer that lines the inside of the eyelids and the outer surface of the eye.

Lacrimal apparatus

A constant flow of tears washes over the eyes to keep the conjunctiva moist and clean. Tears have several functions:

- Reduce friction
- Remove debris
- Prevent bacterial infection
- Provide nutrients and oxygen to parts of the conjunctiva.

The lacrimal apparatus produces, distributes and removes tears. It consists of:

- A lacrimal gland
- Lacrimal canaliculi
- Lacrimal sac
- Nasolacrimal duct.

The lacrimal gland (tear gland) creates most of the content of tears (about 1 ml per day). Once the lacrimal secretions reach the eye they mix with the products of the accessory glands and the tarsal glands. This results in a mixture that lubricates the eye and reduces evaporation. The nutrient and oxygen demands of the corneal cells are supplied by diffusion from the lacrimal secretions. The secretions also contain antibacterial enzymes and antibodies to attack pathogens before they enter the body.

Blinking sweeps the tears across the ocular surface and they accumulate at the medial commissure from where they are drained by the lacrimal canaliculi into the lacrimal sac and from there into the nasal cavity through the nasolacrimal duct.

The eye

The wall of the eye

The wall of the eye has three layers (Figure 16.14):

- Fibrous tunic
- Vascular tunic
- Neural tunic.

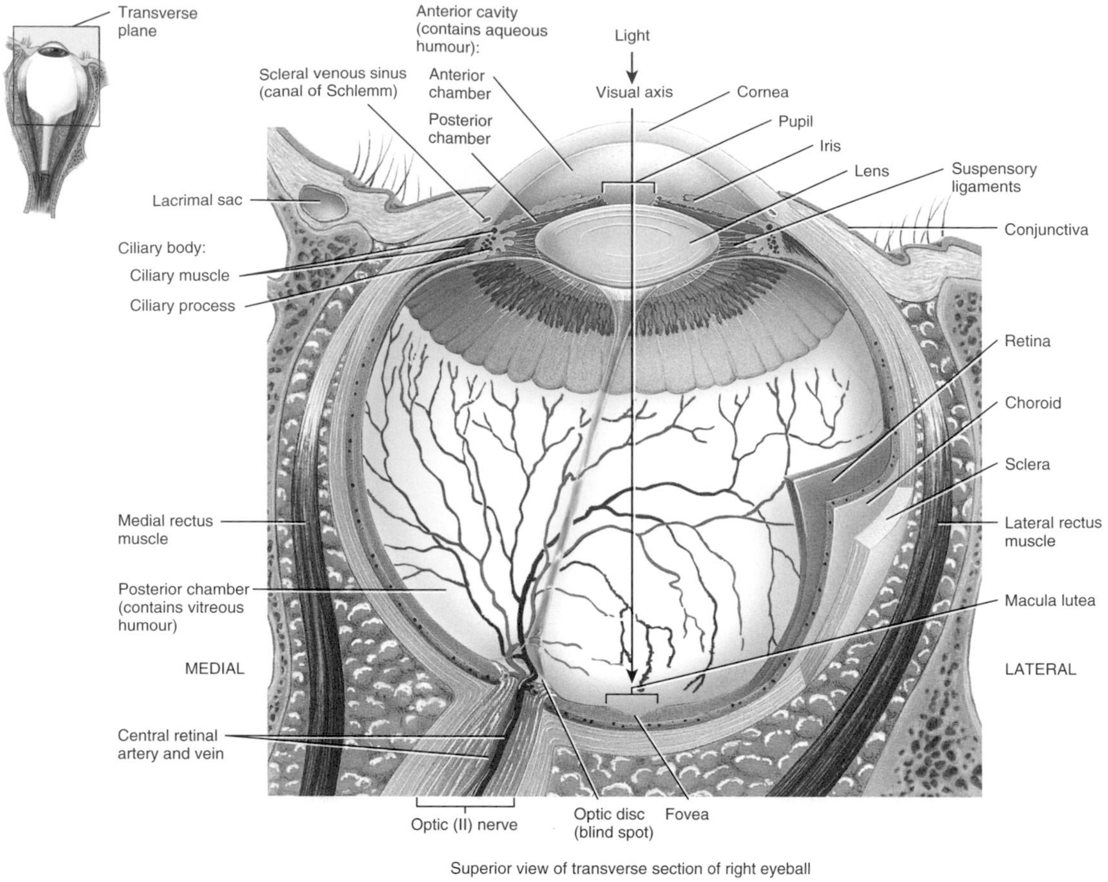
Transverse plane
Anterior cavity (contains aqueous humour):
Light
Scleral venous sinus (canal of Schlemm)
Anterior chamber
Visual axis
Cornea
Posterior chamber
Pupil
Iris
Lens
Suspensory ligaments
Lacrimal sac
Conjunctiva
Ciliary body:
Ciliary muscle
Ciliary process
Retina
Choroid
Sclera
Medial rectus muscle
Lateral rectus muscle
Posterior chamber (contains vitreous humour)
Macula lutea
MEDIAL
LATERAL
Central retinal artery and vein
Optic (II) nerve
Optic disc (blind spot)
Fovea
Superior view of transverse section of right eyeball

Figure 16.14 Anatomy of the eye (Tortora and Derrickson 2009)

Fibrous tunic

The fibrous tunic is the outermost layer of the eye and consists of the sclera and the cornea, it has three main functions:

- Provides support and some protection
- Is the attachment site for the extrinsic muscles
- Contains structures that assist in the focussing process.

Most of the ocular surface is covered by the sclera (the 'white' of the eye) which is made up of dense fibrous connective tissue containing collagen and elastic fibres. The surface of the sclera contains small blood vessels and nerves. The transparent cornea is continuous with the sclera and is made up of a dense matrix of fibres laid down in such a way that they do not interfere with the passage of light.

Vascular tunic (uvea)

The vascular tunic is the middle of the three layers of the eye and contains numerous blood vessels, lymph vessels and the smooth muscles involved in eye functioning. The functions of this layer include:

- Providing a structure for the blood and lymph vessels that supply the tissues of the eye
- Regulating the amount of light that enters the eye
- Secreting and reabsorbing the aqueous humour
- Controlling the shape of the lens.

The vascular tunic is made up of:

- Iris
- Ciliary body
- Choroid.

Iris

The iris is the central, coloured portion of the eye (Figure 16.13) and regulates the amount of light entering the eye by adjusting the size of the central opening (the pupil). It is formed of two layers of pigmented cells and fibres and two layers of smooth muscle (the pupillary muscles):

- Pupillary constrictor muscles
- Pupillary dilator muscles.

Both sets of muscles are controlled by the autonomic nervous system, activation of the parasympathetic nervous system leads to constriction of the pupil in response to bright light. Activation of the sympathetic nervous system leads to the dilation of the pupil in response to dim light levels. At its edge the iris attaches to the anterior part of the ciliary body.

Ciliary body

The greatest part of the ciliary body is made up of the ciliary muscle, a smooth muscular ring that projects into the interior of the eye. The epithelial covering of this muscle has many folds called ciliary processes. The suspensory ligaments of the lens attach to the tips of these processes.

Choroid

The choroid is a vascular layer that separates the fibrous and neural tunics. It is covered by the sclera and attached to the outermost layer of the retina. The choroid contains an extensive capillary network that delivers oxygen and nutrients to the retina.

Neural tunic (retina)

This is the innermost layer of the eye, consisting of a thin, outer layer called the pigmented part and a thicker inner layer called the neural part.

- Pigmented part of the retina absorbs the light that passes through the neural part; this prevents light bouncing back through the neural part and causing 'visual echoes'
- Neural part of the retina contains light receptors, support cells and is responsible for the preliminary processing and integration of visual information.

Organisation of the retina

Figure 16.15 shows the two types of receptor cells contained within the outermost layer of the retina (closest to the pigmented part). These receptor cells are the cells that detect light (photoreceptors).

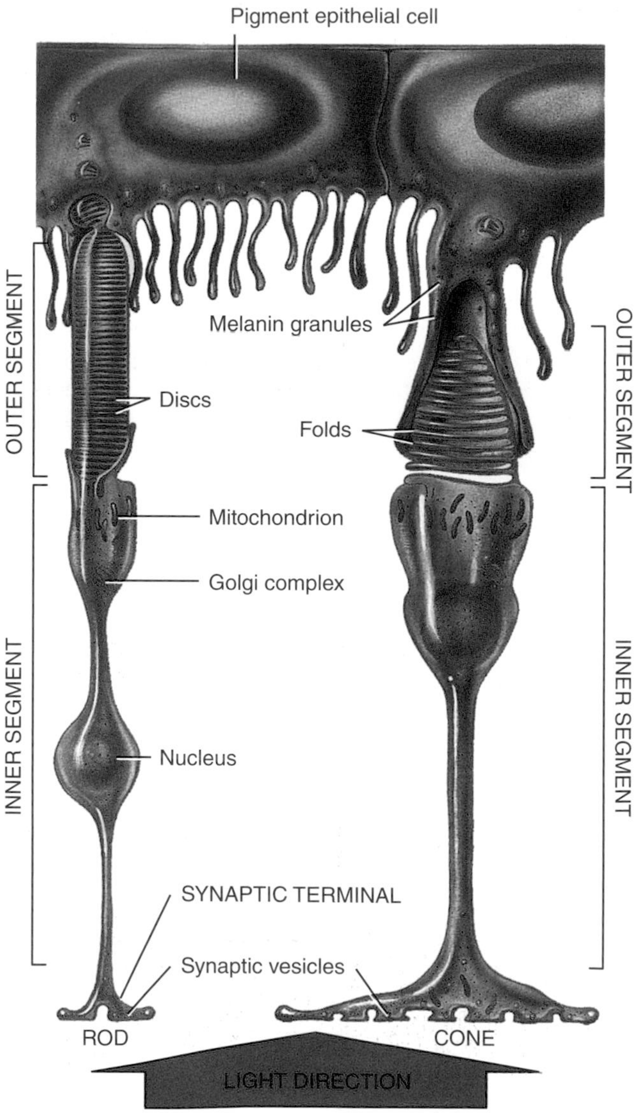
Pigment epithelial cell
OUTER SEGMENT
Melanin granules
Discs
Folds
OUTER SEGMENT
Mitochondrion
Golgi complex
INNER SEGMENT
Nucleus
INNER SEGMENT
SYNAPTIC TERMINAL
Synaptic vesicles
ROD
CONE
LIGHT DIRECTION

Figure 16.15 Cross-section of the retina (Tortora and Derrickson 2009)

- Rods – these photoreceptors do not discriminate between colours. They are very sensitive and enable us to see in very low light levels. Rods are mostly concentrated in a band around the periphery of the retina and this density reduces towards the centre of the eye
- Cones – these photoreceptors provide colour vision and give sharper, clearer images than the rods do but they require more intense light. Cones are mostly situated in the macula lutea and particularly at its centre in an area called the fovea (Figure 16.14).

The elongated outer section of the rods and cones contain hundreds to thousands of flattened membranous discs. In the rods the discs are separate and form the shape of a cylinder. In cones the discs are in fact folds of the plasma membrane and the outer segment tapers to a blunt point.

There are three types of cone, red, blue and green, and colour discrimination is based on the integration of information received from the three types of cones. For instance, yellow is shown by highly stimulated green cones, less strongly stimulated red cones and a relative lack of stimulation of the blue cones.

A narrow connecting stalk links the outer segment to the inner segment, which is the part of the cell that contains all the usual cellular organelles. The inner segment is also the area where synapses with other cells are made and neurotransmitters are released.

The rods and cones synapse with neurones called bipolar cells which in turn synapse within a layer of neurones called ganglion cells. At both these synapse areas there are associated cells that can stimulate or inhibit the communication between the two cells and therefore alter the sensitivity of the retina (for instance, in response to very bright, or dim, light levels).

Axons from approximately one million ganglion cells converge on the optic disc, at which point they turn and penetrate the wall of the eye and proceed to the diencephalon of the brain as the optic nerve. The central retinal artery and vein pass through the centre of the optic nerve. The optic disc contains no photoreceptors and thus this area is known as the blind spot, however we do not notice the blind spot in our vision as involuntary eye movements keep the visual image moving and the brain can thus supply the missing information.

The chambers of the eye

The eye is divided into two main cavities: a large posterior cavity and a smaller anterior cavity. The anterior cavity is further divided into the anterior chamber and the posterior chamber (Figure 16.14).

- Anterior cavity, which is filled with a substance called aqueous humour that circulates between the anterior and posterior chambers by passing through the pupil and performing a vital role as a transport medium for nutrients and waste products. The fluid pressure created by the aqueous humour in the anterior cavity helps to maintain the shape of the eye. Aqueous humour is produced by the epithelial cells of the ciliary body and within a few hours is drained through the canal of Schlemm to the sclera to be recycled.
- Posterior cavity, which is the larger of the two cavities of the eye and is filled with a gelatinous mass known as vitreous humour. The vitreous humour helps to stabilise the shape of the eye as the activity of the extra-ocular muscles would otherwise distort the shape of the eye. Unlike aqueous humour the vitreous humour is created during the development of the eye and is never replaced. A thin film of aqueous humour infiltrates the posterior chamber bathing the retina, supplying nutrients and removing waste. The pressure it creates also helps to keep the neural part of the retina against the pigmented part; though the two are close together they are not fixed to each other and thus this external pressure is required.

Focusing images onto the retina

In order for a visual image to be useful it must be focused onto the retina; this is the purpose of the lens of the eye. First, the light entering the eye is subject to refraction and the lens provides the additional, adjustable refraction required to focus the image onto the retina.

Refraction

Light is refracted (bent) when it passes from one medium to another medium with a different density (Figure 16.16).

The majority of the refraction in the eye happens when light enters the cornea from the air, additional refraction occurs when light passes from the aqueous humour into the lens. The lens provides the extra refraction to focus the light onto the retina and can adjust this refraction according to the focal length.

Focal length is the distance between the focal point (e.g. on the retina) and the centre of the lens (Figure 16.17).

Focal length is dependent on:

- The distance from the object to the lens, the further away an object is the shorter the focal length
- The shape of the lens, the rounder the lens the more refraction occurs. A very round lens has a shorter focal length than a flatter lens.

The lens lies behind the cornea and is held in place by ligaments that are attached to the ciliary body. It is made up of concentric layers of cells that are precisely organised and are covered by a fibrous capsule. Many of the capsule fibres are elastic and if it wasn't subject to external forces by the ligaments the lens would be spherical. Within the lens are lens fibres, specialised cells that

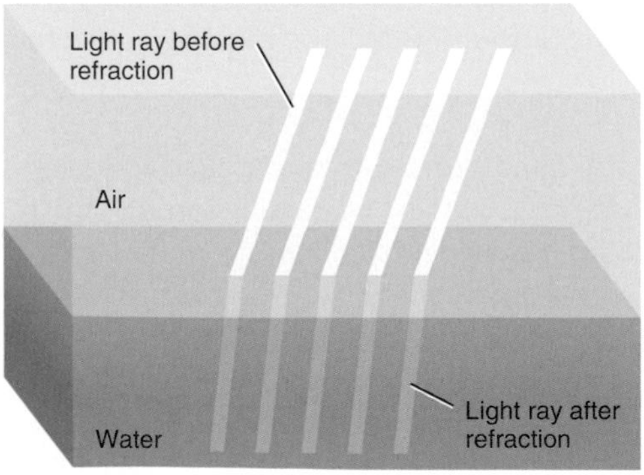
Light ray before refraction
Air
Water
Light ray after refraction
Refraction of light rays

Figure 16.16 Refraction of light passing from air (less dense) to water (dense) (Tortora and Derrickson 2009)

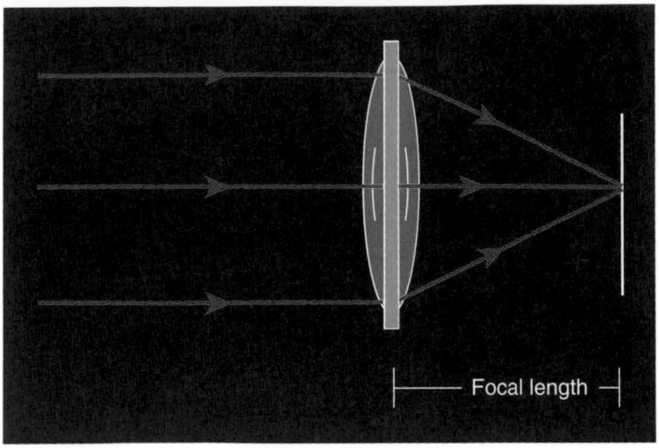
Focal length

Figure 16.17 Focal length

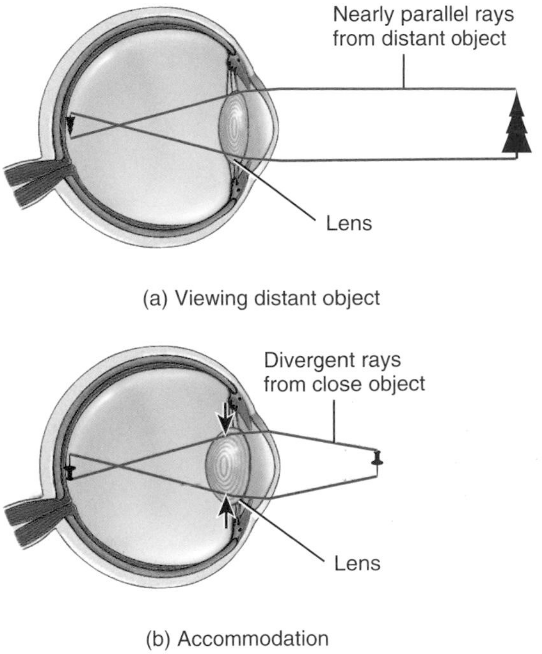
Nearly parallel rays
from distant object
Lens
(a) Viewing distant object
Divergent rays
from close object
Lens
(b) Accommodation

Figure 16.18 Accommodation to near and far objects (Tortora and Derrickson 2009)

have lost their nucleus and other organelles. They are filled with a protein called crystallin which is responsible for the transparency and the focusing power of the lens.

The process of changing the shape of the lens to focus an image onto the retina is known as accommodation. The shape of the lens is altered by tension being applied to or relaxed on the suspensory ligaments by smooth muscles within the ciliary body (Figure 16.18).

Myopia, hyperopia and presbyopia

In a person who has myopia (short-sightedness) the lens is unable to focus the image onto the retina and the focus of the image falls short (Figure 16.19). With myopia people can see objects close to them but those that are far away are blurred. Myopia is easily corrected for by the use of corrective lenses either in the form of glasses or contact lenses.

In the person with hyperopia (long-sightedness) the image is focused onto a point behind the retina (Figure 16.20), therefore these people can see things at a distance but not near to them.

Clinical considerations

20/20 vision

The term 20/20 vision refers to a measure of visual acuity. The meaning is that the person being tested can see the same detail from 20 feet away as a person with normal eyesight would see from 20 feet. In other words 20/20 vision is normal vision. If a person has 20/40 vision they are only able to see detail at 20 feet that a person with normal vision can see at 40 feet. A person with a visual acuity of 20/70 can only see detail at 20 feet that a person with normal sight could see at 70 feet and so on. The visual acuity is not a direct correlation with the prescription for eyeglasses, but the prescribed glasses are intended to achieve 20/20 vision. Visual acuity is tested using a standard size Snellen chart at 20 feet and lit to a standard brightness.

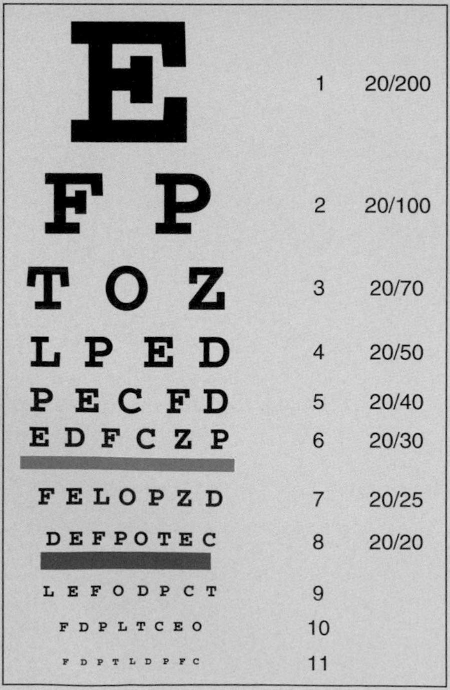
E 1 20/200
F P 2 20/100
T O Z 3 20/70
L P E D 4 20/50
P E C F D 5 20/40
E D F C Z P 6 20/30
F E L O P Z D 7 20/25
D E F P O T E C 8 20/20
L E F O D P C T 9
F D P L T C E O 10
F D P T L D P F C 11

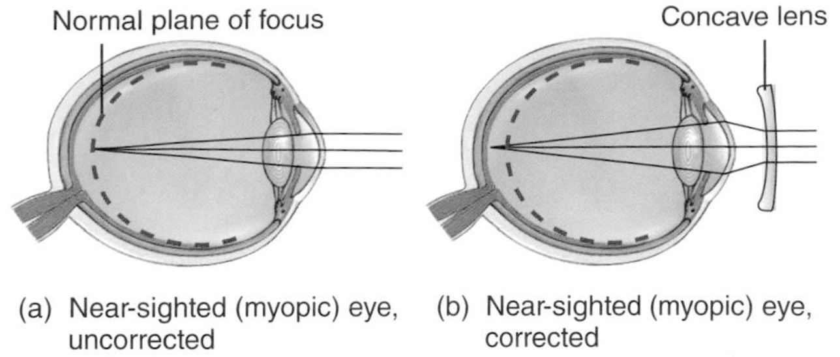
Normal plane of focus
Concave lens
(a) Near-sighted (myopic) eye, uncorrected
(b) Near-sighted (myopic) eye, corrected

Figure 16.19 (a) Myopic eye uncorrected and (b) corrected by a concave lens (Tortora and Derrickson 2009)

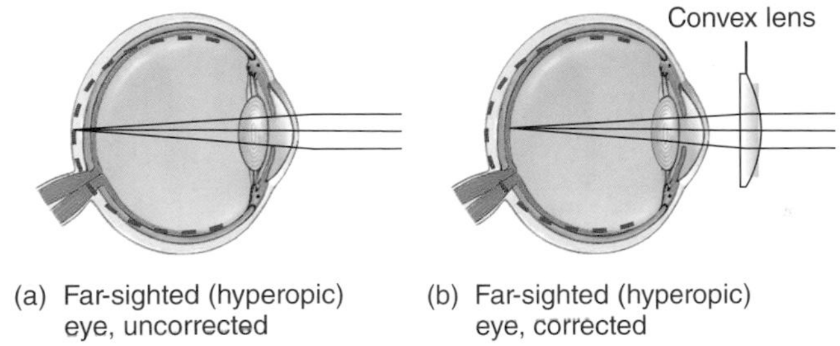
Convex lens
(a) Far-sighted (hyperopic) eye, uncorrected
(b) Far-sighted (hyperopic) eye, corrected

Figure 16.20 (a) Hyperopic eye uncorrected and (b) corrected by a convex lens (Tortora and Derrickson 2009)

Presbyopia is the loss of the ability to focus on close objects as the person ages; the most common theory for this is the loss of elasticity in the lens. The loss of the ability to focus on near objects occurs in everyone but at different rates and with different effects on vision. The onset of presbyopia is most commonly noticed at 40 to 50 years of age. Presbyopia is treatable with corrective glasses (usually known as reading glasses, though they are corrective for all tasks that require near vision).

The processing of visual information

The ganglion cells that monitor the rods in the retina (M cells) supply information about the general form of an object, motion and shadows in dim light. As many as 1000 rods may pass information to one M cell and this convergence leads to a loss of specific information and the activation of an M cell indicates that light has struck a general area rather than a specific point. This loss of specific location-based information is partially compensated for by the fact that the M cells activity varies depending on the pattern of stimulation in their specific field (area of retina). So, for instance, an M cell would react differently to a stimulus at the edge of its receptive field from one at its centre.

Cone cells show very little convergence, for instance in the fovea the ratio of cones to ganglion is 1 to 1 (Martini and Nath 2009). The ganglion cells that monitor cones (P cells) are more numerous than M cells and because there is little convergence these cells provide location-specific information. As a result of this cones supply more precise information about a visual image than do rods.

Central processing of visual information

Once axons from the ganglion cells have exited the eye through the optic disc they proceed to the diencephalon as the optic nerves (cranial nerve II). The two optic nerves (one for each eye) reach the diencephalon at the optic chiasm. From there half the nerves go to the lateral geniculate nucleus on the same side of the brain and the other half cross over and proceed to the lateral geniculate nucleus on the opposite side. From each lateral geniculate nucleus visual information also travels to the occipital cortex of the cerebral hemisphere on the same side. Involuntary eye control (such as pupillary reflexes etc.) is processed in the diencephalon and the brain stem.

Conclusion

In this chapter there has been a review of the special senses:

- Olfaction (smell), which is based in the olfactory receptors of the nose
- Gustation (taste), which is partially based in the gustatory receptors on the tongue but also has a large input from the olfactory receptors
- Equilibrium, which is a part of the sense of balance and is based in the hair cells of the semicircular canals and the vestibule
- Hearing, which is based in the hair cells in the organ of Corti in the cochlea of the inner ear
- Sight which is based in the photoreceptors of the eye.

With the exception of smell, all the information generated by the special senses is processed in the thalamus before being transmitted on to the higher brain centres. Some of the senses (smell and taste) also have direct input into other centres of the limbic system such as the hypothalamus and this is an indication of both how ancient they are in evolutionary terms and the fact that certain smells and tastes can evoke subconscious responses, such as salivation and emotions.

Glossary

Afferent: Heading towards a centre (for instance, the brain).

Ampulla: A sac-like enlargement of a canal or duct.

Anterior: Located at, or related to, the front of a structure.

Antibody: Proteins in the blood that are used by the immune system to identify and destroy pathogens.

Autonomic nervous system: The part of the nervous system that controls involuntary functions, made up of the parasympathetic and sympathetic nervous systems.

Axon:	Extension of a nerve cell that conducts impulses.
Balance:	The ability to control equilibrium.
Cartilage:	A supporting connective tissue made up of various cells and fibres.
Cilia:	Small, hair-like processes on the outer surface of some cells.
Connective tissue:	Tissue that supports and binds other body tissue.
Convergence:	The movement of the eyes inwards to see an object close to the face.
Efferent:	Heading away from a centre.
Endolymph:	GT the fluid in the membranous labyrinth of the inner ear.
Enzyme:	A protein that increases the rate of a chemical reaction.
Equilibrium:	Stability at rest or when moving.
Ethmoid bone:	A bone in the skull that separates the nasal cavity from the brain.
Extrinsic:	Not inherent to the process or object, external.
Focal length:	The distance between the focal point (e.g. on the retina) and the centre of the lens of the eye.
Fovea (fovea centralis):	A small depression in the retina containing cones and where vision is the most acute.
Ganglion:	A mass, or group, of nerve cells.
Glomeruli (singular – glomerulus):	In the olfactory pathway a structure containing a mass of synapses.
Gustatory:	Relating to the sense of taste.
Hyperopia:	Long-sightedness.
Iris:	The central, coloured portion of the eye.
Lacrimal:	Relating to tears.
Lateral:	Away from the midline of the body (to the left or right).
Ligament:	Fibrous tissue that binds joints together and connects bones and cartilage.
Limbic system:	A group of structures/centres in the brain associated with various emotions and feelings such as anger, fear, sadness and pleasure.
Lipid:	A group of organic compounds, including the fats, oils, waxes, sterols and triglycerides.
Medial:	Towards the midline of the body.

Medulla oblongata:	A part of the brainstem which contains the cardiac and respiratory centres.
Microvilli (microvillus – singular):	Protrusions of the cell membrane which increase its surface area.
Myopia:	Short-sightedness.
Nasopharynx:	The part of the airway that begins in the nose and ends at the soft palate.
Neurone:	Nerve cell.
Olfaction:	The sense of smell.
Olfactory:	Pertaining to the sense of smell.
Olfactory bulb:	A structure of the brain involved in olfaction, the perception of odours.
Papilla (plural – papillae):	Small, nipple-shaped projection.
Parasympathetic nervous system:	Part of the autonomic nervous system.
Pathogen:	An infectious agent that causes disease (for instance, bacteria or virus).
Perilymph:	The clear fluid found between the bony labyrinth and the membranous labyrinth in the inner ear.
Photoreceptor:	Light-sensing neurone.
Pons:	Part of the brainstem, the pons contains centres that deal with sleep, swallowing, hearing, equilibrium, taste, eye movement and many other functions.
Posterior:	Located at, or related to, the rear of a structure.
Presbyopia:	The loss of the ability to focus on close objects as the person ages.
Pupil:	The opening in the centre of the iris of the eye that allows light to enter.
Pupillary constrictor muscles:	Smooth muscles contained within the iris of the eye when stimulated they lead to the constriction of the pupil.
Pupillary dilator muscles:	Smooth muscles contained within the iris of the eye; when stimulated they lead to the dilation of the pupil.
Reflex:	Involuntary function or movement in response to a stimulus.
Refraction:	The change of direction of light as it passes from one medium to another with a different density.

Snellen Chart: Standardised chart for testing visual acuity.

Sympathetic nervous system: Part of the autonomic nervous system.

Synapse: A gap between two neurones or a neurone and an organ across which neurotransmitters diffuse to transmit a nerve impulse.

Synovial joint: A freely moving joint in which bony surfaces are covered with cartilage and connected by ligaments lined with a synovial membrane. The membrane secretes a lubricating fluid and keeps it around the joint.

Thalamus: A pair of structures in the brain that relay messages from most of the special senses.

Transparent: Clear, can see through it.

Umami: The 'fifth taste' related to proteins found in meat and fish.

Visual acuity: Detailed central vision.

References

Jenkins, G.W., Kemnitz, C.P. and Tortora, G.J. (2007) *Anatomy and Physiology: From Science to Life.* Hoboken, NJ: John Wiley & Sons.

Marieb, E.N. and Hoehn, K. (2007) *Human Anatomy and Physiology. International Edition*, 7th edn. San Francisco: Pearson Benjamin Cummings.

Martini, F.H. and Nath, J.L. (2009) *Fundamentals of Anatomy and Physiology. Pearson International Edition*, 8th edn. San Francisco: Pearson Benjamin Cummings.

Smith, D.V. and Margolskee, R.F. (2001) Making sense of taste. *Scientific American* 284(3):32–39.

Tortora, G.J. and Derrickson, B.H. (2009) *Principles of Anatomy and Physiology. Volume 1. Organization, Support and Movement, and Control Systems of the Human Body. International Student Version*, 12th edn. Hoboken, NJ: John Wiley & Sons.

Activities

www.wiley.com/go/peate

Multiple choice questions

1. What percentage of inhaled air passes the olfactory organs?

   (a) 2%
   (b) 4%
   (c) 5%
   (d) 10%

2. What is the purpose of the eustachian tube?

   (a) to equalise the pressure between the outer ear and the nasopharynx
   (b) to equalise the pressure between the inner ear and the nasopharynx
   (c) to equalise the pressure between the middle ear and the nasopharynx
   (d) to equalise the pressure between the inner ear and middle ear

3. The utricle and saccule of the ear are stimulated by:

   (a) gravity
   (b) linear acceleration
   (c) rotation of the head
   (d) vertical acceleration

4. The organ of Corti is found in:

   (a) the vestibulocochlear duct
   (b) the tympanic duct
   (c) the vestibular duct
   (d) the cochlear duct

5. Information about the volume and pitch of a sound are transmitted to the brain via a branch of which cranial nerve:

   (a) VI
   (b) VIII
   (c) IX
   (d) X

6. The eyelids are made of:

   (a) elastic cartilage
   (b) connective tissue
   (c) muscle tissue
   (d) epithelial tissue

7. The coloured part of the eye is known as:

   (a) uvea
   (b) cornea
   (c) iris
   (d) choroid body

8. Photoreceptors are found in:

   (a) the fibrous tunic
   (b) the neural part of the neural tunic
   (c) the vascular tunic
   (d) the pigmented part of the neural tunic

9. Rods are mostly found where in the retina:
   (a) centre
   (b) periphery
   (c) optic disc
   (d) fovea

10. The majority of the refraction of light in the eye happens:
   (a) when the light enters the lens of the eye
   (b) when the light enters the pupil
   (c) when the light enters the posterior cavity
   (d) when the light enters the cornea of the eye

Test your learning

1. Name the five basic tastes.
2. Name the three types of papillae that contain taste buds.
3. Describe the mechanism for sensing gravity and linear acceleration.

Label the diagram

From the lists of words, label the diagrams below:

Eyelash, Eyebrow, Pupil, Iris, Upper eyelid (palpebra), Lacrimal caruncle, Lateral commissure, Palpebral fissure, Lower eyelid (palpebra), Conjunctiva (over sclera), Medial commissure

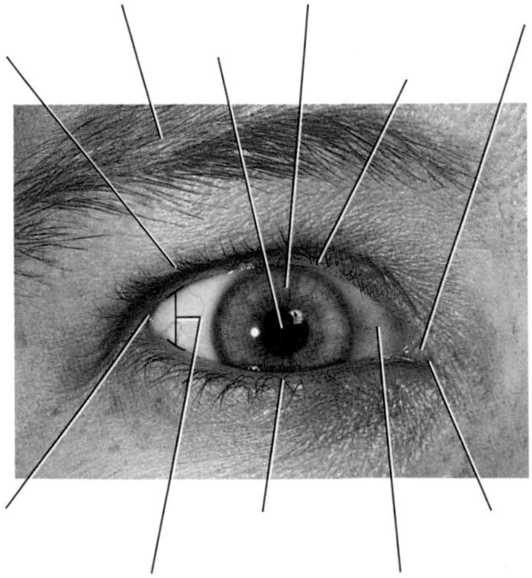

Light ray before refraction, Air, Water, Light ray after refraction

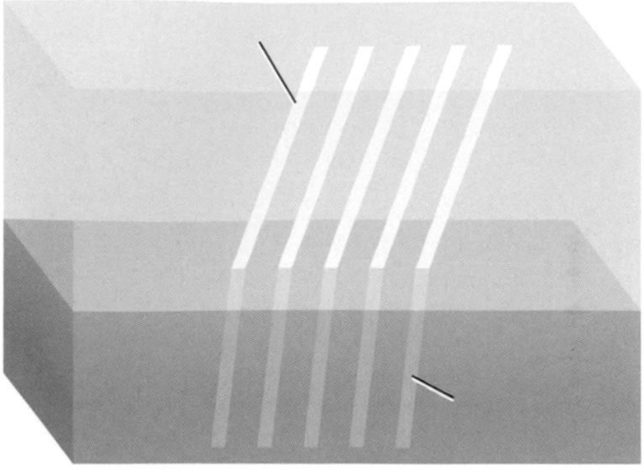

Crossword

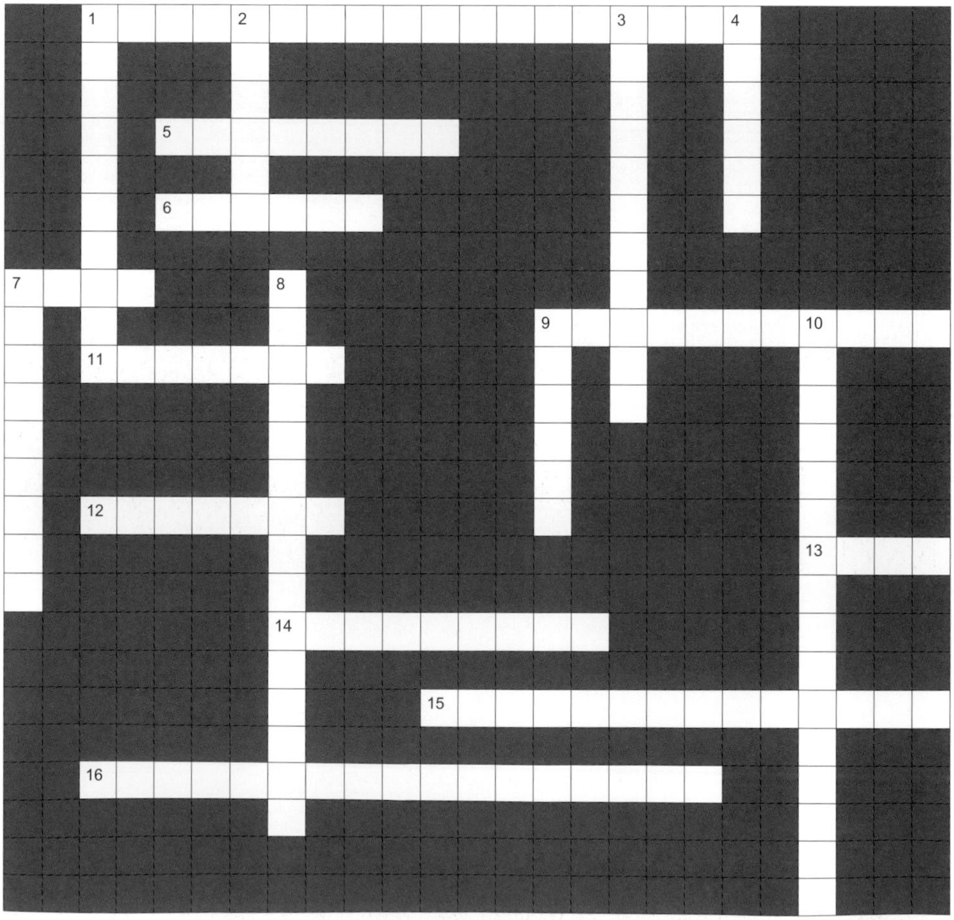
1
2
3
4
5
6
7
8
9
10
11
12
13
14
15
16

Across:

1. Structures of the inner ear that contain the ducts that respond to rotational movement of the head (12, 6).
5. The bones of the middle ear (8).
6. 'Stirrup', one of 5 across (6).
7. The adjustable focusing structure of the eye (4).
9. Epithelial cell layer that lines the outer surface of the eye (11).
11. Structure of the inner ear that contains 2 down (singular) (7).
12. Spiral-shaped bony chamber of the inner ear (7).
13. Central, coloured part of the eye (4).
14. Clear fluid found between the bony labyrinth and the membranous labyrinth (9).
15. Gel-like substance found in the posterior cavity of the eye (8, 6).
16. Reduced perception of a persistent smell (7, 10).

Down:

1. Calcium carbonate crystals found in the utricle and saccule (10).
2. Area of the wall of the ampulla of the inner ear that contains the receptors (6).
3. Retina (6, 5).
4. The 'white' of the eye (6).
7. Fibrous tissues that bind joints together (9).
8. Largest of the peg-like structures containing taste buds, found at the back of the tongue (plural) (7, 8).
9. The majority of the refraction of light in the eye happens here (6).
10. Eardrum (8, 8).

Look at the following diagrams:

1. Which of the diagrams shows an eye with myopia?
2. Which of the diagrams shows an eye with corrected myopia (using a lens)?
3. Which of the diagrams shows an eye with hyperopia?
4. Which of the diagrams shows an eye with corrected hyperopia (using a lens)?

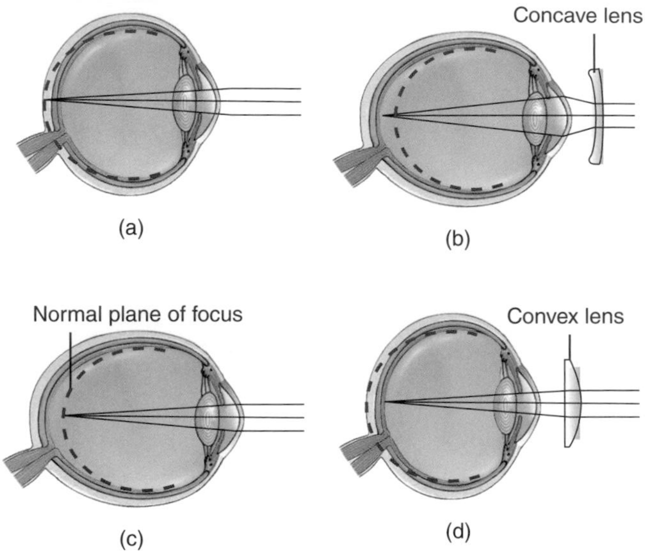
Concave lens
(a)
(b)
Normal plane of focus
Convex lens
(c)
(d)

Conditions

Below is a list of conditions that are associated with the special senses. Take some time and write notes about each of the conditions. You may make the notes taken from text books or other resources, for example, people you work with in a clinical area, or you may make the notes as a result of people you have cared for. If you are making notes about people you have cared for you must ensure that you adhere to the rules of confidentiality.

Anosmia	
Ageusia	
Ménière's disease	
Otosclerosis	
Tinnitus	
Glaucoma	
Macular degeneration	
Retinal detachment	
Cataracts	
Retinopathy	

Answers

MCQs

1a; 2c; 3a; 4d; 5b; 6d; 7c; 8b; 9b; 10d

Crossword

Across:		**Down:**	
1.	Semicircular canals	**1.**	Statoconia
5.	Ossicles	**2.**	Crista
6.	Stapes	**3.**	Neural tunic
7.	Lens	**4.**	Sclera
9.	Conjunctiva	**7.**	Ligaments
11.	Ampulla	**8.**	Vallate papillae
12.	Cochlea	**9.**	Cornea
13.	Iris	**10.**	Tympanic membrane
14.	Perilymph		
15.	Vitreous humour		
16.	Central adaptation		

Look at the following diagrams:

1. Which of the diagrams shows an eye with myopia? c
2. Which of the diagrams shows an eye with corrected myopia (using a lens)? b
3. Which of the diagrams shows an eye with hyperopia? a
4. Which of the diagrams shows an eye with corrected hyperopia (using a lens)? d

17

Genetics

Peter S Vickers

Contents

Introduction	*552*
The double helix	**552**
Nucleotides	553
Bases	553
Chromosomes	**554**
From DNA to proteins	**557**
Protein synthesis	557
Transcription	557
Translation	559
Protein synthesis	559
Summary of protein synthesis	562
The transference of genes	**563**
Mitosis	563
Interphase	564
Prophase	565
Metaphase	565
Anaphase	565
Telophase	565
Cell division	565
Meiosis	565
First meiotic division	567
Second meiotic division	568
Mendelian genetics	**569**
Dominant genes and recessive genes	570
Autosomal dominant inheritance and ill health	571
Autosomal recessive inheritance and ill health	571
Morbidity and mortality of dominant versus recessive disorders	573
X-linked recessive disorders	574
Spontaneous mutation	**575**
Conclusion	*575*
Glossary	*575*
References	*578*
Activities	*579*

Test your knowledge

- Name the components of a chromosome.
- Which process is involved in genetic knowledge transfer from parents to children, and which from cell to cell?

Fundamentals of Anatomy and Physiology for Student Nurses, First Edition. Edited by Ian Peate, Muralitharan Nair.

- Name the stages of mitosis.
- Haemophilia is an inherited X-linked genetic disorder. Who are carriers of the faulty gene, and who can have the disease?

Learning outcomes

On completion of this chapter, you will be able to:

- Understand what a gene is and its importance to our health
- Describe the double helix, including the bases
- Know the difference between DNA and RNA, and their roles in genetics
- Describe the anatomy and functions of a chromosome
- Understand and describe protein synthesis
- Explain cell division
- Understand mendelian genetics and how it relates to gene transfer from parents to children
- Explain the three modes of inheritance – dominant, recessive and X-linked

Anatomical map

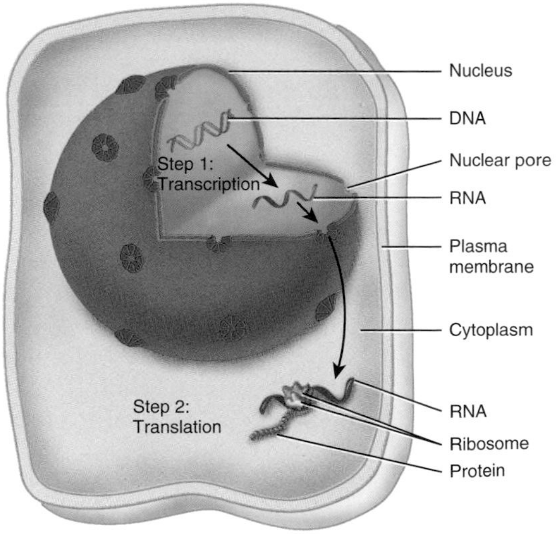
Nucleus
DNA
Nuclear pore
RNA
Plasma membrane
Cytoplasm
RNA
Ribosome
Protein
Step 1: Transcription
Step 2: Translation

Figure 17.1 The cell nucleus (Tortora and Derrickson 2009)

Introduction

Genetics is a very important and endlessly fascinating subject, because we are what our genes make us and many health problems are linked to genes. This chapter will explore just what genes are and their importance to us.

Genes are sections of DNA carried within our **chromosomes**, and these genes contain particular sets of instructions related to our:

- growth
- development
- reproduction
- functioning
- ageing.

and a whole lot of other things.

Basically, we cannot function without our genes, and our genes make us what we are – human for a start. We inherit all our genes from our parents, who in turn inherited theirs from their parents. Our grandparents inherited theirs from their grandparents, and so on.

Already in this chapter various technical terms have been mentioned, so it will help to define what we mean by them. This will help in the understanding of the chapter.

- **DNA** deoxyribonucleic acid – part of the double helix/chromosome
- **RNA** ribonucleic acid, transcribed from DNA
- **mRNA** messenger ribonucleic acid and **tRNA** transfer ribonucleic acid – both these work together with **ribosomes** to produce proteins from **amino acids** which have been coded for by the DNA/gene.

DNA, the essential ingredient of heredity, makes all the basic units of hereditary material – the genes. The capacity of DNA to replicate itself constitutes the basis of hereditary transmission and it provides our genetic code by acting as a template for the synthesis of mRNA.

RNA and mRNA determine the amino acid composition of proteins, which in turn determines the function of those proteins and therefore the function of a particular cell.

Each chromosome, a complicated strand of DNA and protein, is made up of two **chromatids** joined by a **centromere**. Each nucleated cell in our body contains, within its genes, all the genetic material to make an entire human being. Normally, a human has 46 chromosomes (23 pairs) in each nucleated cell – 22 pairs of autosomes, and either two X chromosomes (female) or one X chromosome and one Y chromosome (male). The exception to this are the cells involved in reproduction (gametes – ovum and spermatozoa), which have one copy of each chromosome (23 chromosomes). However, some people have more than 46 chromosomes (e.g. people with Down syndrome have 47 chromosomes, with three copies of chromosome 21 – a condition known as trisomy 21), while others have fewer (e.g. people with Turner's syndrome have 45 chromosomes, because they only have only one X chromosome, and do not have either a second X chromosome or a Y chromosome).

The double helix

The **double helix** was famously discovered in the 1950s by two Cambridge scientists, James Watson and Francis Crick, who were awarded a Nobel prize for their work (although due regard

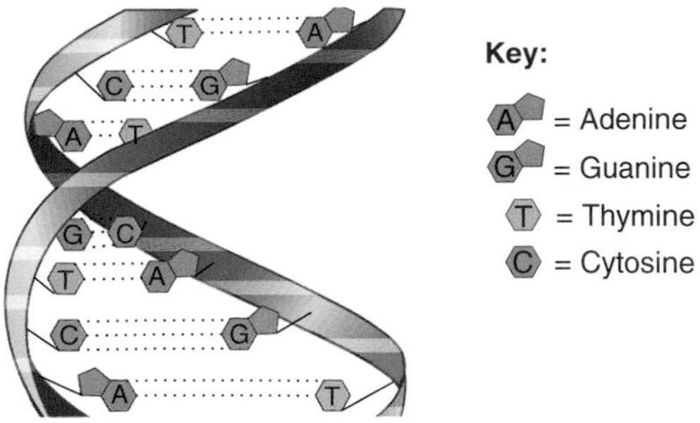
Key:
= Adenine
= Guanine
= Thymine
= Cytosine

Figure 17.2 A pictorial representation of a portion of the double helix (Tortora and Derrickson 2009)

must be paid to Rosalind Franklin who led the way with x-ray crystallography of genes, and who unfortunately died before she could be considered for the Nobel prize). So what exactly is the double helix and why is it important? Well, first of all look at the drawing (Figure 17.2) of part of the double helix.

The double helix is made up of two strands of DNA. It is a spiral molecule, resembling a ladder, with rungs built up of pairs of **bases**. To be more precise, the genetic information is encoded in a linear sequence of chemical subunits, called **nucleotides**.

Nucleotides

Nucleotides consist of three molecules:

- **Deoxyribose** – a 5-carbon cyclic sugar
- **Phosphate** – an inorganic, negatively charged molecule
- **Base** – a nitrogen-carbon ring structure.

The biochemistry of DNA can become quite complex, but remember that the double helix is like a ladder and consists of two parallel **deoxyribose** and **phosphate** supports and a series of bases which make up the rungs of the ladder (known as **strands** – so they are really deoxyribose-phosphate strands).

But what are the bases? It is necessary to explore these next because the bases are those elements of the double helix that carry the genetic code and determine what we look like and how we function.

These bases are arranged in different sequences along the deoxyribose-phosphate supports of the ladder-like double helix, and it is these different sequences that determine the gene sequences.

Bases

There are four bases found in DNA:

- **Adenine** (A)
- **Thymine** (T)

- **Guanine** (G)
- **Cytosine** (C).

As stated above, it is the order of the bases along the length of the DNA molecule that provides the variation, which in turn allows for the storage of genetic information. More important than the order of the individual bases is the order of the pairs of bases.

Look again at the drawing of the double helix (Figure 17.2): each ladder support carries different bases. However, because there are two parallel supports, the bases join together and make the molecule stable. Imagine climbing a ladder where the rungs were all cut and separated in the middle – it would not be very stable, would it? Well, it is the same with the DNA molecule.

However, these bases do not pair haphazardly. Each base is very particular as to which other base it will pair with, and there is a golden rule for you to remember.

Golden Rule

- **Adenine** always pairs with **thymine**
- **Guanine** always pairs with **cytosine**
- So, if one half of the DNA has a base sequence AGGCAGTGC then the opposite side of the DNA will have a complementary base sequence TCCGTCACG.

It is important that you remember this fact, just as it is also very important that you understand two more facts:

- The bases are joined by means of hydrogen/polar bonding (see Chapter 1)
- The individual bases are connected to the deoxyribose of the strand (or support of the ladder) by means of covalent bonds (see Chapter 1).

The reason why this is important is that, as discussed in Chapter 1, hydrogen bonds are not as strong as covalent bonds and so can separate more easily. The importance of this biochemical fact will become apparent when we discuss DNA replication and protein synthesis (Jorde *et al.* 2006).

Chromosomes

Now we can turn our attention to chromosomes.

There is already a brief definition of chromosomes to be found near the beginning of this chapter, so what else can be said about them? Well, the first thing to say is that the chromosome does not consist only of DNA. Rather, the nuclear DNA (also known as **nucleic acid**) of eukaryotes is combined with some protein molecules known as **histones**.

The DNA and histones together make up the **nucleosomes** contained within the cell nucleus. This nucleic acid – histone complex is known as **chromatin**.

Now we run into a problem: if we unravelled all the nucleic acid from every cell in a human adult body, it would stretch to the moon and back about 8,000 times. So how do we manage to package that number of DNA and histone molecules into our rather small bodies? The answer, of course, is that we have to fold them so that they fit into each cell of the body – just like having to fold clothes to ensure that they fit into a suitcase when going on holiday. And just as clothes often will only fit in the suitcase if they are neatly folded, the same applies to the chromatin in our cells. It cannot just be pushed in haphazardly – it would never fit and there would be a great chance of things going wrong.

Consequently, the chromosomes twist on one another, then are arranged in loops, before finally assuming the shape that is commonly recognised as a chromosome – the X shape which is easily seen in a human cell (Figure 17.3) (Jorde *et al.* 2006).

Let us look in more detail at chromosomes. Each chromosome is made up of two chromatids joined by a centromere. Looking at Figure 17.3, you can see that one half of the chromosome is a chromatid, and where they join near the top of the X, that is the centromere (Figure 17.3).

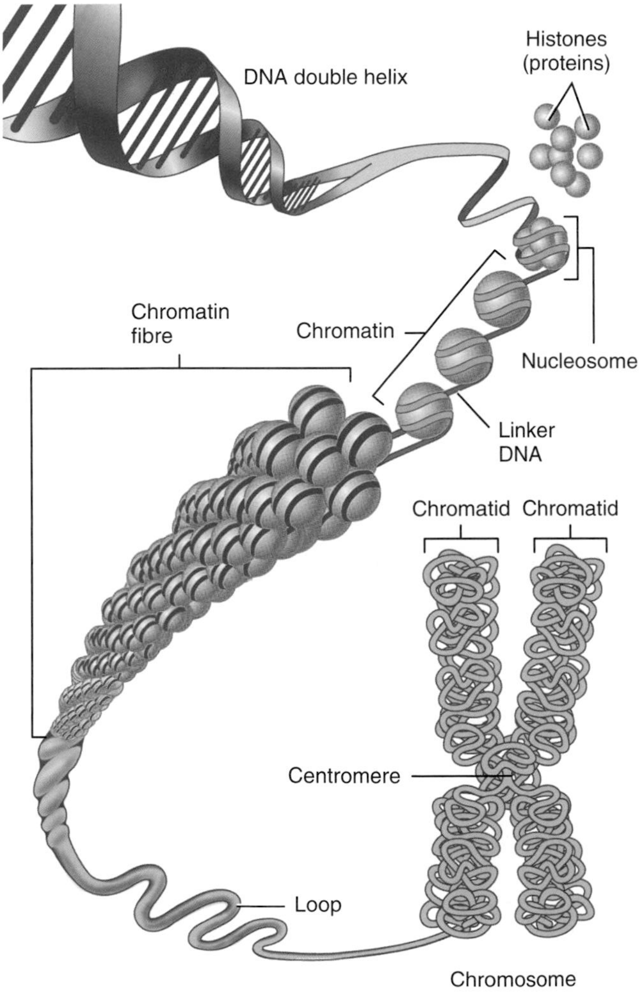
DNA double helix
Histones (proteins)
Chromatin fibre
Chromatin
Nucleosome
Linker DNA
Chromatid
Chromatid
Centromere
Loop
Chromosome

Figure 17.3 DNA from double helix to chromosome (Tortora and Derrickson 2009)

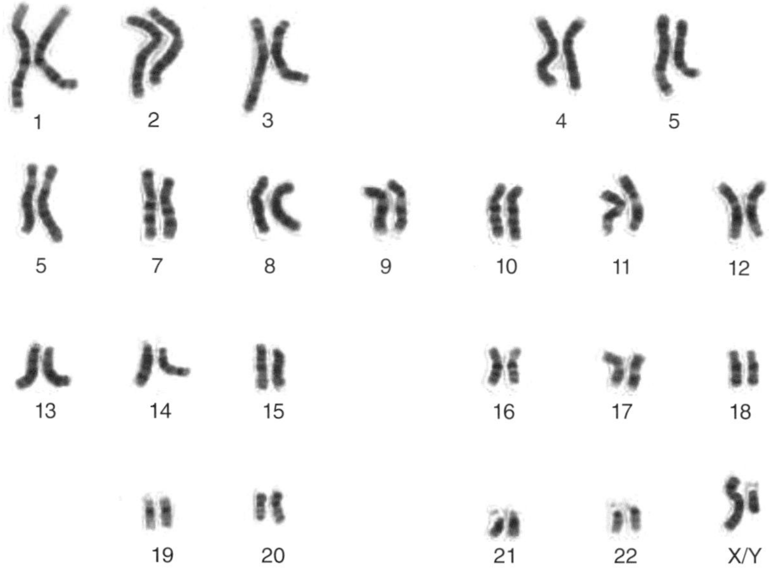
1
2
3
4
5
5
7
8
9
10
11
12
13
14
15
16
17
18
19
20
21
22
X/Y

Figure 17.4 Male human chromosomes (Lister Hill National Center for Biomedical Communications (2010) Genetics Home Reference: Your Guide to Understanding Genetic Conditions (p. 19) http://ghr.nlm.nih.gov/handbook.pdf)

In most humans, each nucleated body cell (i.e. each body cell with a nucleus) has 46 chromosomes, arranged in 23 pairs (Figure 17.4). Of those 23 pairs, one pair determines the gender of the person.

- Females have a matched **homologous** pair of X chromosomes.
- Males have an unmatched **heterologous** pair – one X and one Y chromosome.

Homologous means 'the same'; heterologous means 'different'.

- The remaining 22 pairs of chromosomes are known as **autosomes**. In biology the word 'some' means body, so autosome means 'self body'. This word, 'autosome', can be defined as the chromosomes that determine physical/body characteristics – in other words, all the characteristics of a person that are not connected with gender.

The position a gene occupies on a chromosome is called a **locus**, and there are different **loci** for colour, height, hair, etc. ('loci' is the plural of 'locus'). Think of the locus as the address of that particular gene on Chromosome Street – just like your address signifies that that is where you live.

Genes that occupy corresponding loci are called **alleles**. In other words, the gene for the same characteristic on each of the two chromatids is an allele. Alleles are found at the same place in each of the two corresponding chromatids, and an allele determines an alternative form of the same characteristic. Remembering that one of your chromatids comes from your mother and the other corresponding chromatid comes from your father may be of help in understanding this. As an example, think of the colour of eyes. There is one particular gene that determines eye colour and it is found at the same place on each of the two chromatids of one chromosome. One gene will come from the father and the other from the mother. If parents of a child have different coloured eyes from each other, perhaps the mother has green eyes and the father brown eyes, then the child may have green or brown eyes, depending upon factors that will be discussed later in this chapter.

So each of the genes at that same point (or locus) on each chromatid determines eye colour. This applies to each of a person's characteristics. A person with a pair of identical alleles for a particular gene locus is said to be **homozygous** for that gene, whilst someone with a dissimilar pair is said to be **heterozygous** for that gene.

This section on the chromosome will finish by mentioning a couple of things about genes – and that is that some genes are **recessive** and some genes are **dominant**.

- A dominant gene (known as the **genotype**, i.e. type of gene) is one that exerts its effect and is physically manifested (known as the **phenotype**) when it is present on only one of the chromosomes.
- A recessive gene (genotype) has to be present on both chromosomes in order to manifest itself physically (phenotype).

This will be explained more fully later in this chapter, but it is very important because of the significance that it has in hereditary disorders.

From DNA to proteins

As explained earlier in this chapter, nucleic acids are components of DNA and they have two major functions:

- The direction of all protein synthesis (the production of protein)
- The accurate transmission of this information from one generation to the next (from parents to their children), and from one cell to its daughter cells.

Protein synthesis

Synthesis simply means 'production', so we are talking about the production of protein from raw materials. All the genetic instructions for making proteins are found in DNA, but in order to synthesise these proteins, the genetic information encoded in the DNA has first to be translated.

The first thing that happens in this process is that the DNA has to separate to allow for all of the genetic information in a region of DNA to be copied onto RNA (Figure 17.5). (RNA stands for 'ribonucleic acid, just as DNA stands for deoxyribonucleic acid).

Then, through a complex series of reactions, the information contained in RNA is translated into a corresponding specific sequence of amino acids in a newly produced protein molecule.

So we will look at this process in more detail. To make it easier to understand, we will break the process into two sections – **transcription** and **translation**.

Transcription

In transcription, the DNA has to be transcribed into RNA because our bodies cannot work with DNA as it stands. By using a specific portion of the cell's DNA as a template, the genetic information stored in the sequence of bases of DNA is rewritten so that the same information appears in

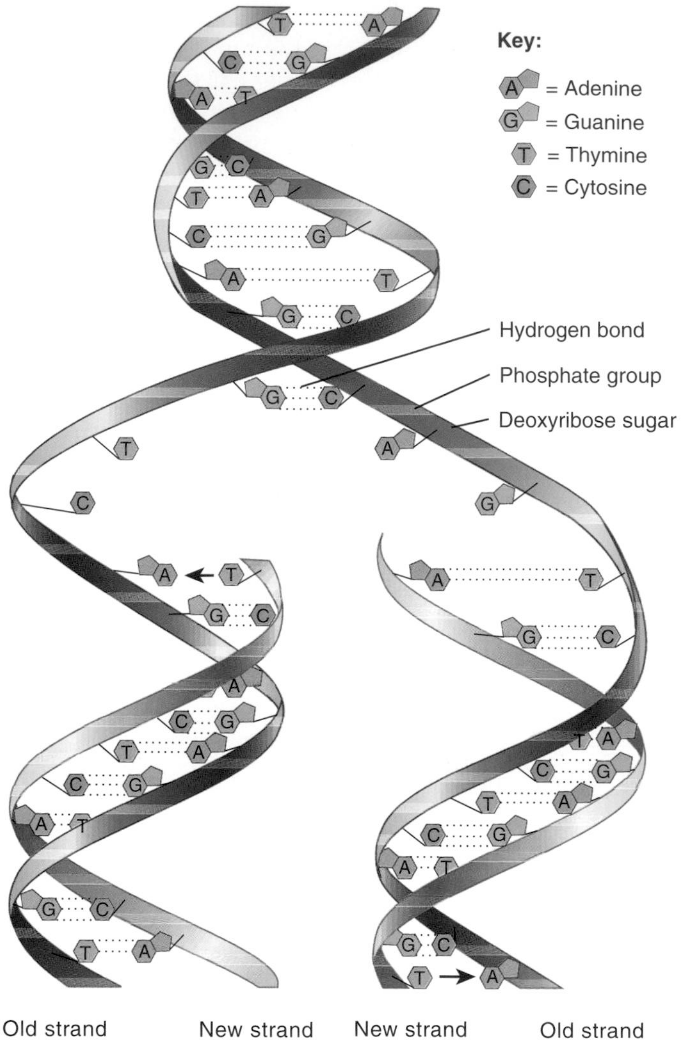
Key:
A = Adenine
G = Guanine
T = Thymine
C = Cytosine
Hydrogen bond
Phosphate group
Deoxyribose sugar
Old strand
New strand
New strand
Old strand

Figure 17.5 The separation of DNA (Tortora and Derrickson 2009)

the bases of RNA. To do this, the two strands of the DNA have to separate, and the bases that are attached to each strand then pair up with bases that are attached to strands of RNA. As with the two strands of DNA, the bases of DNA can only join up with a specific base of RNA (think back to the Golden Rule).

- As with DNA, guanine can only join up with cytosine in RNA.
- But whilst the thymine in DNA can only join to adenine in the RNA, there is no thymine in RNA.
- So, adenine joins to a new base called uracil (U) in mRNA.

DNA mRNA

guanine (G) – cytosine (C)
cytosine (C) – guanine (G)
thymine (T) – adenine (A)
adenine (A) – uracil (U)

For example, if DNA has a base sequence AGGCAGTGC, then mRNA will have a complementary base sequence UCCGUCACG.

Figure 17.4 shows the way in which the DNA separates and makes more DNA. The same process occurs during transcription, except the new strand with its bases is RNA rather than DNA.

Question: In the DNA sequence below, what should the RNA bases be?

C A G C T G C A

Answer: **G U C G A C G U**

So, in the process of transcription, DNA acts as a template for mRNA. However, in addition to serving as the template for the synthesis of mRNA, DNA also synthesises two other kinds of RNA – rRNA and tRNA:

- rRNA = ribosomal RNA – rRNA, together with the ribosomal proteins, makes up the ribosomes.
- tRNA = transfer RNA – this is responsible for matching the code of the mRNA with amino acids.

Once prepared and ready, mRNA, rRNA and tRNA leave the nucleus of the cell and in the cytoplasm of the cell commence the next step in protein synthesis, namely **translation**.

Translation

Translation allows us to make sense of what we have before us. In genetics, translation is the process by which information in the bases of mRNA is used to specify the amino acid of a protein (proteins are composed of amino acids). This involves all three types of RNA, as well as ribosomal proteins.

The key steps are shown in the next section.

Protein synthesis

The key steps of protein synthesis (the production of proteins from DNA) are shown in Figure 17.6 and Figure 17.7.

- In the cytoplasm, a small ribosomal subunit (see Chapter 2, Cells) binds to one end of the mRNA molecule
- There is a total of 20 different amino acids in the cytoplasm that may take part in protein synthesis

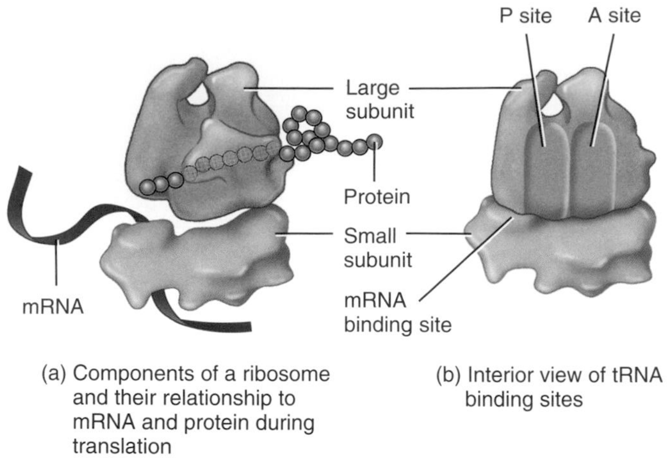
P site
A site
Large subunit
Protein
Small subunit
mRNA
mRNA binding site
(a) Components of a ribosome and their relationship to mRNA and protein during translation
(b) Interior view of tRNA binding sites

Figure 17.6 mRNA becomes associated with small ribosomal subunit (Tortora and Derrickson 2009)

- The amino acid comes from the food that we eat, and is then taken up by the cells
- For each amino acid there is a different small tRNA strand of just three bases (known as a **triplet**).

Now follow the rest of this description of translation alongside Figure 17.5:

- A tRNA triplet picks up the selected amino acid
- This triplet is known as an **anticodon** – an important word to remember
- One end of the tRNA anticodon couples with a specific amino acid – it has receptors on it that only allow it to couple with that particular type of amino acid
- The other end of the tRNA anticodon has a specific sequence of bases
- That tRNA anticodon then seeks out the corresponding three bases on the mRNA strand that is bound to the small ribosomal subunit
- These three bases are known as a codon
- By means of base pairing, the anticodon of the specific tRNA molecule recognises the corresponding codon of the mRNA strand and attaches to it. For example, if the anticodon is **UAC**, then the mRNA **codon** is **AUG**
- In the process of attaching itself to the mRNA codon, the tRNA anticodon brings the specific amino acid with it
- This base pairing of codon and anticodon only occurs when the mRNA is attached to a ribosome
- Once the first tRNA anticodon attaches to the mRNA strand, the ribosome moves along the mRNA strand and the second tRNA anticodon, along with its specific amino acid, moves into position
- The two amino acids that are attached to the two tRNA anticodons (which in turn are paired to the mRNA codons) are joined by a peptide bond
- The larger ribosomal subunit contains the enzymes that organise the joining of the amino acids together

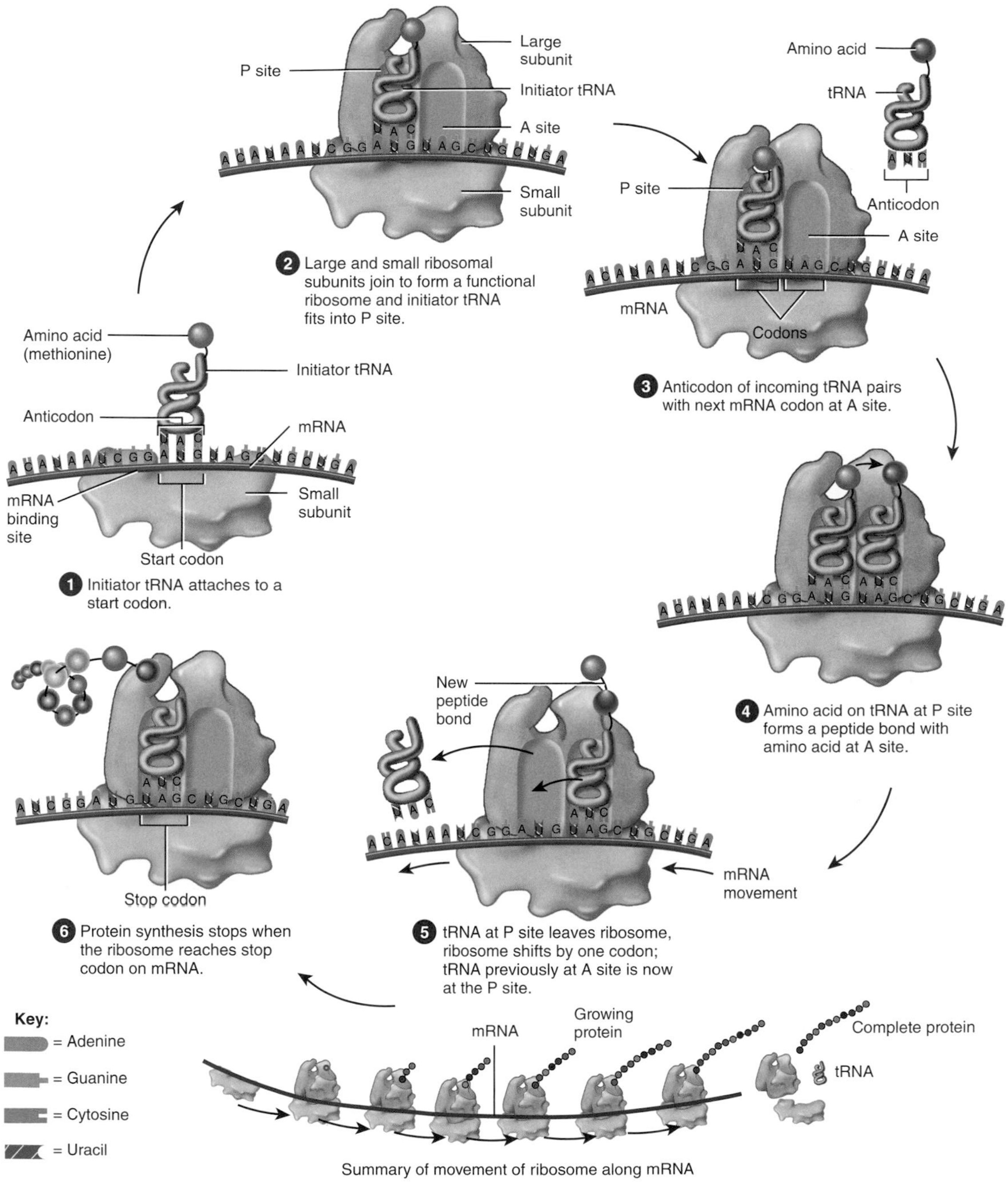

Large subunit
P site
Initiator tRNA
A site
Small subunit
2 Large and small ribosomal subunits join to form a functional ribosome and initiator tRNA fits into P site.
Amino acid
tRNA
Anticodon
P site
A site
mRNA
Codons
3 Anticodon of incoming tRNA pairs with next mRNA codon at A site.
Amino acid (methionine)
Initiator tRNA
Anticodon
mRNA
mRNA binding site
Small subunit
Start codon
1 Initiator tRNA attaches to a start codon.
4 Amino acid on tRNA at P site forms a peptide bond with amino acid at A site.
New peptide bond
mRNA movement
5 tRNA at P site leaves ribosome, ribosome shifts by one codon; tRNA previously at A site is now at the P site.
Stop codon
6 Protein synthesis stops when the ribosome reaches stop codon on mRNA.
Key:
= Adenine
= Guanine
= Cytosine
= Uracil
mRNA
Growing protein
Complete protein
tRNA
Summary of movement of ribosome along mRNA

Figure 17.7 Summary of the movement of the ribosome along mRNA (Tortora and Derrickson 2009)

- Once this has happened, the first tRNA anticodon detaches itself from the mRNA strand and then goes back into the body of the cell to pick up another molecule of its specific amino acid
- Meanwhile, the ribosome moves along the strand of mRNA
- The smaller ribosomal subunit then moves along the mRNA strand and the process keeps continues in the same way
- As more amino acids are detached by their tRNAs, the protein becomes increasingly longer
- As the correct amino acids are brought into line, one by one, peptide bonds are formed between them and the protein becomes progressively larger
- This process is continued until the protein specified by the mRNA strand (which was initially specified by the genes on the DNA strand) is complete – in other words, the correct number of amino acids have been joined together in the correct order
- Once the specified protein is completed, further synthesis of amino acids/protein is stopped by a special codon known as a **termination codon**
- This effectively blocks any further codon/anticodon base pairing
- A termination codon is a combination of three bases that signal the end of the protein synthesis process for that particular protein
- When the termination codon occurs, the assembled new protein is released from the ribosome, and the ribosome separates again into its two discrete component subunits.

Although this process of protein synthesis has probably taken a long time to work through, the process is actually very quick. In fact, protein synthesis progresses at the rate of about 15 amino acids per second.

Summary of protein synthesis

- As each ribosome moves along the mRNA strand, it 'reads' the information coded in the mRNA and synthesises a protein according to that information
- The ribosome synthesises the protein by translating the codon sequence into an amino acid sequence
- As the ribosome moves along the mRNA, and before it completes translation of the first gene into protein, another ribosome may attach to the beginning of the mRNA strand and begin translation of the same strand to form a second copy of the protein. So, several ribosomes moving simultaneously in tandem along the same mRNA molecule permit the translation of a single mRNA strand into several identical proteins simultaneously
- Thus we can now define a gene as a group of nucleotides on a DNA molecule that serves as the master mould for manufacturing a specific protein
- Genes average about 1,000 pairs of nucleotides, which appear in a specific sequence on the DNA molecule
- No two genes have exactly the same sequence of nucleotides, and this is the key to heredity.

Remember now that:

- The base sequence of the gene determines the sequence of bases in the mRNA
- The sequence of the bases in the mRNA determines order and types of amino acids that will form the protein (Figure 17.8).
- Each gene is responsible for making a particular protein, and the process is in the following order:

(Jorde *et al.* 2006)

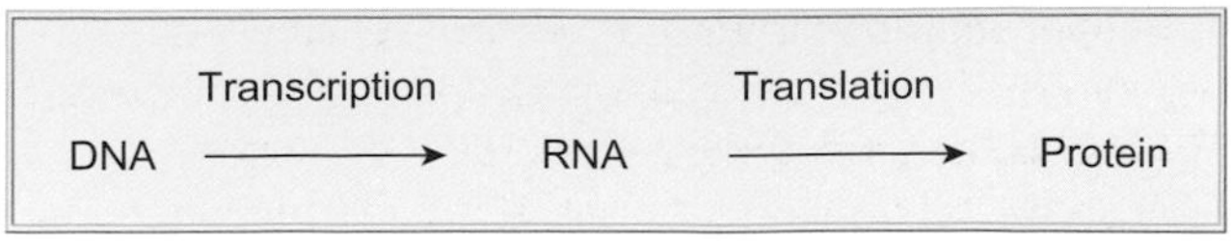
Transcription
Translation
DNA
RNA
Protein

Figure 17.8 Brief summary of protein synthesis

The transference of genes

This section discusses how genetic information is transferred from cells to new cells, and also from parents to children. The first thing to do is to look at how cells pass on genetic information to new cells.

In order for the body to grow, and also for the replacement of body cells that die, our cells must be able to reproduce themselves, but in order for genetic information not to be lost, they must be able to reproduce themselves accurately. They do this by cloning themselves.

In some organisms this occurs by simple fission, whereby the nucleus in a single cell becomes elongated and then divides to form two nuclei in the same cell, each of which carries identical genetic information. The cytoplasm then divides in the middle between the two nuclei, and so two identical daughter cells result, each with its own nucleus and other essential organelles.

The process of transference of genes (or reproduction of cells carrying genetic information) is divided into two stages – **mitosis** and **meiosis**.

Mitosis

This section commences by looking at the way that cells reproduce, particularly how they reproduce their genetic material.

In humans, cell reproduction takes place using a complex process called **mitosis**, in which the number of chromosomes in the daughter cells has to be the same as in the original parent cell.

In the figures below, only a few of the chromosomes are depicted in order to improve the clarity of the figures.

Mitosis can be divided into four stages:

- Prophase
- Metaphase
- Anaphase
- Telophase.

Before and after it has divided, the cell enters a stage known as **interphase**.

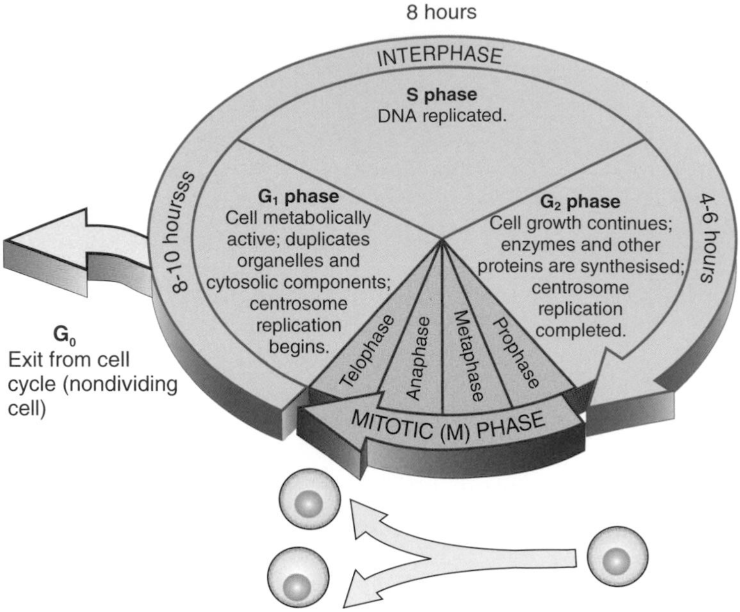
8 hours
INTERPHASE
S phase
DNA replicated.
8-10 hoursss
G$_1$ phase
Cell metabolically active; duplicates organelles and cytosolic components; centrosome replication begins.
G$_2$ phase
Cell growth continues; enzymes and other proteins are synthesised; centrosome replication completed.
4-6 hours
G$_0$
Exit from cell cycle (nondividing cell)
Telophase
Anaphase
Metaphase
Prophase
MITOTIC (M) PHASE

Figure 17.9 The cell cycle (Tortora and Derrickson 2009)

Interphase

Mitosis begins with interphase. This was often thought to be a resting period for the cell, but the cell is actually very busy during this period because it has to get ready for replication. If we look at the **cell cycle** and suppose that one full cycle represents 24 hours, then the actual process of replication (mitosis) would only last for about one of those 24 hours (Figure 17.9). During the rest of the time the cell is undertaking DNA synthesis (i.e. producing DNA). During this period of interphase the cell has to produce two of everything, not just DNA, but all the other organelles in the cell (see Chapter 2, Cells), such as the mitochondria. In addition, the cell has to go through the process of obtaining and digesting nutrition so that it has the raw materials for this duplication and also for the energy that will power the various functions of the cell.

During interphase, the chromosomes in the nucleus are very difficult to see because they are in the form of long threads – they have not yet become super-coiled. They need to be in this state so that they can be duplicated. During the process of duplication, the cells have to ensure that there will be sufficient and accurate genetic material for each of the two daughter cells. The strands of DNA separate and reattach to new strands of DNA. Because of the selectivity of the bases as to which other base they will join in this process, an exact replication of the DNA occurs (Figure 17.5).

In addition, extra cell **organelles** are manufactured or produced by the replication of existing organelles. Also during Interphase, the cell builds up a store of energy, which is required for the process of division.

Prophase

The first stage after interphase is prophase. During prophase, the chromosomes become shorter, fatter and more visible. Each chromosome now consists of two chromatids, each containing the same genetic information (in other words, the DNA has exactly replicated itself during Interphase). These two chromatids are joined together at an area known as the centromere. The two centrosomes move to opposite ends of the cell (the **poles**) and are joined together by the **nuclear spindle**, which stretches from end to end (or pole to pole) of the cell. The centre of the cell is now called the **equator**. Finally, the **nucleolus** and **nuclear membrane** disappear, leaving the chromosomes in the cytoplasm.

Metaphase

During metaphase, the 46 chromosomes (2 of each of the 23 chromosomes) each consisting of two chromatids move to the equator of the nuclear spindle, and here they become attached to the spindle fibres.

Anaphase

During anaphase, the chromatids in each chromosome are separated, and one chromatid from each chromosome then moves towards each pole of the spindle.

Telophase

There are now 46 chromatids at each pole, and these will form the chromosomes of the daughter cells. The cell membrane constricts in the centre of the cell dividing it into two cells. The nuclear spindle disappears, and a nuclear membrane forms around the chromosomes in each of the daughter cells. The chromosomes become long and threadlike again, and are very difficult to see.

Cell division

Cell division is now complete (Figure 17.10) and the daughter cells themselves enter the Interphase stage in order to prepare for their replication and division.

This process of cell division explains how we grow by producing new cells as well as replacing old, damaged and dead cells.

Meiosis

Mitosis is concerned with the reproduction of individual cells, whilst meiosis is concerned with the development of whole organisms – e.g. human beings.

The reproduction of a human being depends upon the fusion of reproductive cells (known as **gametes**) from each of the parents. These gametes are:

- **Spermatozoa** (sperm) from the male
- **Ova** (eggs) from the female.

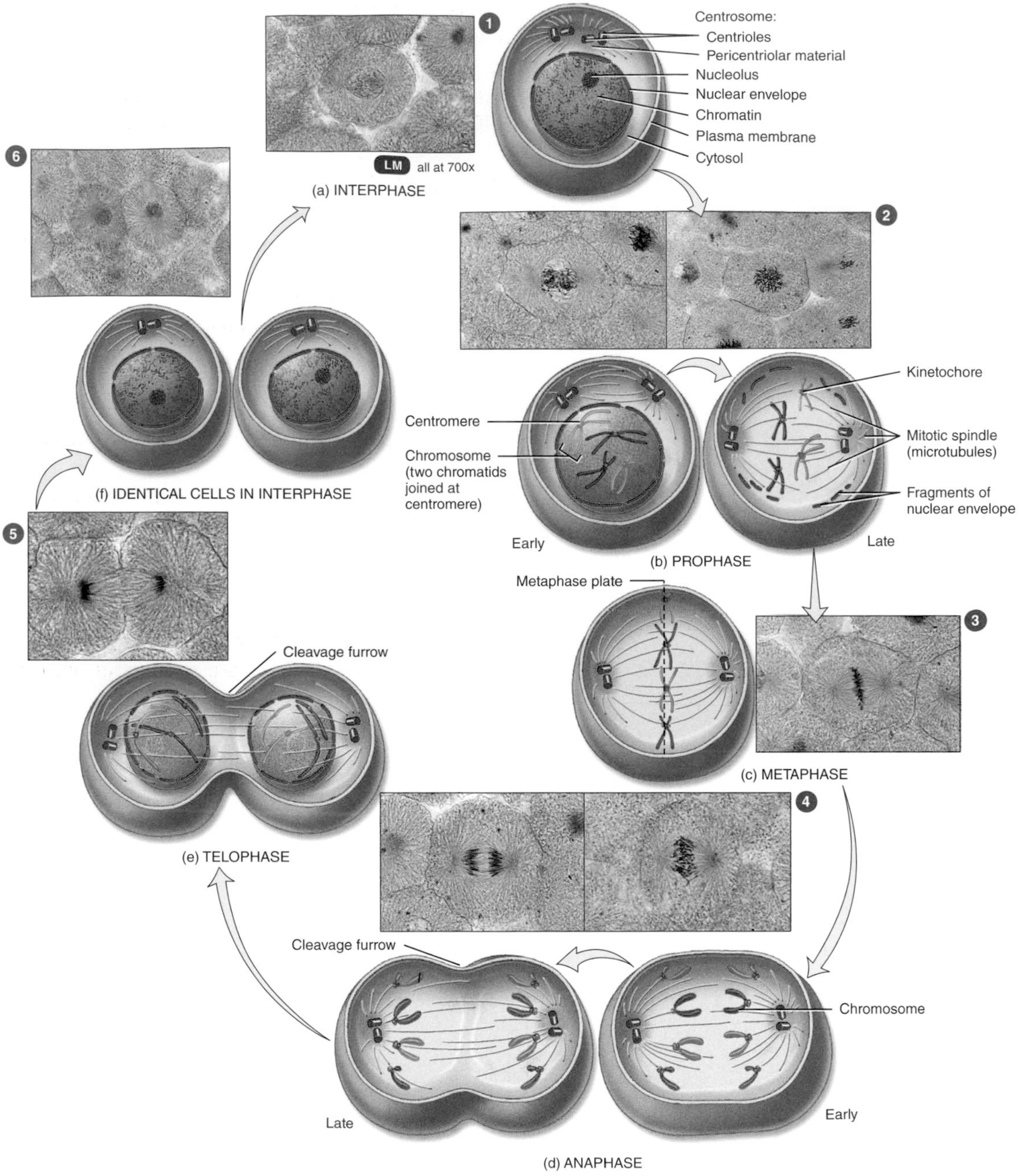
Centrosome:
Centrioles
Pericentriolar material
Nucleolus
Nuclear envelope
Chromatin
Plasma membrane
Cytosol
LM all at 700x
(a) INTERPHASE
Centromere
Chromosome (two chromatids joined at centromere)
Kinetochore
Mitotic spindle (microtubules)
Fragments of nuclear envelope
Early
Late
(b) PROPHASE
Metaphase plate
(c) METAPHASE
Chromosome
Cleavage furrow
Late
Early
(d) ANAPHASE
Cleavage furrow
(e) TELOPHASE
(f) IDENTICAL CELLS IN INTERPHASE
1
2
3
4
5
6

Figure 17.10 Mitosis (Tortora and Derrickson 2009)

Each cell of the human body contains 23 pairs of chromosomes (i.e. 46 in total). It is very important that during the process of human reproduction the cell formed when the gametes fuse has the correct number of chromosomes for a human being (23 pairs). Therefore, each gamete must possess only 23 single chromosomes because when gametes fuse during reproduction, all their chromosomes remain intact in the new life form. If each gamete had a full complement of 46 chromosomes, then the resulting fused cell would possess 92 chromosomes – or four copies of each chromosome rather than the two that a human cell should possess. From then on, each succeeding generation would have double the number of chromosomes, so that after several generations humans would have cells that possess millions and millions of copies of the 23 chromosomes. To stop this happening, the gametes only possess one copy of each chromosome, so that the resulting fused cell has 46 chromosomes, like the parents.

Now you have two new terms to learn and understand – **diploid** and **haploid** cells.

- **Diploid cell:** a cell with a full complement of 46 chromosomes (that is, 23 pairs)
- **Haploid cell:** a cell with only half that number of chromosomes (i.e. 23 single chromosomes).

Gametes are therefore haploid cells, because they only possess one copy of each chromosome, whilst all other cells of the body are diploid cells.

Gametes actually develop from cells with 46 chromosomes, and it is through the process of meiosis that they end up with just 23 chromosomes. Basically, the way that meiosis works is that the cells actually divide twice, without the replication of DNA occurring again before the second division.

For descriptive purposes, meiosis can be divided into eight stages (not the four of mitosis), but rather two meiotic divisions each with four stages. However, they do have the same names, but are given the number I or II. As with mitosis, these stages are continuous with one another.

First meiotic stage

- Prophase I
- Metaphase I
- Anaphase I
- Telophase I

Second meiotic stage

- Prophase II
- Metaphase II
- Anaphase II
- Telophase II

However, there are differences between what happens during the process of mitosis and what happens during meiosis, as well as many similarities.

First meiotic division

Prophase I

Prophase I is similar to the stage of prophase in mitosis. However, instead of being scattered randomly, the chromosomes (consisting of two chromatids) are arranged in pairs – 23 in all. For

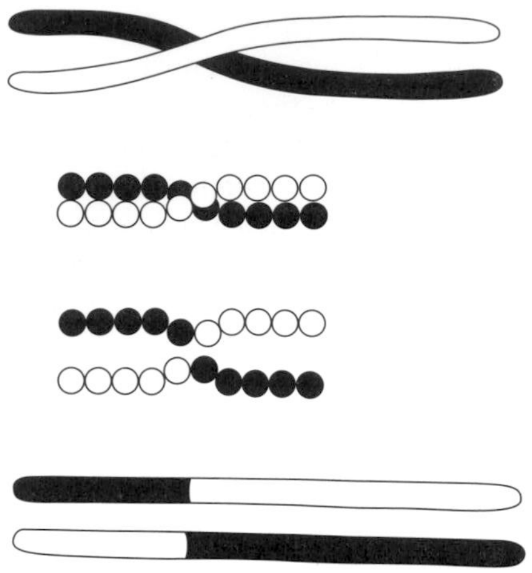

Figure 17.11 Gene crossover

example, the two chromosome ones will pair up, as will the two chromosome twos, and so on. Each pair of chromosomes is called a **bivalent**. Within each pair of chromosomes, genetic material may be exchanged between the two chromosomes, and it is these exchanges that are partly responsible for the differences between children of the same parents. This process is called **gene crossover** (Figure 17.11).

The important point to remember about meiosis is that the DNA is not replicated during the first meiotic division.

Metaphase I

As in mitosis, the chromosomes become arranged on the spindles at the equator. However, they remain in pairs.

Anaphase I

One chromosome from each pair moves to each pole, so that there are now 23 chromosomes at each end of the spindle.

Telophase I

The cell membrane now divides the cell into two halves, as in mitosis. Each daughter cell now has half the number of chromosomes that each parent cell had (Jorde *et al.* 2006).

Second meiotic division

During the second meiotic division, both of the cells produced by the first meiotic division now divide again.

Prophase II, metaphase II, anaphase II and telophase II are all similar to their equivalent stage in mitosis, with the exception that the chromosomes are not replicated, before prophase II, so there are only 23 single chromosomes in each of the granddaughter cells. That way, when the gametes fuse during reproduction, there are still only 23 pairs of chromosomes per human cell, rather than the 46 pairs if the chromosomes had replicated during the **first meiotic division**.

Of the 23 pairs of chromosomes, 22 pairs are autosomal and two chromosomes (i.e. one pair) are the sex chromosomes. Remember, autosomal means 'of the self body' (auto = self; somatic = of the body). In other words, autosomal chromosomes are concerned with the body. On the other hand, the sex chromosomes determine the gender of a person. Male sex chromosomes are designated by the letter Y, and female chromosomes are designated by the letter X. A male will carry the chromosomes XY (an X chromosome from the mother and a Y chromosome from the father), while a female will carry the chromosomes XX (an X chromosome from both the father and the mother).

Mendelian genetics

So far this chapter has examined the biology of genetics, and now it is going to look at the role of genetics in inheritance. This is very important because, as stated early in the chapter, what we are is designated to a large extent by our genetic makeup – which is inherited from our parents. The caveat 'to a large extent' is because as well as being a product of our genes, we are also a product of our environment – time, space, relationships, education, etc.

So how do we inherit our genes from our parents? To understand this we have to return to the 1860s. In Brno (which is now a large town in the Czech Republic but was then a small, sleepy town in Bohemia) there was a monastery, and in that monastery there lived and worked a monk with a very inquiring mind. His name was **Gregor Mendel** and he worked in the monastery gardens where he put his mind to good use trying to perfect the ideal pea. As part of this work, he experimented with cross-breeding. Now, at that time, cross-breeding went on everywhere – on farms and in gardens – and of course we humans cross-breed as well. However, what was different about Mendel was that not only did he experiment with cross-breeding different peas, but he also made notes on his experiments and observations. He introduced three novel approaches to the study of cross-breeding – at least novel for his time, because no one else was doing this. Not only did he observe, but he experimented and observed. Having observed and experimented he then used statistics. He ensured that the original parental stocks, from which his crosses were derived, were pure breeding stocks. (The use of statistics was not at that time fully part of the tradition of biology.)

The phenomena that Mendel discovered/observed were statistical in form: the now famous ratios made sense only in the context of counting large numbers of specimens and calculating averages. However, the methods for evaluating and statistical data did not exist then and were not to be developed for a further 30 years or so. It was only much later that the validity of such an approach could be accepted.

In 1866, Mendel wrote and published a paper on his experiments and the response from the scientific community to this paper was deafening in its silence – his observations and theories were completely ignored until their 'rediscovery' in the early 1900s.

In addition, Mendel's work was carried out not in one of the main centres of science, but at the periphery and it was obscurely published. In science, as in the rest of life, who expresses an idea and where they work affects its reception. This is as true today as it was in 1866. The science of inheritance is based upon what Mendel discovered all those years ago.

So, what did Mendel discover? Well he demonstrated that members of a pair of alleles separate clearly during meiosis (remember that alleles are different sequences of genetic material occupying the same gene locus or place on the DNA, but on different chromosomes).

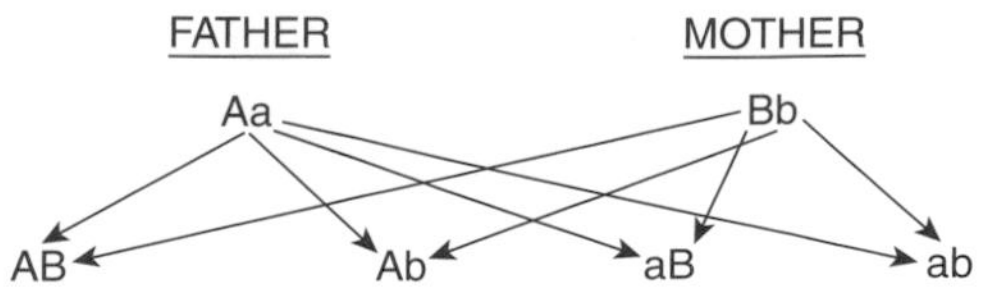
FATHER
MOTHER
Aa
Bb
AB
Ab
aB
ab

Figure 17.12 Genetic inheritance

Remember that we all have a pair of genes (alleles) at each locus, but because of the process of meiosis (discussed above) we can only pass one of those genes to our child.

Figure 17.12 makes things clearer.

At the same locus on a chromosome, the father has the two alleles Aa and the mother has the two alleles Bb. When they reproduce, the father can pass either **gene A** or **gene a** (both are at the same locus and are therefore alleles) and the mother can pass on either **gene B** or **gene b** (again both at the same locus). However, each child can only inherit one of gene A or gene a from the father and one of gene B or gene b from the mother.

What the child cannot do is inherit both gene A and gene a or gene B and gene b. Only one allele from each parent can be inherited by a child. This is known as **Mendel's first law.**

What are the statistical chances of a child inheriting any one of those sets of genes from the parents **AB, Ab, aB, ab**? The answer is 1 in 4 (or 1:4). In other words, there is a 25% chance that any child will inherit one of those pairs of genes from his parents.

So, that brings us to Mendel's second law which asserts that members of different pairs of alleles sort independently of each other during gametogenesis (the production of gametes), and each member of a pair of alleles may occur randomly with either member of another pair of alleles. Note that **gametogenesis** is the production of haploid sex cells which each carry one half the genetic makeup of the parents.

This now brings us to the concept of dominant and recessive genes. This has a great bearing on many health disorders that we may encounter, as well as determining such characteristics as eye colour and hair colour, etc.

Dominant genes and recessive genes

At each locus, the two alleles (genes) can be either dominant or recessive. A **dominant** gene is an allele that will be reflected in the phenotype (the physical manifestation) no matter what the other allele does. By contrast, a recessive gene is one that will only appear in the phenotype if the corresponding allele is also recessive and has the same characteristic as the first allele.

Note that in genetic representations, dominant genes are usually given capital letters, whilst recessive genes are usually given lower-case letters – but not always. Therefore in the figures above and below, one gene is dominant and one is recessive.

Look again at Figure 17.12 – suppose parents had four children and they all had different genotypes (genetic makeup), so that they each were represented by one of the pairs of genes. How many of the offspring would carry at least one dominant gene, and how many would carry only recessive genes at this locus?

The answer is that three of the four children (75%) would carry at least one dominant gene, and one of the four children (25%) would carry both recessive genes. Of course, all four children may inherit the same pair of genes at this locus, or maybe two will inherit the same genes. Mendel's first law is relevant only in saying that there is a 1 in 4 chance at each pregnancy that the children will carry a certain genotype.

Another example – a man with red hair marries a woman with brown hair. As time goes by, they have several children, all of whom have brown hair. Which is the dominant gene for hair colour and who carries it?

The gene for brown hair carried by the mother is the dominant gene in this instance. Their offspring all marry partners with brown hair, but some of their offspring have red hair, like their maternal grandfather. How can this be explained?

There are two possible explanations:

- Some of the children carry the red hair recessive gene from their father and their partners also carry a recessive red hair gene – this is most likely
- The father was not the genetic father of those children.

Autosomal dominant inheritance and ill health

If the dominant gene of one of the parents is one that causes a medical disorder, for example Huntington's disease or neurofibromatosis, what is the risk of any child of those parents having the disease?

The answer is 50% or a one in two risk of a child having an **autosomal dominant disorder**.

Why is this? Look at Figure 17.12, and assume that the father (genes **A** and **a**) carries the mutant gene on gene **A.** As a dominant gene is always expressed in the phenotype, then statistically there will be a 50% chance of any child having the disease, because the child could inherit gene **a**. Of course, any child who carries gene **A** will have a 100% chance of having the disease, there is no escaping it.

Autosomal recessive inheritance and ill health

Autosomal recessive diseases occur when both parents are carrying the same defect on a recessive gene at the same locus. Both parents have to carry the defective gene otherwise the child cannot be affected by the disease.

In autosomal recessive diseases, if the child (or parent) only carried the defect on one gene, then he (or she) is a carrier of that disease and can pass on that defective gene to his (or her) children. They in turn could pass it on to their children, who, if they inherit it, would also be carriers, and this situation could continue through many generations until the carrier has children with someone who is also a carrier of that mutant gene. There is then a risk of their children being either a carrier or having the disorder.

So, then, what are the risks of:

- A child being a carrier of the recessive gene?
- A child having the disease caused by this mutated/abnormal gene?

To work this out, look again at Figure 17.12. In this case, the lower-case letter '**a**' represents the abnormal recessive gene. As can be seen, both parents carry this abnormal gene, for example, for cystic fibrosis – this is a well-known disease that is inherited as an autosomal recessive disorder.

If one of the two recessive genes (**a** or **b**) that code for cystic fibrosis is carried by each of the parents, then the chances at each pregnancy of:

- Having an affected child are 1 in 4 (or 25%)
- Having a child who is a carrier are 2 in 4 (or 50%)
- Having a child who is neither affected nor a carrier is 1 in 4 (or 25%).

Why is this? Look at Figure 17.12 again.

- Only one child has two affected genes (**a** and **b**), and because both affected genes have to be present in order for the disease to appear, this is one child out of four, or 25%
- Only one child does not have an affected gene (**a** and **b**), and so the disease cannot occur, neither can the child be a carrier, because there is no affected gene to be carried, so this is one child out of four, or 25%
- Two children have an affected gene (either **a** or **b**), but they also have an unaffected dominant gene (**A** or **B**).

Whenever there is a dominant gene, the affected recessive gene cannot be expressed in the phenotype (physically) as the dominant gene blocks the action of the affected recessive gene. So, there are two children out of four that lead to the carrier state (or 50%). However, always remember that children who are carriers can pass on the affected gene to their children.

It is important to remember that these odds occur for each pregnancy, so you could have four children and have:

- 1 affected
- 2 carriers and 1 unaffected
- 4 carriers, 3 affected and 1 carrier
- and so on.

Remember that the odds are the same for each child born to those parents (LeMone and Burke 2008).

Clinical considerations

Genetic counselling

Most of the clinical application of genetics in health is, at the moment, the responsibility of doctors and scientists. However, there is one extremely important aspect of genetics in ill health that is within the nurse's scope of practice and that is genetic counselling.

A genetic counsellor has to provide information, offer support to the patient and family, as well as being able to attempt to deal with a patient and family's specific questions and concerns. The inclusion of the family is very important when dealing with genetic illnesses because, particularly if the illness is an inherited one, that has ramifications for the family as a whole. However, if requested, the patient will be seen separately from the family – and indeed, the family may wish to have individual consultations with the genetic counsellor as they may have questions that are particularly relevant to them.

For a consultation, a genetics counsellor will need:

- Knowledge of genetics and genetic diseases
- Knowledge of the variety of treatments available for genetic diseases

- Empathy and respect for the patient and family
- Time and patience
- A box of tissues.

During a consultation, the genetics counsellor will:

- Start to build up a rapport and trust with the patient and family members
- Explain in terms appropriate for the patient/family complex medical and scientific information
- Help the patient/family to make informed and independent decisions concerning the present and future implications of the genetic illness
- Give the patient/family the time to start to come to terms with the information they have received, and help them by repetition and innovative explanations until they have absorbed and understood the situation
- Respect the patient's/family member's individual beliefs and feelings and not attempt to impose their own feelings and beliefs on the situation
- NOT tell anyone what they should do, e.g. advise a couple not to have children, end a pregnancy, undergo testing for a genetic disorder or have specific treatment
- Maintain privacy and confidentiality at all times
- Be truthful as to potential consequences, but emphasise any positives over negatives, for example, if a couple are found to carry an autosomal recessive gene, explain that there is a 1 in 4 chance that any children will be affected and a 2 in 4 chance that any children will be a carrier of the disease, but then tell them that this means that, in fact, there is a 3 in 4 chance that any children will not have the genetic disease. Also, it is important to stress that these odds apply to every pregnancy, so a couple could have four children and all be affected, or they could have four children and none of them be affected
- Allow the patient/family members time to go away and think about the information and its potential ramifications, and arrange for them to be seen again in the near future, as well as be available to answer queries as and when they crop up.

Morbidity and mortality of dominant versus recessive disorders

Autosomal dominant disorders are generally less severe than recessive disorders because if someone carries the affected gene they would have that disorder, whereas with autosomal recessive disorders a person can be a carrier but not have the disease.

If autosomal dominant disorders were as severe and fatal as autosomal recessive disorders, then the disease would die out as all the people with an affected autosomal dominant gene would normally die before being old enough to pass it on to their offspring.

As exception is Huntington's disease, which is a fatal autosomal dominant disorder, but it survives because the symptoms do not usually become apparent until the person with it is in their 30s, by which time they could have passed on the affected gene to their children.

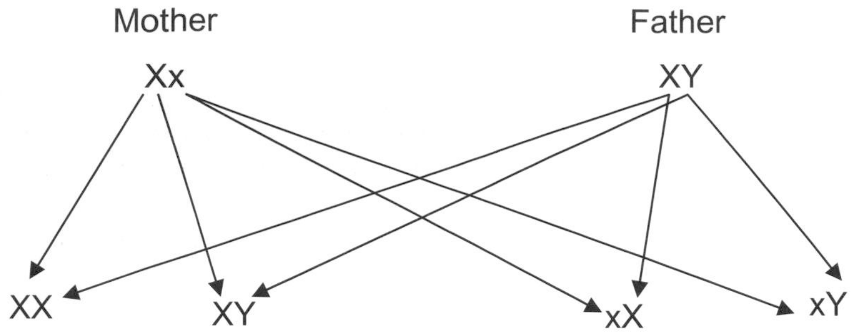
Mother
Xx
Father
XY
XX
XY
xX
xY

Figure 17.13 X-linked inheritance

X-linked recessive disorders

As well as autosomal inheritance, we can also inherit disorders via the sex chromosomes. The main role of these chromosomes is to determine the gender of the baby:

- **XX** = girl
- **XY** = boy.

First of all, look at the possibilities of having a boy or a girl when you decide to have a baby.

From Figure 17.13, it can be seen that the chances for each pregnancy of a boy or a girl are 50%.

Some disorders are only passed on via the X chromosome. Examples are haemophilia and Duchenne muscular dystrophy. With these disorders, only boys are affected and only girls are carriers but are unaffected.

If we consider that the lower-case '**x**' is the affected gene for haemophilia, then what is going to happen?

- The first child is a girl who does not carry the affected gene, but two normal genes, so she is neither a carrier nor affected
- The second child carries a normal X and a Y, so he is a boy who does not carry the abnormal gene – consequently he is neither a carrier nor affected
- The third child is a girl who carries the abnormal gene, but the action of that gene is blocked by the other normal X gene, so she is not affected, but is a carrier
- The fourth child is a boy who carries an abnormal X gene and a normal Y gene. Unfortunately, the Y gene is unable to block the action of the abnormal gene, so he is a carrier and is also affected.

Consequently, we can say that there is a chance that:

- 1 out of 2 girls (50%) will be a carrier
- 1 out of 2 boys (50%) will be affected.

Spontaneous mutation

Now to briefly mention another way in which an unusual or abnormal gene can occur in someone and cause genetic disorders. This is known as **spontaneous mutation**. Because of the great speed and precision needed at each replication of DNA of the germ cells, or of protein synthesis, it is possible for mistakes to occur, and in this way genetic mutations arise.

Finally, there are also the problems of chemical/trauma mutations to consider.

Conclusion

This completes the chapter on basic genetics. Although genetics may appear complicated, it is a very important subject because our genes make us what we are, but also they can leave us susceptible to certain diseases and have a say in how we respond to treatment for diseases, and indeed, how we live our lives, work, develop relationships, and indeed survive in the world.

Glossary

Adenine: One of the four nitrogen – carbon bases of DNA.

Allele: The place on the chromosomes where genes which code for the same function are to be found.

Amino acid: Amino acids, which are coded for by genes, can be considered as the building blocks of proteins.

Anaphase: The stage in cell division where the chromosome separates and moves to the **poles** of the cells.

Anticodon: A triplet of bases on tRNA encoding for **amino acids** that join with other triplets (or anticodons) to produce the appropriate proteins.

Autosome: The name given to chromosomes that are not one of the two sex chromosomes.

Autosomal dominant disorder: A medical disorder caused by a faulty dominant gene inherited from one of the parents.

Autosomal recessive disorder: A medical disorder caused by the same fault on recessive genes inherited from both parents.

Base: Part of the double helix, bases are the code which will eventually lead to the formation of protein.

Bivalent:	A pair of associated homologous chromosomes formed after replication of the chromosomes, with each replicated chromosome consisting of two chromatids.
Cell cycle:	The process by which a cell prepares for, and undertakes, cell growth and division.
Chromatid:	One half of a chromosome.
Centromere:	The point at which two chromatids become attached to form a **chromosome**.
Chromosome:	Mixture of DNA and protein – contains our genetic makeup.
Codon:	A triplet of **bases** on mRNA which encodes for a particular **amino acid**.
Cytosine:	One of the four nitrogen – carbon bases of DNA.
Deoxyribose:	A major part of DNA, deoxyribose is derived from a sugar known as ribose but has lost an atom of oxygen – which leads to its name.
Diploid cell:	A cell which contains two sets of identical chromosomes. See haploid.
DNA:	Deoxyribonucleic acid – part of the double helix.
Dominant gene:	A gene which can exert its effects on the body on its own. In other words, it dominates the recessive gene at the same **locus**.
Double helix:	Two strands of DNA joined together in a spiral formation.
Equator of the cell:	The centre of the cell during cell division.
Gamete:	A reproductive cell, e.g. **spermatozoon** or **ovum**.
Gametogenesis:	The production of gametes.
Gene:	A unit of heredity in a living organism.
Gene crossover:	The process at the commencement of meiosis whereby genetic material may be transferred between chromosomes.
Genotype:	The genotype of a person is her or his genetic makeup. See phenotype.
Guanine:	One of the four nitrogen-carbon bases of DNA.
Haploid cell:	A cell which contains just one set of chromosomes. See diploid.
Heredity:	The passing down of genes from generation to generation.
Heterologous:	'Different' as opposed to **homologous** which means 'the same'.
Heterozygous:	A pair of dissimilar alleles for a particular gene locus. See homozygous.
Histone:	Proteins found in cell nuclei, which package and order the DNA into nucleosomes – so making it possible for the **chromosomes** to be fitted into a cell without becoming tangled.

Homologous: 'The same' – see heterologous.

Homozygous: A pair of identical alleles for a particular gene locus. See heterozygous.

Interphase: The longest stage of the cell cycle, during which the cell is growing and preparing for replication.

Locus: A gene's position on a chromosome.

Meiosis: Concerned with the development of whole organisms and is a process in which diploid cells become haploid cells, so ensuring that the correct number of chromosomes are passed to the offspring.

Mendelian genetics: The genetics of inheritance (named after Gregor Mendel).

Mendel's first law: Only one allele from each parent can be inherited by their child.

Mendel's second law: During gametogenesis, members of different pairs of **alleles** are randomly sorted independently of each other.

Metaphase: The stage in the **cell cycle** when the chromosomes move to the equator of the cell preparatory to separating.

Mitosis: The process by which chromosomes are accurately reproduced in cells during cell division.

mRNA: Messenger ribonucleic acid; it is important in the production of proteins from amino acids.

Nucleic acid: A mixture of phosphoric acid, sugars, and organic bases, nucleic acids direct the course of protein synthesis (or production), so regulating all cell activities. DNA and RNA are nucleic acids.

Nucleosome: The basic unit of DNA once it is packaged in a cell's nucleus; it consists of a segment of DNA wound around a **histone**.

Nucleotide: The name for the parts of DNA consisting of sugar (deoxyribose) and one of the four bases (adenine, thymine, guanine and cytosine). In other words, it is the basis of our genes.

Ova: Female reproductive cells (also known as eggs).

Phenotype: The phenotype is the expressed features of a person, and is derived from the interaction of the **genotype** of a person with the environment.

Phosphate: An inorganic molecule forming part of the double helix.

Poles of the cell: The ends of a cell during the stages of cell division.

Prophase: The first stage of cell division where chromosomes fold together and become more visible.

Recessive gene: A recessive gene requires another recessive gene at the same **locus** before it can have an effect on the body. In other words, it is not dominant over another gene at the same locus.

Ribosomes: Small, bead-like structures in a cell that, along with RNA, are involved in making proteins from amino acids (see Chapter 2, Cells).

RNA: Ribonucleic acid – transcribed from DNA.

Spermatozoa: Male reproductive cells.

Spontaneous mutation disorder: A medical disorder caused by a new fault that has developed on a gene, i.e. neither of the parents carries that faulty gene.

Strand: The long parts of the double helix, consisting of deoxyribose and phosphate.

Telophase: The stage in cell division where the cell actually divides and forms two identical daughter cells.

Termination codon: A triplet of bases that stop the synthesis of amino acids once the specified protein of that sequence have been produced.

Thymine: One of the four nitrogen-carbon bases of DNA.

Transcription: The process by which something with which we cannot work is changed into something that we can. In genetics, this is the changing of DNA into RNA.

Translation: The process that allows us to make sense of what we have in front of us. In genetics, translation is the process by which information in the bases of mRNA is used to specify the amino acid of a protein

Triplet: Sequences of three RNA bases that code for different amino acids.

tRNA: Transfer ribonucleic acid; it is important in the production of proteins from amino acids.

X-linked recessive disease: A medical disorder caused by a fault on the X gene (one of the sex genes). Only females are carriers and only males can have these disorders.

References

Jorde, L.B., Carey, J.C., Bamshad, M.J. and White, R.L. (2006) *Medical Genetics*, 3rd edn. St. Louis, MO: Mosby.

LeMone, P. and Burke, K. (2008) *Medical-Surgical Nursing: Critical Thinking in Client Care*, 4th edn. Upper Saddle River, NJ: Pearson Prentice Hall.

Tortora, G.J. and Derrickson, B.H. (2009) *Principles of Anatomy and Physiology*, 12th edn. Hoboken, NJ: John Wiley & Sons.

Activities

www.wiley.com/go/peate

Multiple choice questions

1. A chromosome is made up of:
   (a) DNA and RNA
   (b) RNA and protein
   (c) DNA and protein
   (d) protein and gene

2. The double helix consists of:
   (a) chromatids and genes
   (b) bases and genes
   (c) bases and nucleotides
   (d) nucleotides and chromatids

3. A person with a pair of identical alleles for a particular gene locus is:
   (a) heterosexual
   (b) homozygous
   (c) homosexual
   (d) heterozygous

4. The two principal steps in protein synthesis are:
   (a) transubstantiation and transmogrification
   (b) translation and transmogrification
   (c) transcription and translation
   (d) transubstantiation and translation

5. For reproduction to take place, the cells need to undergo:
   (a) osmosis
   (b) mitosis
   (c) stenosis
   (d) meiosis

6. The sex chromosomes for a boy are:
   (a) YY
   (b) XX
   (c) XY
   (d) YX

7. Under mendelian genetics, the odds that an affected child will be born to parents who each carry the same defective recessive gene will be for each pregnancy:

   (a) 1:2
   (b) 1:4
   (c) 1:1
   (d) 1:3

8. In the double helix, adenine always pairs with:

   (a) guanine
   (b) cytosine
   (c) uracil
   (d) thymine

9. tRNA is responsible for:

   (a) matching the code of mRNA with amino acids
   (b) producing the bases of the double helix
   (c) pairing with DNA to form a chromosome
   (d) mitosis

10. The phases of mitosis are:

   (a) metaphase, anaphase, gene crossovers, interphase
   (b) metaphase, S phase, prophase, telophase
   (c) S phase, metaphase, prophase, interphase
   (d) prophase, metaphase, anaphase, telophase

Test your learning

1. Describe DNA, RNA, chromosome.
2. Explain how the chromosome is organised so that it can fit in a cell.
3. Explain dominant and recessive genes.
4. List the bases of DNA and their corresponding RNA bases.
5. Describe in your own words the process of protein synthesis.
6. List the stages of mitosis and meiosis.
7. Explain the important of gene crossover during meiosis.
8. Discuss autosomal dominant and autosomal recessive genes in relation to ill health.

Label the diagram

From the lists of words, label the diagrams below:

Nucleus, DNA, Nuclear pore, RNA, Plasma membrane, Cytoplasm, RNA, Ribosome, Protein

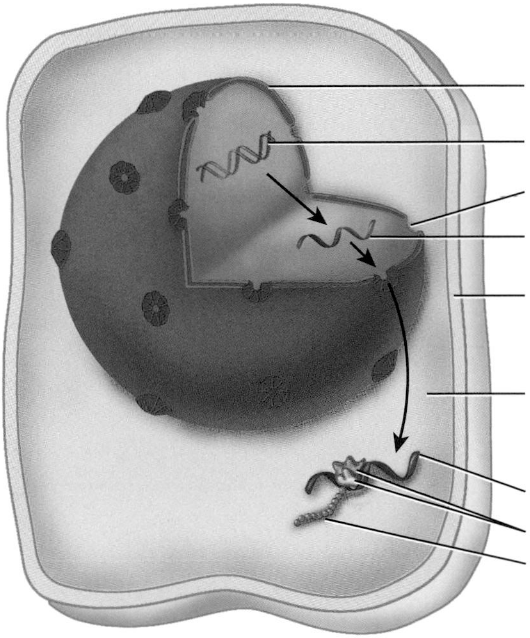

Transcription, Translation, DNA, RNA, Protein

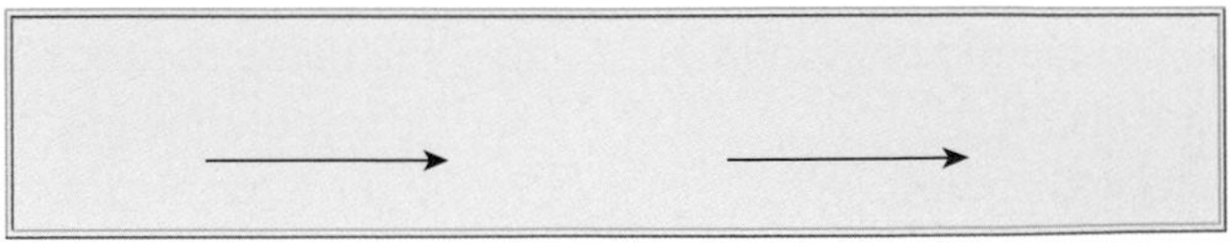

Crossword

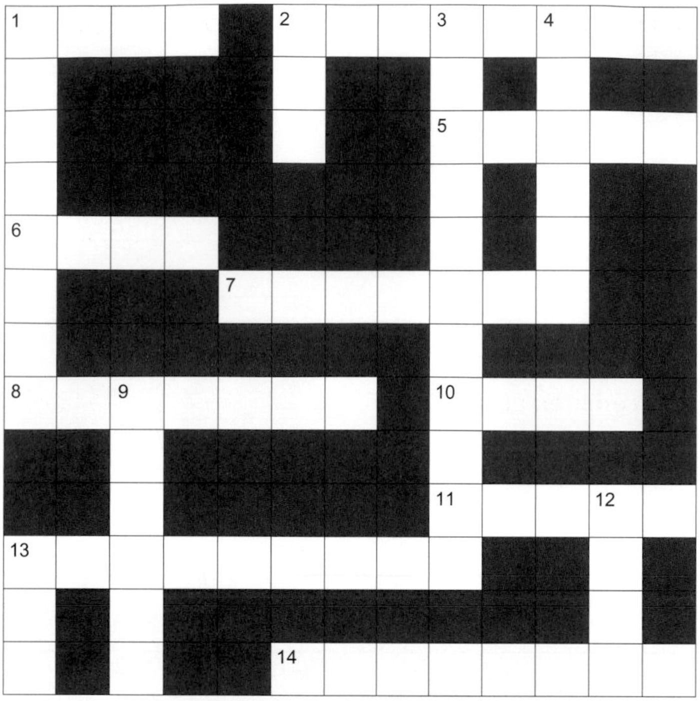

Across:

1. The basic unit of genetics (4).
2. A gene always expressed in the phenotype (8).
5. The double _____ – discovered by Crick and Watson (5).
6. Helps in the production of protein from amino acids (4).
7. A base – pairs with cytosine (7).
8. The middle of a cell (7).
10. An amino ____ builds up protein (4).
11. A triplet on mRNA (5).
13. The opposite of 2 across (9).
14. A chromosome that is not a sex chromosome (8).

Down:

1. Genetic makeup of a person (8).
2. Part of the double helix – codes for genes (3).
3. The common name for the process by which we receive our parents' genes (11).
4. The name for genes that occupy corresponding loci on a chromosome (6).
9. An RNA base – pairs with DNA adenine (6).
12. One female gamete (4).
13. Transcribed from DNA (3).

Words

Find the words linked to genetics that are hidden in each of these sentences: e.g. Sheila sighed to see Neil = cytosine.

1. To get the right total you need to add a nine to your present total.
2. He shouted at his sister when she had made a mistake and put salt in the tea rather than sugar 'my, my, oh sis what have you done?'.
3. Paul McCartney used to play the bass guitar in the Beatles.
4. The crew of the ship had a special ceremony when they were crossing the Equator.

Conditions

Below is a list of common genetic conditions. Take some time and write notes about each of the conditions. You may make the notes taken from text books or other resources, for example, people you work with in a clinical area, or you may make the notes as a result of people you have cared for. If you are making notes about people you have cared for you must ensure that you adhere to the rules of confidentiality.

Cystic fibrosis	
Huntington's disease	
Inherited breast cancer	
Haemophilia	
X-linked agammaglobulinaemia	
Duchenne's muscular dystrophy	

Answers

MCQs

1c;2c;3b;4c; 5f+h;6c;7b; 8d;9a;10d

Crossword

Across:		**Down:**	
1.	Gene	**1.**	Genotype
2.	Dominant	**2.**	DNA
5.	Helix	**3.**	Inheritance
6.	TRNA	**4.**	Allele
7.	Guanine	**9.**	Uracil
8.	Equator	**12.**	Ovum
10.	Acid	**13.**	RNA
11.	Codon		
13.	Recessive		
14.	Autosome		

Words

1 adenine; 2 meiosis; 3 base; 4 equator

Index

Page numbers in *italics* denote figures, those in **bold** denote tables.

abdominopelvic cavity 117, 122
abduction 247, **273**, 284, **284**
ABO blood groups 384–5, *384*, **385**, 397
absorption 2, 144, 146, 435
accessory muscles 339, 351
accessory structures
  eye *530*
  skin
    glands 140–1, *141*
    hair 139–40, *140*, 146
accommodation *537*
acetylcholine 161, 178, 266, 286
acetylcholinesterase 267, 286
acid base balance 23, 348–50, 351
  maintenance of 373
acids 16–18, 23
acini glands 422, 435
acquired immunity 72, 79–82, 92
  cell-mediated immunity 79–80, *79*, 92
  humoral immunity 80–2, *81*, *82*, 92
acquired immunodeficiency syndrome *see* AIDS
actin 264, *268*, 286
action potential 160–1, *162*, 180, 317
  cardiac 299, 318, *318*
  conduction of 267
active immunity 90–1, 92
active transport 38, 41–2, *41*, 52
Adam's apple *202*, 332
adduction *245*, 247
adenine 553, 575
adenosine diphosphate (ADP) 41, 52
adenosine triphosphate (ATP) 41, 52, 286
  muscle energy *270*, 397
adipose tissue 50, 113, 132, 211–12
adrenal glands 205–8, *206*
  adrenal cortex 207–8, *207*, 498
  adrenal medulla 206–7
adrenaline *see* epinephrine
adrenocorticotrophic hormone (ACTH) **200**, 201–2
adventitia 416, 438
aerobic respiration 269, *270*, 286
afferent fibres 160, 180
afterload 314, 317
ageing, effects on muscle 285
agglutination 384, 397
AIDS 64, 90
albumin 370–1
aldosterone 50, 208, *209*, 461
alkalis 16–18, 23
alleles 556, 570, 575
alveolar minute ventilation 341, **342**, 351
alveoli 105, 334, *335*, 340
amino acids 196, 214, 575
ampulla 540
  of ear *525*
amylase 411, 435, 438
anaemia 230, 348, 372
anaerobic respiration 269, 286
anaphase 563, 565, 575
anatomical dead space 341, 351
anatomy 2, 23, 247
androgens 484, 490, 498
angiogenesis 231
angiotensin 50, 208, 455, 461
antagonists (muscle) 271, 284, 286
anterior median fissure 172
antibiotics, prophylaxis 123
antibodies 9, 20, 23, 74, 83, *85*, 92, 397, 540
  see also immunoglobulins
anticholinesterases 267, 268
anticodons 560, 575
anticytokine drugs 87
antidiuretic hormone (ADH) 50, 180, 199, 461
antigens 70, *85*, 92, 397
antihaemophilic factor A **383**
antihaemophilic factor B **383**
antihaemophilic factor C **383**

anus 72, *407*, *425*, 435
aorta 317, 352, 397
aortic valve 301, 317
apical surface 122
apneustic centre 343, 352
apocrine glands 141, 146
aponeurosis *279*, *282*, 286
apoptosis 146
appendicitis 426
arachnoid mater 163, *165*, 171, 180
areola 500
areolar tissue 113
argon, atmospheric **338**
arrector pili 146
arterial blood 317
arterial blood gases 348
arteries 247, 317, 385–6, *388*, **388**, 397
  tunica externa 385, *388*, 397
  tunica media 385, *388*, 398
arterioles 50, 78, 237, 260, *386*, 397
articulation 229, 241, 247
arytenoid cartilage 333, 352
aspiration 333, 352
assimilation 4
asthma 84, 211, 267, 333, 340, 352
astrocytes 163, *164*, 180
atmospheric gases **338**
atomic number 6, 23
atoms 4–5, *5*, 23
  carbon 6–7, *6*
  ionic bonding 7, *8*
atopy 92
atria 299–301, *300*, 317
atrial natriuretic peptide 50, 461
atrioventricular bundle 317
atrioventricular node 307, 308, 317
atrioventricular valves 300, 301, 318
auditory (Eustachian) tubes 330, 352
auricle of ear 520–1
autocrine 194, *195*
autoimmune diseases 86–7
automaticity 306, 318
autonomic nervous system 157, 176–8, 180, 540
  heart rate regulation 314–15
  parasympathetic nervous system 178, **178**, *179*
  sympathetic nervous system 176–8, *177*, **178**
autoregulation 166, 389
autosomal dominant disorders 575
  and ill health 571
  morbidity and mortality 573
autosomal recessive disorders 575
  and ill health 571–2
  morbidity and mortality 573
autosomes 556, 575
axons 119, 158, 180, 541

B-lymphocytes 66, 70, 92, 397
  see also humoral immunity
bactericidal 72, 92
balance 541
ball and socket joints **245**, 247
baroreceptor reflex *316*
baroreceptors 315, 318, 390, 397
basal surface 104, 109, 122
bases 16–18, 24, 553–4, 575
basophils 92, 380, *381*
bicarbonate **49**, 348
bicuspid valve 300, 318
bifurcation 463, 469
bile 418, 423, 435
  production 423–4, *424*
bile duct 435
bilirubin 376, *378*, 397, 423
bivalent chromosomes 576
bladder 464, *465*
blast cells **112**
blood
  composition of 368–9, *368*, *369*
  functions of 371–2
  pH values 18
  properties of 369–70
  transportation in 372
blood cells *66*
  development 64–5, *65*
  formation of 374, *374*
  innate immunity 73
  multipotent stem cells 64
  platelets 66, 95, 382, 397
  red blood cells 66, 368, 374–8, *375*, 397
  white blood cells 93, 368, 378–82, 398
blood groups, ABO 384–5, *384*, **385**, 397
blood pressure 389–91, 397
  control of 390
  factors regulating 389–90

recording 391
taking 390
blood vessels 385–9, *386*, *387*
arteries 247, 317, 385–6, *388*, **388**, 397
capillaries 388, *389*
veins 385–6, *388*, **388**
blood–brain barrier 163, *164*
bodily requirements 4
body fluids 46–7
body temperature, maintenance of 372, *373*
bonds 24
chemical 7, 24
covalent 8–9, *10*, 24
hydrogen 9, *11*
ionic 7, *8*, 24
polar 9, *11*, 24, 25
bone 115, 226
flat bones 238, *241*
formation 230–3, **231**, *232*, *233*
fractures 235–6, *235*, 248
functions 226, 229
irregular bones 241, *242*
length and thickness 234
long bones 237, *239*
sesamoid bones 241, *243*
short bones 238, *240*
structure and blood supply 236–7, **236**
see also skeleton
bone marrow 66, 248
development of 232
red 230
bone remodelling 234, 249
Bowman's capsule 452, *453*
Boyle's law **337**, *338*
brain 166–70
structures of *167*
see also central nervous system; and individual areas
brain stem 169, 180
breast milk 73
breasts 497, *498*
breathing
control of 342–3, *343*
mechanics of 337–9, *339*
work of 339–40, *340*
broad ligaments 499
bronchi 331, 334–5, *335*
bronchial artery 352
bronchial tree 334–5, *335*
bronchial veins 336, 352
bronchioles 334, 352
brush border 420, 454
bundle of His 307, 318

calcification 231, 247
calcitonin 146
calcitriol 145, 205
calcium **49**, **434**
calcium pump 42
calyces 451, 469
cancellous bone 237, 247
canine teeth 410, 435
capillaries 388, *389*
carbohydrates 19, 214, 429–30, 435
carbon atom 6–7, *6*
carbon dioxide
atmospheric **338**
transport 347–8, *349*
carbonic acid 348
carbonic anhydrase 348
cardiac action potential 299, 318, *318*
cardiac cycle 309–12, *311*, 318
diastole 310–11, 318
electrocardiogram 312, *312*
systole 310–11, 320
cardiac muscle 118, 260
cardiac notch 334, 352
cardiac output 312–13, 318
cardioinhibitory centre 315, 318
cardiovascular centre 315, 318
cardiovascular system 294–327
see also individual parts
carotid artery 352
cartilage 114–15, 122, 247, 352, 541
sites of *116*
cartilaginous joints 242, 247
catabolism 429, 435
catecholamines 206–7, 214
see also individual substances
cations 180
cell adhesion proteins 112
cell cycle *564*, 576
cell division 565, *566*
cell membrane *see* plasma membrane
cell-mediated immunity 79–80, *79*, 92

cells 34–5, *34*, *35*
  compartments **36**, 52
  structure *35*
cementum 410
central nervous system 157, 180
centrioles **36**
centromere 552, 555, 565, 576
cerebellum 169, 180
cerebral cortex 168
cerebral hemispheres *168*, 180
cerebrospinal fluid 164, 166, 180, 352
cerebrum 167–9, 180
cerumen 146
cervix 496–7
chemical barriers 73
chemical bonds 7, 24
chemical equations 13–16, *14*
  product 13, 25
  reactants 13, 25
chemical properties 13
chemical reaction 24, 52
chemoreceptors 352, 390, 512
chemotaxis *77*, 379
chief cells 417, *418*, 435
chloride **49**
chlorine **434**
cholecystokinins 423, **427**, 435
chondroblasts 231
chondrocytes 231–2, 234
chondroitin sulphate 114
choroid 541
choroid plexus 164
chromatids 552, 555, *555*, 565, 576
chromatin **36**, 554
chromosomes 552, 554–7, *555*, *556*, 567
chronic obstructive pulmonary disease 352
chyme 122, 417, 435
chymotrypsinogen 422, 423
cilia **36**, 73, 330, 352, 541
  of ear 524
  of nose 513
ciliary body 532, 541
circle of Willis *166*, 180
circulation 2
circulatory system 366–405
clavicle 352
clitoris 467, 488, 497
clotting system 77, 92
coagulation 383, **383**, 397
  clotting factors **383**
cochlea 523, *524*, *528*, *529*
cochlear ducts 528, *528*
codons 560, 576
collagen 112, 146, 247
collecting ducts 454, **460**
colloid osmotic pressure 45
colloids 46
common bile duct 418
compartments **36**, 52
complement system 74, 77, 92
compounds 13, 24
conducting zone 352, 363
condyloid joints **246**, 247
cone cells 535, 539–40
conjunctiva *530*, 531
connective tissue 110–15, *111*, *112*, **112**, *113*, 122, 499, 541
  dense 113–14
  liquid 115
  loose 113
  types of **114**
constipation 426
control centres 18
convergence 541
corniculate cartilage 353
coronary arteries 302, *302*, **303**, 318
coronary sinus 300, 318
corpus albicans 499
corpus luteum 490, 499
cortex 214
corticosteroids 208, 214
corticotropin releasing hormone **200**
cortisol 210, 214
  stress response *210*
coughing 73
covalent bonds 8–9, *10*, 24
cranial nerves 170, *171*, **172**, 180
craniosacral division *see* parasympathetic nervous system
creatine phosphate 269
cremasteric reflex 486
cribriform plate 514, *515*
Crick, Francis 552
cricoid cartilage 332, 353
cricothyroid ligament 332, 353
cross-infection, prevention by hand washing 88

crypts of Lieberkühn 420
crystalloids 46
cuneiform cartilage 333, *334*, 353
cutaneous sensation 147
cyanosis 145, 146
cystic fibrosis 571
cystitis 465–6
cytokines 78, 92
cytoplasm **36**, 52, 214
cytosine 554, 576
cytoskeleton **36**
cytotoxicity 74, 76, 80, 92

Dalton's law **337**
defaecation reflex 426
deglutition *413*, 414, 435
dehydration 47, 144
dendrites 119, 158, 180
dentine 410
deoxyribose 553, 576
depolarisation 161, 312, 318
dermatitis 146
dermis 137–9
  papillary and reticular aspects 138–9
desmosomes 318
diabetic foot ulcers 121
diaphragm 353
diaphysis 232, 237, 247
diarrhoea 48, 51, 90, 267, 426
diastole 310–11, 318
dicrotic notch 311, 318
diencephalon 169, 180
diet, balanced 428, *428*
diffusion 38–9, *39*, 52, 122, 353
  facilitated 39, *40*, 52
  factors affecting 344–5
digestion 2, 435
digestive system 406–45, *408*
  activity of 408–9
  hormones of 427, **427**
  structure 414–16, *415*
  see also individual parts
diploid cells 567, 576
disease-modifying anti-rheumatoid drugs (DMARDs) 87
dissociation 16
distal convoluted tubule 454, **460**
diuresis 461, 469
DNA 552, *555*, 576
  double helix 552–3, *553*, 576
  separation of *558*
dominant genes 557, 570–1, 576
dopamine 163, 206
double helix 552–3, *553*, 576
Down syndrome (trisomy 21) 552
down-regulation 197, 214
drug administration, cutaneous 145
duodenum 418, 435
dura mater 163, *165*, 171, 180

ear 520–3, *520*
  inner 523, *524*
  middle 521–2
  noise damage 522–3
  outer 520–1
eccrine glands 140, *141*
effectors 19, 180
efferent fibres 160, 181
ejaculatory duct *479*, 484, 488
elastic cartilage 115
elastic fibres 112, 113
elastin 113
electrocardiogram 312, *312*
electrolytes 9, 24, 47–51, *48*, 52, 214
  functions of 47–9, **49**
  hormone regulation 50
  see also individual electrolytes
electrons 5
elements 10–13, 24
  classes of 11–12
  properties of 13
embolism 345, 353
emotional brain *see* limbic system
enamel 410, 435
end diastolic pressure 310, 318
end diastolic volume 310, 318
endocardium 299, 302, 318
endocrine glands 122, 192, 194, *195*
  physiology 198–204
  see also individual glands and hormones
endocrine system **192**
  organs of 193–4, *193*, *194*
  stress response *210*
  see also individual glands and hormones
endocytosis 42–3, *42*, 52
endolymph 541

endometrium 495, **496**, 499
endoplasmic reticulum **36**
endothelial cells 68
energy, units of measurement **22**
enteroendocrine cells 417, 420
enzymes 9, 20, 24, 38, 541
  see also individual enzymes
eosinophils 92, 379–80, *380*
ependymal cells 163, 181
epidermis 132–4, *135*
  layers of **137**
  stratum basale 134–5
  stratum corneum 136
  stratum granulosum 135–6
  stratum lucidum 136
  stratum spinosum 135
epididymis 483, 487–8
epiglottis 332, 353, 413, 435
epinephrine 181, 206
  heart rate regulation 315
epiphysis 247
epithalamus 169, 181
epithelial tissue 104–10, *105*, 122
  glandular epithelia 110, *111*
  simple epithelia 105–8, *106–8*
  stratified epithelia 108–10, *109*, *110*
epithelium 318
epitopes *85*, 92
eponychium 142
equator (of cell) 576
equilibrium 523–7, *525*, 541
  nerve pathways 526–7
erythema 146
erythrocytes *see* red blood cells
erythropoietin 376, *377*, 469
ethmoid bone 330, 353, 514, *515*, 541
eustachian tube 521
excretion 4, 144, 146, 469
exercise, effect on bone structure **236**
exocrine glands *111*, 122, 194
exocytosis 43, *43*, 52
expectorate 353
expiration *340*
expiratory reserve volume 341, 353
external respiration 336, 343–4, *345*, *350*, 353
extracellular fluid 44
extracellular matrix 122
extracellular space 52
extrinsic pathway 384
eye
  accessory structures *530*
  chambers of *532*, 535
  choroid 541
  ciliary body 532, 541
  conjunctiva *530*, 531
  iris 533, 541
  pupil 542
  retina 533–5, *534*
  wall of 532–4, *533*
eyelashes 531
eyelids 531

facilitated diffusion 39, *40*, 52
faeces 426, 435
faecoliths 426
fallopian tubes 495, *495*
fascia 146
fats 19, 215, 430, 435, 541
fatty acids 214
fauces 330, *332*, 353
female
  reproductive system 488–98, *489*
    see also individual parts
  urethra 467, *468*
female sex hormones 490, 492
fibres 112, *113*
fibrin 382, 383
fibrin stabilising factor **383**
fibrinogen 371, **383**
fibrocartilage 115
fibrosis 121, 285
fibrous joints 242, 247
fibrous pericardium 320
Fick's law **337**, 344
fight or flight *see* sympathetic nervous system
filtration 40, 469
fimbriae *489*, 495, 499
flat bones 238, *241*
flexion 248
fluid balance
  hormonal control 460–1
  hormone regulation 50
  regulation of 373
fluid compartments 43–5, *44*
  movement between 44–5, *45*
  see also individual compartments

focal length *537*, 541
foetus 499
follicle stimulating hormone 201, 499
follicles, ovarian 489–90, 499
follicular development *492*
food 4
foot, diabetic ulcers 121
fovea 541
fractures 235–6, *235*, 248
Frank-Starling law 313
Franklin, Rosalind 553
frenulum 409, 435

gall bladder 425, *425*
gametes 499, 565, 576
gametogenesis 570, 576
ganglia 181, 214
  of eye 535
gap junctions 320
gas exchange 343–4, *345*
gas laws **337**
gas transport 345–9, **346**, 356
  carbon dioxide 347, *349*
  oxygen 345–7, *349*
gastrin **427**
gene crossover *568*, 576
genes 552, 576
  transference 563–9
genetic counselling 572–3
genetic inheritance *570*
genetics 550–84
genotype 557, 576
glands 122, 214
  endocrine 122, 192, 194, *195*, 198–202
  exocrine *111*, 122, 194
glandular epithelia 110, *111*
glans penis 487, 499
gliding joints **246**, 248
globulins 371
glomeruli 541
glomerulus 457, 469
glossopharyngeal nerve 353
glucagon 211, 212–13, *212*, 422
glucocorticoids 208–10, 214
  and inflammatory diseases 211
gluconeogenesis 214, 435
glycogen 215, 286
glycogen granules **36**
glycogenolysis 215
glycolysis 435
glycoproteins 122
glycosaminoglycans 112
goblet cells 353, 420, 426, 435
Golgi complex **36**
gonadotrophic hormone 499
gonadotropin releasing hormone **200**, 484
gonads 499
  female 488–98, *489*
  male 478–88, *479*
graafian follicles 490
granulation 121
granulocytes 92
ground substance 112, *113*
growth 2
growth hormone 200
growth hormone release inhibiting factor **200**
growth hormone releasing factor **200**
guanine 554, 576
gustatory pathway 519–20

haematocrit 368
haematopoiesis 229, 248
haemoglobin 375, *376*, 397
haemostasis 382
  platelet aggregation 382
  vasoconstriction 147, 382
Hageman factor **383**
hair 139–40, *140*, 146
hair cells *526*
hand washing 88
haploid cells 499, 567, 576
haustrum 426, 435
haversian canals 237, *238*
head, muscles of 271, **272**, *276*
hearing 527–30
  ear 520–3
  mechanism of 529–30
heart 296
  blood flow through 304–6, *305*, *306*
  blood supply 302–4, *302*, **303**
  chambers of 299–301, *300*
  electrical pathways 306–9, *307*, *308*, *309*
  size and location 296–7, *296*
  structures 297–301
  see also cardiac; and individual parts
heart rate, regulation of 314–15

heart wall 297–9, *297*
  endocardium 299, 318
  myocardium 298–9, *299*, 320
  pericardium 297–8, 317, 320
heat 4
Henry's law **337**
hepatic portal vein 436
hepatocytes 423, 436
hepatopancreatic ampulla 418, 436
hepatopancreatic sphincter 436
heredity 556–7, 570, 576
heterologous 556, 576
heterozygous 557, 576
hilus 469
hinge joints **244**
histology 248
histones 554, 576
HIV 90
homeostasis 18–19, 24, 146, 192, 248, 397
homologous 556, 577
homozygous 557, 577
hormonal stimulation 198, 215
hormones 122, 194–8, 215, 248, 320
  and bone structure **236**
  control of release 197–8, *197*
  destruction and removal 197
  effects of 196–7
  heart rate regulation 315
  target cells *196*
  transport of *194*
  see also individual hormones
human chorionic gonadotrophin 499
human immunodeficiency virus *see* HIV
humoral immunity 80–2, *81*, *82*, 92
humoral stimulation 197, 215
Huntington's disease 573
hyaline cartilage 114
hydrochloric acid 417, 436
hydrogen 12
hydrogen bonds 9, *11*
hydrogen-linked cotransporter 42
hydrolysis 436
hydrophilic 52
hydrophobic 52
hyoid bone 436
hyperglycaemia 215
hyperkeratosis 146
hyperopia *539*, 541, 542
hypersensitivity 93
hyperthyroidism 204
hypertonic solutions 52
hypochondriac region 436
hypoglycaemia 213, 215
hyponatraemia 51
hypothalamus 169, 181, 198–9, *198*, 353, 390
hypothyroidism 204
hypotonic solutions 52
hypoventilation 353
hypovolaemia 215
hypoxaemia 347, 353
hypoxia 347, **349**, 353

ileocaecal valve 418, 425
ileum 418, 436
immune memory 80
immune system 64
  blood cells of 73–4
  control of 92
  organs of 67–8, *67*
  primary immune response 86–7, 94
  secondary immune response 88–9, *89*, 94
immunisation 89–90, 93
  active 90
  passive 89–90
immunity 93
  acquired *see* acquired immunity
  active 90–1, 92
  innate *see* innate immunity
  passive 94
immunodeficiency
  importance of hand washing 88
  secondary 90–1
immunoglobulins 66, 74, 77, 83, 93
  role of 84–5, *85*
immunoglobulin A 83–4
immunoglobulin D 84
immunoglobulin E 84
immunoglobulin G 83
immunoglobulin M 84
immunology 64
in utero 248, 499
incisors 410, 436
incus 521
inferior vena cava 300, 320
inflammation 74, 76–8, *77*, 93
ingestion 436

inguinal canal 499
inhibin 499
innate immunity 72, 93
  blood cells 73
  chemical barriers 73
  mechanical barriers 73
  physical barriers 72
innervation 122, 146
inorganic substances 19, 20, 24
inspiration *340*
inspiratory reserve volume 341, 353
insulin 211–12, *212*, 422
insulin-like growth factor 248
integumentary 146
interatrial septum 300, 320
intercostal nerves 342, 353
intercostal spaces 339, 353
intermediate filament **36**
internal respiration *350*, 351, 354
interphase 564, 577
interstitial fluid 112, 122
interstitial space 44, 53
interventricular septum 301, 320
intervertebral foramen 173
intestinal crypts 436
intracellular fluid 44
intracellular space 53
intramuscular injection 265
intrapulmonary pressure 354
intravenous infusion 46
intrinsic factor 417, 436
intrinsic pathway 382, 383
iodine **434**
ionic bonding 7, *8*, 24
ions 7–8, 24, 215, 320
iris 533, 541
iron **434**
islets of Langerhans 211, 422
isovolumetric 320
isthmus 500

jejunum 418, 436
joints 241–3, **244–6**
  cartilaginous 242, 247
  fibrous 242, 247
  synovial 243, **244–6**

keratin 122, 146
keratinocytes 133
kidney 469
  blood supply 456–7
  Bowman's capsule 452, *453*
  collecting ducts 454, **460**
  distal convoluted tubule 454, **460**
  external structures 449, *449*
  functions 455, **455**
  glomerulus 457, 469
  internal structures 450–1, *450*, *451*
  loop of Henle 453, **460**
  proximal convoluted tubule 453, **459**
  see also renal
kinesiology 248
kinin system 77, 93
kinins 93
Kupffer cells 423, 436
kwashiorkor 90

labia 497
labyrinth of ear 523, *524*
lacrimal 541
lacrimal apparatus 531
lacrimal caruncle 531
lacteals 420, 436
lacuna 248
lamellae 248
lamina propria 117, 415, 436
Langerhans cells 133
lanugo 146
large intestine 425–6, *425*
laryngopharynx 330, 354, 413, 436
larynx 330, 331, 332–3, *334*, 354
length, units of measurement **22**
leucocytes *see* white blood cells
levels of organisation 2, *3*
Leydig cells 480, 500
life, characteristics of 2–4
ligaments 248, 286, 500, 541
limbic system 169–70, 181, 354, 514, 541
lingual tonsils 354
lipase 436
lipids *see* fats
liquid connective tissue 115
liver 423–4, *424*, 436
  functions 424
  lobules *424*
  sinusoids 423, 436

lobes 181, 354
lobules 334, *335*, 354
  liver *424*
  testes 480, *480*
locus 556, 577
long bones 237, *239*
longitudinal cerebral fissure 167
loop of Henle 453–4, **460**
lotions 145
lower limbs, muscles of **275**, *280–1*
lower respiratory tract 330–1, 354
lung capacities 340–2, *341*, **342**
lung compliance 354
lung volumes 340–2, *341*, **342**
lungs 331, *333*, 334
  blood supply 336, *336*
  surfactant 340, 356
lunula 142, 146
luteinising hormone 201, 484, 500
lymph 68, 93, 391, 397
lymph capillaries 391, *393*
lymph nodes 68, 70, *71*, 93, 122, 394, *395*, 397
lymph nodules 331, 354
lymph vessels 68, 93, 334, 354, 391, *393*
lymphatic organs 394
lymphatic system 68–72, *69*, 93, 391–6, *392*, *393*
  functions of 394, 396
lymphocytes 68, 93, 380–2, *381*
lymphoid cells 64
lymphoid tissue 68, 70–1, *71*
lysosomes **36**
lysozyme 436

M cells 539
macronutrients 436
macrophages 70, 93, 123, 248
magnesium **49**, **434**
male
  reproductive system 478–88, *479*
    see also individual parts
  urethra 466–7, *467*
malleus 521
mast cells 93
  degranulation 77
  histamine release 78
mastication 437
meatus 500
mechanical barriers 73
mediator cells 74
medulla 70, 93, 215
medulla oblongata 169, 181, 315, 320, 354
meiosis 482, 500, 563, 565, 567–9, 577
  first meiotic division 567–8, *568*
  second meiotic division 568–9
Meissner's plexus 415, 437
melanin 146
melanocytes 133
membranes 115, 117, *117*, 123
  cutaneous 115
  mucous 115, 117
  serous 117
  synovial *117*, 118
Mendel, Gregor 569
mendelian genetics 569–72, 577
Mendel's first law 577
Mendel's second law 577
meninges 163, *165*, 171, 181
meningitis 166
menopause 500
menstrual cycle 492–3, *493*
Merkel cells 133–4
mesenchyme 248
mesenteric plexus 437
mesothelium 117
metabolism 146, 437
metalloids 11–12
metals 11–12
metaphase 563, 565, 577
metaphysis 248
microfilaments **36**
microglia 163, 181
micronutrients 437
microtubules **36**
microvilli **36**, 437, 542
micturition 467–8
midbrain 169, 181
mineralocorticoids 208, 215
minerals 431, **434**, 437
  and bone structure **236**
minute volume 341, **342**, 354
mitochondria **36**
mitosis 123, 563, *566*, 577
mitral valve 320
mixed nerves 170

molars 410, 437
mole 16, 24
molecules 7
monocytes 66, 94, 380, *381*
mononuclear phagocytes 74
mons pubis 497
motor area 181
motor end plate 266
motor nerves 157–9, *159*, 160, 170, 181
motor unit *266*
mouth 409, *410*, 437
movement 2, 271, 284, **284**
mRNA 552, *560*, 577
mucosa 437
mucosal membranes 72
mucous membranes 115, 117
mucous neck cells 437
multiple sclerosis 160
multipotent stem cells 64
muscle 118, *119*, 260–1, **261**
  cardiac 118, 260
  functions of 260–1
  skeletal 118, 260, 261–85
  smooth 118, 260
muscular dystrophy 285
muscularis mucosa 415, 437
myasthenia gravis 267, 286
myelin sheath 158, 181
myeloid cells 64
myenteric plexus 415
myocardial infarction 303–4
myocardium 298–9, *299*, 317, 320
myocytes 50, *298*, 320
myofibrils 264, **265**, 286
myofilaments **265**
myoglobin **265**, 286
myometrium **496**, 500
myopia 538, *539*, 542

nails 141–2, *142*, 146
nasal cavity 330, 354
nasal conchae 330, *332*
nasal meatus 330, 354
nasal septum 330, 354
nasopharynx 330, 354, 437, 542
natural killer (NK) cells 86, 94
neck, muscles of 271, **272**, *276*
negative feedback 197–8, *197*, *204*
nephron 451–2, *452*, *458*, 469
nerve impulse, propagation of 161
nerves 158
  cranial 170, *171*, **172**, 180
  mixed 170
  motor 157–9, *159*, 160, 170, 181
  sensory 157, 160, 170, 182
  spinal 173–6, *174–6*, 182
  see also individual nerves
nervous system
  central nervous system 157, 180
  motor division 157–9, *159*
  organisation of 156, *156*
  parasympathetic 178, **178**, *179*, 542
  sensory division 157
  sympathetic 176–8, *177*, **178**, 543
  see also individual parts
nervous tissue 118–19, *120*, *121*
neural stimulation 198, 215
neuroglia 119, 123, 163, 181
neuromuscular junction 181
neurones 123, 157–8, 181
  axon 119, 158, 180, 541
  cell body 158
  dendrites 119, 158, 180
neurotransmitters 161, 163
neutral solutions 16, 24
neutrons 5, 24
neutropenia 379
neutrophils 74, 94, 379, *379*
nipple 500
nitrogen, atmospheric **338**
nodal cells 308, 320
nodes of Ranvier 158
noise exposure 522–3
non-keratinised stratified squamous
    epithelium 330, 354
non-self cells 68
noradrenaline *see* norepinephrine
norepinephrine 161, 176, 206
nuclear membrane 565
nuclear spindle 565
nuclei 24
nucleic acids 554, 577
nucleolus **36**, 565
nucleosomes 554, 577
nucleotides 553, 577
nucleus **36**

null cells *see* natural killer (NK) cells
nutrient groups 429–31
nutrients 428, 437
nutrition 427–31
  see also individual nutrients

obesity 429
oedema 94
oesophageal sphincters 436, 439
oesophagus 354, 413, 437
  peristalsis *414*
oestrogens 490, 500
olfaction 354, 512–16, *513*, 542
olfactory bulb 514, 542
olfactory discrimination 514, 516
olfactory pathway 514, *515*
olfactory receptors 513–14
oligodendrocytes 24, 163
oncotic pressure 45
oocytes 123, 500
oogenesis 490, *491*, *492*, 500
oogonia 490
opsonins 94
oral cavity 409, *410*, 437
organ of Corti 528, *529*
organelles 2, 20, 25, 53, 564
organic substances 19–20, 25
organism 147
organs 147
oropharynx 330, 355, 413, 437
osmosis 9, 25, 39–40, 53, 215
osmotic pressure 40, *41*, 53
osseous 248
ossicle 248
ossification 230, **231**, 248
  embryonic 231
  endochondral 231–3, *233*
  intramembranous 231, *232*
osteoarthritis 234–5
osteoblasts 234, 236, 248
osteoclasts 215, 234, 236, 248
osteocytes 234, 235, 248
osteon *238*, 249
osteophytes 249
otoliths *526*
  action of gravity on *527*
ova 500, 565, 577
ovarian cycle 492–3, *493*, 500
ovarian follicle 500
ovaries 489, 500
  cortex 490
  medulla 490
oxygen 4, 19
  arterial
    content **346**
    partial pressure **346**
  atmospheric **338**
  measurement 348
oxygen capacity **346**
oxygen consumption **346**, 351
oxygen debt 269
oxygen delivery **346**
oxygen extraction ratio **346**, 351
oxygen saturation **346**, 348
oxygen transport 345–7, *349*
oxyhaemoglobin 377
  dissociation curve 355
oxytocin 199

pacemaker cells 308, 320
pacemakers 309, *309*
pain 78
palate 409, 437
palatine tonsils 331, 355
pancreas 211, 421–3, *422*
pancreatic duct 418, 437
pancreatic juice 418
Paneth cells 420, 437
papillae 409, 437
  tongue 516, *517*
paracrine 194, *195*
parasympathetic fibres 437
parasympathetic nervous system 178, **178**, *179*, 542
parathyroid glands *202*, 205
parathyroid hormone 205
parenchyma 123
parietal cells 417, 437
parietal pericardium 320
parietal pleura 334, 355
parotid glands 410, *412*, 437
passive immunity 94
passive transport 38, 53
pathogens 147, 542
peak expiratory flow rate 342
penis 486–7, *487*, 500

pepsin 417, 437
pepsinogen 417, 437
percutaneous coronary intervention 303–4, *304*
perfusion 345
pericardial fluid 320
pericardium 297–8, 317, 320
perichondrium 114
perilymph 542
perimetrium **496**
Periodic Table 11
periosteum 249
peripheral nervous system 24, 170
peristalsis *414*, 416, 437, 500
peritoneum 416, 437
peritonitis 117
peroxisomes **36**
personal hygiene 134
pessaries, insertion of 494
Peyer's patches 420, 437
pH 16–18, *17*, 25, 500
  blood 18
phagocytes 74, *74*, 94
  migration to injury site 77, *77*
phagocytosis 42, *42*, 70, 73, 74–5, *74*, *75*, 94, 147, 500
pharyngeal phase 437
pharyngeal tonsil 355
pharynx 330, 355, 413, *413*, 437
phenotype 557, 577
pheromones 147
phosphate **49**, 553, 577
photoreceptors 542
phrenic nerve 355
physical barriers 72
physical properties 13
physiology 2, 25
pia mater 24, 163, *165*, 171
pilosebaceous unit *140*
pineal gland 24
pinocytosis 42, *42*
pituitary gland 182, 198–9, *198*
  anterior 199–202, **200**
  posterior 199
pivot joints **244**, 249
placenta 500
plasma 368, 370–1, 397
  properties of 369–70
  water in 371
plasma cells 66, 94
plasma membrane 35, **36**, 37, *37*, 53, 565
  functions of 37–8
plasma proteins 370–1
platelet aggregation 382, 397
platelets 66, 95, 382, 397
pleural space 355
plicae circularis 420, 438
pneumotaxic centre 355
pneumothorax 118
polar bonds 9, *11*, 24, 25
polarity 9
poles (of cell) 577
polymorphonuclear leucocytes 66
polymorphonuclear phagocytes 74
polypeptides 397
pons 169, 355, 542
portal fissure 438
portal triad 423, 438
posterior median sulcus 172
potassium **49**, **434**
potassium chloride 12
preload 313
premolars 410, 438
prepuce 487
presbyopia *539*, 542
pressure 4
primary immune response 86–7, 94
proaccelerin **383**
procarboxypeptidase 422, 423
proconvertin **383**
product 25
progesterone 490, 500
prognosis 147
prolactin 200–1, 497, 500
prolactin inhibiting hormone **200**
prolactin releasing hormone **200**
proliferation 147
prophase 563, 565, 577
propulsion 438
prostaglandins 78, 94
prostate gland 484, 488
protective function of skin 143
proteins 19, 430–1, 438
  synthesis 557, *558*, 559–63, *560*, *561*, *563*
prothrombin **383**
protons 5, 25
proximal convoluted tubule 453, **459**

pruritus 147
pseudopodia 75, 94
pseudostratified ciliated columnar epithelium 330, 355
pulmonary artery 355
pulmonary circulation 305, 320
pulmonary oedema 355
pulmonary valve 301, 320
pulmonary veins 320, 336, 355
pulmonary ventilation 336, 337–9, **338**, *339*, 355
pulp cavity of tooth 410, 438
pulse oximetry 348
pupil 542
pupillary constrictor muscles 542
Purkinje fibres 307, 317, 320
pyloric canal 417, 438
pyloric region 438
pyloric sphincter 417, 438
pyramidal tracts, decussation 169
pyrexia 355
pyridostigmine 267

reactants 13, 25
receptors 18, 182
recessive genes 557, 570–1, 578
rectum 438
red blood cells 66, 368, 374–8, *375*, 397
  formation 375–6, *377*
  gas transport 377–8
  haemoglobin 375, *376*, 397
  life cycle 376–7, *378*
reflexes 542
refraction 536, *536*, 542
refractory period 161, 182
regeneration 121
renal artery 469
renal colic 463
renal cortex 450, 469
renal failure 456
renal medulla 450, 469
renal papilla 450
renal pelvis 469
renal pyramids 450, 469
renal stones 463
renal system 446–75, *448*
renal vein 469
renin 469
renin–angiotensin system *209*, 220, 390
repolarisation 320
reproduction 2
reproductive system 476–509
  female 488–98, *489*
  male 478–88, *479*
residual volume 341, 355
respiration 3, 336–7
respiratory centres *343*
respiratory rate 343
respiratory system 328–65
  lower respiratory tract 330–1, 354
  organisation of 330, *331*
  upper respiratory tract 330–1, *332*, 356
  see also individual parts
respiratory zone 355
responsiveness 2
rete testis 483, 500
reticular activating system 169–70
reticular fibres 112
reticular formation 170, 182
reticular tissue 113
retina 533–5, *534*
  focusing images onto 536–7, *536*, *537*
rheumatoid disease 86
ribosomes **36**, *561*, 578
RNA 552, 578
rod cells 535, 539
rRNA 559
rugae
  bladder 464
  stomach 417, 438

saddle joints **245**, 249
saliva 73, 411
salivary amylase 411, 438
salivary glands 410–12, *412*
  calculi 412
saltatory conduction 161, 182
sarcolemma 264, **265**, 286, 320
  conduction of action potentials 267
sarcomere 264
sarcoplasm 264, **265**, 286
sarcoplasmic reticulum **265**
scar tissue 121
Schwann cells 158
scrotum 484, *486*, 500
sebum 144, 147
secondary immune response 88–90, *89*, 94

secretin 423, **427**, 438
secretory vesicles **36**
segmentation 425, 438
self cells 68
semen 73, 500
semicircular canals 523, *524*
semilunar valves 320
seminiferous tubules *480*
sensation 143
sensory area 182
sensory nerves 157, 160, 170, 182
septum 320
serosa 416, 438
serous membranes 117
serous pericardium 320
Sertoli cells 480
sesamoid bones 241, *243*
shell (of atom) 5–7, *6*, 9, 25
short bones 238, *241*
SI units **21**, **22**
sight 530–40, *530*
simple epithelia 105–8, *106–8*
columnar 107–8, *107*, *108*
cuboidal 105, *107*
sinoatrial node 307, 308, 315, 317, 320
skeletal muscle 118, 260, 261–85
ageing effects 285
anatomical organisation 270–1, **271**, *282–3*
head and neck 271, **272**, *276*
lower limbs **275**, *280–1*
nomenclature **271**
trunk **274**, *279*
upper limbs **273**, *277–9*
blood supply 265–6
contraction/relaxation 266–7, *266*, *268*
energy sources 267, 269
endomysium 263
epimysium 263
fatigue 269
fibre types 264–5, **265**
gross anatomy 262–3, *262*
microanatomy 263–4, *263*, **265**
myofibrils 264, **265**, 286
myofilaments **265**
myoglobin **265**, 286
sarcolemma 264, **265**, 286
sarcomere 264
sarcoplasm 264, **265**, 286
sarcoplasmic reticulum **265**
T tubules **265**, 286
transverse tubules 264
movement 2, 271, 284, **284**
oxygen debt 269
perimysium 263
skeleton *228*
appendicular 226, **227**
axial 226, **227**
skin 72, 132, *136*, *138*
accessory structures
glands 140–1, *141*
hair 139–40, *140*, 146
dermis 137–9
epidermis 132–6, *135*, **137**
functions of 142–3
small intestine 418, 419–21, *420*
smooth muscle 118, 260
sneezing 73
Snellen chart 538, 543
sodium **49**, **434**
hyponatraemia 51
sodium bicarbonate 12
sodium chloride 8, 12
sodium-potassium pump 42
somatic nervous system 157, 182
somatostatin 213
speaking 333
special senses 510–49
equilibrium 523–7
hearing 520–3, 527–30
olfaction 512–16, *513*, 542
sight 530–40, *530*
taste 516–20
spermatic cord 488
spermatids 483
spermatogenesis 482–3, *482*, 500
spermatozoa 480, 483–4, *483*, 565, 578
sphincter 469
sphincter of Oddi 418, 438
spinal cord 170–6, *173*
functions of 172
spinal nerves 173–6, *174–6*, 182
spirometry 342
splanchnic circulation 438
spleen 67, 68, 71, 94, 123, 394
spongy bone *see* cancellous bone
spontaneous mutation 575, 578

stapedius 522
stapes 521
stem cells 66, 120
stercobilin 398, 426, 438
stereocilia 524
sternum 355
steroid hormones 196
stomach 416–18, *416*, 438, 439
  body 416, 435
  cardia 416, 435
  chief cells 417, *418*, 435
  fundus 416, 435
  gastric juice secretion *419*
  glands *418*
  mucous neck cells 417, *418*, 437
  parietal cells 417, *418*, 437
  pyloric region 416–17
stomach acid 73
strands 553
stratified epithelia 108–10, *109*, *110*
stratum 147
stratum basale 134–5
stratum corneum 136
stratum lucidum 136
stratum spinosum 135
stress response *210*
stroke volume 313–14, 320
stroma 123
Stuart–Prower factor **383**
subcutaneous 123
sublingual glands 438
submandibular glands 438
submucosa of digestive tract 415, 438
substrate 215
sulphate **49**
superior mesenteric artery 438
superior mesenteric vein 438
superior vena cava 300, 320
surface mucous cells 438
surfactant 340, 356
swallowing *413*, 414
sweat 73
sympathetic nervous system 176–8, *177*, **178**, 543
synapse 182
synchondroses 242
synovial cavity 249
synovial fluid 249
synovial joints 243, **244–6**, 543
  see also individual types
synovial membranes *117*, 118
systemic circulation 305, 320, 356
systole 310–11, 320

T tubules **265**, 286
T-effector lymphocytes 66
T-helper lymphocytes 66, 80
T-lymphocytes 66, 67, 94
  development *79*
T-suppressor lymphocytes 66, 80
tactile 147
taeniae coli 426, 439
Tanner scale 481–2, *481*
taste 516–20
  gustatory pathway 519–20
taste buds 516–17, *517*, *518*
taste map *519*
taste receptors 517–18
tears 73
teeth 409, *411*
  canines 410, 435
  cementum 410
  dentine 410
  enamel 410, 435
  incisors 410, 436
  molars 410, 437
  premolars 410, 438
  pulp cavity 410, 438
telophase 563, 565, 578
tendons 286
tensor tympani 522
termination codons 562, 578
testes 479–80, *480*, *486*, 500
  hormonal influences 484
  lobules 480, *480*
  seminiferous tubules 480, *480*
testosterone 484, 500
  negative feedback 484, *485*
tetany 320
thalamus 169, 182
thermoreceptors 147
thermoregulation 143, 147
thoracic cage 356
thoracicolumbar division *see* sympathetic nervous system
thorax 334, 356

thrombin 383
thrombocytes *see* platelets
thrombokinase **383**
thrombolysis 303
thromboplastin 383
thromboplastinogenase 383
thymine 553, 578
thymus 66, 67–8, *67*, 95, 394
thyroid cartilage 332, 356
thyroid gland 202–4, *202*, *204*
thyroid hormone 196, 203, 205
  negative feedback control *204*
thyroid releasing hormone **200**
thyroid stimulating hormone 199, 201
thyrotrophin releasing hormone 199
thyroxine 203, 205
  free 214
  heart rate regulation 315
tidal volume 356
tissue repair 119–21
tongue 409, 516, *517*, *518*
  taste map *519*
tonsillitis 396
tonsils 95, 331, 356
  pharyngeal 355
total lung capacity 340, 356
trabeculae 70, 95, 231, *238*, 249
trachea 331, 333–4
tracheostomy 332, 356
transcription 557–9, 578
translation 559, 578
transport proteins 53
transverse tubules 264
tricuspid valve 300, 320
triglycerides 215
trigone of bladder 464
triiodothyronine 203
triplets 560, 578
tRNA 559, 578
trunk, muscles of **274**, *279*
trypsinogen 422, 423
tunica albuginea 478, 490
tunica externa 385, *388*, 397
tunica intima 397
tunica media 385, *388*, 398
tunica vaginalis 478
tunica vasculosa 478
tympanic duct *529*
tympanic membrane 521

umami 516, 543
units of measurement 20–3
  energy **22**
  length **22**
  SI units **21**, **22**
  volume **22**
  weight **22**
up-regulation 196, 215
upper limbs, muscles of **273**, *277–9*
upper respiratory tract 330–1, *332*, 356
ureters 463, *464*, 469
urethra 466–7, 469, 500
  female 467, *468*
  male 466–7, *467*
urinary tract infection 465–6
urine
  characteristics 462–3
  composition 461–2, **462**
  formation 457–61, **459–60**
    filtration 457
    hormonal control 460–1
    secretion 459
    selective reabsorption 457, 459
urobilin 377
urobilinogen 377, 398
uterus 494–5, *495*, 500
  layers of **496**
uvula *410*, 439

vagina 496, 500
vagus nerve 356, 417
valency 7, 25
Valsalva manoeuvre 426
valvular heart disease 301
  regurgitation 301
  stenosis 301
vas deferens 484, 488, 500
vasoconstriction 147, 382
vasodilation 147
vasomotor centre 320
veins 385–6, *388*, **388**
venous 320
venous blood 320
ventilation 345, 356

ventricles (of brain) 164, *165*, 182
ventricles (of heart) *300*, 301, 320
vermiform appendix 439
vertebrae 123
vestibular duct *529*
vestibule 330, 356
  of ear 523, *524*
villi 420, *421*, 439
visceral pericardium 320
visceral peritoneum 439
visceral pleura 334, 356
vision *see* sight
visual acuity 538, 543
visual processing 539–40
vital capacity 341, *341*, 356
vitamins, and bone structure **236**
vitamin D, synthesis 145
vitamins 431, **432–3**, 439
Volkmann's canals 237
volume, units of measurement **22**
voluntary phase 439
vomer 330, 356
vulva 497, 500

waste products, removal in blood 373
water 4, 19
  deficiency 47, 144
Watson, James 552
weight, units of measurement **22**
white blood cells 93, 368, 378–82, 398
  see also individual cell types
white matter 182

X-linked recessive diseases 574, *574*, 578